Atlas of Common and Rare Genodermatoses

Nayera Moftah • May El Samahy
Nadia Abd El Wadood • Monira Waseef

Atlas of Common and Rare Genodermatoses

Springer

Nayera Moftah
Dermatology and Venereology Department
Faculty of Medicine for Girls
Al-Azhar University
Cairo, Egypt

Nadia Abd El Wadood
Dermatology, Venereology and Andrology
Al-Haud Al-Marsoud Hospital
Cairo, Egypt

May El Samahy
Dermatology and Venereology Department
Faculty of Medicine
Ain Shams University
Cairo, Egypt

Monira Waseef
Dermatology, Venereology and Andrology
Al-Haud Al-Marsoud Hospital
Cairo, Egypt

ISBN 978-3-031-60787-5 ISBN 978-3-031-60788-2 (eBook)
https://doi.org/10.1007/978-3-031-60788-2

This Springer imprint is published by the registered company Springer Nature Switzerland AG
The registered company address is: Gewerbestrasse 11, 6330 Cham, Switzerland

Preface

The fast-moving world of genetic research inspired us to present an atlas containing common and rare genodermatoses. It provides the dermatologists, pediatricians, and internists with about 1000 photos of more than 200 different genodermatoses collected from multicenter medical institutions in Egypt since 2010, some of which very rare.

Consanguinity is high in Egypt; hence, many different varieties of genodermatoses with different presentations are encountered. In this atlas, the reader is presented with photos of affected family members at different ages.

The diagnosis of genodermatoses is not an easy task; key points for a correct diagnosis of each disease are mentioned in a concise manner, while a wealth of photographs will assist the practitioner's review, through their colorful presentation, in giving the most accurate diagnosis of the different genodermatoses and counseling families and patients.

With the advances in genetic studies, further research will be of invaluable support to those studying the expected affected gene, to build what may be the basis of gene therapy.

It is the hope of the authoring team that this atlas will, in the meantime, contribute to a better understanding of genodermatoses, their variability, and thus to sound medical decisions and safer, more effective treatments for patients facing a life with these complex conditions.

Nayera Moftah
May El Samahy
Nadia Abd El Wadood
Monira Waseef

Acknowledgments

We would like to thank all the co-authors who contributed to writing the main criteria of the genodermatoses published in this atlas and to the revision of its chapters.

Co-authors
Nermeen S.A. Abdel Fattah, MD
Professor of Dermatology and Venereology
Faculty of Medicine, Ain Shams University, Cairo, Egypt
Noha H. Moftah, MD
Professor of Dermatology, STDS, and Andrology
Faculty of Medicine, Minia University, Al-Minia, Egypt
Shaimaa Hassan Mohamed, MD
Assistant Professor of Dermatology and Venereology
Faculty of Medicine for Girls, Al-Azhar University, Cairo, Egypt

We would like to thank all the dermatologists who contributed clinical photographs of their patients to this atlas, after obtaining their parents' consent for publication, and who assisted in preparing the chapters.

Contributors (Alphabetically)
Abeer Mostafa, MD
Dermatology and Venereology Department, Faculty of Medicine for Girls, Al-Azhar University, Cairo, Egypt
Ahmed Kamal, MD
Al-Haud Al-Marsoud Hospital, Cairo, Egypt
Ahmed Said Alkasbi, EFB
Al-Haud Al-Marsoud Hospital, Cairo, Egypt
Alfallooji, EFB
Al-Haud Al-Marsoud Hospital, Cairo, Egypt
Aliaa El-Said, MSc
Dermatology and Venereology Department, Faculty of Medicine for Girls, Al-Azhar University
Amjad Saad, EFB
Al-Haud Al-Marsoud Hospital, Cairo, Egypt
Ammar Aldujalli, EFB
Al-Haud Al-Marsoud Hospital, Cairo, Egypt
Asmaa Hamdy, EFB
Al-Haud Al-Marsoud Hospital, Cairo, Egypt
Ayat A. Abo Oun, EFB
Al-Haud Al-Marsoud Hospital, Cairo, Egypt
Belal Muwafak, EFB
Al-Haud Al-Marsoud Hospital, Cairo, Egypt
Doaa Atef, MSc

Al-Haud Al-Marsoud Hospital, Cairo, Egypt
Eman Fathy Gomaa, EFB
Al-Haud Al-Marsoud Hospital, Cairo, Egypt
Fady Waheed, MSc
Al-Haud Al-Marsoud Hospital, Cairo, Egypt
Fatma Abd El Salam, MD
Dermatology and Venereology Department, Faculty of Medicine for Girls, Al-Azhar University, Cairo, Egypt
Ghada Osama Elshahat, EFB
Al-Haud Al-Marsoud Hospital, Cairo, Egypt
Ghada Raslan, MD
Al-Haud Al-Marsoud Hospital, Cairo, Egypt
Hala Fayed, MSc
Al-Haud Al-Marsoud Hospital, Cairo, Egypt
Hanan Hamdy, MSc
Al-Haud Al-Marsoud Hospital, Cairo, Egypt
Hayder Al-Darraji, EFB
Almatareya Educational Hospital
Husham Adnan Abbas, EFB
Al-Haud Al-Marsoud Hospital, Cairo, Egypt
Khadega Husien Fata, EFB
Al-Haud Al-Marsoud Hospital, Cairo, Egypt
Maged Farid, MD
Consultant of Dermatology, Venereology and Andrology
Al-Haud Al-Marsoud Hospital, Cairo, Egypt
May Farook, MD
Consultant of Dermatology, Venereology, and Andrology
Al-Haud Al-Marsoud Hospital, Cairo, Egypt
Mohamed Samir, MSc
El Sinbelaween Hospital, El Sinbelaween, Egypt
Monira Waked, MD
Consultant of Dermatology, Venereology, and Andrology
Al-Haud Al-Marsoud Hospital, Cairo, Egypt
Mostafa Kadry, MD
Consultant of Dermatology, Venereology and Andrology, Al-Haud Al-Marsoud Hospital, Cairo, Egypt
Muath Abkar AL Ahdal, EFB
Al-Haud Al-Marsoud Hospital, Cairo, Egypt
Nada Shaaban Mohamed, MSc
Dermatology and Venereology Department, Faculty of Medicine for Girls, Al-Azhar University, Cairo, Egypt
Rasha Saeed Awad, EFB
Al-Haud Al-Marsoud Hospital, Cairo, Egypt
Samar Ashry, MSc
Al-Haud Al-Marsoud Hospital, Cairo, Egypt
Samir Sabry, MSc
Al-Haud Al-Marsoud Hospital, Cairo, Egypt

Shaimaa Farouk, MSc, EFB
Al-Haud Al-Marsoud Hospital, Cairo, Egypt
Shamil Aljobory, MD
General Mosul Hospital, Iraq
Shaymaa Hosny Elgabry, MSc
Al-Haud Al-Marsoud Hospital, Cairo, Egypt
Wafaa Abd Elbaset, MSc, EFB
Al-Haud Al-Marsoud Hospital, Cairo, Egypt
Youmna El-Sayed, MSc
Dermatology and Venereology Department, Faculty of Medicine for Girls, Al-Azhar University, Cairo, Egypt

Lastly, we would like to thank the Springer team, especially Mrs. Juliette R. Kleemann and Ms. Sharon Spears for their great support during the preparation of this atlas.

Contents

1 Ichthyoses and Ichthyotic Syndromes 1
Hereditary (Primary) Ichthyosis 1
Common Ichthyosis 1
Autosomal Recessive (AR) Ichthyoses 2
Keratinopathic Ichthyoses 12
Ichthyosiform Syndromes 22
Keratitis, Ichthyosis, and Deafness (KID) Syndrome 22
Hystrix-Like Ichthyosis with Deafness (HID) Syndrome (AD) 22
Chanarin-Dorfman Syndrome (AR) Neutral Lipid Storage Disease with Ichthyosis 22
Refsum Syndrome (AR) 24
Sjögren-Larsson Syndrome (AR) 25
Netherton Syndrome (AR) 25
Tay-Sachs Syndrome (PIBIDS) (AR) (Congenital Ichthyosis with Trichothiodystrophy) 26
Rud Syndrome (AR) 28
Laurence-Moon-Bardet-Biedl Syndrome (AR) 28
MEDNIK Syndrome (AR) 29
Conradi-Hünermann-Happle Syndrome (XLD) (XLD Chondrodysplasia Punctata) 29
CHILD Syndrome (XLD) 31
References 38

2 Erythrokeratodermas and Palmoplantar Keratoderma 39
Erythrokeratoderma 39
Erythrokeratoderma Variabilis (AD) 39
Progressive Symmetric Erythrokeratoderma (AD) 39
Palmoplantar Keratodermas (PPK) 42
Punctate PPK Type 1 (AD) (Buschke-Fischer Syndrome) 42
Acrokeratoelastoidosis of Oswald Costa (AD) (Inverse Papular Acrokeratosis) . . 42
Punctate Keratosis of Palmar Creases 45
Cole Disease (AD) 45
PPK Striate (AD) 47
PPK Areata (AD) 47
Carvajal Syndrome (AD) (Cardio-Cutaneous Syndrome) 47
Howel-Evans Syndrome (AD) (Tylosis with Esophageal Cancer) 47
Richner-Hanhart Syndrome (AR) (Tyrosinemia Type II) (Oculocutaneous Tyrosinemia) 47
Pachyonychia Congenita Type 1 (AD) 49
Diffuse Palmoplantar Keratoderma (PPK) 49
Transgredient Keratodermas 53

Mal de Meleda PPK (AR) (Keratosis Extremitatum Hereditaria Trangrediens et Progrediens) . . . 53
Greither's Disease (AD) (Transgrediens et Progrediens PPK) . . . 56
Papillon-Lefèvre Syndrome (AR) . . . 58
Vohwinkel Syndrome (AD) (Keratoderma Hereditaria Mutilans) (PPK with Honeycomb Pattern) . . . 63
Bart-Pumphrey Syndrome (AD) . . . 64
Olmsted Syndrome (AD/R, XLR) (Diffuse Mutilating Keratoderma with Periorificial Plaques) . . . 65
Huriez Syndrome (AD) (Sclerotylosis) . . . 66
Non-Transgredient Keratodermas . . . 66
Unna-Thost Syndrome (AD) . . . 66
Vorner Syndrome (AD) . . . 68
Naxos Disease (AR) . . . 68
References . . . 70

3 Epidermolysis Bullosa . . . 71
Epidermolysis Bullosa Simplex (EBS) . . . 73
Acral Peeling Skin Syndrome (APPS) (AR) . . . 73
Skin Fragility Syndrome . . . 75
Epidermolysis Bullosa Simplex (EBS), Localized Subtype (AD) . . . 75
Epidermolysis Bullosa Simplex (EBS), Generalized Subtype (AD) . . . 75
Epidermolysis Bullosa Simplex (EBS), Severe Subtype (AD) . . . 78
Epidermolysis Bullosa Simplex (EBS) with Mottled Pigmentation (AD) . . . 78
Epidermolysis Bullosa Simplex (EBS)-Ogna (AD) . . . 78
Junctional Epidermolysis Bullosa (JEB) . . . 80
Junctional Epidermolysis Bullosa (JEB)-Severe Subtype (AR) . . . 80
Junctional Epidermolysis Bullosa (JEB)-Intermediate Subtype (AR) . . . 80
Dystrophic Epidermolysis Bullosa (DEB) . . . 83
Recessive Dystrophic Epidermolysis Bullosa (RDEB), Severe Subtype . . . 83
Dominant Dystrophic Epidermolysis Bullosa (DDEB), Intermediate Subtype . . . 86
Dystrophic Epidermolysis Bullosa (DDEB) Pruriginosa . . . 86
Dominant Dystrophic Epidermolysis Bullosa (DDEB) Albopapuloid (AD) . . . 86
Kindler Epidermolysis Bullosa (AR) . . . 88
References . . . 93

4 Pigmentary Genodermatoses . . . 95
Hypomelanosis . . . 95
Hypomelanosis Related to a Defect of Embryological Development of Melanocytes . . . 95
Hypomelanosis Related to a Defect of Melanogenesis . . . 96
Hypomelanosis Related to a Defect of Biogenesis of Melanosomes . . . 100
Hypomelanosis Related to a Defect of Melanosomes Transport . . . 102
Other Hypomelanoses . . . 103
Hypermelanosis . . . 106
Incontinentia Pigmenti (XLD) . . . 106
Linear and Whorled Nevoid Hypermelanosis (LWNH) . . . 107
Dowling-Degos Disease (DDD) (AD) . . . 107
Reticulate Acropigmentation of Kitamura (RAK) (AD) . . . 108
Reticulate Acropigmentation of Dohi (RAD) (AD) . . . 109
Dyschromatosis Universalis Hereditaria (DUH) (AD/AR) . . . 109
Naegeli–Franceschetti–Adassohn Syndrome (NFJS) (AD) . . . 109
Familial Gigantic Melanocytosis (FGM) (AD) . . . 112

McCune–Albright Syndrome (MAS) 113
Peutz–Jeghers Syndrome (AD) 116
Laugier–Hunziker Syndrome 116
References 126

5 Genodermatoses with Malignant Potential 129
Tuberous Sclerosis (AD) 129
Neurofibromatosis (NF) (AD) 137
Von Recklinghausen Syndrome 137
Birt–Hogg–Dubé Syndrome (BHDS) (AD) 145
Cowden Syndrome (AD) 148
Gorlin Syndrome (AD) 149
Nevoid Basal Cell Carcinoma Syndrome 149
Bazex–Dupré–Christol Syndrome (XLD) 150
Rombo Syndrome (AD) 151
Reed Syndrome (AD) 152
Brooke-Spiegler Syndrome (AD) 153
References 155

6 Genodermatoses with Defective Excision Repair 157
Xeroderma Pigmentosum (XP) (AR) 157
Pigmented Xerodermoid 160
DeSanctis–Cacchione Syndrome (DSC) (AR) 161
Cockayne Syndrome (CS) (AR) 162
Dyskeratosis Congenita (DC) (Zinsser-Engman-Cole syndrome) (X-linked Recessive, AD or AR) 163
Rothmund-Thomson Syndrome (AR) 165
References 167

7 Vascular Disorders 169
Capillary Malformations 169
Port-Wine Stain (Nevus Flammeus) 169
Sturge–Weber Syndrome 169
Klippel–Trenaunay Syndrome 171
Proteus Syndrome 172
Fabry Disease 174
Venous Malformations 180
Venous Lake 180
Blue Rubber Bleb Nevus Syndrome (Sporadic/AD) 180
Maffucci Syndrome 181
Osler-Weber-Rendu Syndrome (AD) 184
Hereditary Hemorrhagic Telangiectasia 184
Hemangiomas 186
PHACES Syndrome 187
Lumbar (Sacral) Syndrome (XL) 190
Pelvis Syndrome 190
Lymphangioma Circumscriptum (LC) 191
References 193

8 Acantholytic Genodermatoses 195
Darier Disease (Keratosis Follicularis) (AD) 195
Hailey-Hailey Disease (Benign Familial Chronic Pemphigus) (AD) 199
References 199

9 Dermal Disorders . . . 207
Cutis Laxa (AD, AR, XLR) . . . 207
Ehlers-Danlos Syndrome (EDS) (AD, AR) . . . 209
Pseudoxanthoma Elasticum (PXE) (AR) . . . 211
Marfan Syndrome (AD) . . . 213
Buschke-Ollendorff Syndrome (AD) . . . 214
Lipoid Proteinosis (Hyalinosis Cutis et Mucosae) (AR) . . . 215
Focal Dermal Hypoplasia (Goltz syndrome) . . . 220
Juvenile Hyaline Fibromatosis (JHF) (AR) . . . 226
References . . . 227

10 Ectodermal Dysplasia . . . 229
Hypohidrotic or Anhidrotic Ectodermal Dysplasia (Christ-Siemens-Touraine Syndrome) (XLR) . . . 229
Hidrotic Ectodermal Dysplasia [*3*, *4*] (Clouston Syndrome) (AD) . . . 233
Ankyloblepharon-Ectodermal Dysplasia-Clefting Syndrome (Hay-Wells Syndrome) (AD) . . . 235
Witkop's Syndrome (Tooth-and-Nail Syndrome) (AD) . . . 237
Hallermann-Streiff Syndrome (Oculo-Mandibulo-Facial Syndrome) (Sporadic/AD) . . . 238
Monilethrix (AD) . . . 239
Atrichia with Papular Lesions (AR) . . . 240
Uncombable Hair Syndrome (AD/AR) . . . 241
Björnstad Syndrome (AR) . . . 242
References . . . 243

11 Premature Aging Syndromes (Progeroid Syndromes) . . . 245
Hereditary Conditions with Premature Aging . . . 245
  Progeria (Hutchinson-Gilford Syndrome) (AD) . . . 245
  Adult Progeria (Werner Syndrome) (AR) . . . 245
References . . . 248

12 Genetic Immunodeficiency Disorders . . . 249
Chronic Mucocutaneous Candidiasis (CMC) (AD/AR) . . . 249
Wiskott-Aldrich Syndrome (XLR) . . . 250
Hyper-IgE Syndrome (Job Syndrome) (AD/AR) . . . 251
References . . . 254

13 Miscellaneous . . . 255
Lesch-Nyhan Syndrome (X-Linked Recessive) . . . 255
GAPO Syndrome (AR) . . . 256
Phakomatosis Pigmentokeratotica (PPK) (AR) . . . 257
Aplasia Cutis Congenita (AD, AR) . . . 258
  Membranous Aplasia Cutis Congenita . . . 258
Bart Syndrome [*15*] (Aplasia Cutis + Epidermolysis Bullosa) . . . 259
Adams-Oliver Syndrome (AD, AR or Sporadic) (Aplasia Cutis + Limb Defect) . . . 260
Prolidase Deficiency (Peptidase Deficiency) (AR) . . . 262
Brauer Syndrome (Focal Facial Dermal Dysplasia) (AD, AD) . . . 262
H Syndrome (AR) . . . 263
Epidermodysplasia Verruciformis (AR) (Tree-Man Disease) . . . 264
Turner Syndrome . . . 264
References . . . 265

1 Ichthyoses and Ichthyotic Syndromes

Ichthyosis is commonly inherited as a single entity. However, it may be part of syndromes that induce abnormalities in organs other than the skin. These include KID, HID, Chanarin-Dorfman, Refsum, Sjögren-Larsson, Netherton, Tay-Sachs (PIBIDS), Rud's, Laurence-Moon-Bardet-Biedl, MEDNIK, Conradi-Hünermann-Happle, and CHILD syndrome.

1. **Hereditary (Primary) Ichthyoses**
   (a) Common Ichthyoses
   - Ichthyosis Vulgaris
   - X-linked Recessive (XLR) Ichthyosis

   (b) Autosomal Recessive (AR) Ichthyoses
   Major Forms
   - Non-Bullous Congenital Ichthyosiform Erythroderma.
   - Lamellar Ichthyosis
   - Harlequin Ichthyosis

   Minor Forms
   - Self-healing Collodion Baby
   - Acral self-healing Collodion Baby
   - Bathing-suit Ichthyosis

   (c) Keratinopathic Ichthyoses
   - Epidermolytic Ichthyosis
   - Superficial Epidermolytic Ichthyosis (of Siemens)
   - Ichthyosis Hystrix Curth-Macklin
   - Ichthyosis en Confetti
2. **Ichthyosiform Syndromes**
   (a) KID Syndrome
   (b) HID Syndrome
   (c) Chanarin-Dorfman Syndrome
   (d) Refsum Syndrome
   (e) Sjögren-Larsson Syndrome
   (f) Netherton Syndrome
   (g) Tay-Sachs Syndrome (PIBIDS)
   (h) Rud's Syndrome
   (i) Laurence-Moon-Bardet-Biedl Syndrome
   (j) MEDNIK Syndrome
   (k) Conradi-Hünermann-Happle Syndrome
   (l) CHILD Syndrome

Hereditary (Primary) Ichthyosis

Common Ichthyosis

Ichthyosis Vulgaris (AD) [1, 2] (Figs. 1.1, 1.2, and 1.3)

- The most common disorder of cornification.
- Autosomal dominant inheritance: mild ichthyosis with a heterozygous filaggrin (*FLG*) mutation and more severe ichthyosis with mutations in both *FLG* alleles.
- Onset: during infancy and most patients exhibit clear clinical manifestations by the age of 5 years.
- Clinical characteristics:
  - Skin: dry, fine, small, white, flaky scales. The extensor surfaces of the upper and lower extremities are the initial target with sparing of the flexural creases.
  - In most cases, no extracutaneous involvement of the eyes, ears, skeletal, and the nervous systems.
- Associations:
  - Atopic dermatitis, asthma, allergic rhinitis.
  - Palmoplantar hyperlinearity and hyperkeratosis (keratosis punctata).
  - Keratosis pilaris and furrowed heels.
- Prognosis: improves with age and summer.
- Treatment: emollients, humectants, and keratolytics (e.g., urea, lactic, and salicylic acids); the latter group may be irritating in patients with coexistent atopic dermatitis.

X-Linked Recessive Ichthyosis [3] (Figs. 1.4 and 1.5)

- Absence of steroid sulfatase (STS) activity due to the deletion of the entire *STS* gene.
- Almost exclusively affects boys and men, with transmission by asymptomatic female carriers.
- Onset: skin findings usually appear within the first year of life, 15–20% have manifestations at birth.
- Clinical characteristics:
  - Widespread polygonal large dark brown plate-like adherent scales on the anterior aspect of lower legs and trunk with fine-scale on the scalp.

N. Moftah et al., *Atlas of Common and Rare Genodermatoses*, https://doi.org/10.1007/978-3-031-60788-2_1

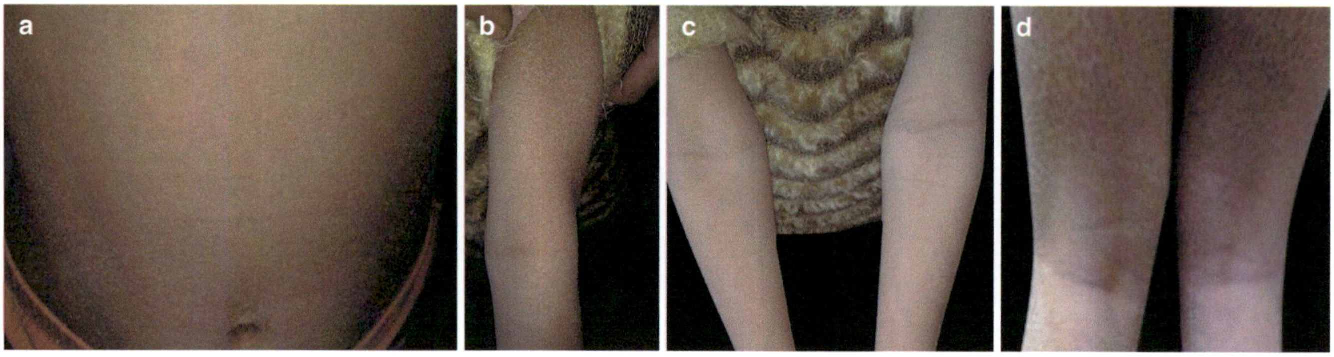

Fig. 1.1 Ichthyosis vulgaris. Fine white scales on the abdomen (**a**) on the limbs (**b**, **c**, **d**), sparing flexures (**c**, **d**)

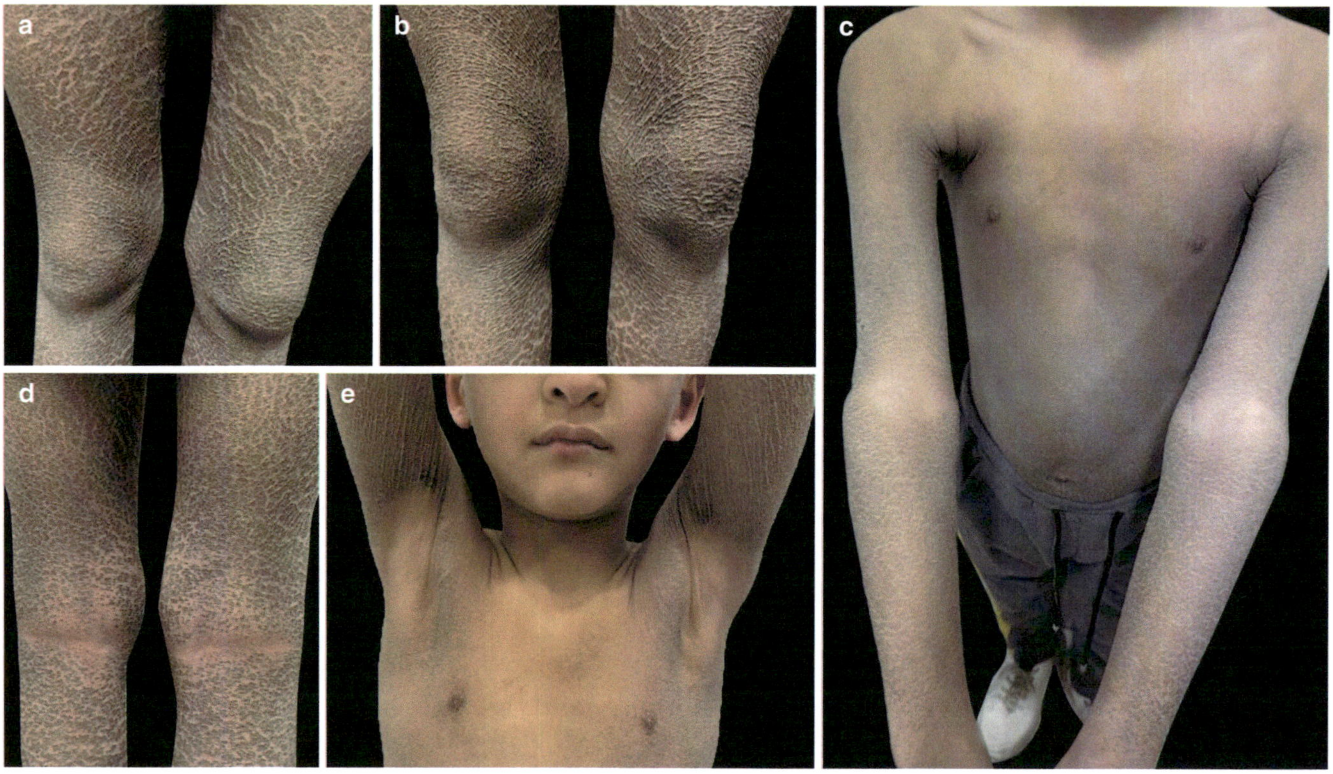

Fig. 1.2 Ichthyosis vulgaris. Large adherent scales, grayish tessellated (tile-like), similar to fish skin on the lower legs (**a**, **b**), sparing flexures (**c**–**e**)

  - Dirty neck appearance and affection of axillae.
  - Face (except pre-auricles), palms, and soles are spared. Flexor areas are variably involved.
- Associations:
  - Corneal opacities.
  - Cryptorchidism.
  - Prolonged labor due to low placental estrogen production (may result in birth via cesarean section).
- Prognosis: improves with summer, worsens with age.
- Treatment: topical humectants, keratolytics, and retinoids.

Autosomal Recessive (AR) Ichthyoses

Non-Bullous Congenital Ichthyosiform Erythroderma (AR) [4] (Figs. 1.6 and 1.7)

- Mutations in Transglutaminase 1 (*TGM1*), *ALOXE3*, *ALOX12B*, and *NIPAL4* genes.
- Onset: at birth.
- Clinical Characteristics:
  - Scales: at birth with collodion membrane, generalized erythroderma with fine, flaky white, powdery scales. Flexures, face, palms, and soles are involved.

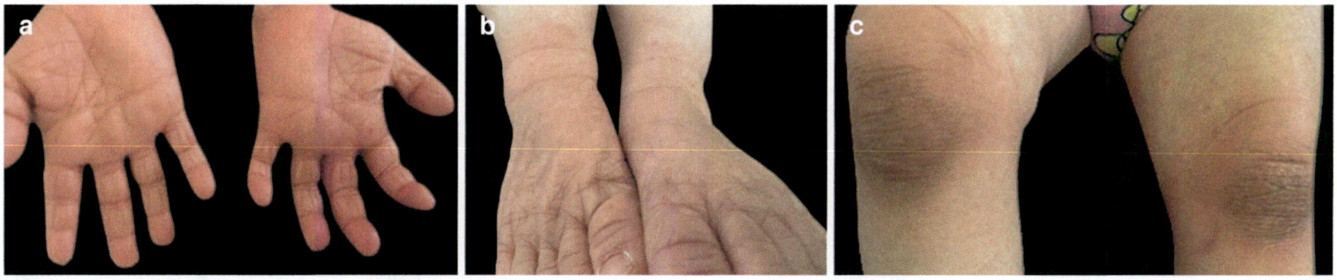

Fig. 1.3 Ichthyosis vulgaris. Hyperlinearity of the palms (accentuated skin marking) (**a**), dorsum of feet (**b**), knees (**c**)

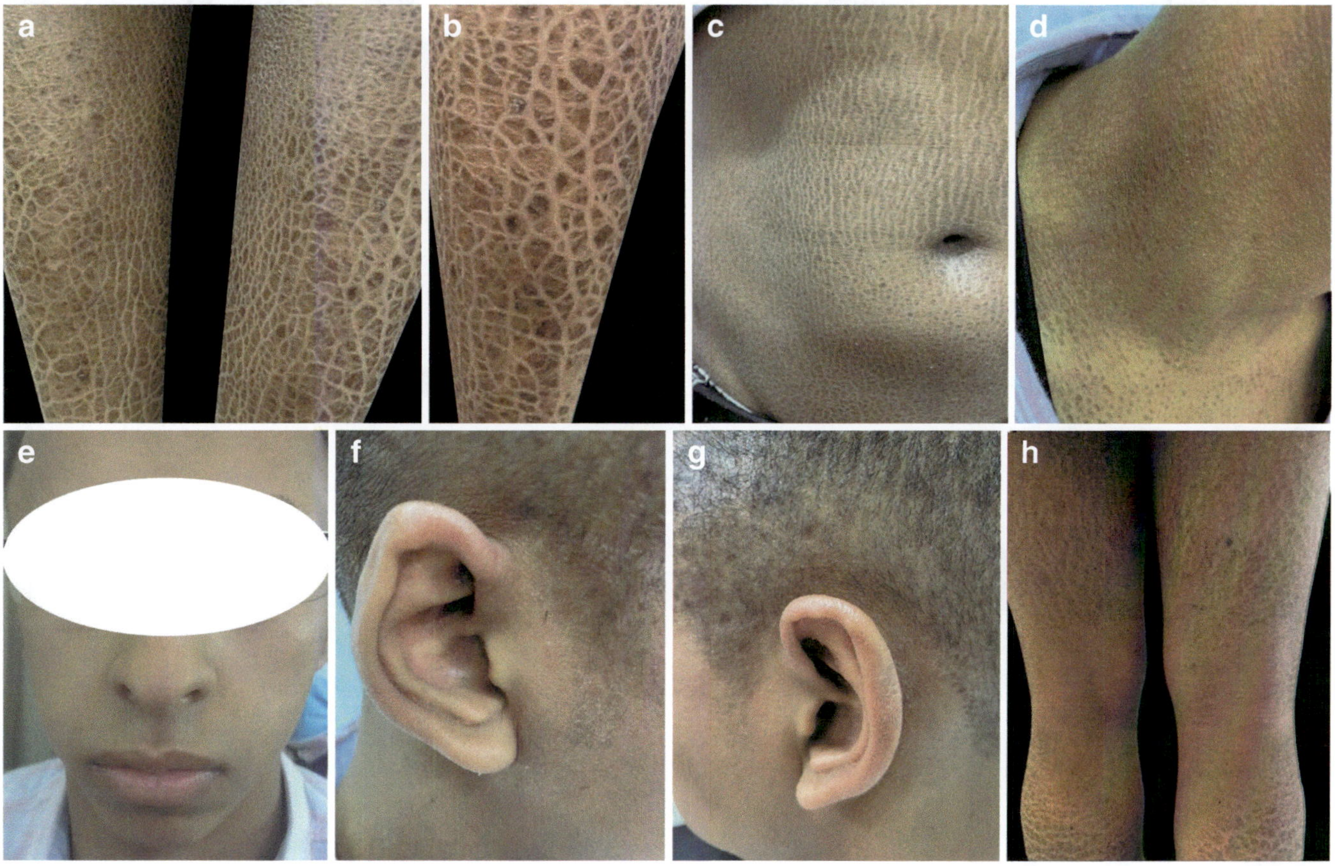

Fig. 1.4 X-linked ichthyosis. Large prominent dark dirty brown scales on limbs (**a**, **b**) smaller light brown on trunk (**c**), Dark scales on the neck 'dirty neck' (**d**), face spare (except pre-auricles) (**e–g**), with sparing flexures (**h**)

  - Mild form of lamellar ichthyosis.
  - Hearing impairment due to accumulation of scales in external ear ± scarring alopecia.
  - Hyperkeratotic lesions on joints.
  - Ectropion, palmoplantar hyperkeratosis, heat intolerance, and hypohidrosis due to obstruction of sweat ducts and nail dystrophy may occur.
  - Severe exfoliative erythroderma may cause metabolic stress or mild growth retardation.
- Treatment: oral retinoids are more beneficial for scaling than for the associated erythema; increased intake of fluids, calories, and protein is required for erythrodermic patients.

Lamellar Ichthyosis (AR) [5, 6] (Figs. 1.8, 1.9, 1.10, 1.11 and 1.12)

- Mutation in *TGM-1* and *ABCA12* genes.
- Onset: at birth.
- Clinical Characteristics:
  - Usually a collodion-like membrane is present at birth.
  - During the first week of life, the membrane cracks and peels off in sheets then forms generalized large thick,

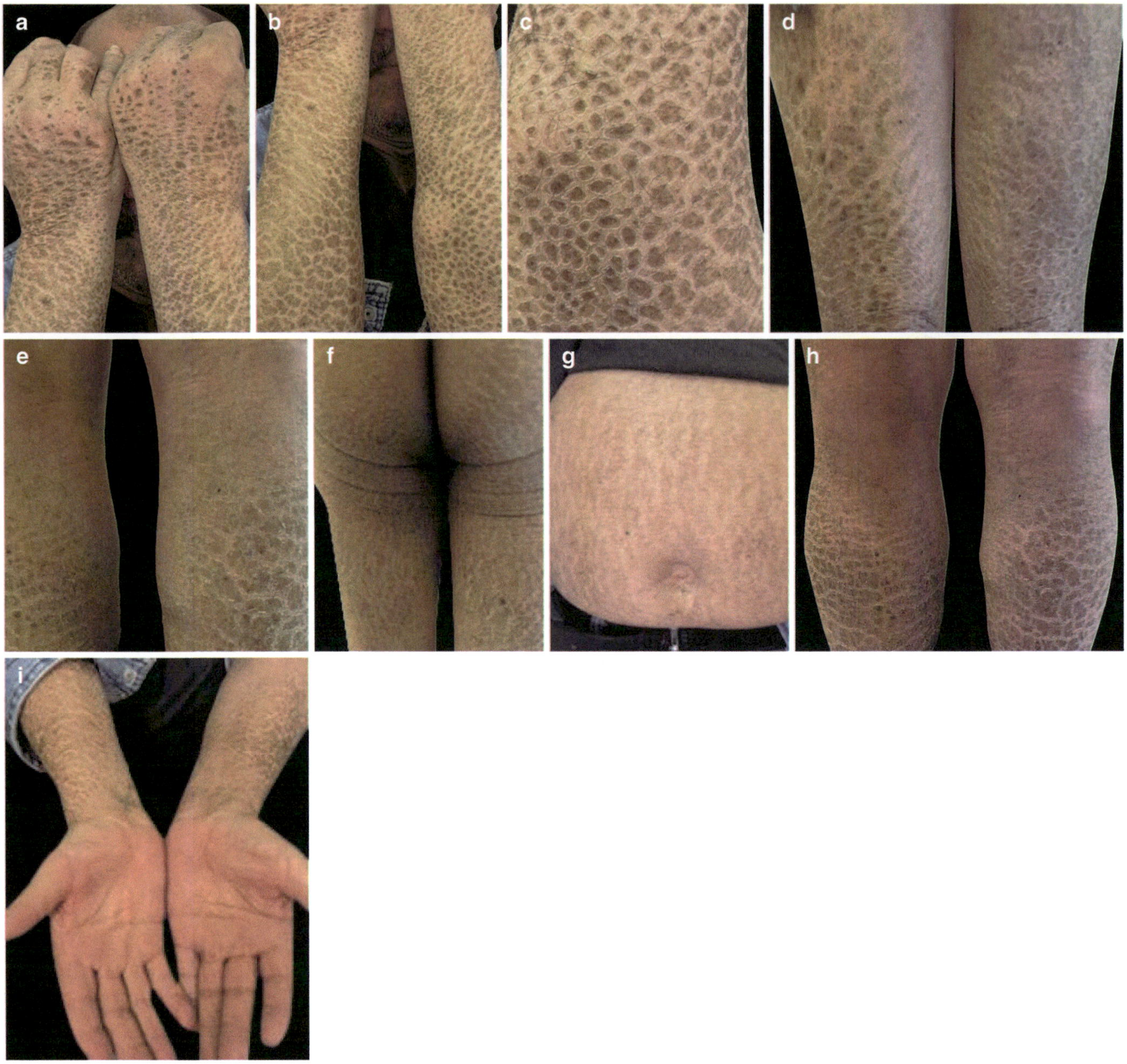

Fig. 1.5 X-linked ichthyosis in adult male. Large prominent dark dirty brown scales on upper limbs (**a**–**c**), lower limbs (**d**, **e**), buttocks (**f**), abdomen (**g**). Flexor areas and palms are spared (**h**, **i**)

dark, brown plate-like adherent scales, which are quadrilateral, adherent in the center, and free at the edge with raised border often leading to superficial fissures, forming a mosaic or bark-like pattern. Erythroderma is either absent or minimal.

- Heat intolerance (heat stroke) and hypernatremia.
- Scarring alopecia especially at the periphery of the scalp (tautness of facial skin) and sparse scalp hair.
- Marked ectropion due to taut skin as well as plate-like scales around eyes associated with madarosis, conjunctivitis and keratitis, eclabium, hypoplasia of nasal and auricular cartilage (crumbled).
- Ears are small and deformed. Accumulation of scales in the ear may lead to recurrent infection.
- "Bathing-suit ichthyosis" caused by temperature sensitive *TGM-1* mutation affects primarily trunk and scalp with a higher incidence in the South African population.
- Palmoplantar hyperkeratosis range from accentuating skin markings to severe thickened skin with cracking and fissuring.
- Hypotrichosis and nail dystrophy with thickening and ridging.
- Prognosis: persistent.

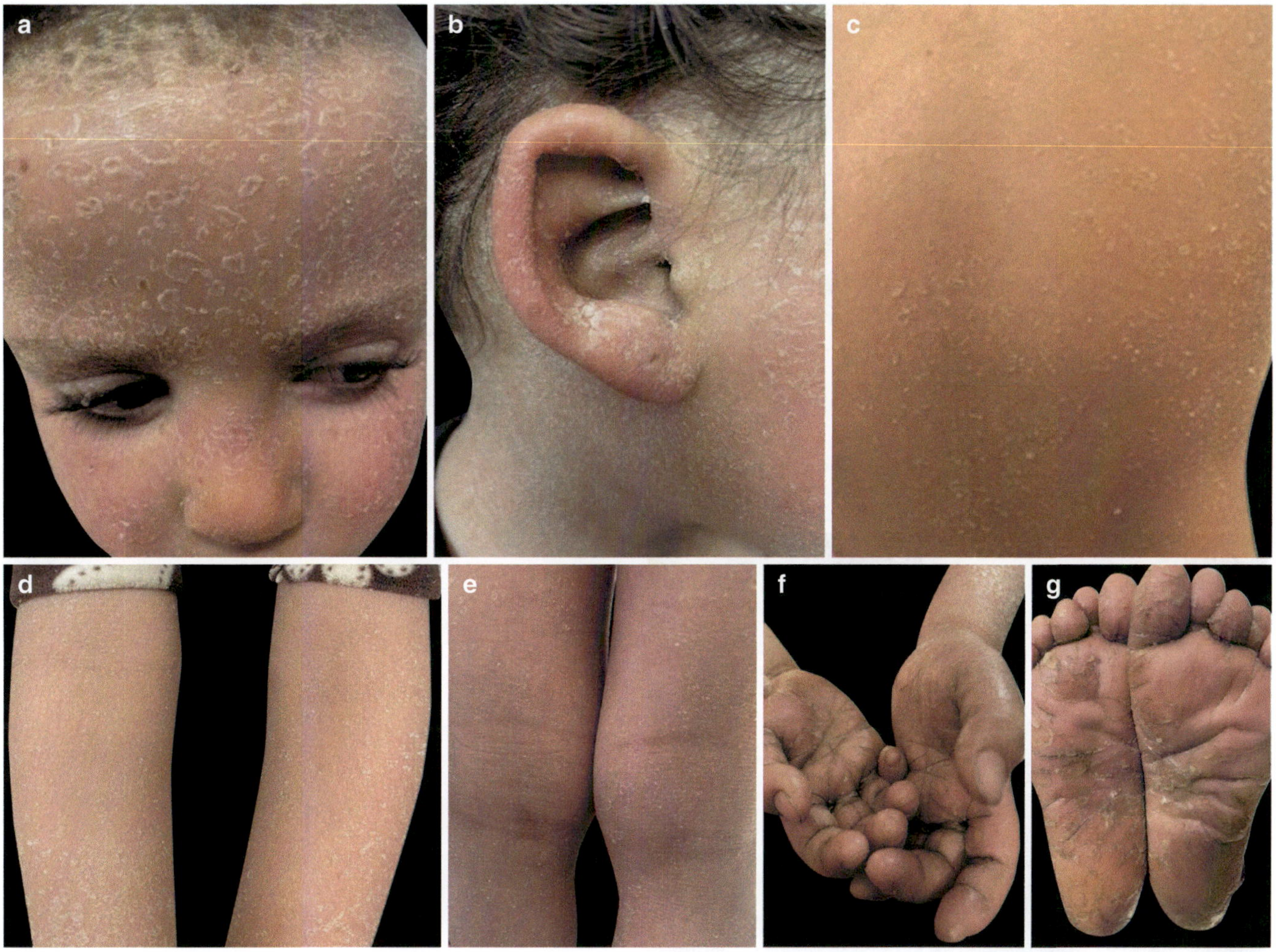

Fig. 1.6 Non-Bullous congenital ichthyosiform erythroderma. Generalized Fine, flaky white, powdery scales with dry skin and persistent generalized erythroderma on face with ear affection (**a**, **b**), back (**c**), limbs with flexures (**d**, **e**), and palmoplantar hyperkeratosis (**f**, **g**)

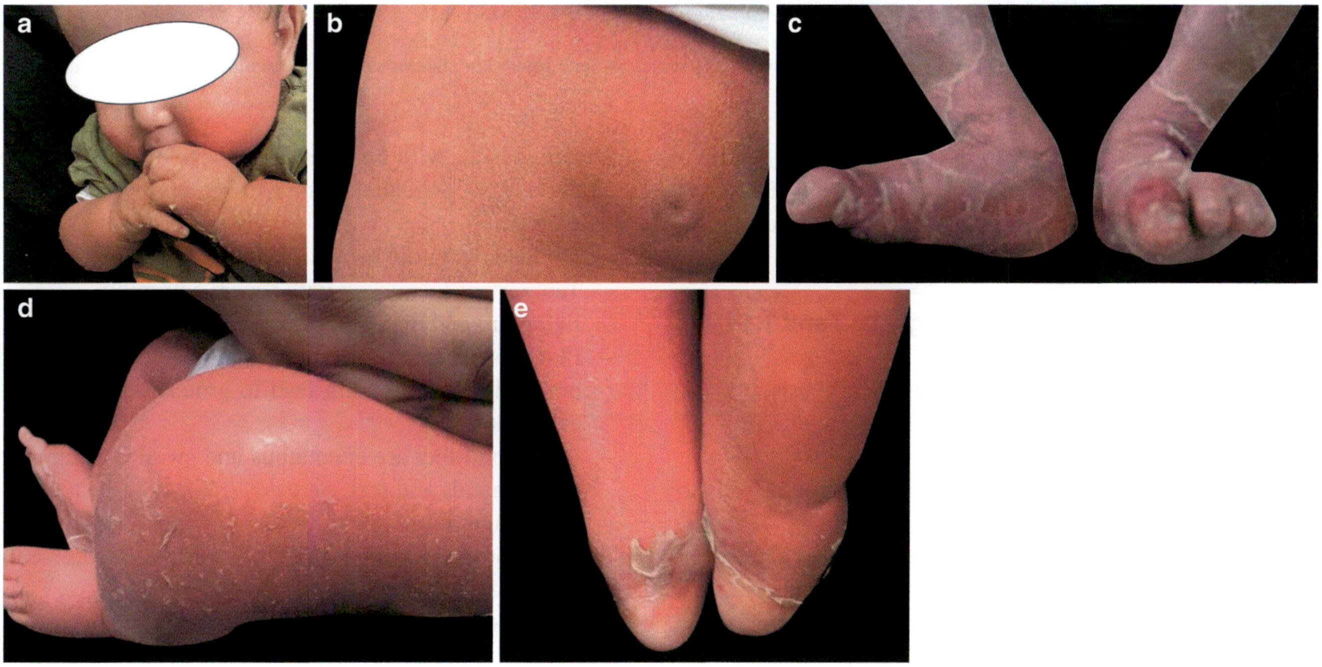

Fig. 1.7 Non-bullous congenital ichthyosiform erythroderma. Generalized fine, flaky white, powdery scales with dry skin and persistent generalized erythroderma on face (**a**), trunk(**b**) and limbs (**c**–**e**)

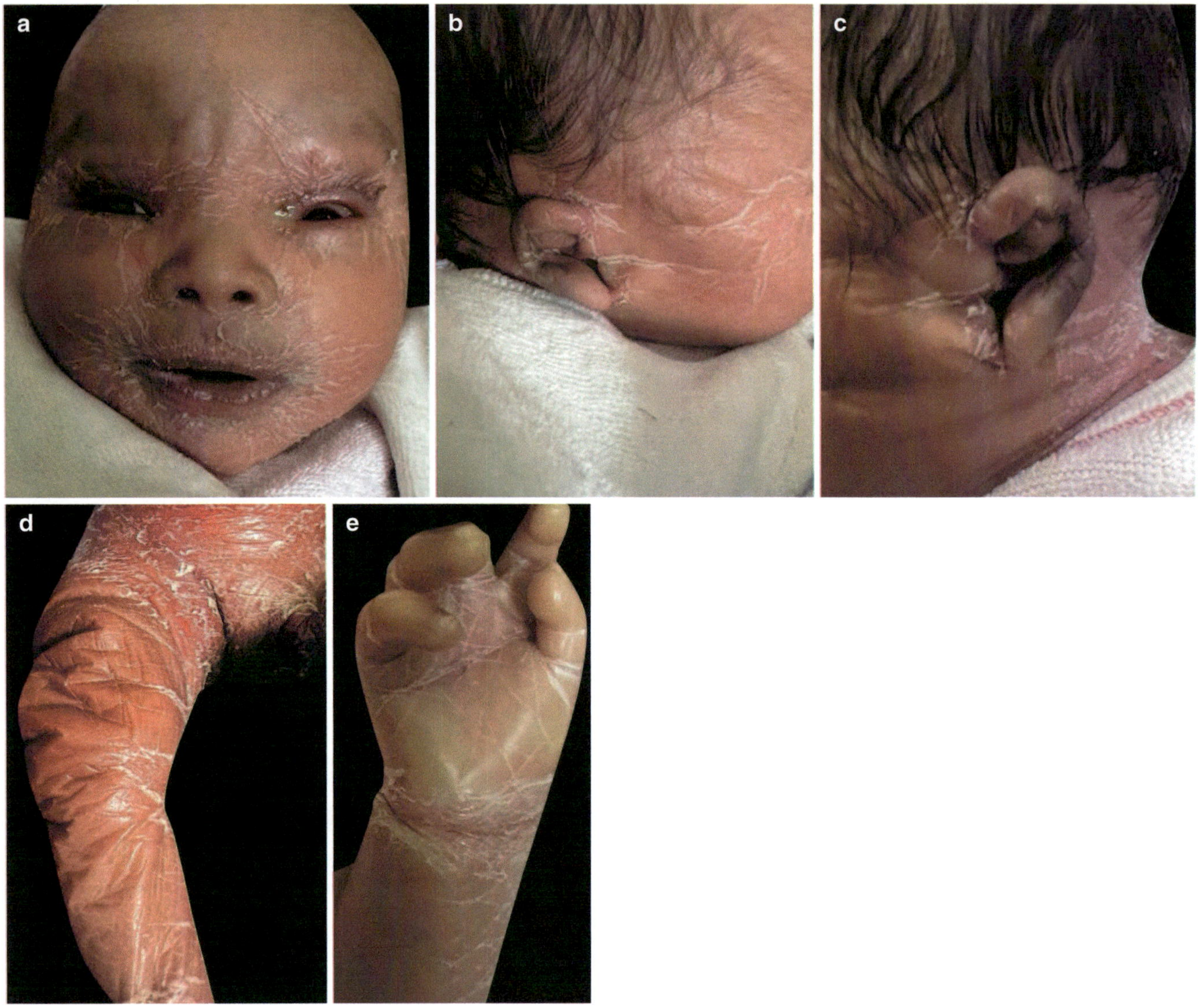

Fig. 1.8 Lamellar ichthyosis. 2 weeks neonate with large, plate-like scales on face (taut skin causing ectropion), scalp, ear deformity and accumulation of scales in the ear (**a**–**c**), limbs and extremities (**d**, **e**)

- Treatment: acitretin use during early childhood is effective for hyperkeratosis and scaling. Acitretin improves ectropion and avoid eye complications and eyelid surgery.

Harlequin Ichthyosis (AR) [7, 8] (Figs. 1.13 and 1.14)

- Mutation in *ABCA12* gene.
- It is a severe and usually fatal form of ichthyosis.
- Onset: infant born premature.
- Tightly encased neonate.
- Encasement of hard thickened stratum corneum leads to hyperkeratotic cast (cracks).
- Scales: large, yellow, brown adherent plate, separated by broad deep intensely red fissures gives armor-like plaques. Baby is stillborn or dies soon after delivery. Acitretin may allow survival, with treatment may develop into lamellar ichthyosis or congenital ichthyosiform erythroderma-like phenotype.
- Complications in the neonatal period:
  - Tautness of facial skin with severe ectropion.
  - Eclabium and microcephaly.
  - Flat ears, rudimentary or absent, and deformities of the nose (all with taut skin lead to grotesque appearance and distortion).
  - Hands and feet are edematous and swollen leading to mitten hands and feet.
  - Autoamputation.
  - Eyelashes/eyebrows are usually missing (spare scalp hair).
  - Erythroderma.

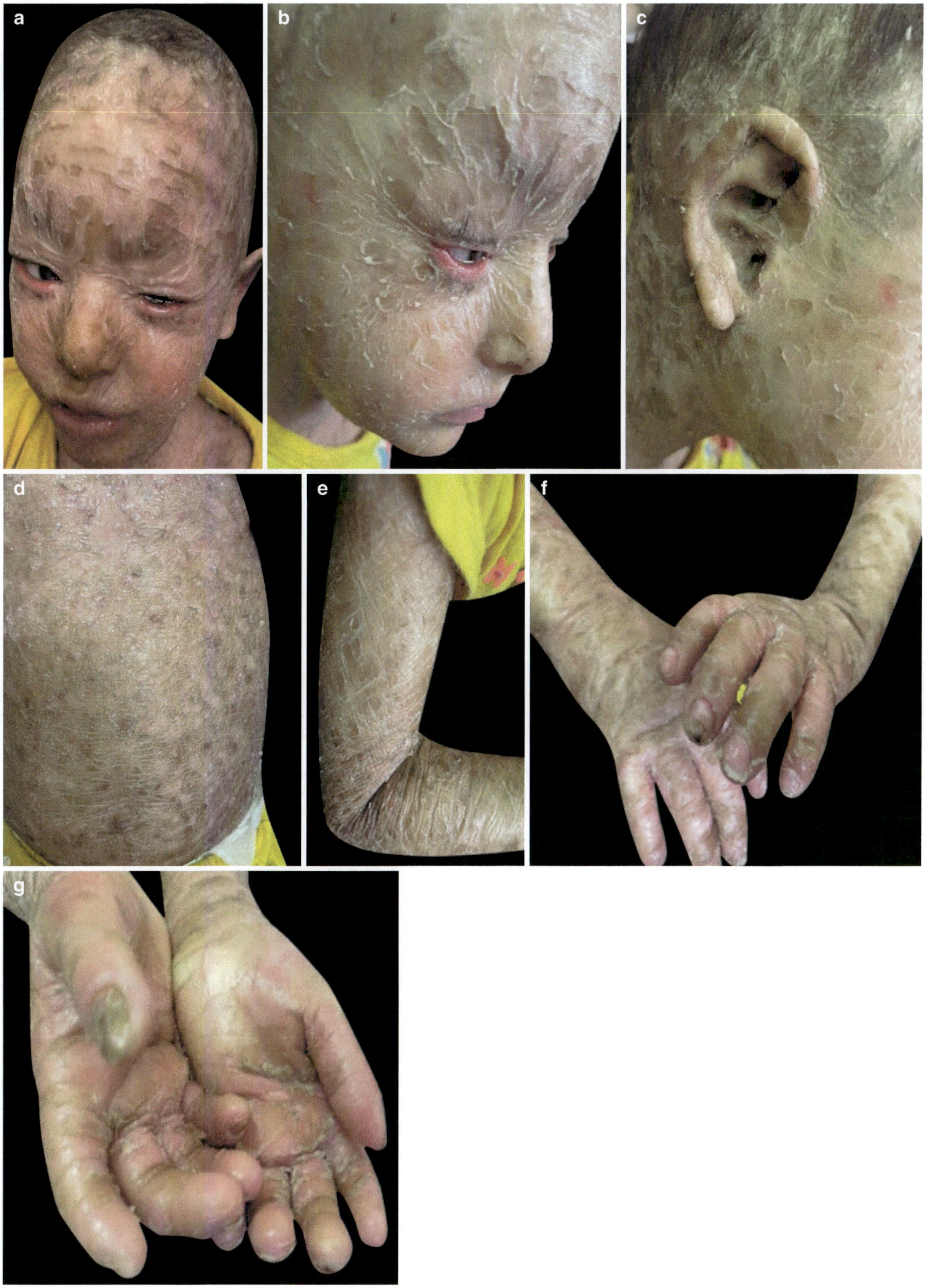

Fig. 1.9 Lamellar ichthyosis. Female patient with large, plate- like scales on face with obvious ectropion, scarring alopecia with ear deformity and accumulation of scales in ear (recurrent infection) (**a–c**), plate-like scales with mosaic pattern on trunk (**d**), upper limb and extremities (**e**, **f**). Hyperkeratosis of the palms and nail dystrophy (**f**, **g**)

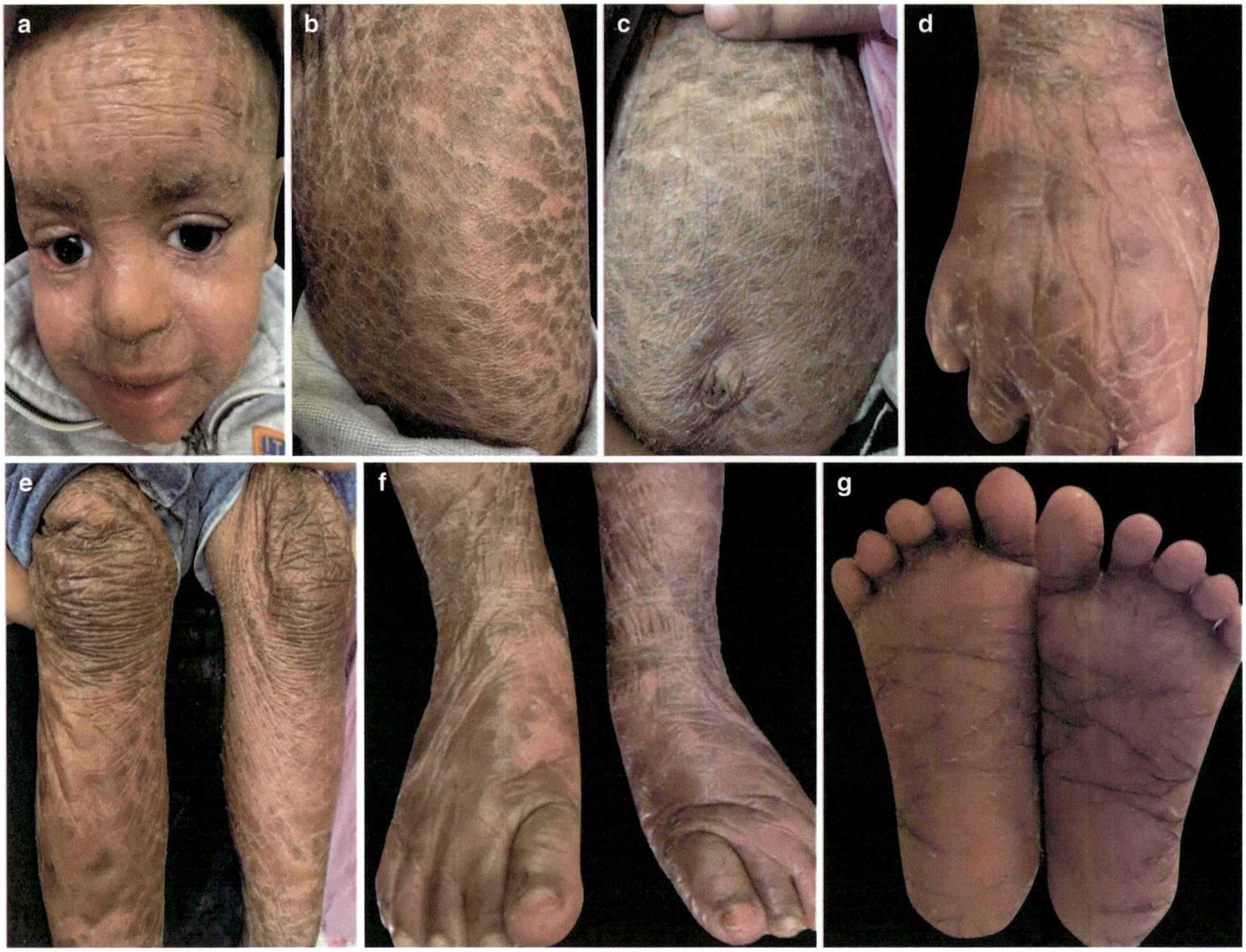

Fig. 1.10 Lamellar ichthyosis. A male patient with large, plate-like scales on face with ectropion, scarring alopecia, eclabium (**a**). Large thick, dark plate-like adherent scales in the center and free at the edge and form a mosaic pattern (reptilian scales) on trunk (**b**, **c**), limbs and extremities (**d**–**f**). Hyperkeratosis of the soles (**g**)

  - Dies within days due to respiratory failure and sepsis.
  - Taut facial skin prevents the infant from suckling.
- Treatment: systemic retinoid and advanced neonatal intensive care (life-threatening and often fatal disorder).

Collodion Baby (AR) [9] (Figs. 1.15 and 1.16)

- Onset: these babies are often premature with low birth weight.
- Born covered with a taut, yellow, shiny, transparent membrane resembling plastic wrap, a cellophane-like membrane. Within 2–3 weeks, the membrane peels off in sheets, leading to erythema, mild scaling, ectropion, eclabium, and distortion of nose and ears (misshapen or crumbled ears), hypoplastic fingers, nose, and anonychia.
- Complications: impaired suckling, restricted ventilation, fluid and electrolyte imbalances, dehydration, skin infection, and sepsis.
- Prognosis:
  - Collodion baby is the usual presentation for Harlequin ichthyosis and congenital ichthyosiform erythroderma. AD lamellar ichthyosis, Sjögren-Larsson syndrome, trichothiodystrophy, neutral lipid storage disease, Conradi-Hünermann-Happle syndrome, Hays-Wells syndrome, and ectodermal dysplasia may also occasionally present as collodion baby.
  - A subset of collodion babies with underlying mutations in *TGM1, ALOX12B*, or *ALOXE3* have a "self-healing" phenotype (self-healing collodion baby) where the skin is fairly normal in appearance when the membrane resolves.
- Treatment: humidified incubator, emollients, and monitoring for complications; keratolytics and manual debridement of the membrane are not advised due to risk of systemic absorption and infection, respectively.

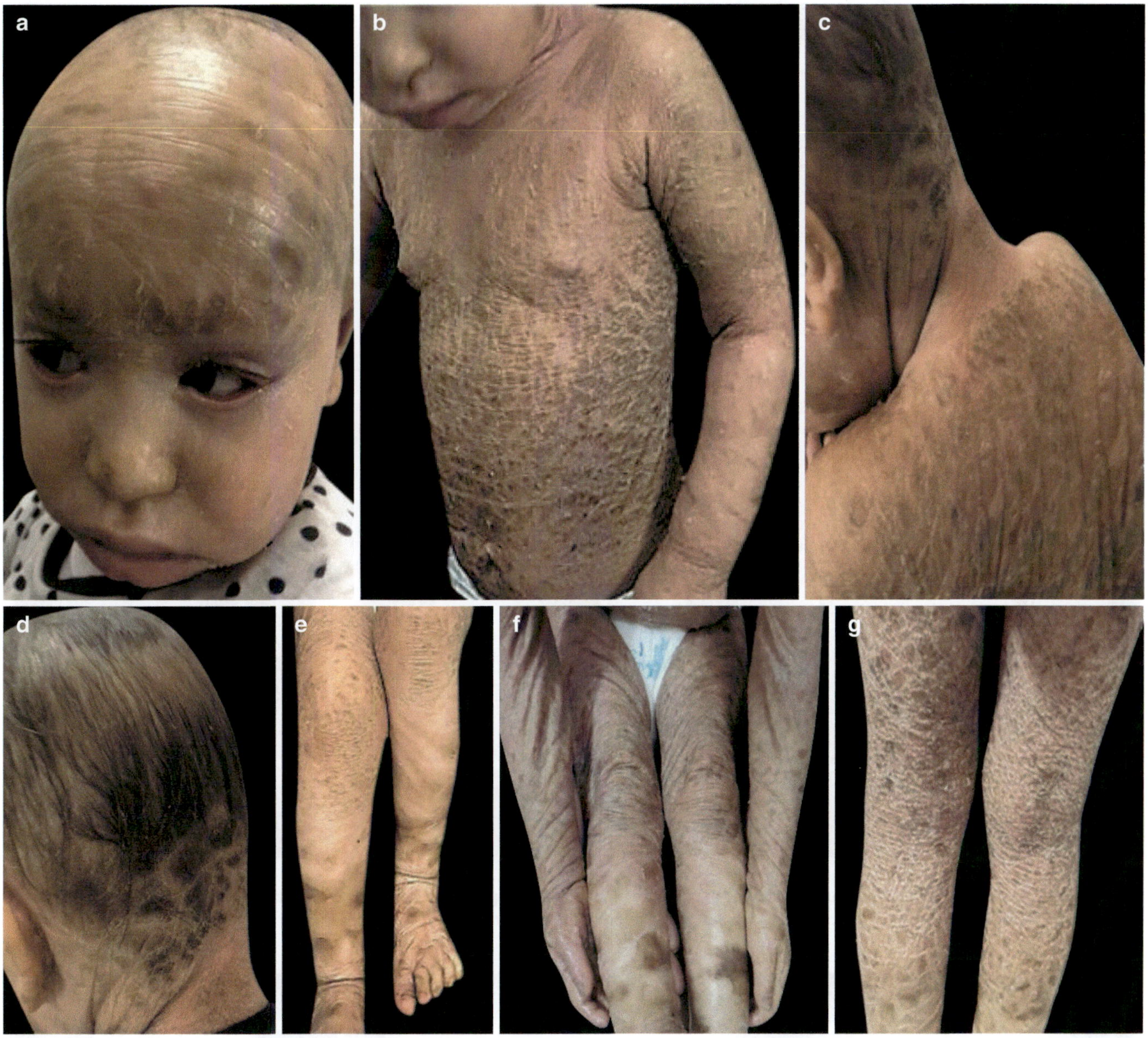

Fig. 1.11 Lamellar ichthyosis. Large thick brown plate-like scales on face with obvious ectropion, scarring alopecia (periphery of scalp) (**a**). Large, plate-like scales forming a mosaic pattern on trunk (**b**, **c**), scalp (**d**), and limbs with significant flexural involvement (**e**–**g**)

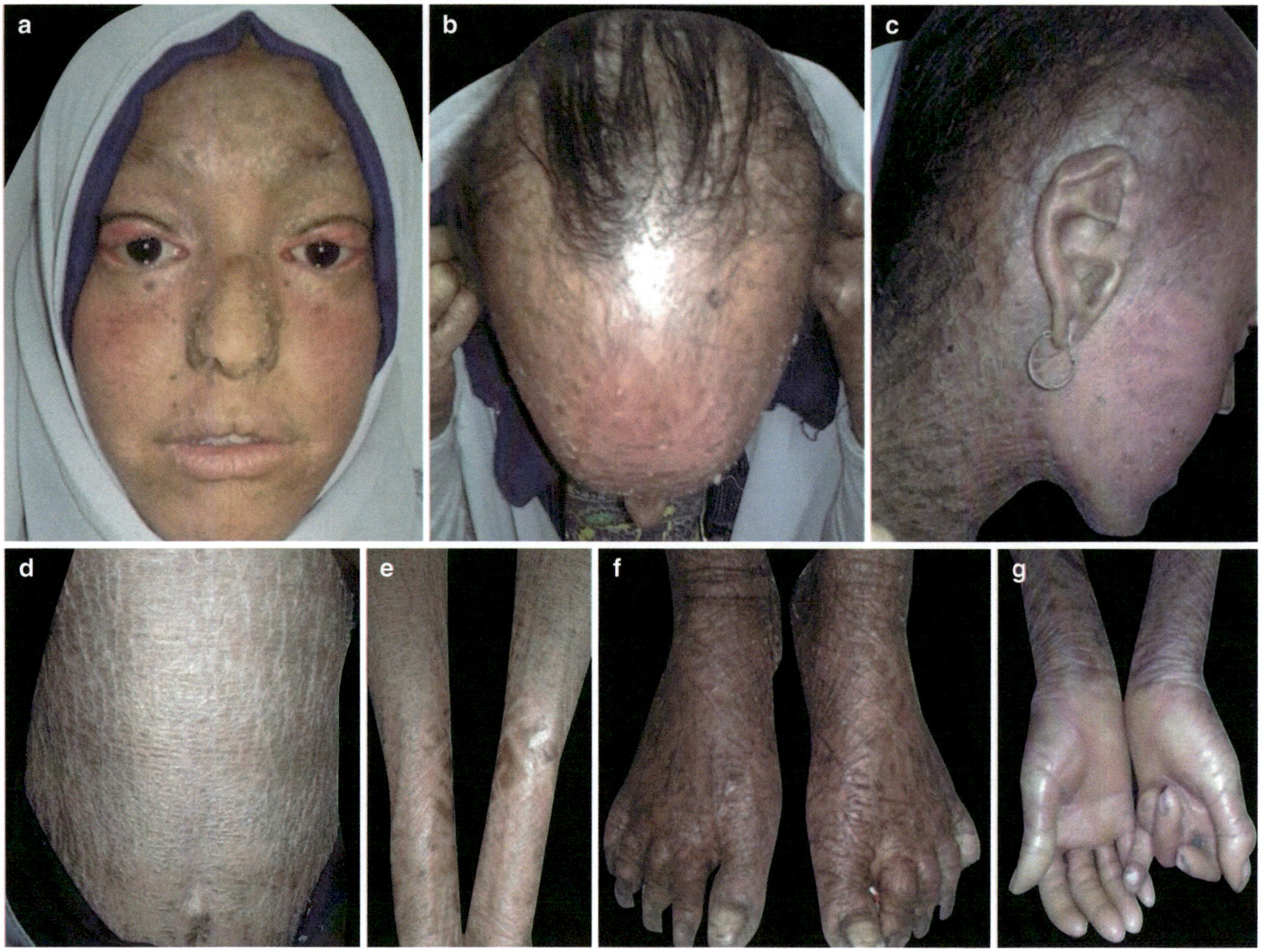

Fig. 1.12 Lamellar ichthyosis in an adult female. Adult patient with obvious ectropion with large, plate-like scales on face, scarring alopecia with ear deformity (**a**–c). Large, plate-like scales forming a mosaic pattern on neck, trunk, limbs, extremities (**c**–**f**), and palmar hyperkeratosis (**g**)

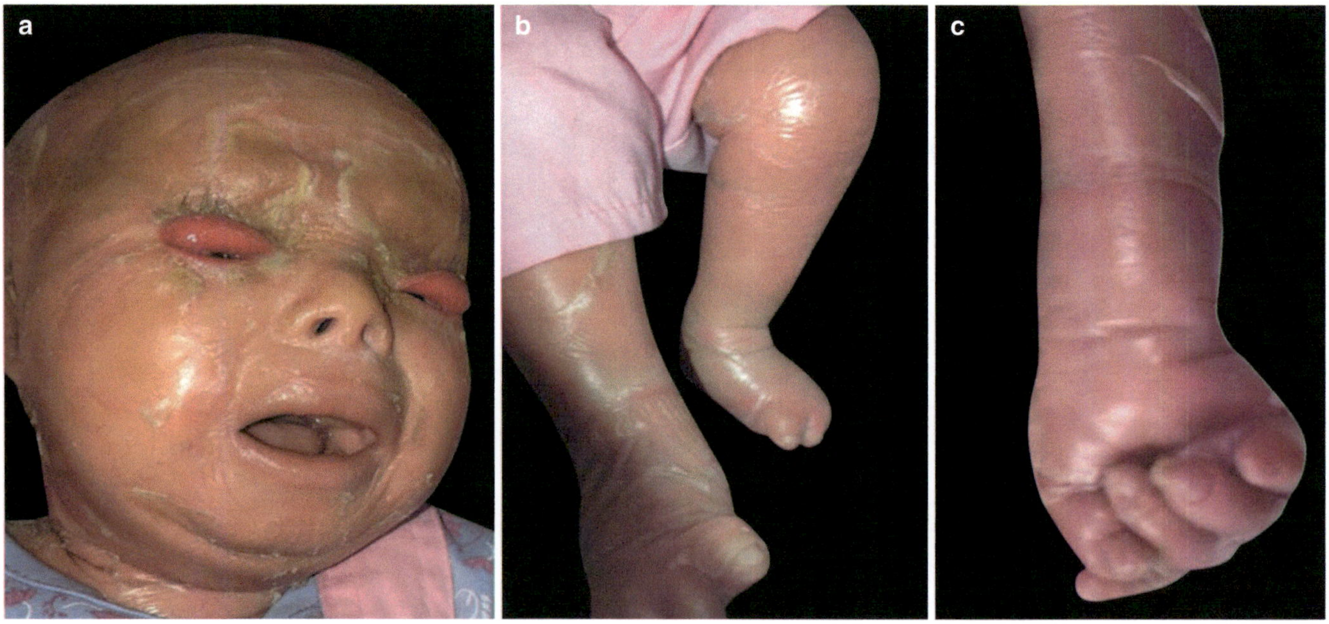

Fig. 1.13 Harlequin Ichthyosis. Obvious ectropion with large, yellow, horny, extremely thickened armor-like plaques on face associated with eclabium and scarring alopecia (**a**), mitten hands and feet (**b**, **c**)

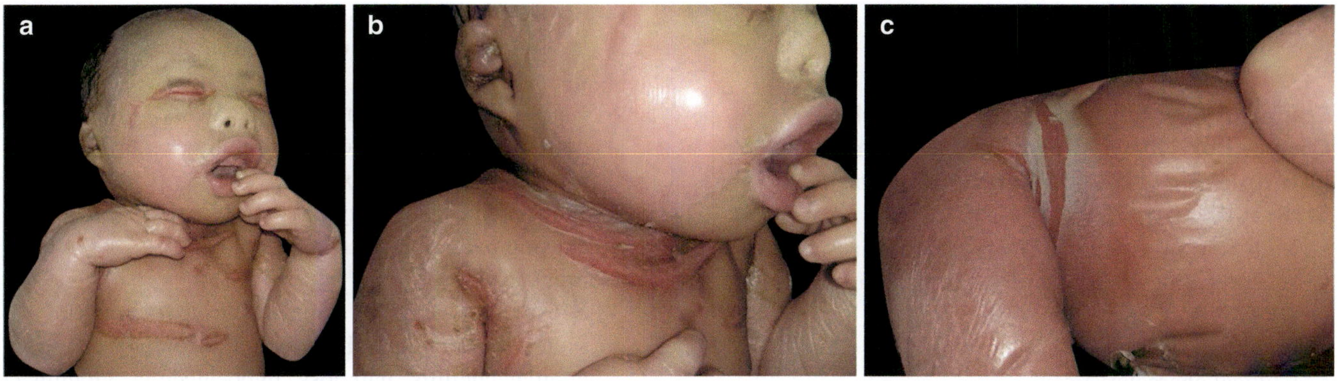

Fig. 1.14 Harlequin Ichthyosis. Eclabium and obvious ectropion with extremely thickened scales with red deep fissures on face, neck, upper chest (**a**, **b**) and lower trunk (**c**)

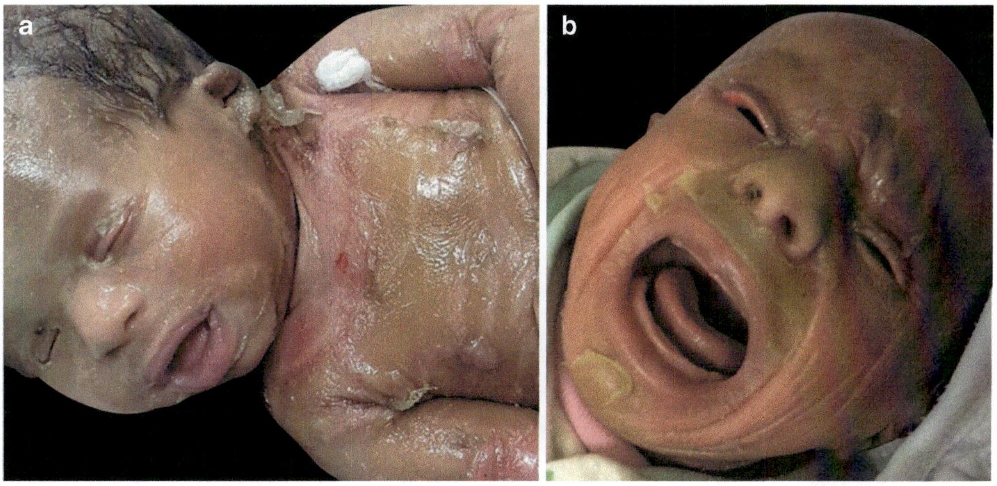

Fig. 1.15 Collodion baby. Day 1 with shiny, transparent membrane resembling plastic wrap, ectropion, eclabium with deformed ears (**a**). Day 5 with erythema, diffuse mild scaling, ectropion, eclabium (**b**)

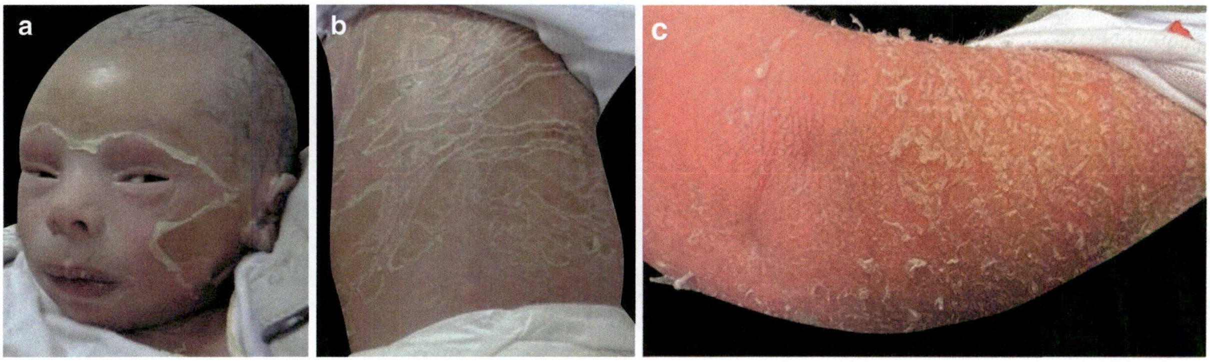

Fig. 1.16 Collodion baby. Baby with a taut, shiny, transparent membrane resembling plastic wrap with erythema on desquamation (**a**–**c**)

Keratinopathic Ichthyoses

Epidermolytic Ichthyosis (AD) [10] (Bullous Congenital Ichthyosiform Erythroderma) (Multiple-Ridged Hyperkeratosis) (Figs. 1.17, 1.18, 1.19, and 1.20)

- Mutation in Keratin *(KRT1)* gene is associated with severe palmoplantar hyperkeratosis while mutation in *KRT10* spare palms and soles.
- Onset: at birth.
- Clinical characteristics:
  - Erythroderma, peeling, erosions, denuded skin, and multiple blisters (misdiagnosed as epidermolysis bullosa in newborns).
  - Later (First few months): decrease skin fragility, with the development of widespread erythema, hyperkeratosis, and focal erosions that form yellow-brown, thick, warty, corrugated ridges and furrows on flexors, joints, and neck, also form cobblestone pattern on extensors surface of joints and dorsal surface of hands and feet.
  - Multiple blisters occur due to skin friction.
  - Severe hyperkeratosis leads to the shedding of scales in the superficial epidermis revealing a tender erythematous base.
  - Carpus-like scales and hyperkeratosis on the trunk, anterior neck, and flexors sometimes may outgrow into Ichthyosis Hystrix.
  - Thickened horny warty or spine-like scales on creases causing palmoplantar hyperkeratosis.
- Complications:
  - Sepsis and electrolyte imbalance (hypernatremia).
  - Foul odor (a pungent body odor), secondary infection, angular cheilitis, hair loss, hypocalcemia, vitamin D resistance, severe palmoplantar hyperkeratosis leading to severe digital contractures and deformities, and gait posture abnormalities due to excessive keratinization.
- Histopathology: (Epidermolytic Hyperkeratosis) (Diagnostic).
  - Massive orthokeratotic hyperkeratosis.
  - Hypergranulosis.
  - Lysis of keratinocytes of the granular cell layer.
- Treatment: keratolytics, topical retinoid and vitamin D preparation with the treatment of secondary bacterial infection.

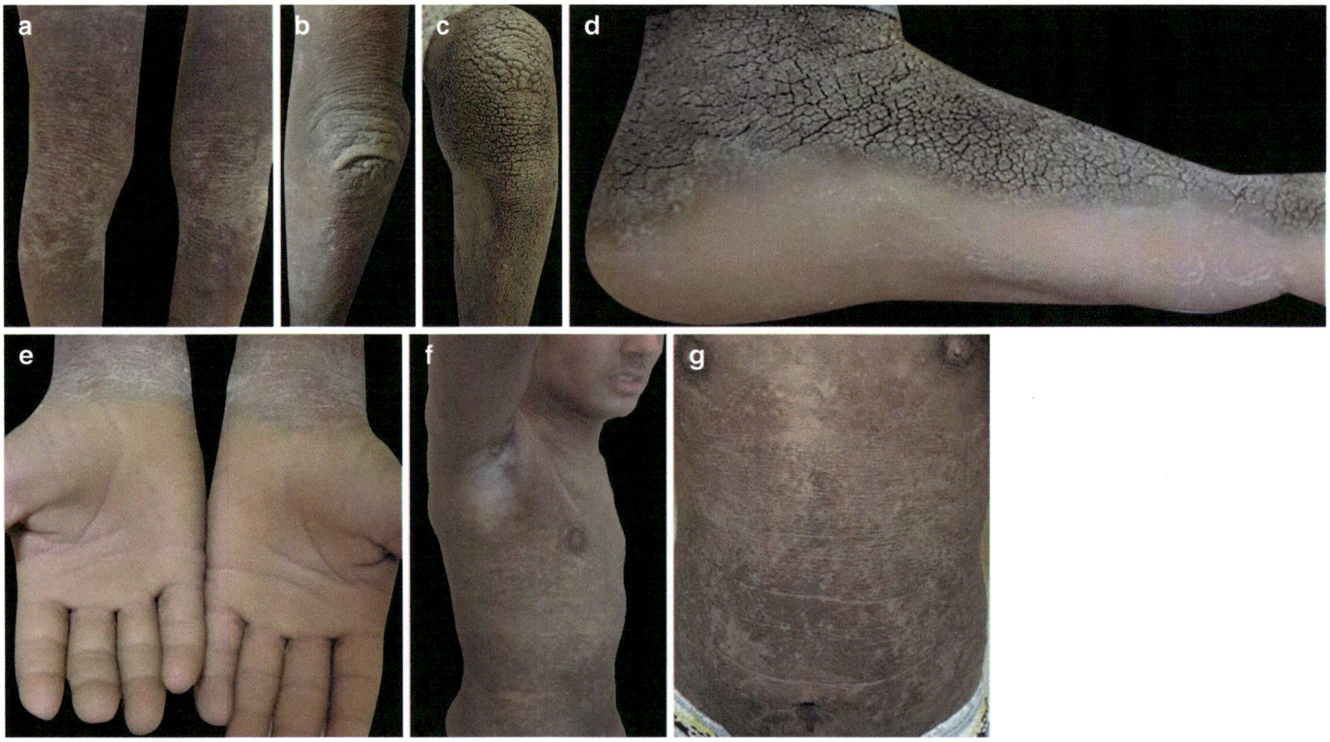

Fig. 1.17 Epidermolytic ichthyosis. Hyperkeratosis with corrugated ridges and furrows on flexors (**a**). Hyperkeratosis with a cobblestone pattern on extensors surface of joints (**b**, **c**) on dorsa of feet (**d**), palmar hyperkeratosis (**e**), carpus-like scales on trunk with focal erosions (**f**, **g**)

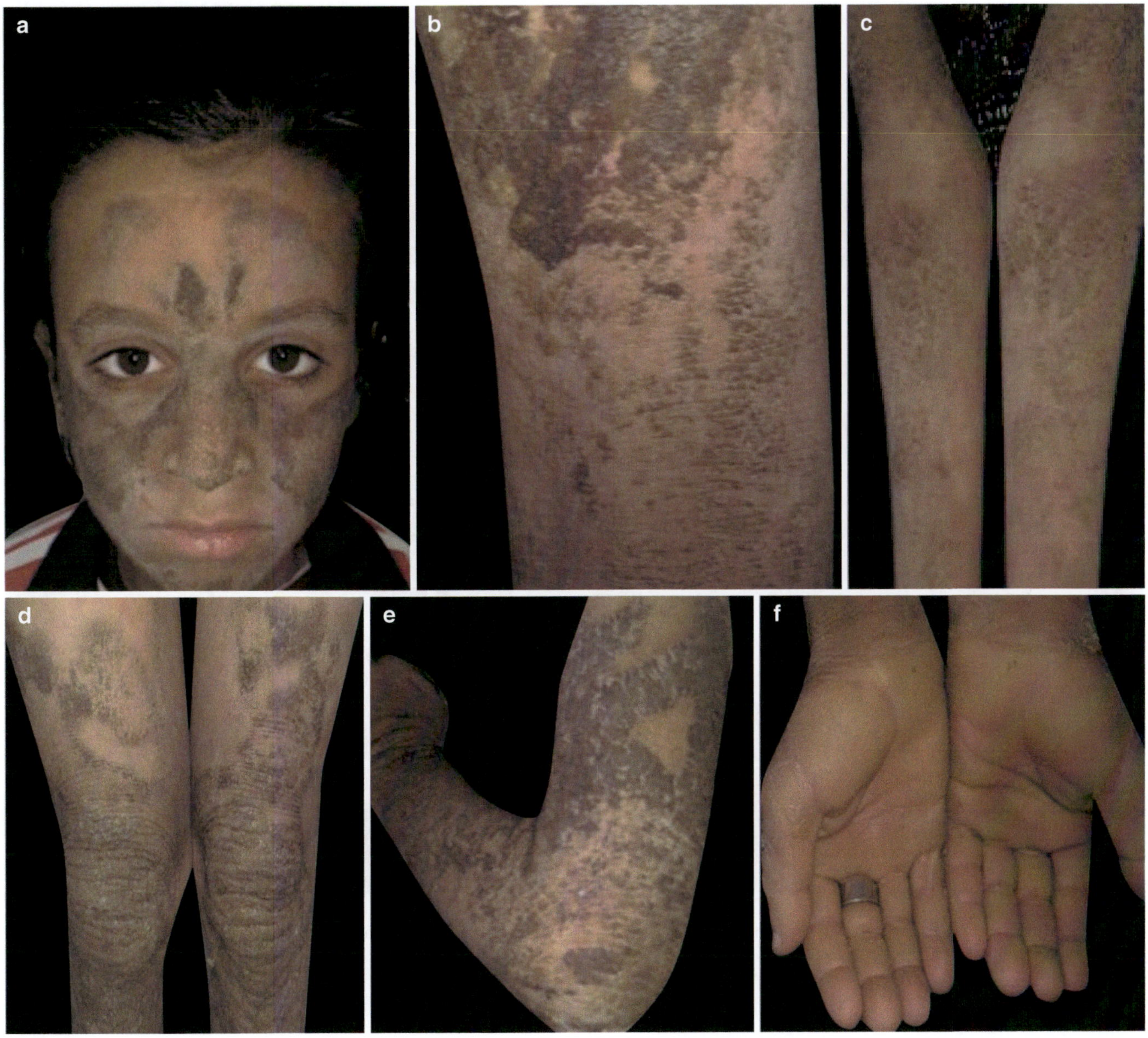

Fig. 1.18 Epidermolytic Ichthyosis. Male patient, showing hyperkeratosis with corrugated ridges and furrows on face (**a**), flexors (**b**, **c**), extensors (**d**, **e**) with palmar hyperkeratosis (**f**)

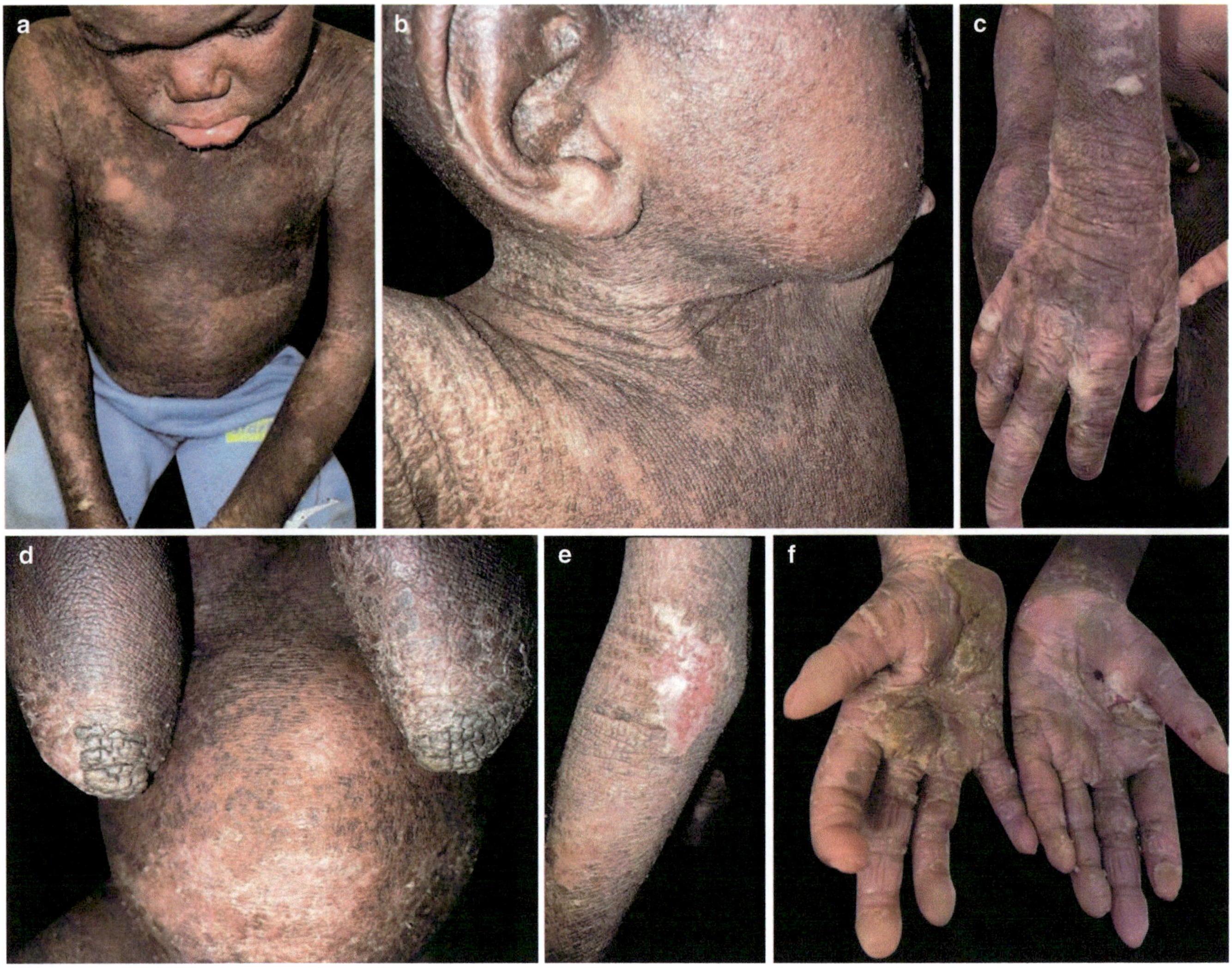

Fig. 1.19 Epidermolytic ichthyosis. Male patient, showing hyperkeratosis with corrugated ridges and furrows on face (**a**), neck (**b**), extensors (**c**, **d**) with maceration (**e**) and palmar hyperkeratosis (**f**)

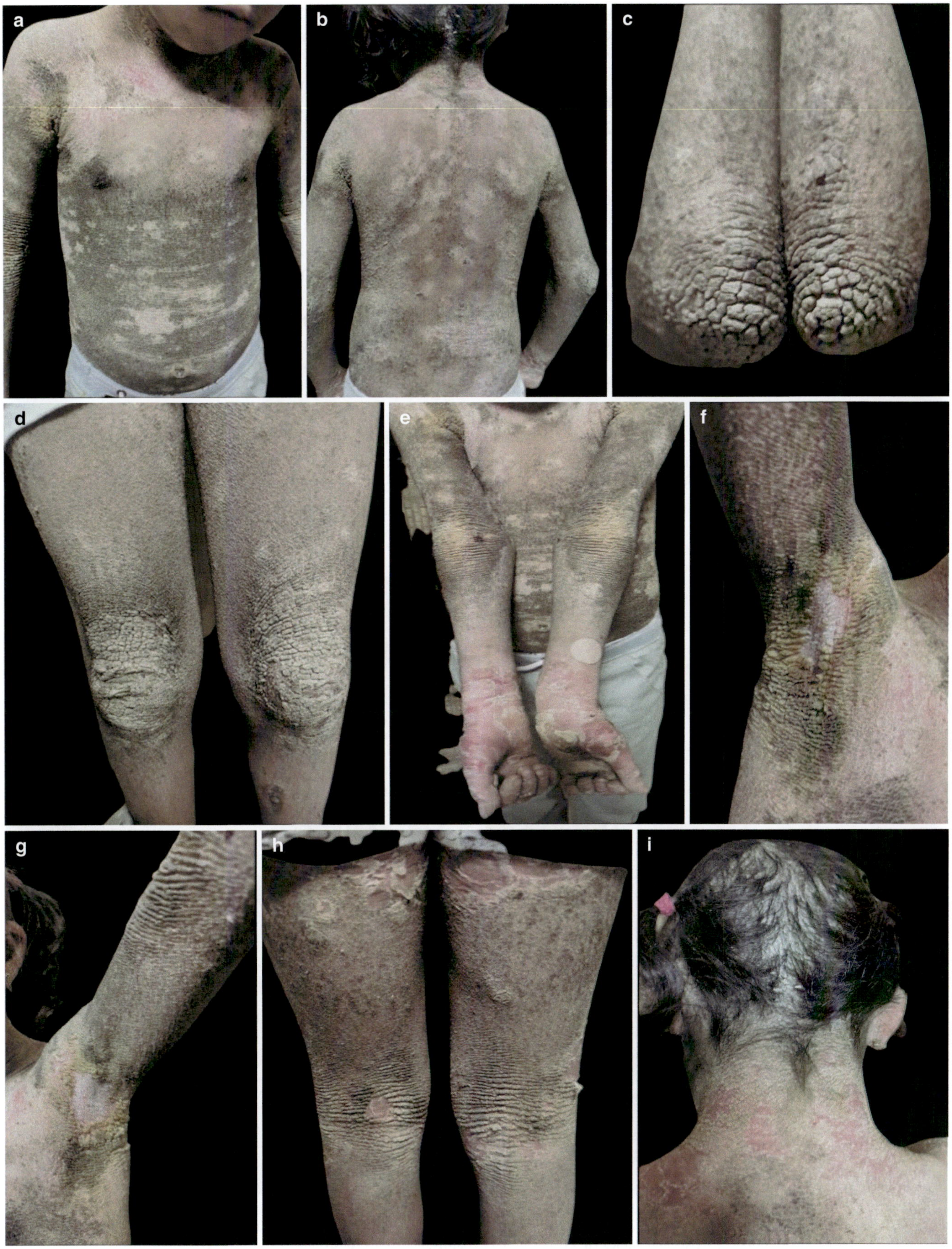

Fig. 1.20 Epidermolytic ichthyosis. Female patient showing hyperkeratosis with corrugated ridges and furrows on trunk (**a**, **b**), limbs with increasing severity on elbows and knees (**c**, **d**). Maceration is marked in hands and flexures (**e**–**i**)

- Oral retinoid: low initial dose then gradually increasing dose and careful monitoring until the lowest maintenance dose has been determined.

Superficial Epidermolytic Ichthyosis (Ichthyosis Bullosa of Siemens) [10] (Figs. 1.21, 1.22, and 1.23)

- Mutation in *KRT2* gene.
- Onset: at birth.
- A mild form of classic Epidermolytic Ichthyosis.
- Normal at birth or mild superficial blisters with mild erythema.
- At infancy: trauma leads to the formation of small blisters characterized by superficial denuded areas with collarette-like borders known as molting or mauserung phenomenon (characteristic). The latter appears as small patches of apparently normal skin in the middle of areas of hyperkeratosis. No palmoplantar hyperkeratosis.
- In childhood: a form of hyperkeratosis (ridged, dirty rippled), and lichenification on joints, flexures, dorsal of hands, and feet sparing face, palms, and soles and is associated with mild blisters leading to brown hyperkeratotic plaques.

Hystrix [11] (Figs. 1.24, 1.25, and 1.26)

- Massive hyperkeratosis with spiny scales (verrucous porcupine scales).
- Descriptive term, not a clinical entity.
- Can be seen in:
  - Epidermolytic ichthyosis: it starts as bullae/erosion, fragile skin, and increased hyperkeratosis.
  - Ichthyosis hystrix of verrucous epidermal nevi: it starts as epidermal nevus then systematized epidermal verrucous nevus (massive hyperkeratosis with spiny scales, linear, elevated, bilateral, and symmetrical) with multiple swirled patterns on both sides.
  - Ichthyosis hystrix of Curth-Macklin: it starts as massive hyperkeratosis with spiny scales at birth.
  - HID Syndrome: **H**ystrix-like **I**chthyosis with **D**eafness.

Ichthyosis Hystrix of Curth-Macklin (AD) [11] (Figs. 1.27 and 1.28)

- Mutation in *KRT1* gene.
- Onset: at birth.

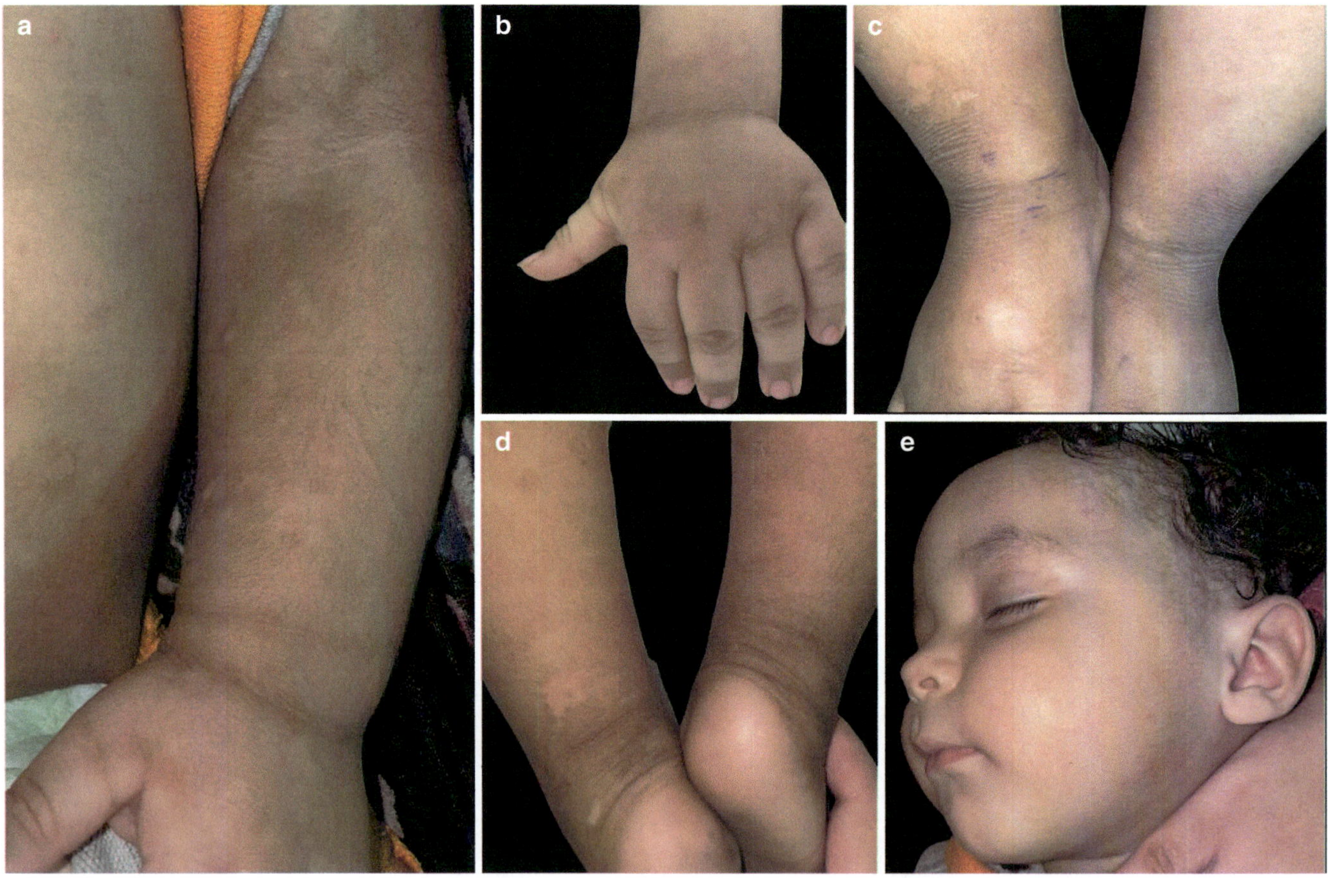

Fig. 1.21 Superficial epidermolytic ichthyosis (Ichthyosis bullosa of Siemens). Hyperkeratosis with slight corrugated ridges and furrows on flexors as cubital fossa (**a**), dorsa of wrists and ankles (**b**, **c**) sparing face, palms, and soles (**d**, **e**)

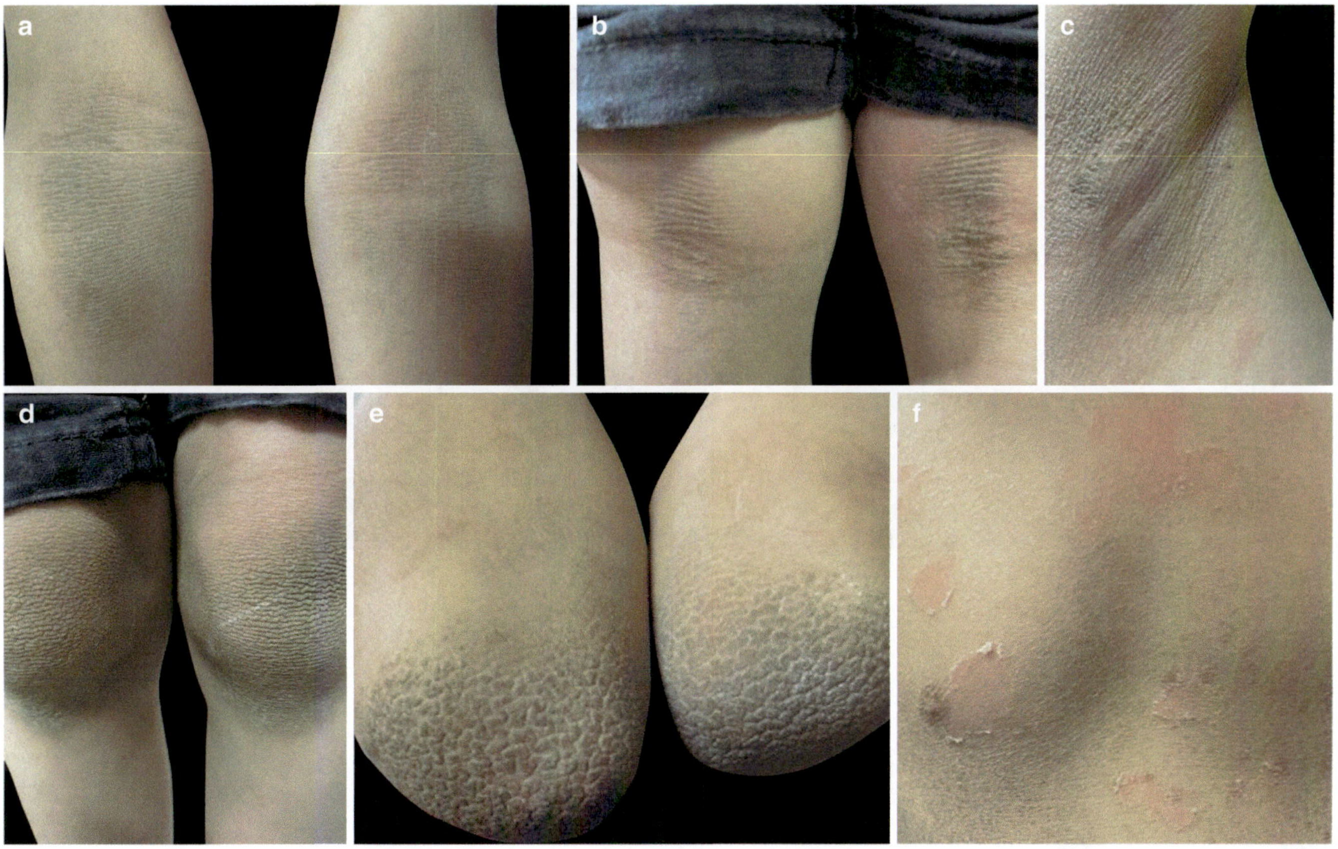

Fig. 1.22 Superficial epidermolytic ichthyosis (Ichthyosis Bullosa of Siemens). Mild hyperkeratosis with corrugated ridges and furrows on flexors (**a**–**c**), extensors (**d**, **e**). Molting or Mauserung phenomenon on chest (**f**)

Fig. 1.23 Superficial epidermolytic ichthyosis in an infant (Ichthyosis Bullosa of Siemens). Molting or mauserung phenomenon (**a**, **b**)

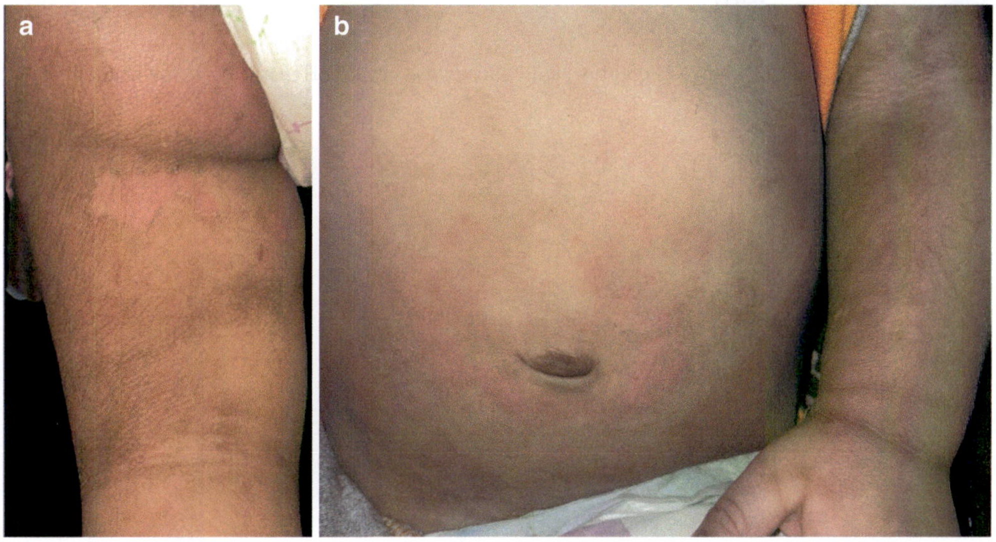

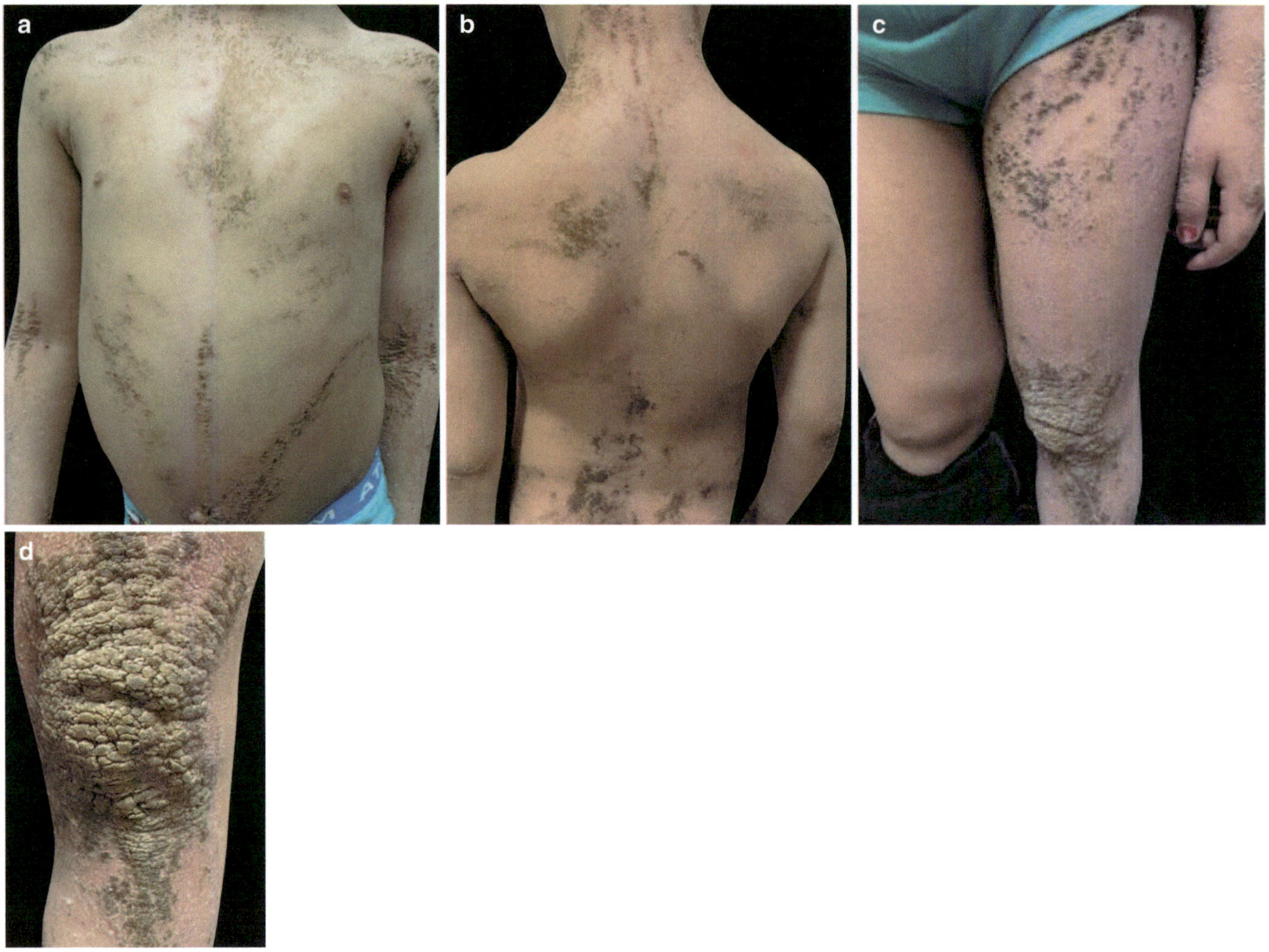

Fig. 1.24 Epidermolytic ichthyosis outgrowing into ichthyosis hystrix. Hyperkeratosis on abdomen (**a**), nape of the neck, back (**b**), and limbs (**c**, **d**)

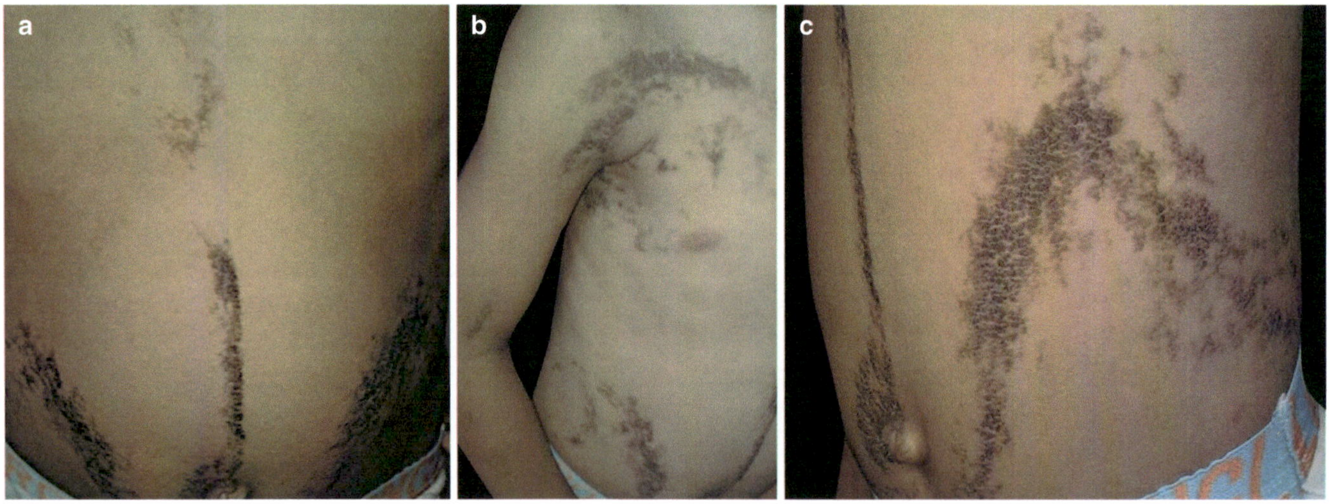

Fig. 1.25 Ichthyosis Hystrix of verrucous epidermal Nevus. It starts as epidermal nevus then systematized epidermal nevus. Massive spiny brownish black hyperkeratosis (muddy) (**a**–**c**)

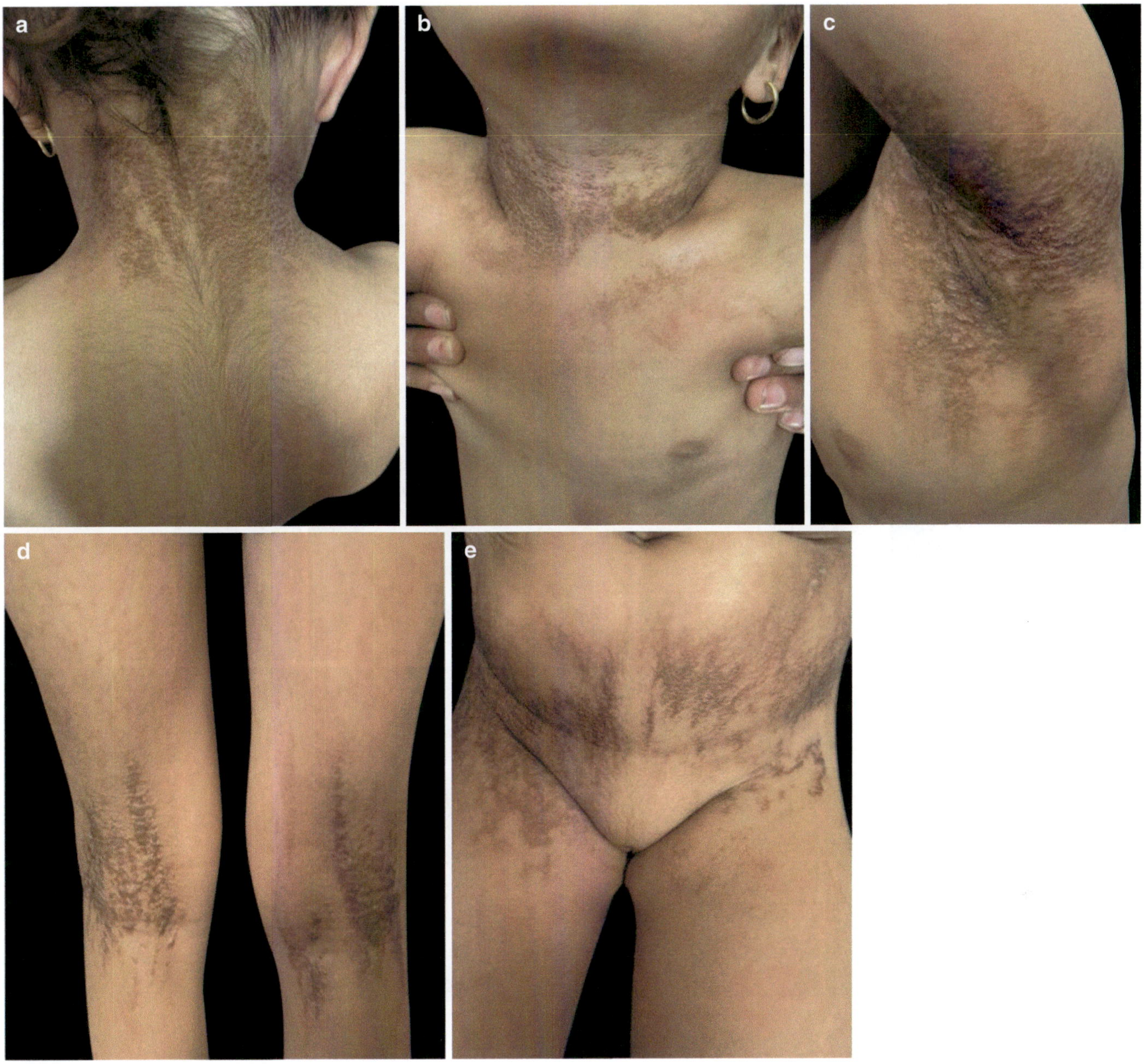

Fig. 1.26 Ichthyosis Hystrix of verrucous epidermal nevus. Systematized, linear, verrucous, hyperkeratotic brownish black (muddy) dermatomal lesion on back (**a**), neck (**b**), skin folds (**a**–**d**), abdomen and groin (**e**)

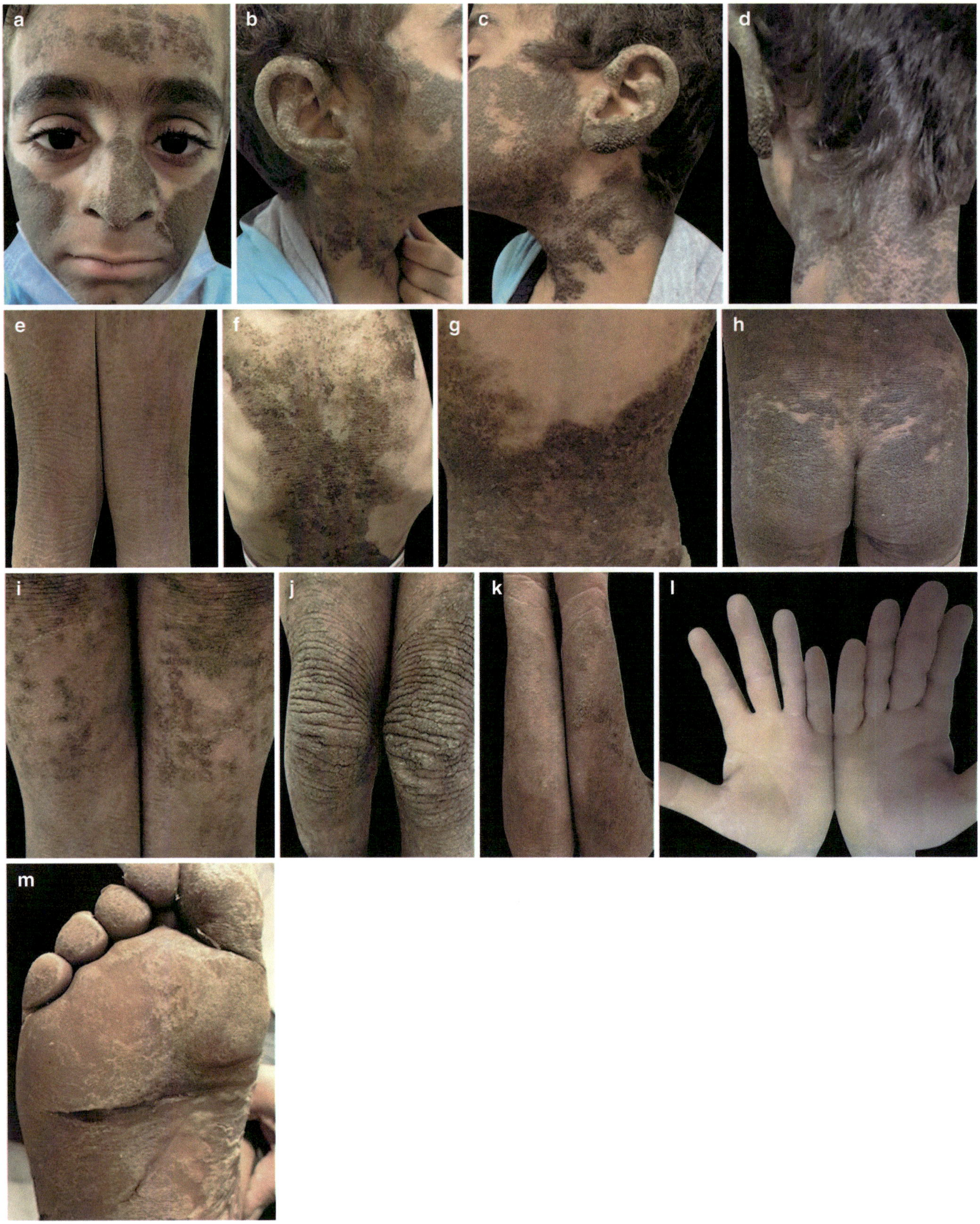

Fig. 1.27 Ichthyosis Hystrix of Curth-Macklin. Hyperkeratosis with horny, rigid spikes on face (**a**), ears (**b**, **c**), back of the neck (**d**), back of lower limbs (**e**), trunk (**f**, **g**), buttocks (**h**), thighs (**i**), and over the knees (**j**). Hyperkeratosis on forearms (**k**) with palmoplantar hyperkeratosis (**l**, **m**)

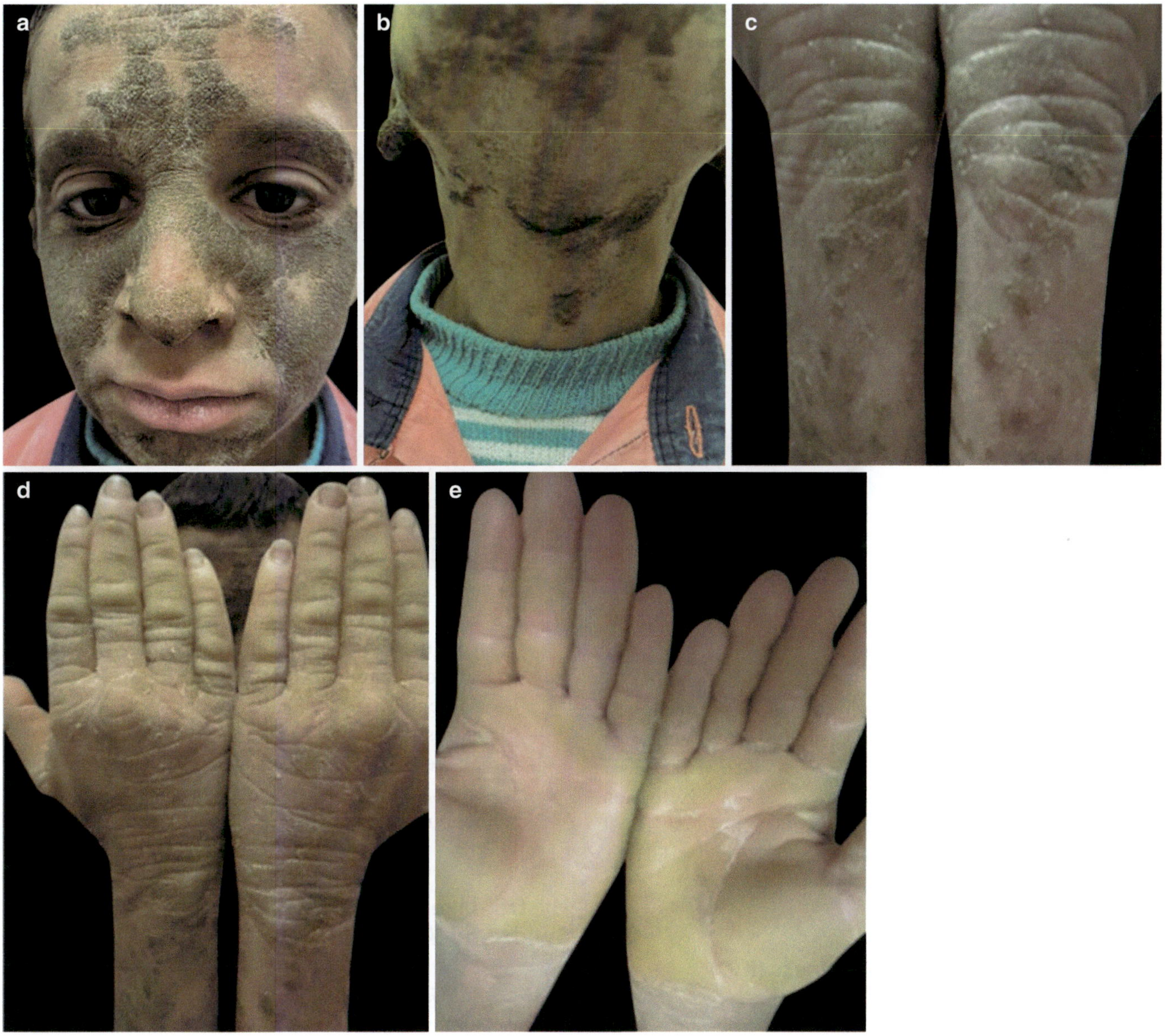

Fig. 1.28 Ichthyosis Hystrix of Curth-Macklin (brother of Fig. 1.27). Hyperkeratosis with horny, rigid spikes on face (**a**), chin (**b**), over the knees (**c**), over the wrists (**d**) with palmoplantar hyperkeratosis (**e**). It is less severe than his brother

- Can initially mimic epidermolytic ichthyosis with no skin fragility.
- Characterized by generalized hystrix-like hyperkeratosis with horny, rigid spikes on extremities, large joints, skin folds, and trunk (cobblestone-like).
- Mild to severe mutilating palmoplantar hyperkeratosis (isolated).
- Pseudo-ainhum (circular construction band), flexural digital contractures, starfish-like keratosis, knuckle pads, and secondary bacterial infection may occur.

Ichthyosis En Confetti (AD) [12] (Fig. 1.29)

(Ichthyosis variegata or congenital reticular ichthyosiform erythroderma)

- Mutation in *KRT10* or *KRT1* genes.
- Onset: at birth.
- Major clinical features:
  - Ichthyosiform erythroderma.
  - Confetti-like spots of healthy skin mainly on the trunk reflecting revertant mosaicism.
- Associations: ear deformities, mamillae hypoplasia, palmoplantar hyperkeratosis, hypertrichosis, and ectropion.

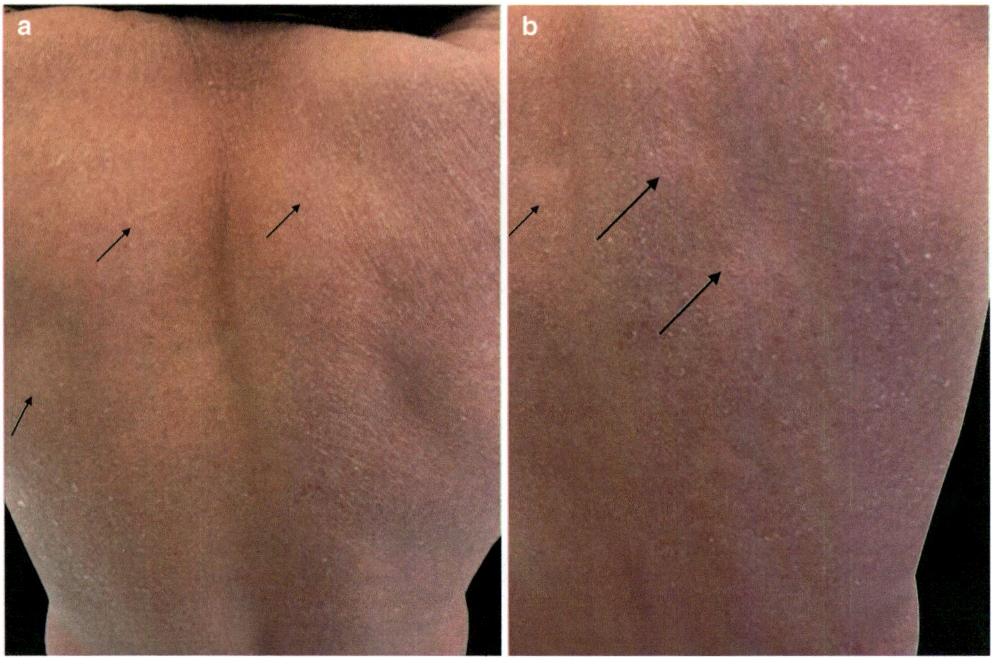

Fig. 1.29 Ichthyosis en Confetti. Ichthyosiform erythroderma, confetti islands of normal skin on trunk (arrow) (**a**, **b**)

Ichthyosiform Syndromes

Among diseases that cause ichthyosis as one of the symptoms, there are some diseases that induce abnormalities in organs other than the skin. These include KID, HID, Chanarin-Dorfman, Refsum, Sjögren-Larsson, Netherton, Tay-Sachs (PIBIDS), Rud's, Laurence-Moon-Bardet-Biedl, MEDNIK, Conradi-Hünermann-Happle and CHILD syndrome.

Keratitis, Ichthyosis, and Deafness (KID) Syndrome [13, 14] (Fig. 1.30)

- Defect in *GJB2* and Connexin (*Cx26*) genes.
- Onset: at birth with transient neonatal erythema.
- Clinical characteristics:
  - Progressive keratitis (photophobia), blepharitis, conjunctivitis, and secondary night blindness.
  - Ichthyosis: well-demarcated hyperkeratotic plaques with erythematous base and rough-ridged verrucous surface "erythrokeratoderma" on the knees, elbows, face, ear helices, scalp, and groin with a radial deep furrow on the face (around mouth and chin) and prominent follicular keratosis. Lastly, diffuse palmar hyperkeratosis with coarse-grained leather, reticulated stippled surface associated with nail dystrophy and leukonychia. Erythroderma may develop.
  - Deafness (sensorineural).
  - Hair is lusterless with bright-dark bands, hypotrichosis, alopecia, absent eyebrows and eyelashes, folliculitis, follicular triad occlusion, and pilar cyst tumor.
  - Anhidrosis.
  - Small teeth and excessive caries.
  - Cheilitis, chronic mucocutaneous candidiasis and squamous cell carcinoma.

Hystrix-Like Ichthyosis with Deafness (HID) Syndrome (AD) [13, 14] (Fig. 1.31)

- Defect in *GJB2* and *Cx26* genes.
- Onset: at birth.
- Increased risk of squamous cell carcinoma.
- Clinical characteristics:
  - Skin: all features of KID, however, with more severe skin involvement with mild keratitis. Newborns early developed red skin then dry, thick, and spiky scales (porcupine quills) all over the body appear. Palms and soles are mildly affected.
  - Deafness.

Chanarin-Dorfman Syndrome (AR) [15] Neutral Lipid Storage Disease with Ichthyosis (Fig. 1.32)

- Defect in abhydrolase domain containing 5, lysophosphatidic acid acyltransferase (*ABHD5*) gene.

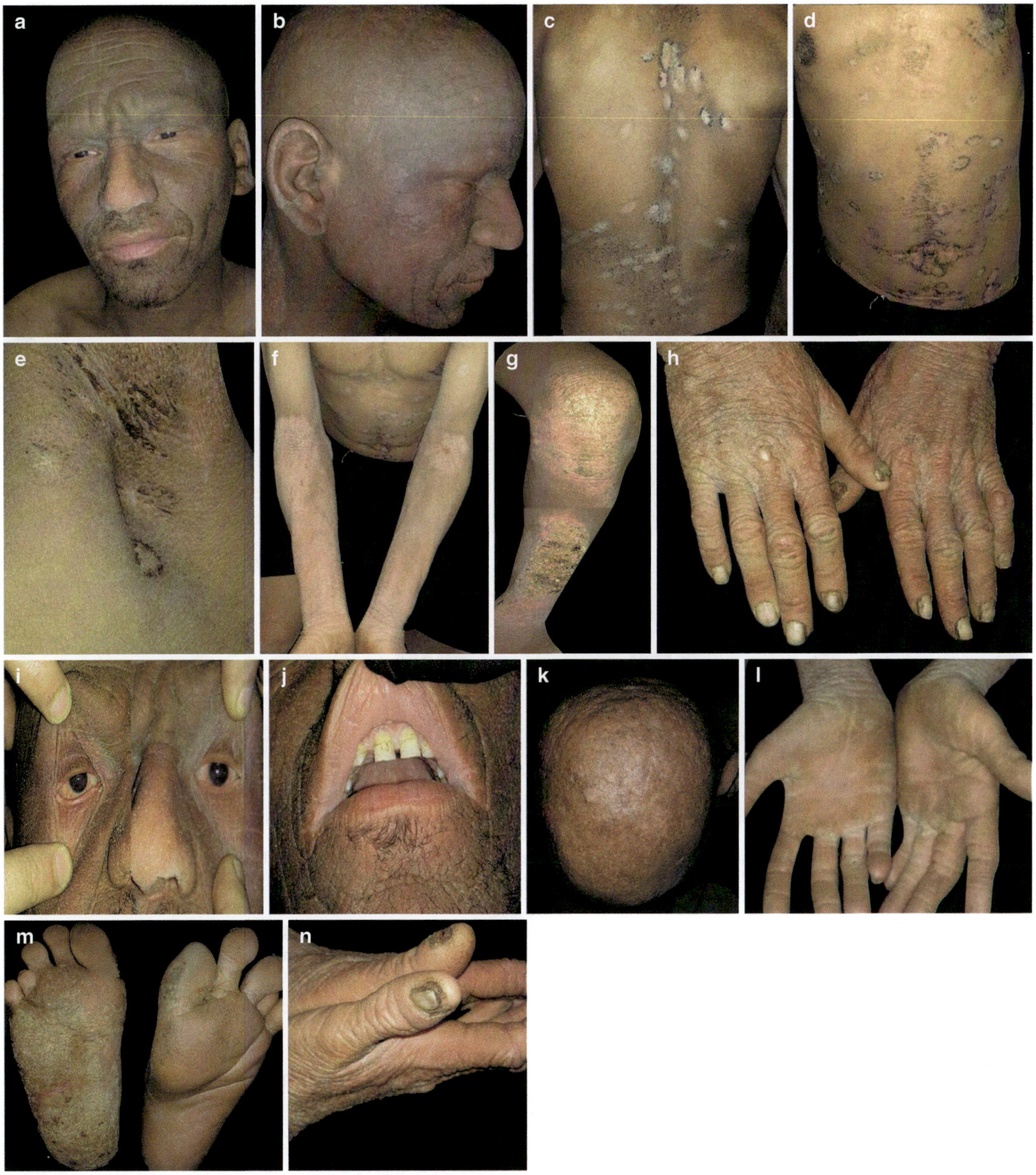

Fig. 1.30 KID syndrome. Symmetrical well demarcated hyperkeratotic plaques with rough-ridged verrucous surface on the face (**a**), helices (**b**), trunk (**c**, **d**), axilla (**e**), flexors (**f**), lower limb (**g**), and on skin overlying small joints of hands (**h**) Keratitis, conjunctivitis, absent eyebrows and eyelashes (**i**). Radial furrows around the mouth, small teeth and caries (**j**), alopecia (**k**), palmoplantar hyperkeratosis (**l**, **m**), and nail dystrophy (**n**)

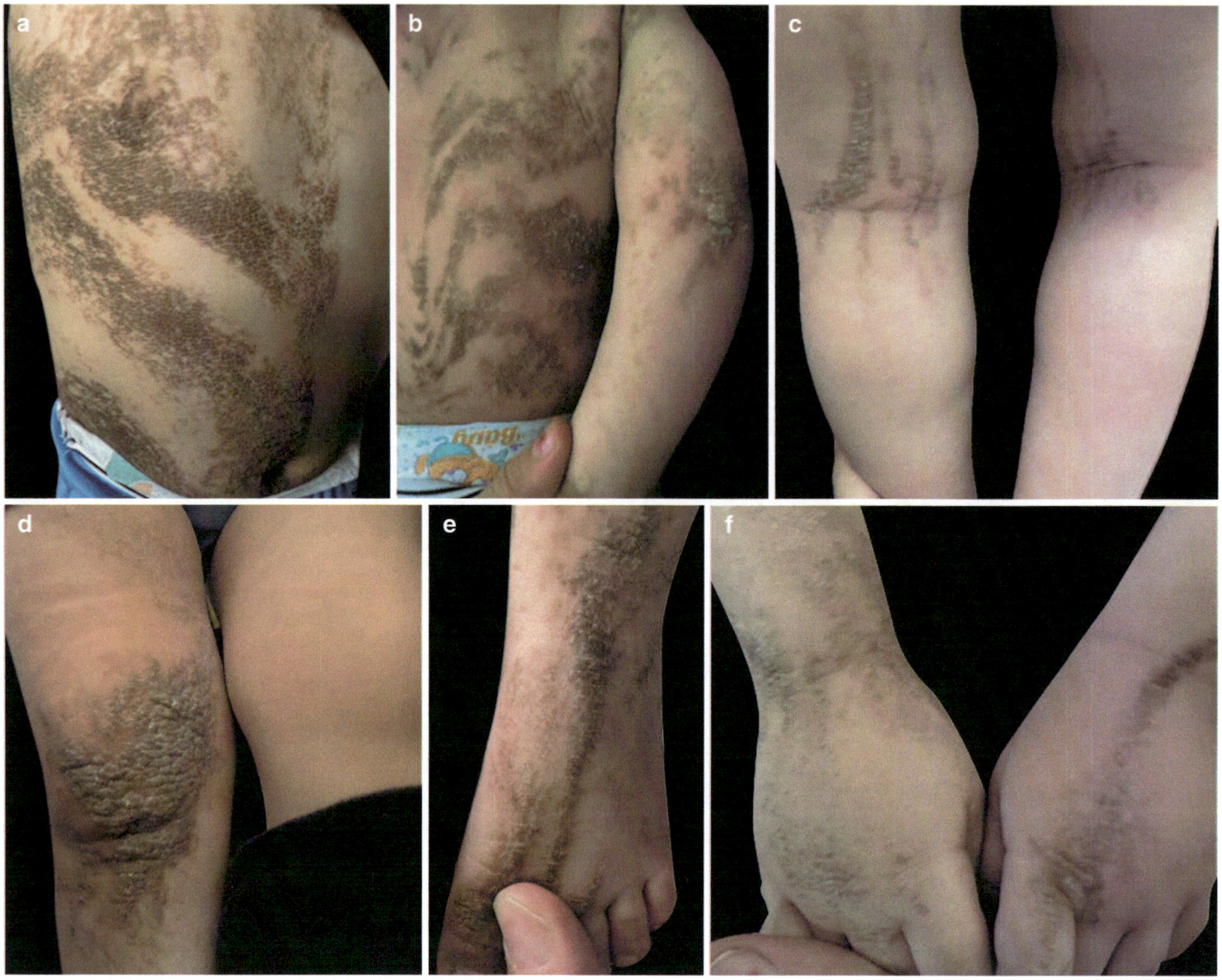

Fig. 1.31 HID syndrome. Hyperkeratosis with spiny scales (porcupine quills), linear brownish black (muddy), linear, elevated lesions on trunk (**a**, **b**) and limbs (**c**–**f**)

- Onset: at birth.
- Rare collodion baby.
- Mutation in this gene leads to abnormal fatty acid (triglyceride) deposition in organs.
- Clinical characteristics:
  - Skin: collodion baby, ichthyosiform erythroderma (CIE-like), fine white-grayish plate scale, poikiloderma atrophicans vascular, eclabium, alopecia, and shiny skin.
  - Neurological: ataxia, microcephaly, mental retardation, myopathy, myalgia, progressive weakness of proximal arms and legs.
  - Eyes: Cataract, myopia, dryness, and ectropion.
  - Ears: sensorineural deafness 15%.
  - Neurological problems.
  - Interstitial malabsorption, fatty liver, and steatorrhea.
- Laboratory findings: lipid vacuoles in white blood cells with granulocytes, monocytes, and eosinophils (Jordan's anomaly).
- Treatment: early intervention with a fat restricted diet.

Refsum Syndrome (AR) [16, 17] (Fig. 1.33)

- Defects in Phytanoyl-Co-A Hydroxylase (*PHYH*) or *PEX7* genes lead to phytanic acid accumulation.
- Onset: early childhood.
- Clinical characteristics:
  1. Neurocutaneous disorder:
     - Ichthyosis vulgaris-like in adults: Whitish fine scales on trunk and extremities, palmoplantar hyperkeratosis, and hyperlinear palms.
     - Cerebellar ataxia (difficult walking).

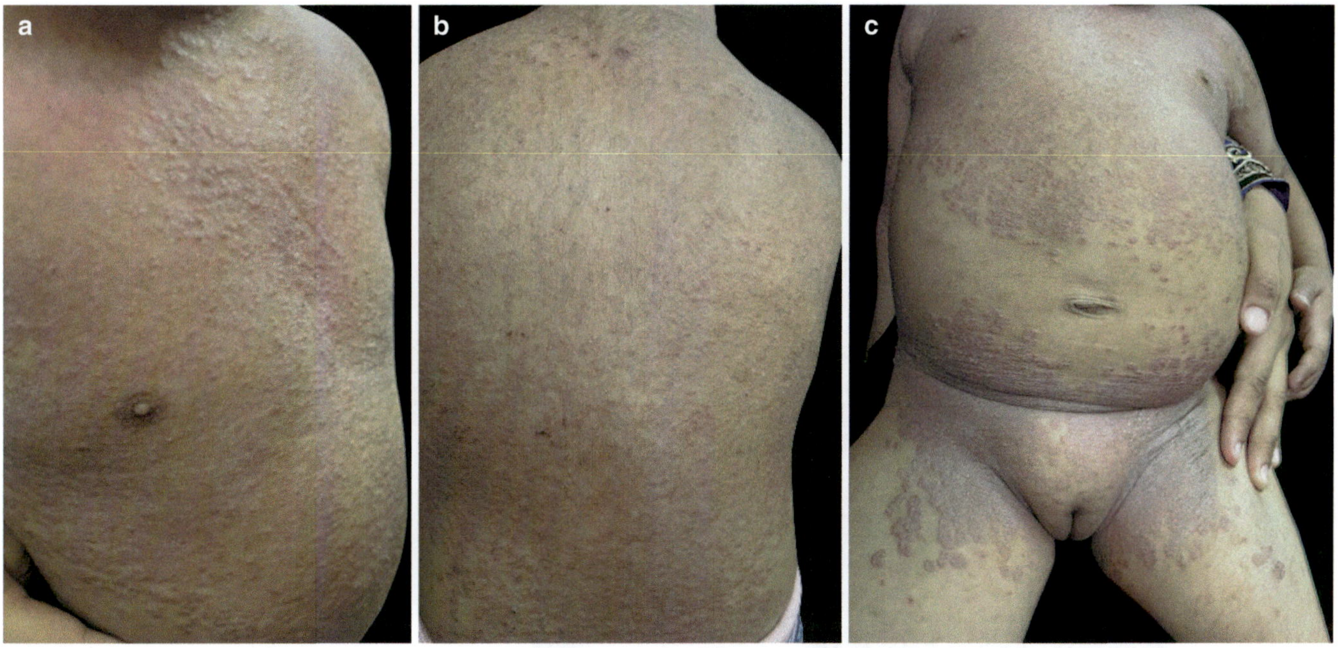

Fig. 1.32 Chanarin-Dorfman Syndrome. Ichthyosiform erythroderma (congenital ichthyosiform erythroderma-like), fine grayish plate-like scale on trunk and intertriginous area (**a**–**c**)

  - Peripheral neuropathy.
  - Atypical retinitis pigmentosa (diagnostic), salt pepper pigmentation, cataract, and poor night vision.
  - Sensorineural deafness.
  - Anosmia (diagnostic) or reduced smelling.
2. Cardiac: muscle wasting, cardiac myopathy, and abnormal electrocardiographic (ECG) findings (arrhythmia and heart block) which may lead to sudden death.

- Phytanic acid dietary restriction (animal product) leads to improvement of the neurological disorder.

2. Eyes: perifoveal glistening white dots in the fundus (retinal degeneration) which is considered a pathognomonic sign, corneal defect, photophobia, and hypertelorism.
3. Central nervous system affection starts during the first year of life in form of white matter disease of the brain, progressive spasticity di or tetraplegia with contractures more on the lower limb.
4. Abnormal gait (stiff movement with scissor type of gait) (pyramidal sign), speech defects, seizure in 40%, intellectual disability, and mental retardation.
5. Teeth: enamel hypoplasia (pits).

Sjögren-Larsson Syndrome (AR) [18, 19] (Figs. 1.34 and 1.35)

- Defect in *FALDH* gene.
- Onset: at birth.
- Collodion baby.
- Clinical characteristics:

  Skin: congenital ichthyosis, eyes: retinal glistening white dots, and CNS: spasticity are diagnostic.

1. Skin:
   (a) Pruritic non-scaling hyperkeratosis more than scaling (fine to plate-like); favors abdomen, neck, flexures.
   (b) Persistent pruritus and excoriation with accentuated skin marking and palmoplantar hyperkeratosis.

Netherton Syndrome (AR) [20] (Figs. 1.36, 1.37 and 1.38)

- Defect in *SPINK5/LEKT1* genes.
- Onset: at birth or during infancy.
- Collodion baby.
- **Triad: Ichthyosis linearis circumflexa, hair shaft anomalies, pruritus**
  1. Skin manifestations:
     - At birth congenital ichthyosiform erythroderma and peeling, then after 2 years ichthyosis linearis circumflexa appears "erythematous polycyclic and serpiginous migratory plaques with double-edged scales in the periphery" on trunk and extremities.

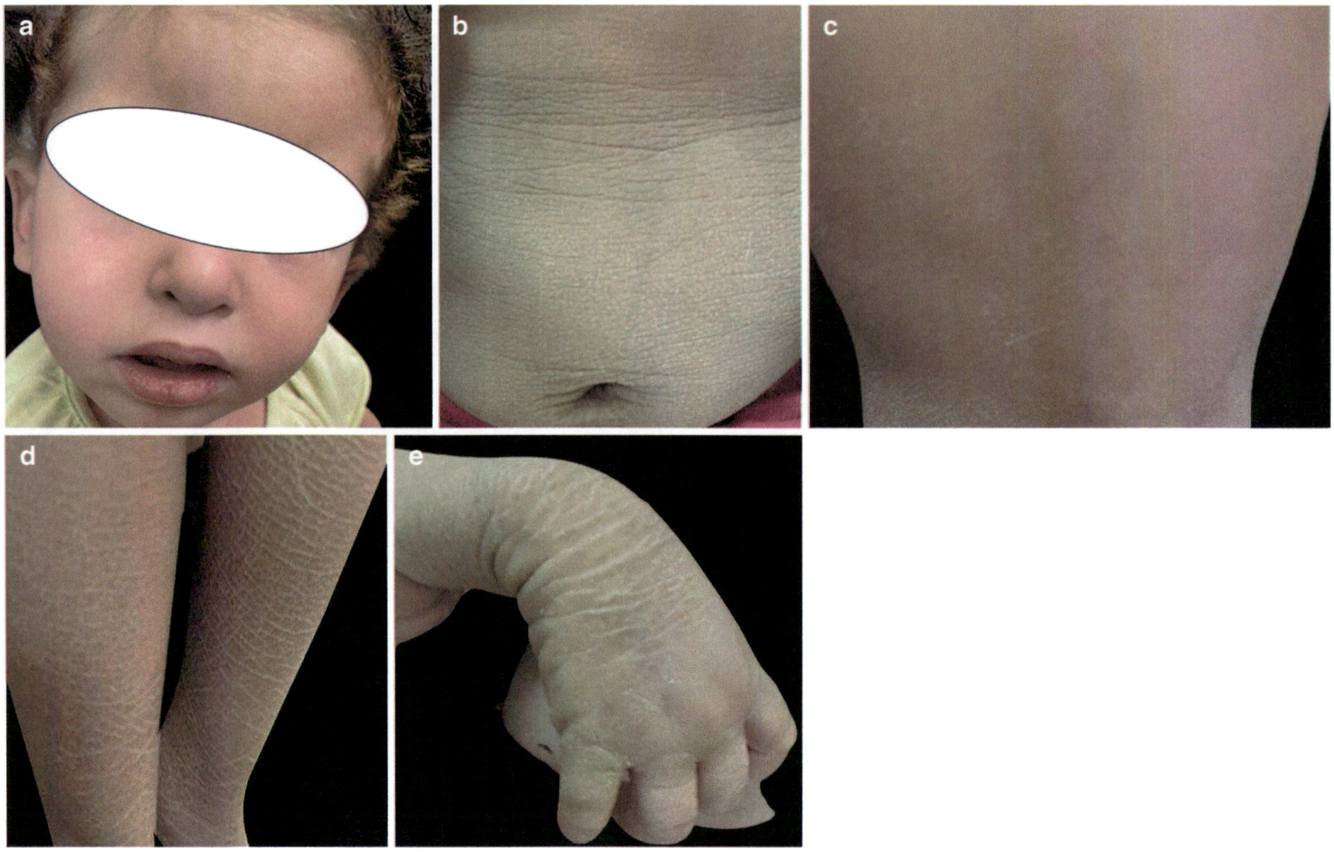

Fig. 1.33 Refsum Syndrome. Ichthyosis vulgaris-like (whitish fine scales) on trunk and limbs (**a–d**) and hyperlinear dorsum of wrist joint and hand (**e**)

   - Lichenification in flexors, wrists and antecubital popliteal fossae.
   - Scalp with thick scales, erythroderma, ichthyosis, and eczematous lesions in childhood.
2. Hair affection:
   - Trichorrhexis invaginata: intussusception of hair shaft into itself (microscopy: Bamboo hair, and ball and socket-type hair shaft deformity) with short, brittle sparse hair.
   - Trichorrhexis nodosa (hair intermittent nodule).
   - Pili torti: short thin hair.
   - The eyelashes and eyebrows may be affected.
   - The hair abnormality may not be noticed in infancy because babies often have sparse hair.
3. Atopy, eosinophilia, allergic reaction to foods, pruritus, urticaria, angioedema, anaphylaxis, and asthma.

- Associations: recurrent skin and chest infections, squamous cell carcinoma in the skin or vulva, poikiloderma, dehydration, aminoaciduria, and electrolyte imbalance (hypernatremia).

Tay-Sachs Syndrome (PIBIDS) (AR) [20] (Congenital Ichthyosis with Trichothiodystrophy) (Figs. 1.39, 1.40 and 1.41)

(P: photosensitivity, I: ichthyosis, B: brittle hair, I: intellectual impairment, D: decreased fertility, and S: short stature)

- Defect in *ERCC2* and *ERCC3* genes.
- Onset: at birth.
- Collodion baby.
- Clinical characteristics:
- Hair: brittle short sparse fragile hair (low sulfur content).
  - Sulfur defect leads to:
  - In light microscopy: Trichoschisis + Trichorrhexis nodosa + pili torti.
  - In polarizing light microscopy: Trichothiodystrophy, tiger tail (zigzag) banding.
- Nail: thinning, longitudinal ridging, yellow, splitting onychogryphosis.
- Eye: photosensitivity in half of the patients and hyperpigmentation of eyelids.

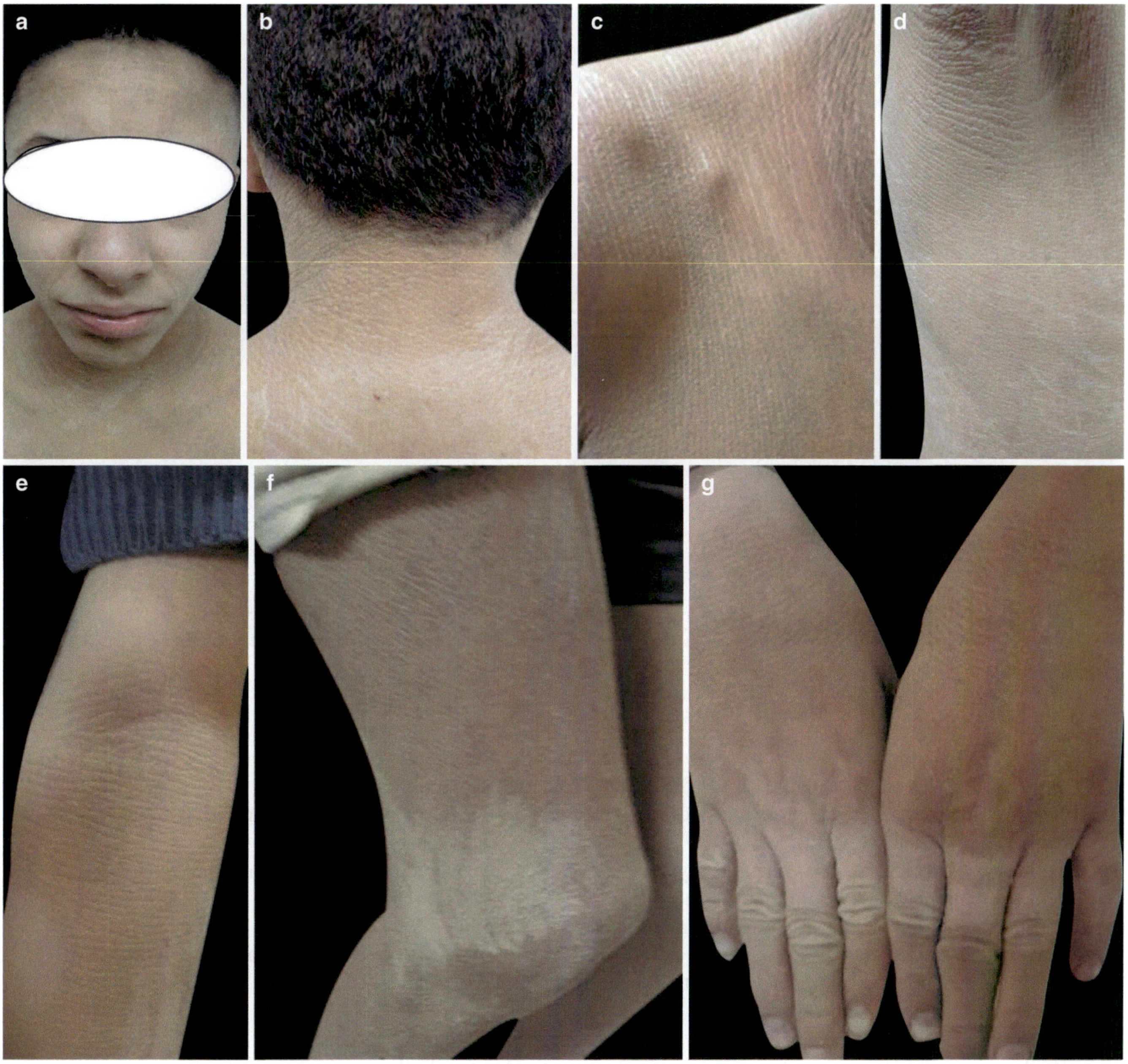

Fig. 1.34 Sjögren-Larsson Syndrome. Lamellar ichthyosis (plate-like scale) with increase skin markings on neck (**a**–**c**), trunk (**d**, **e**), limbs (**f**), dorsum of hands (**g**) with scratch marks due to pruritus (**f**, **g**). White matter disease of brain (**h**)

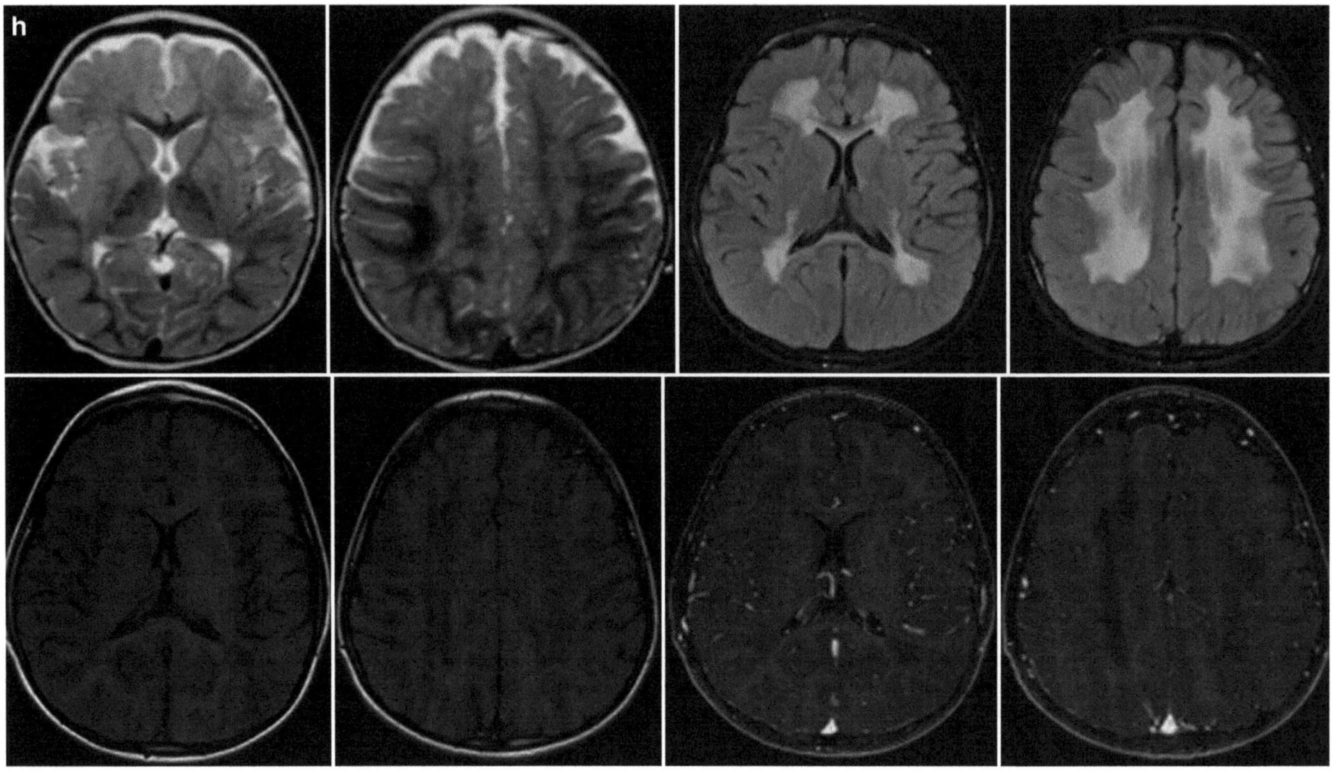

Fig. 1.34 (continued)

- Skin:
  - Erythroderma decreased with age.
  - Ichthyosis (generalized fine large translucent to dark scale with minimal erythema).
  - Folliculitis, atopic-like skin, cheilitis, hypohidrosis, pruritus, lentigines, hypopigmented macules, telangiectasia, poikiloderma, lipoatrophy, pyoderma, and palmar pustules.
- CNS: intellectual impairment (mental retardation), microcephaly, ataxia, and spastic paralysis.
- Brain MRI: demyelination, cerebellar atrophy, and dilated ventricles.
- Skeletal: short stature.
- Others: decreased fertility due to hypogonadism, recurrent infection, and progeria-like.

Rud Syndrome (AR) [21] (Fig. 1.42)

- Defect in Steroid Sulfatase *(STS)* gene.
- Onset: at birth.
- Clinical characteristics:
  - Skin: lamellar ichthyosis-like.
  - CNS: mental retardation, epilepsy.
  - Peripheral neuropathy.
  - Eye: retinitis pigmentosa.
  - Endocrinal: acanthosis nigricans, dwarfism, and hypogonadism.
  - Hematology: macrocytic anemia.

Laurence-Moon-Bardet-Biedl Syndrome (AR) [22] (Fig. 1.43)

- Defect in *LMBBS* gene.
- Onset: at birth.
- Occurs at birth and develops during the first year of life.
- Clinical characteristics:
  - Polydactyly.
  - Ichthyosis.
  - Pseudo-acanthosis nigricans.
  - Retinitis pigmentosa.
  - Hypogonadism.
  - Obesity.
  - Mental retardation.
  - Diabetes insipidus.
  - Some patients may suffer from calcification on the skin and tendons.

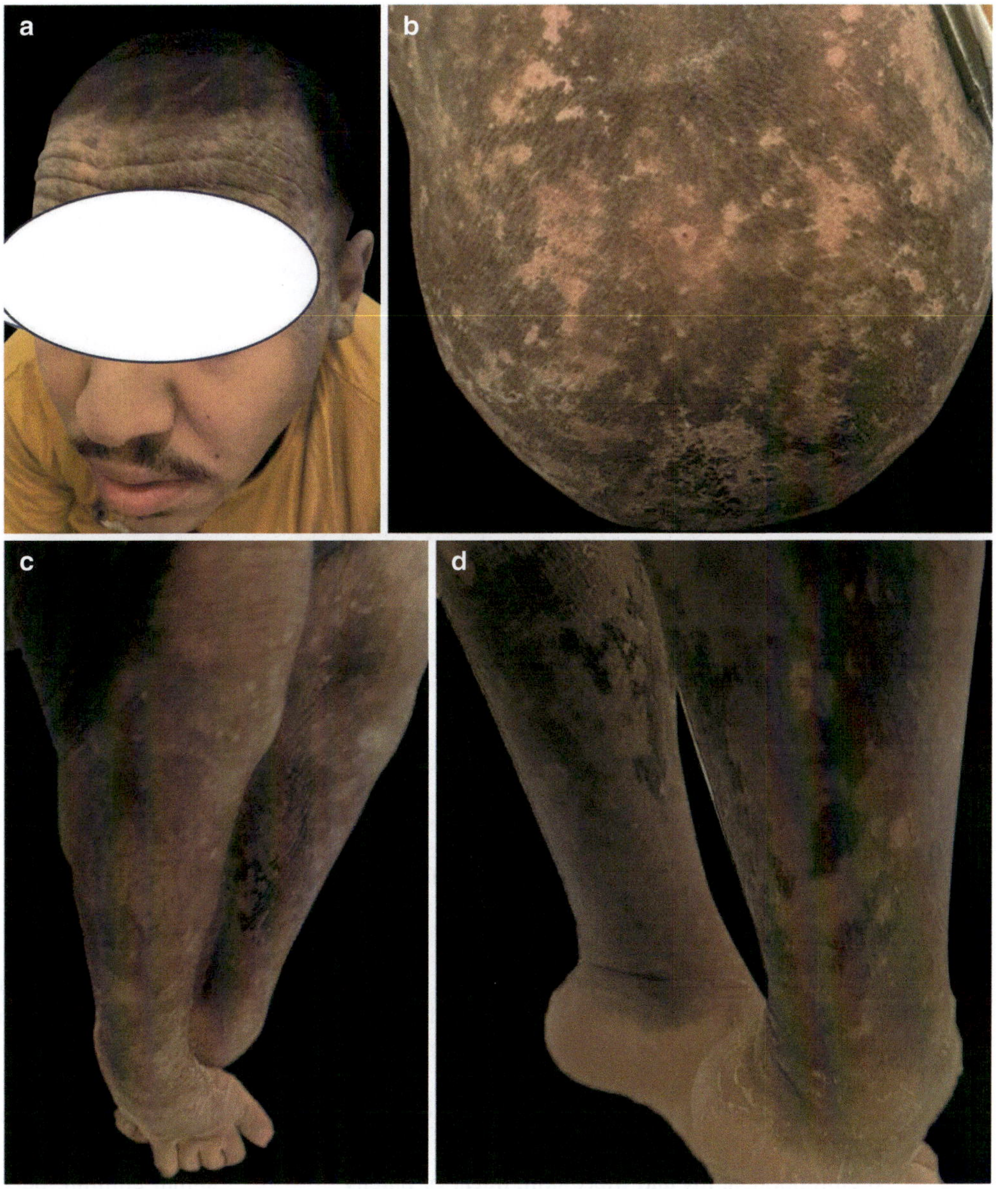

Fig. 1.35 Sjögren-Larsson Syndrome. Lamellar ichthyosis (plate-like scale) on face (**a**), trunk (**b**), and lower limbs (**c**, **d**) with increased skin markings. Abnormal gait (stiff movement with scissor type of gait) with inability to stand on his heel due to spasticity (**c**, **d**)

MEDNIK Syndrome (AR) [23] (Fig. 1.44)

- Defect in *AP1S1* gene leading to copper metabolism disorder.
- Onset: at birth.
- Clinical characteristics:
  - M: mental Retardation.
  - E: enteropathy.
  - D: deafness.
  - N: neuropathy (peripheral).
  - I: ichthyosis.
  - K: keratoderma.

Conradi-Hünermann-Happle Syndrome (XLD) (XLD Chondrodysplasia Punctata) [12] (Fig. 1.45)

- Defect in Emopamil binding protein (*EBP*) gene which plays a role in cholesterol biosynthesis.
- A form of chondrodysplasia punctata, a group of rare genetic disorders of skeletal development involving abnormal accumulation of calcium salts within the growing ends of long bones.
- Onset: at birth.
- Collodion baby.

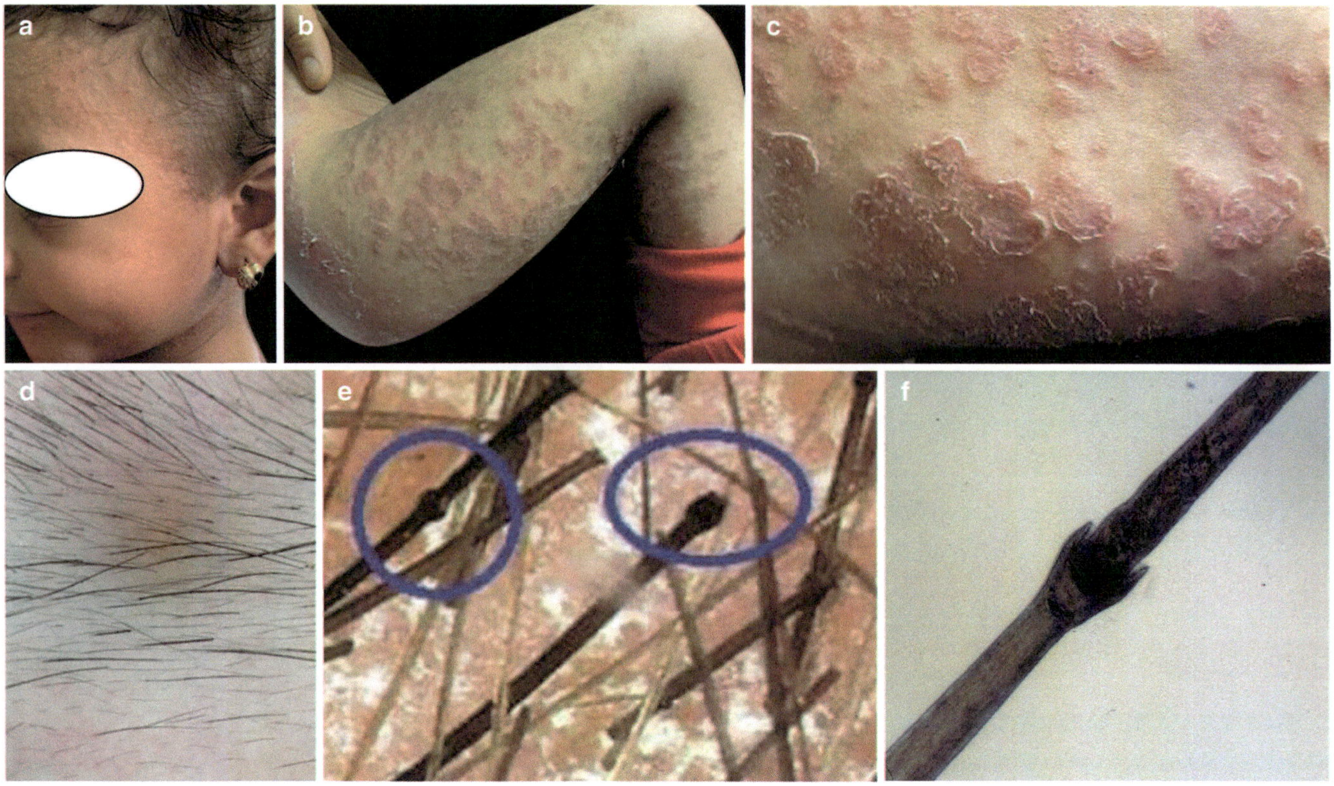

Fig. 1.36 Netherton Syndrome. Ichthyosis linearis circumflexa: circular scaling with thickened horny margin (erythematous polycyclic and serpiginous migratory plaques with double-edged scales in the periphery) on face (**a**), limbs (**b**, **c**). Hair abnormality (Trichorrhexis invaginata) (**d**–**f**)

- Clinical characteristics:
  1. Skin: congenital ichthyosiform erythroderma-like:
     - At birth: generalized erythema with thick adherent feathery scales.
     - At first week to months: streaks and whorly hyperkeratosis following Blaschko's lines.
     - At childhood: shiny and waxy skin, linear or patchy follicular atrophoderma with a dilated follicular opening on the forearm and dorsal hands (ice pick-like scars), sparing palms and soles, healed with hypopigmentation and hyperpigmentation.
  2. Facial asymmetry (frontal bossing, malar hypoplasia, and flat nasal bridge), with a short neck.
  3. CNS: mental retardation, hydrocephalus, and dandy-walker malformation.
  4. Ear: sensorineural deafness.
  5. Hair: sparse coarse hair with cicatricial alopecia.
  6. Nail: onychoschizia and flat nails.
  7. Eye: unilateral cataract.
  8. Skeletal:
     - Chondrodysplasia punctata of head of long bones. Punctate calcifications may develop throughout the spinal column, pelvis, frontal ends of the ribs, and in rare cases in (the larynx and trachea).
     - Scoliosis, asymmetrical limb shortening (rhizomelia), and short stature.
     - X-Ray finding: chondrodysplasia punctata (epiphyseal bone stippling and crippled).
  9. System affection: renal (congenital renal anomalies), and CVS abnormalities (congenital heart defect) associated with myopathy and fatty liver.

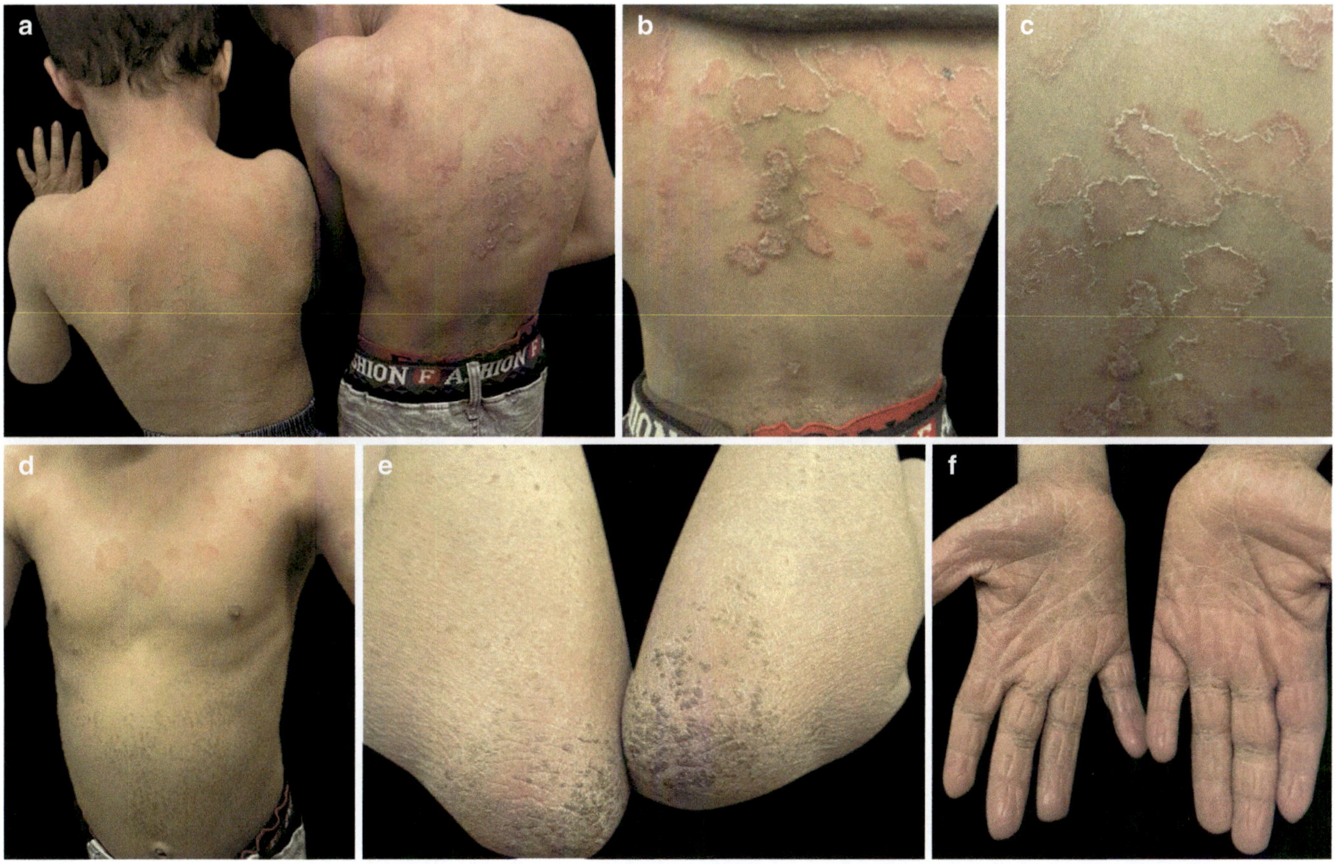

Fig. 1.37 Netherton Syndrome. Ichthyosis linearis circumflexa: circular scaling with thickened horny margin (erythematous polycyclic and serpiginous migratory plaques with double-edged scales in the periphery) on back (**a–c**). Dryness (atopic-like) on forearms with hyperkeratosis on abdomen (**d**), elbows (**e**), associated with palmar hyperkeratosis (**f**)

CHILD Syndrome (XLD) [12] (Fig. 1.46)

(**C**ongenital **H**emidysplasia with **I**chthyosiform Erythroderma and **L**imb **D**efect)

- Defect in *NADPH* steroid, dehydrogenase-like protein (*NSDHL*) gene, almost exclusively in females since it is X-linked dominant.
- Onset: at birth.
- Clinical characteristics:
  - **C**ongenital **H**emidysplasia, ipsilateral alopecia and skeletal abnormalities (hypoplasia of digits and ribs associated with organ hypoplasia (brain, renal and heart).
  - **I**chthyosiform erythroderma:
    Unilateral erythema and thickened skin with waxy adherent scale.
    The erythema is sharply demarcated at the anterior and posterior midline of the trunk.
    The face is typically spared.
  - **L**imb **D**efect: scoliosis and stippled epiphysis.
- It is commonly associated with hearing loss, cleft palate, and verrucous xanthoma.

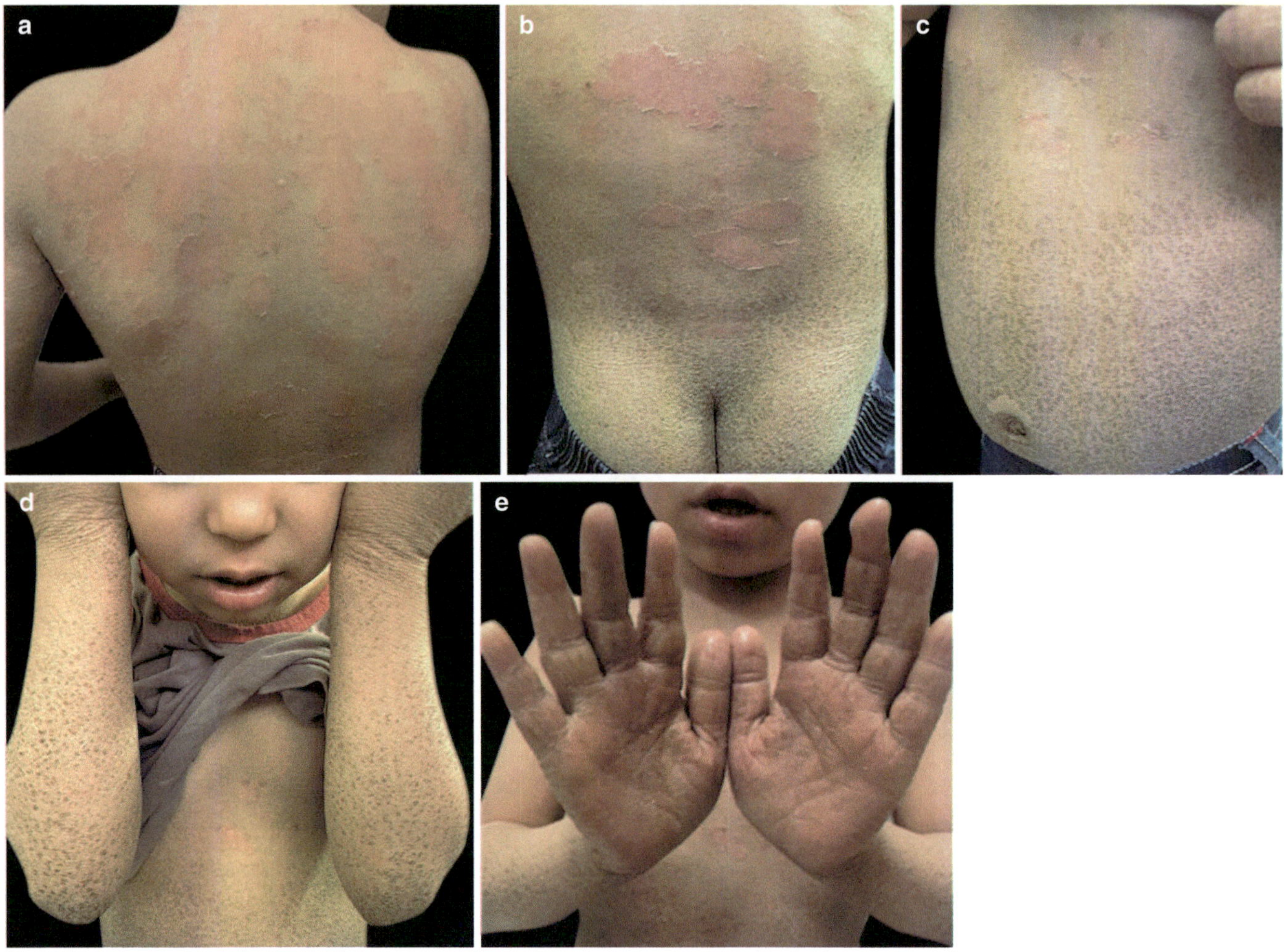

Fig. 1.38 Netherton Syndrome (brother of the previous patient of Fig. 1.37). Ichthyosis linearis circumflexa: circular scaling with thickened horny margin (erythematous polycyclic and serpiginous migratory plaques with double-edged scales in the periphery) on back (**a**, **b**), associated with hyperkeratosis on abdomen (**c**), forearms (**d**), and palmar hyperkeratosis (**e**)

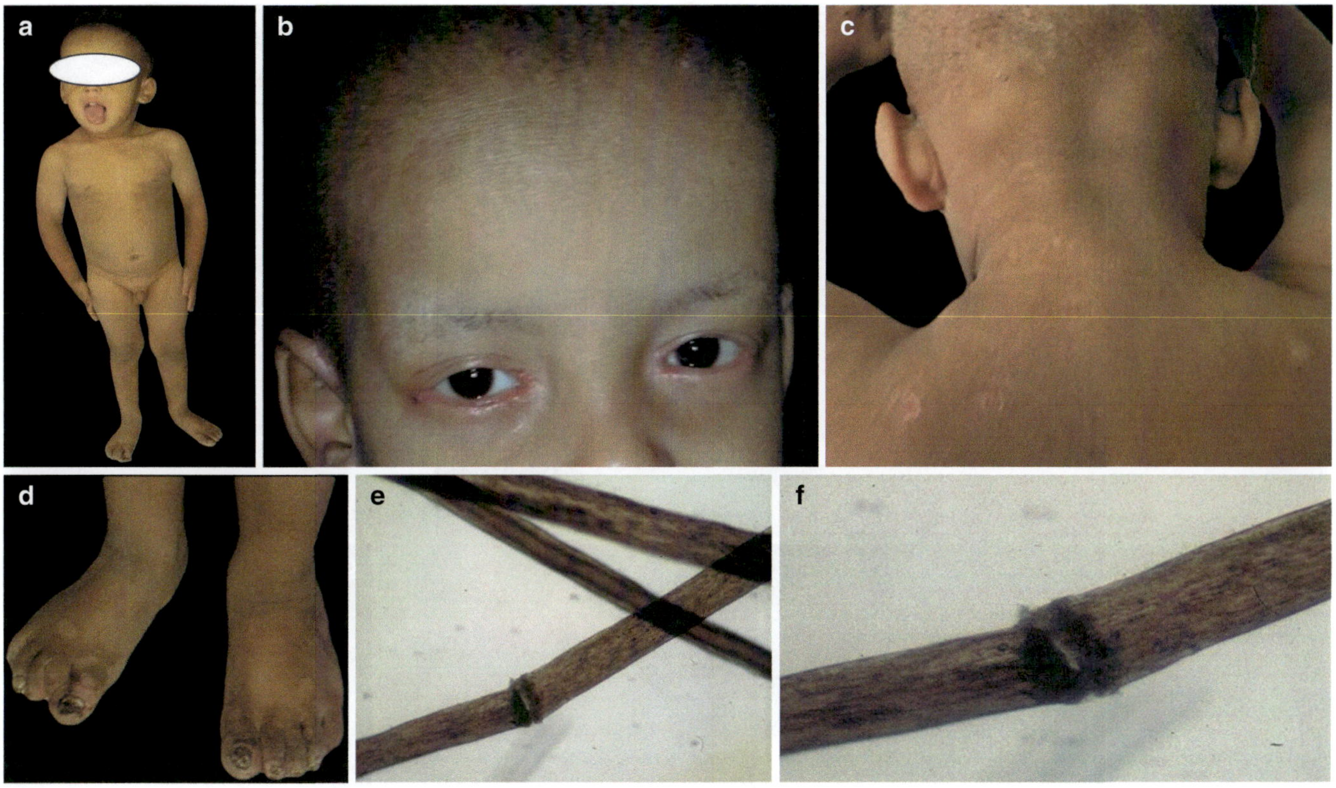

Fig. 1.39 Tay Syndrome (PIBIDS). Short stature and hypogonadism (**a**), brittle short sparse hair and photosensitivity (**b**), generalized fine scale with minimal erythema (atopic-like) (**c**), with nail dystrophy (**d**). Trichorrhexis nodosa (**e**, **f**)

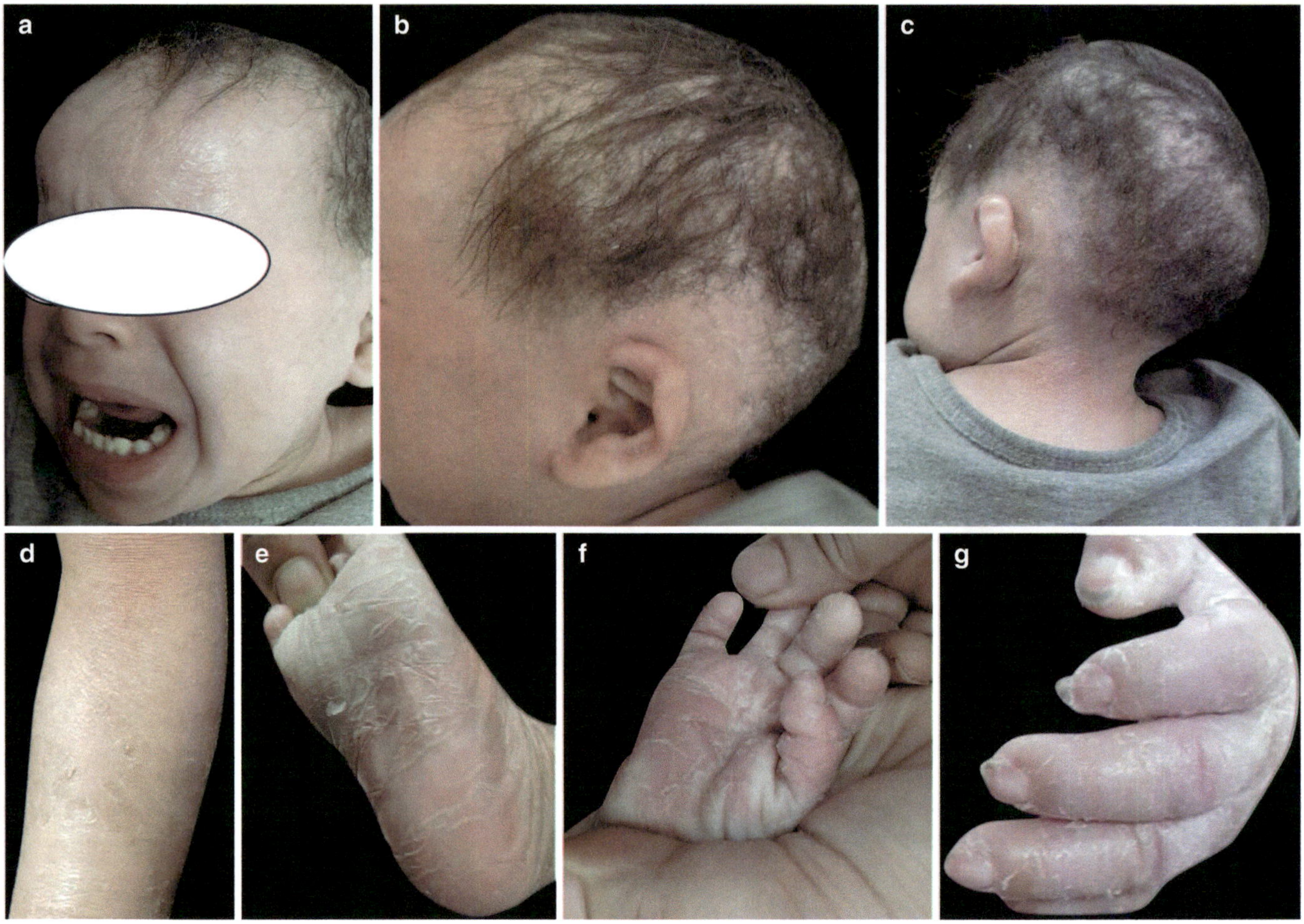

Fig. 1.40 Tay Syndrome (PIBIDS syndrome). Brittle short sparse hair (**a–c**) associated with generalized fine scales with minimal erythema (atopic-like) on face (**a–c**), limbs (**d**, **e**), palmoplantar hyperkeratosis (**f**), and brittle nails with onychogryphosis (**g**)

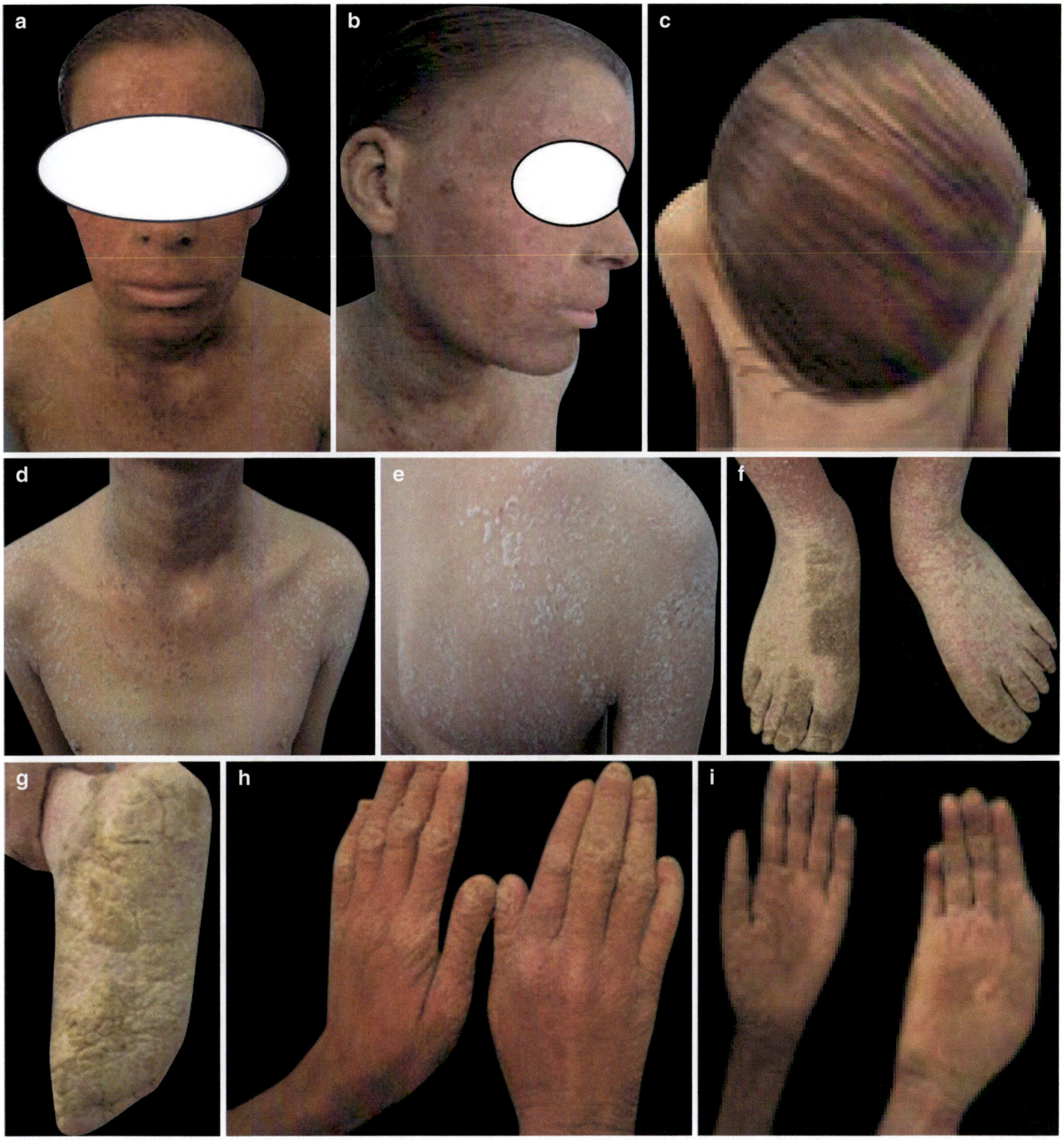

Fig. 1.41 Tay Syndrome (PIBIDS). Ichthyosis (generalized scaling with minimal erythema) associated with photosensitivity (**a**, **b**). Brittle sparse hair (**c**), erythroderma with fine scale on trunk (**d**, **e**), extremities (**f**–**h**), and palmoplantar hyperkeratosis (**g**, **i**)

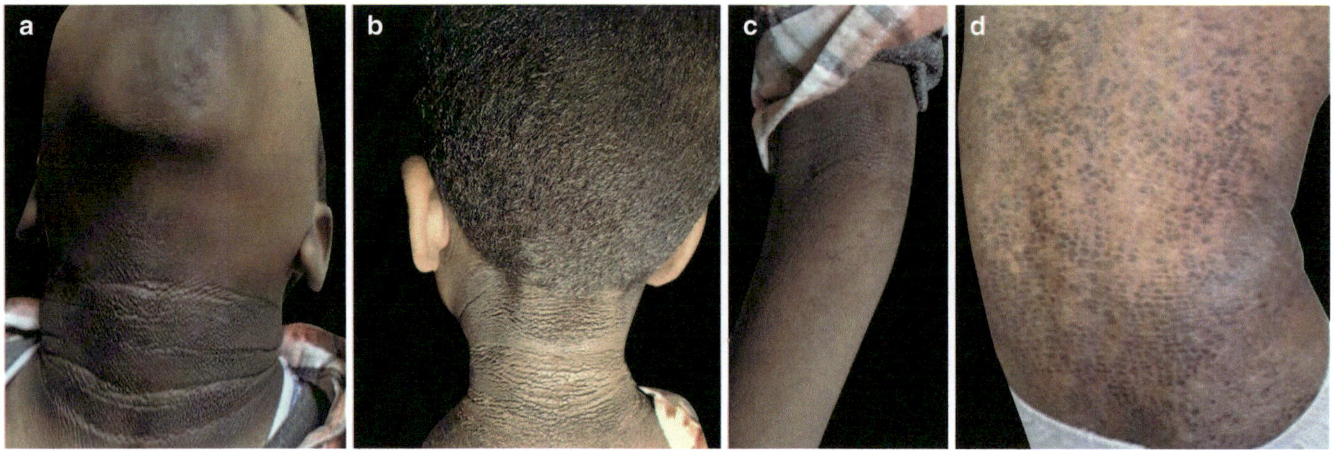

Fig. 1.42 Rud Syndrome. Acanthosis nigricans in the neck, nape of neck (**a**, **b**) and cubital fossa (**c**) with lamellar ichthyosis-like on the trunk (**d**)

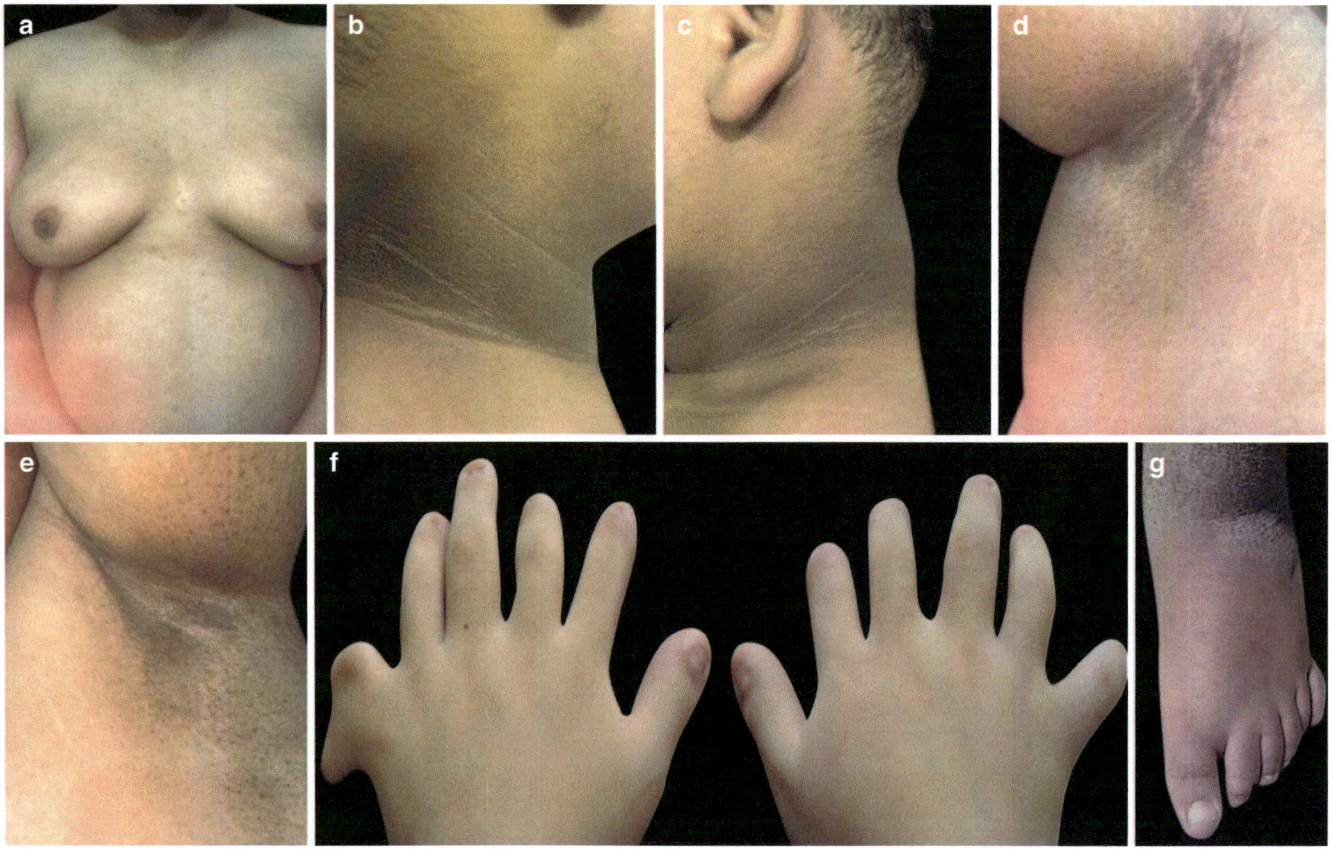

Fig. 1.43 Laurence-Moon-Bardet-Biedl syndrome. Obesity associated with striae alba (**a**), pseudo-acanthosis nigricans on the neck (**b**, **c**), and axilla (**d**, **e**) and polydactyly on hands and feet (**f**, **g**)

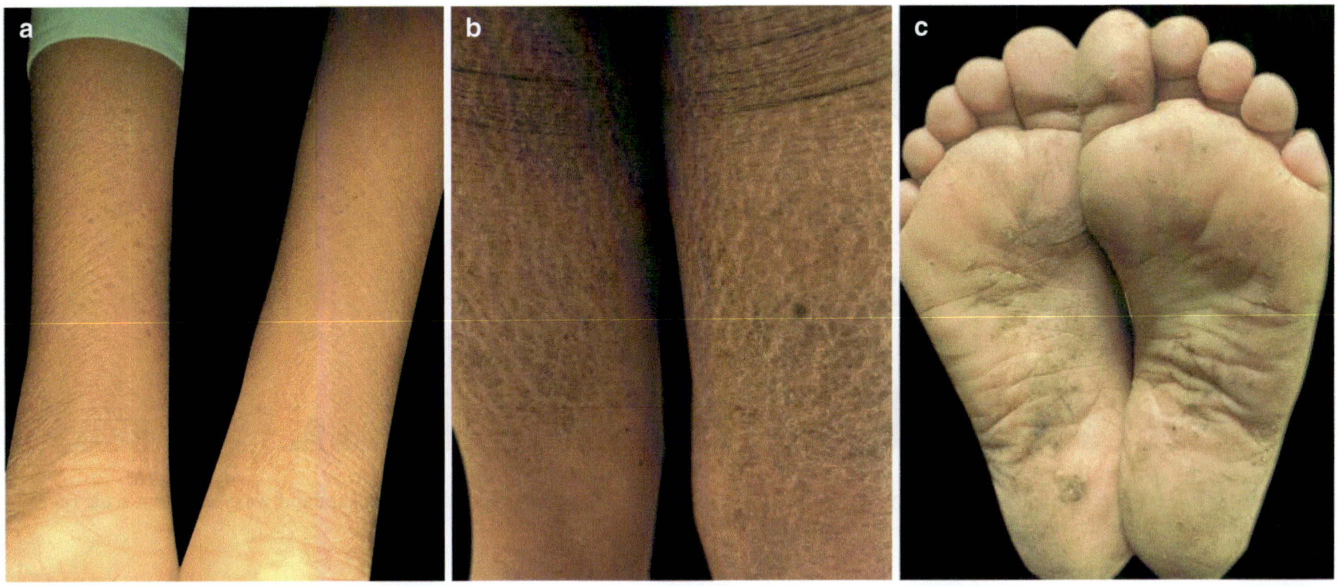

Fig. 1.44 MEDNIK syndrome. Ichthyosis on the limbs and plantar hyperkeratosis (**a**–**c**)

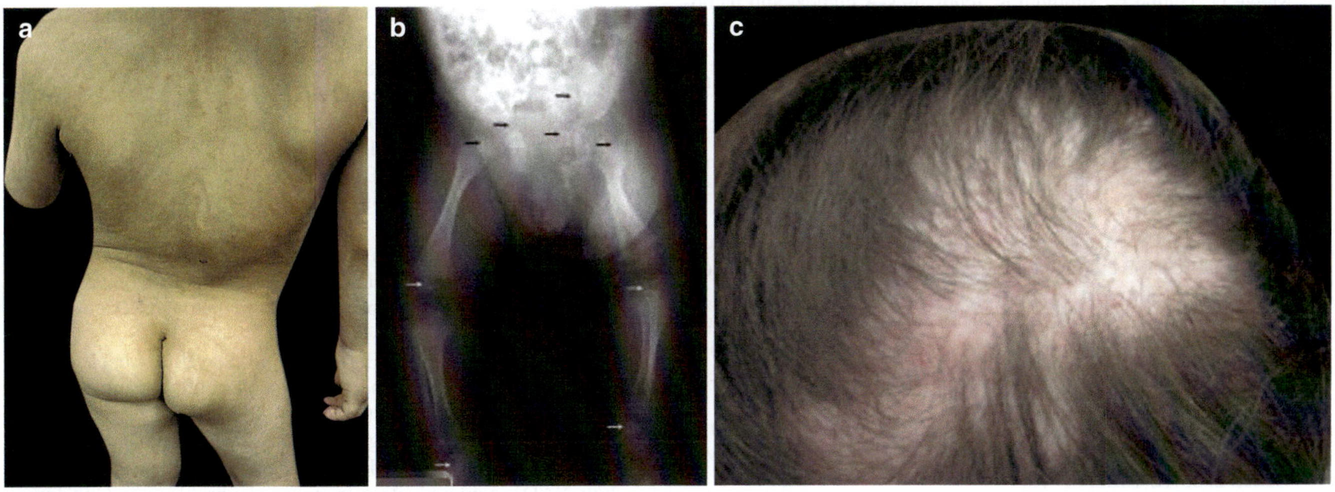

Fig. 1.45 Conradi-Hünermann-Happle Syndrome. Scoliosis, with asymmetrical limb (rhizomelia).Skin shows linear hypopigmentation following Blashko's lines (**a**), punctate stippled calcifications found in hips and in the epiphysis of long bones of lower limbs (**b**), sparce hair and cicatricial alopecia (**c**). (*Courtesy, Hala Abdel Salam Fayed*)

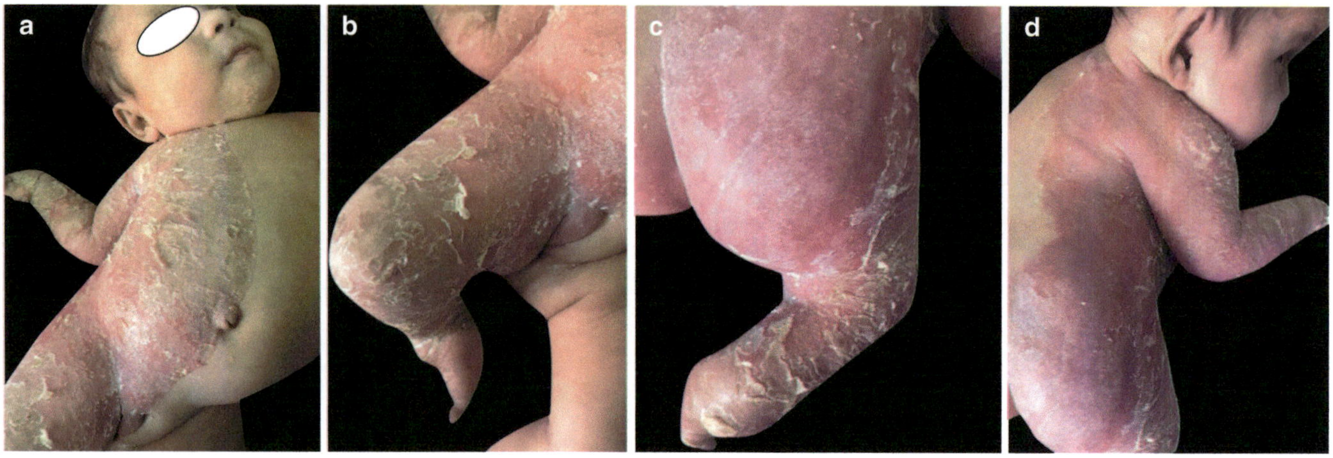

Fig. 1.46 CHILD syndrome. Unilateral sharply demarcated ichthyosiform erythroderma with thickened skin and waxy adherent scale on right side of trunk (**a**), right upper and lower limb (**b–d**), sparing the face

References

1. Metze D, Traupe H, Süßmuth K. Ichthyoses-A clinical and pathological spectrum from heterogeneous cornification disorders to inflammation. Dermatopathol. 2021;8(2):107–23.
2. Jaffar H, Shakir Z, Kumar G, et al. Ichthyosis vulgaris: an updated review. Skin Health Dis. 2022;3(1):e187.
3. Bonifa's JM, Morley BJ, Oakey RE, et al. Cloning of a cDNA for steroid sulfatase: frequent occurrence of gene deletions in patients with recessive X chromosome-linked ichthyosis. Proc Natl Acad Sci USA. 1987;84(24):9248–51.
4. Heinz L, Kim GJ, Marrakchi S, et al. Mutations in SULT2B1 cause autosomal-recessive congenital ichthyosis in humans. Am J Hum Genet. 2017;100(6):926–39.
5. Herman ML, Farasat S, Steinbach PJ, et al. Transglutaminase-1 gene mutations in autosomal recessive congenital ichthyosis: summary of mutations (including 23 novel) and modeling of TGase-1. Hum Mutat. 2009;30(4):537–47.
6. Lefevre C, Audebert S, Jobard F, et al. Mutations in the transporter ABCA12 are associated with lamellar ichthyosis type 2. Hum Mol Genet. 2003;12(18):2369–78.
7. Akiyama M, Sugiyama-Nakagiri Y, Sakai K, et al. Mutations in lipid transporter ABCA12 in harlequin ichthyosis and functional recovery by corrective gene transfer. J Clin Invest. 2005;115(7):1777–84.
8. Martínez-García S, Vera A, Romero J, et al. Feto arlequin. Actas Dermosifiliogr. 2003;94(6):392–4.
9. Heinz L, Kim G-J, Marrakchi S, et al. Mutations in SULT2B1 cause autosomal-recessive congenital ichthyosis in humans. Am J Hum Genet. 2017;100:926–39.
10. Irvine AD, McLean WH. Human keratin diseases: the increasing spectrum of disease and subtlety of the phenotype-genotype correlation. Br J Dermatol. 1999;140(5):815–28.
11. Sprecher E, Miller CJ, Richard G, et al. Evidence for novel functions of the keratin tail emerging from a mutation causing ichthyosis hystrix. J Invest Dermatol. 2001;116(4):511–9.
12. Choate KA, Lu Y, Zhou J, et al. Mitotic recombination in patients with ichthyosis causes the reversion of dominant mutations in KRT10. Science. 2010;330(6000):94–7.
13. van Geel M, van Steensel MA, Küster W, et al. HID and KID syndromes are associated with the same connexin 26 mutation. Br J Dermatol. 2002;146(6):938–42.
14. Todt I, Hennies HC, Küster W, et al. Neurotological and neuroanatomical changes in the connexin-26-related HID/KID syndrome. Audiol Neurootol. 2006;11(4):242–8.
15. El Kabbany Z, Khalifa O, Wafeeq A, et al. A new patient of Chanarin Dorfman syndrome in Egypt. Arch Clin Med Case Rep. 2019;3(6):702–7.
16. Refsum S. Heredopathia atactica polyneuritiformis: phytanic-acid storage disease, Refsum's disease: a biochemically well-defined disease with a specific dietary treatment. Arch Neurol. 1981;38(10):605–6.
17. Baldwin EJ, Gibberd FB, Harley C, et al. The effectiveness of long-term dietary therapy in the treatment of adult Refsum disease. J Neurol Neurosurg Psychiatry. 2010;81(9):954–7.
18. Rizzo WB, Craft DA. Sjogren–Larsson syndrome. Deficient activity of the fatty aldehyde dehydrogenase component of fatty alcohol: NAD+ oxidoreductase in cultured fibroblasts. J Clin Invest. 1991;88:1643–8.
19. Jagell S, Polland W, Sandgren O. Specific changes in the fundus typical for the Sjogren-Larsson syndrome. An ophthalmological study of 35 patients. Acta Ophthalmol. 1980;58(3):321–30.
20. Happle R, Traupe H, Gröbe H, et al. The Tay syndrome (congenital ichthyosis with trichothiodystrophy). Eur J Pediatr. 1984 Jan;141(3):147–52.
21. Pavani K, Reddy BS, Singh BA. Rud's syndrome. Indian Dermatol Online J. 2014;5(2):173–5.
22. Rissardo JP, Caprara AL. Laurence-moon-Biedl-Bardet syndrome: an overview. Taiwan J Ophthalmol. 2020;11(1):108–9.
23. Montpetit A, Côté S, Brustein E, et al. Disruption of AP1S1, causing a novel neurocutaneous syndrome, perturbs the development of the skin and spinal cord. PLoS Genet. 2008;4(12):e1000296.

2 Erythrokeratodermas and Palmoplantar Keratoderma

Erythrokeratodermas constitute erythrokeratoderma variabilis and progressive symmetric erythroderma. Palmoplantar keratodermas are either focal or diffuse. The focal palmoplantar keratoderma may be isolated or syndromic, while the diffuse type is either transgredient or non-transgredient.

Erythrokeratoderma

- **Erythrokeratoderma Variabilis**.
- **Progressive Symmetric Erythrokeratoderma**.

Erythrokeratoderma Variabilis (AD) [1] (Fig. 2.1)

- Due to mutations in genes encoding *Cx31, GJB3,* or *Cx30.3*.
- Onset: at birth or infancy.
  - Erythematous migratory patches: transient variable erythema with facial sparing, burning sensation variable in site, shape, and size.
  - Persistent sharply demarcated, polycyclic hyperkeratotic plaques (bizarre shape and geographic border) surface ridged, verrucous, velvety, collarette like may be with blanched halo and hypertrichosis on extensors, elbow, knee, and feet.
  - Palmoplantar hyperkeratosis in 50% of patients.

Progressive Symmetric Erythrokeratoderma (AD) [2] (Figs. 2.2 and 2.3)

- Defect in *LORICRIN* protein.
- Onset: infancy or childhood.
- Clinical characteristics:
  - Symmetrically distributed, nonmigratory, large, well-defined, erythematous, hyperkeratotic plaques with marked peripheral erythema. The sites of predilection are extensors of extremities and sometimes face. The trunk is usually spared.
  - Palmoplantar hyperkeratosis is common.

N. Moftah et al., *Atlas of Common and Rare Genodermatoses*, https://doi.org/10.1007/978-3-031-60788-2_2

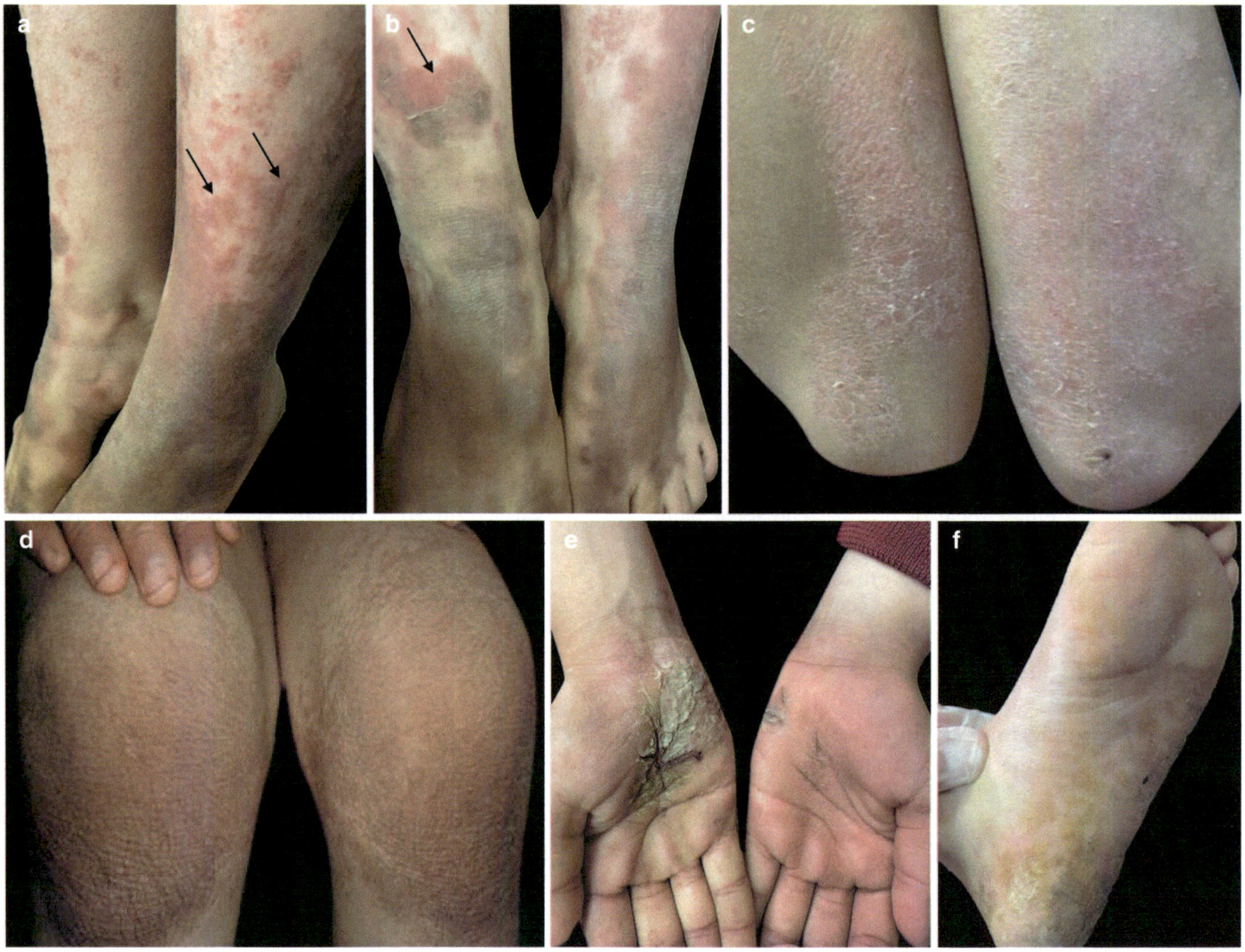

Fig. 2.1 Erythrokeratoderma Variabilis. Transient erythematous patches (**a**, **b** arrows). Sharply demarcated hyperkeratotic red brown plaques on extensors, elbows, knees (**a–d**), palmoplantar hyperkeratosis (**e**, **f**)

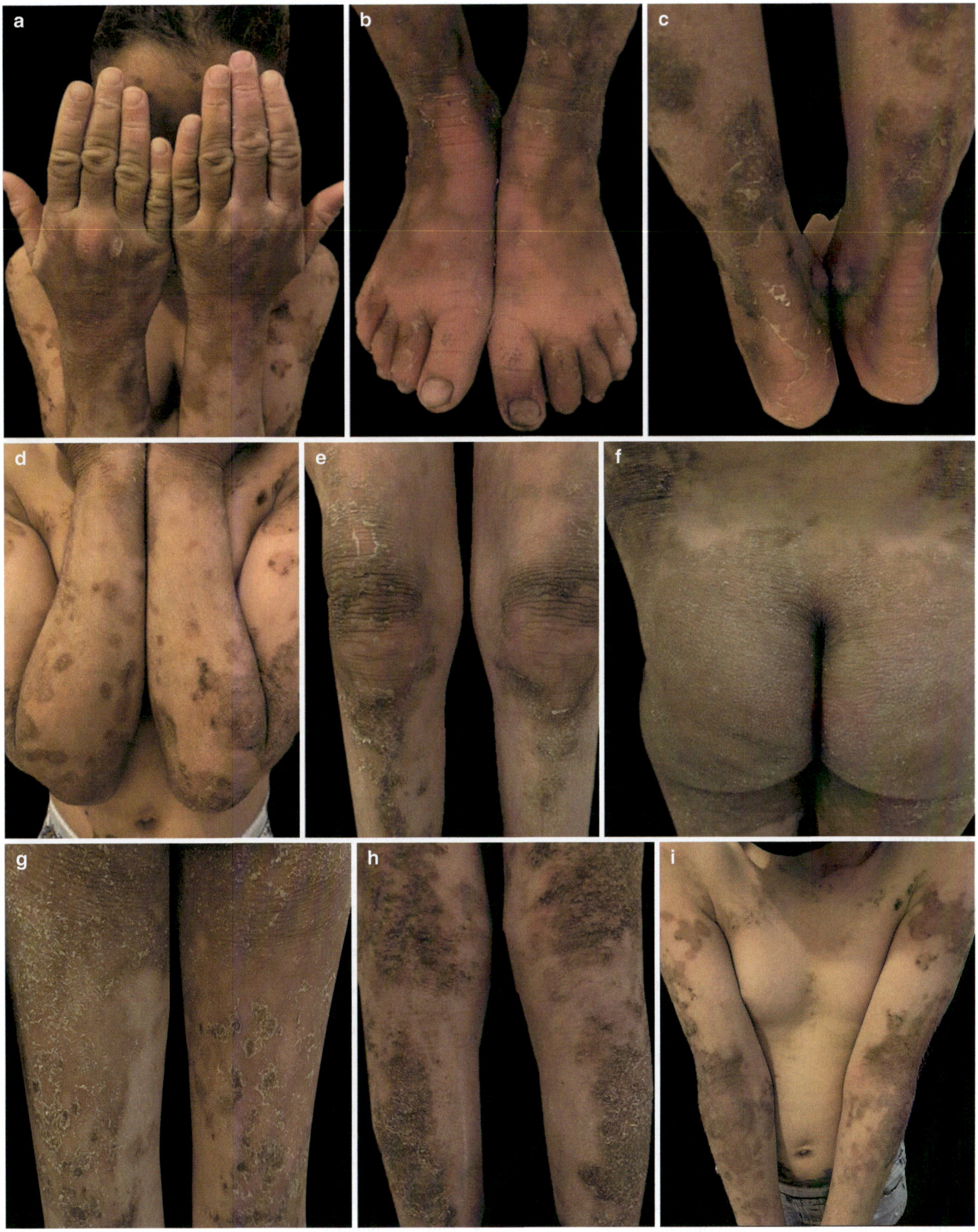

Fig. 2.2 Progressive Symmetric Erythrokeratoderma. Symmetrical persistent erythematous hyperkeratotic plaques on hands (**a**), feet (**b**), tendo Achilles (**c**), elbows (**d**), knees (**e**), buttocks (**f**), thighs (**g**), legs (**h**), and spare the trunk (**i**)

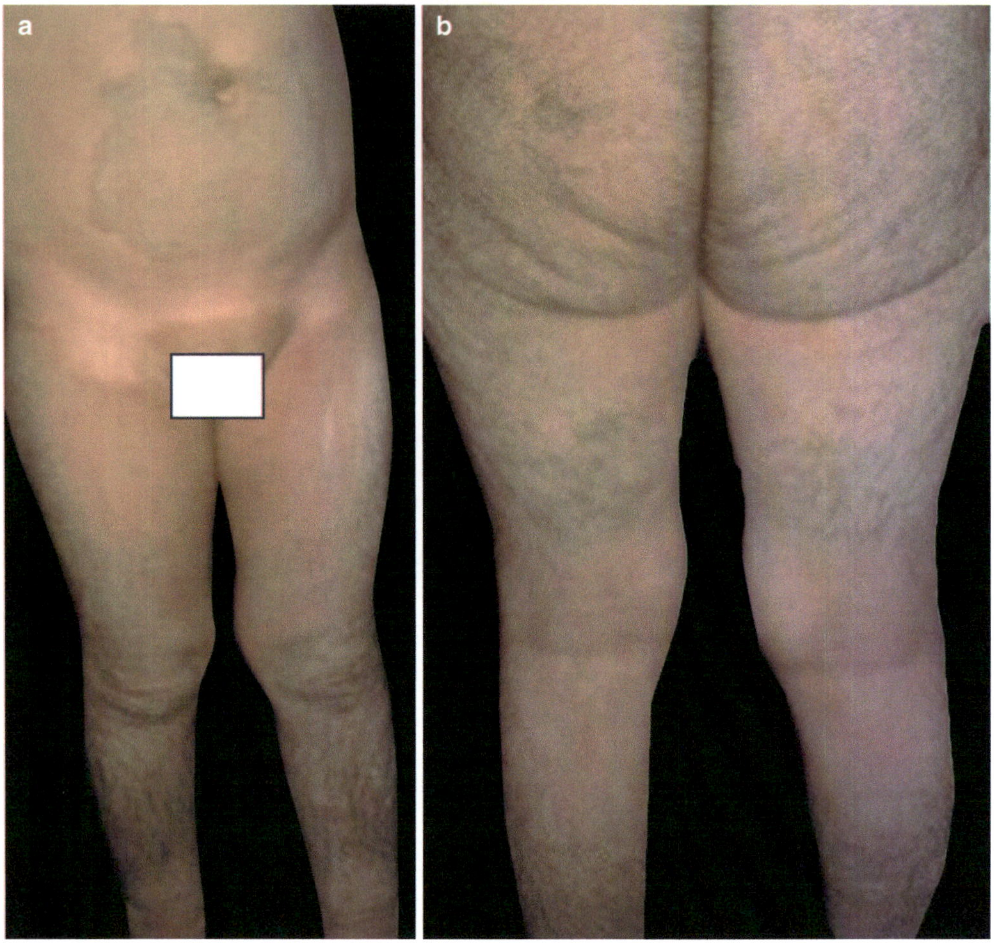

Fig. 2.3 Progressive Symmetric Erythrokeratoderma. Erythematous hyperkeratotic patches on abdomen, buttocks, and lower limbs (**a**, **b**)

Palmoplantar Keratodermas (PPK)

- **Focal PPK**.
- **Diffuse PPK**.

Focal palmoplantar keratoderma are presented as either isolated or syndromic (Table 2.1).

Table 2.1 Focal palmoplantar keratoderma (PPK)

Isolated PPK	Syndromic PPK
• **PPK punctata** – Punctate PPK type 1 (Buschke-Fischer-Brauer disease) – Punctate PPK type 2 (spiny keratoderma) – Punctate PPK type 3 (Acrokeratoelastoidosis) • **Punctate keratosis of palmar creases** • **Cole disease** • **PPK striata** • **PPK areata**	• **Carvajal syndrome** • **Howel-Evans syndrome** • **Richner-Hanhart syndrome (oculocutaneous tyrosinemia II)** • **Pachyonychia congenita type 1**

Punctate PPK Type 1 (AD) (Buschke-Fischer Syndrome) [3] (Figs. 2.4 and 2.5)

- Defect in alpha and gamma adaptin binding protein (*AAGAB*) gene.
- Onset: 12–30 years age.
- Punctate PPK or multiple asymptomatic punctate hyperkeratotic papules involving whole or part of palms and soles. Hyperhidrosis is not a feature.
- Nails may show longitudinal ridging, notching, trachyonychia, onychoschizia, and onychorrhexis.

Acrokeratoelastoidosis of Oswald Costa (AD) (Inverse Papular Acrokeratosis) [4] (Figs. 2.6, 2.7, and 2.8)

- Defect in *GRCh38* gene.
- Onset: at puberty.
- Clinical Characteristics:
  - Marginal papular keratoderma and focal acral hyperkeratosis.

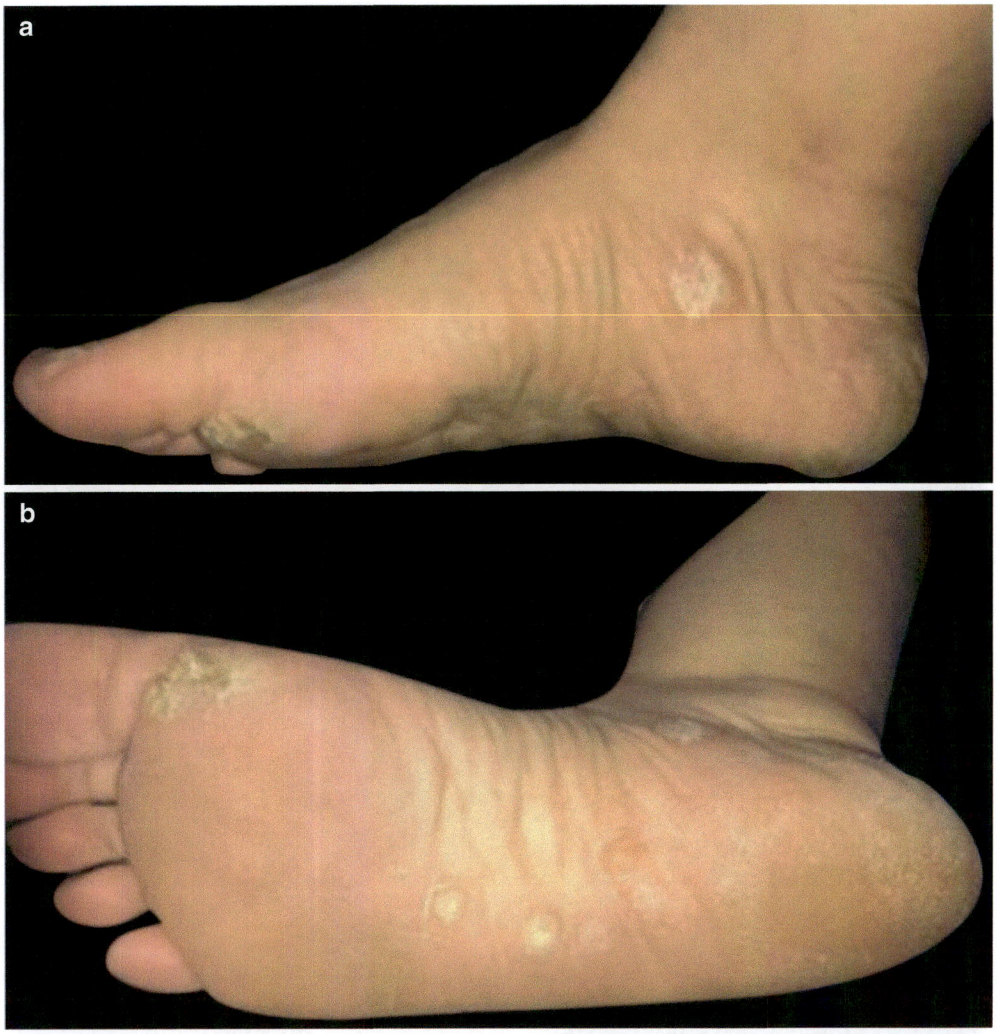

Fig. 2.4 Palmoplantar Punctata of palms and soles in a child. Multiple yellow, punctate, hyperkeratotic, hard, round papules, and plaques on margins of soles (**a**, **b**)

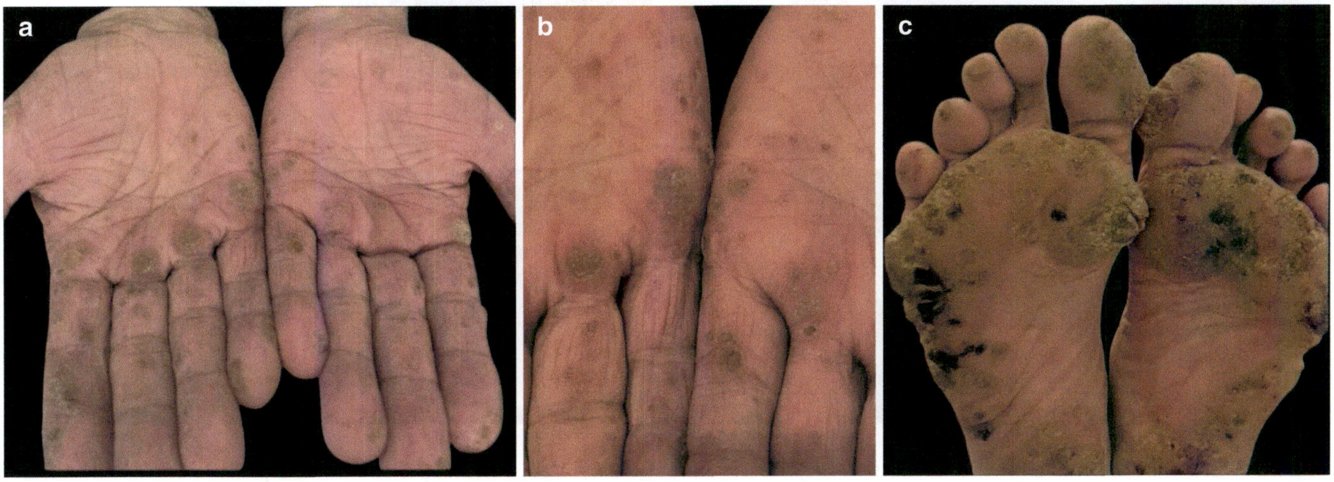

Fig. 2.5 Palmoplantar Punctata of palms and soles in an adult. Multiple yellow rounded punctate spine keratotic papules and plaques (warty like) on palms and soles (**a**–**c**)

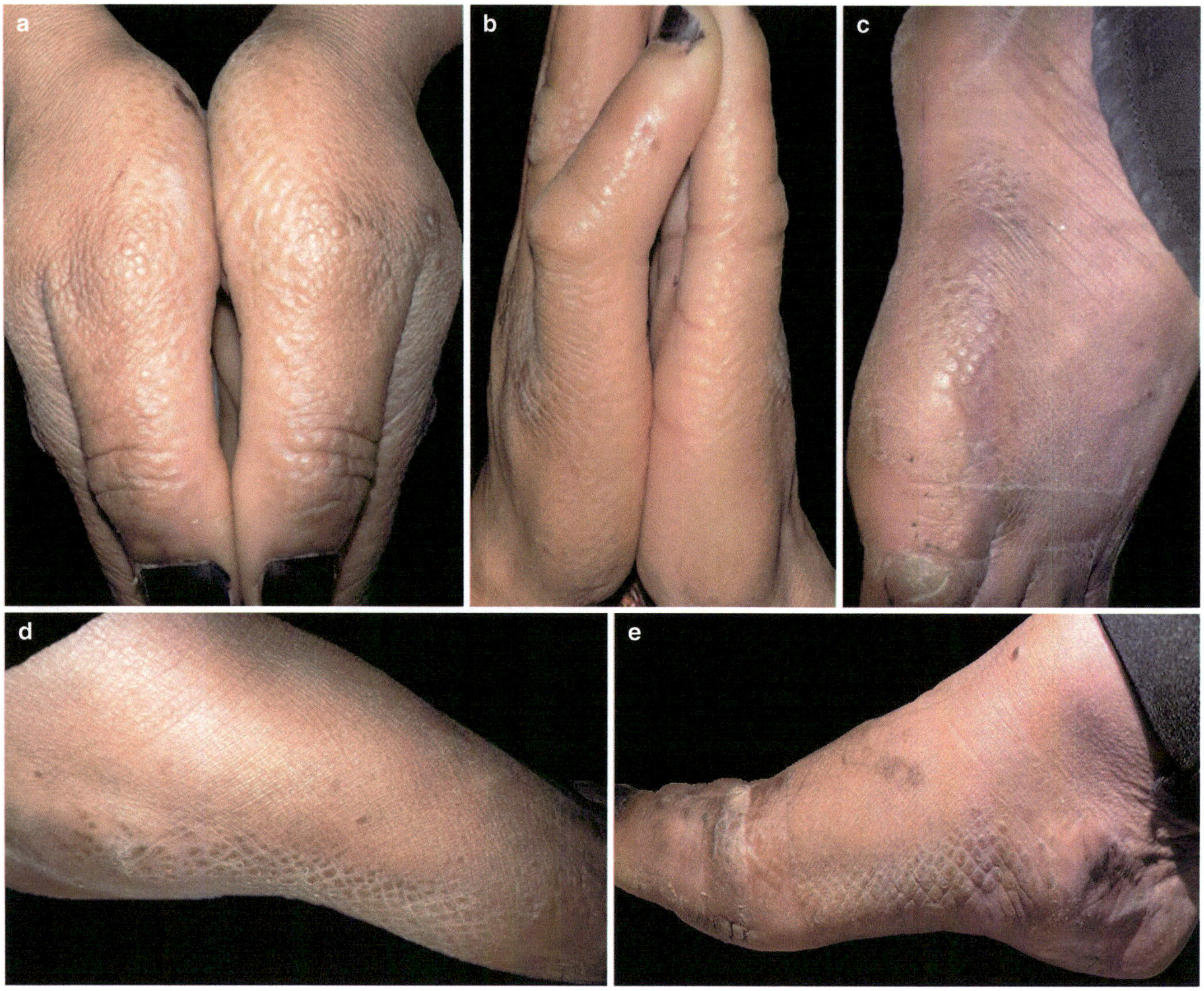

Fig. 2.6 Acrokeratoelastoidosis of Oswald Costa. Multiple focal marginal punctate hyperkeratotic papules on margins of hands (**a**, **b**) and feet (**c**–**e**)

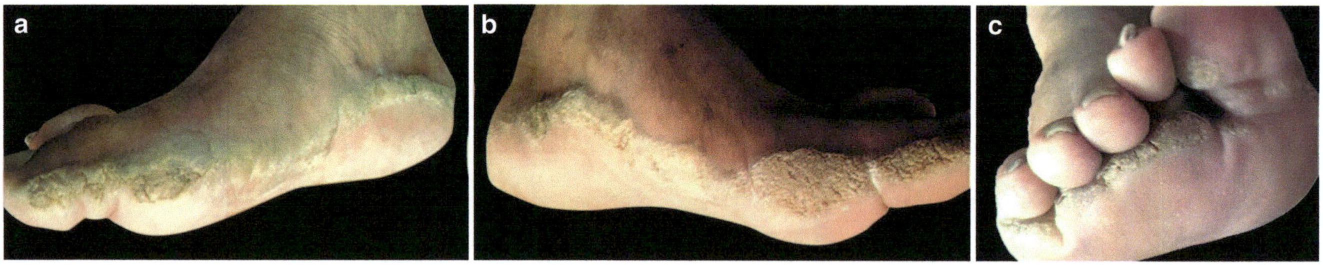

Fig. 2.7 Acrokeratoelastoidosis of Oswald Costa. Warty keratotic papules and plaques on margin of sole with punctate transgredient warty keratotic papules on dorsum of feet (**a**–**c**)

- Multiple skin colored small punctate papules on margins of palms and feet (Wallace line), transgradient keratotic lesion on dorsal of hand, feet, elbows, and knees.

- The histological features are hyalinized and homogenous collagen, hyperkeratosis, and a decrease in, and fragmentation of the elastic fibers (elastorrhexis).

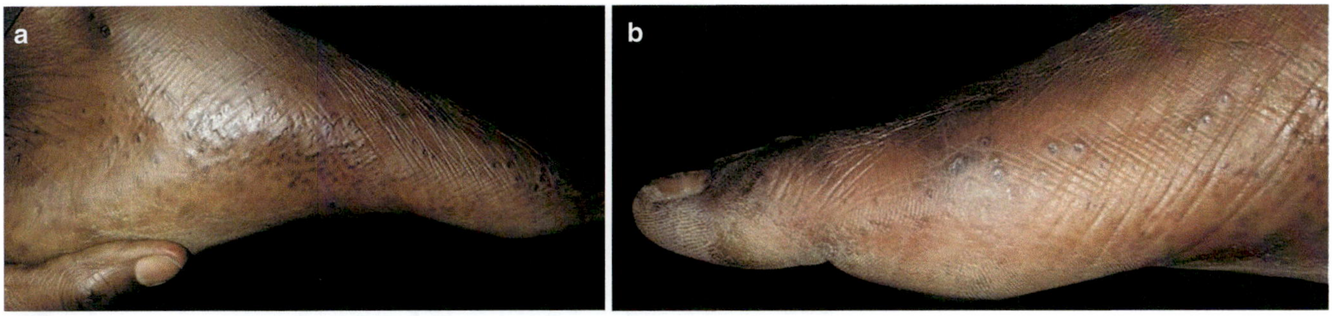

Fig. 2.8 Acrokeratoelastoidosis of Oswald Costa. Warty papules on margin of soles (**a**, **b**)

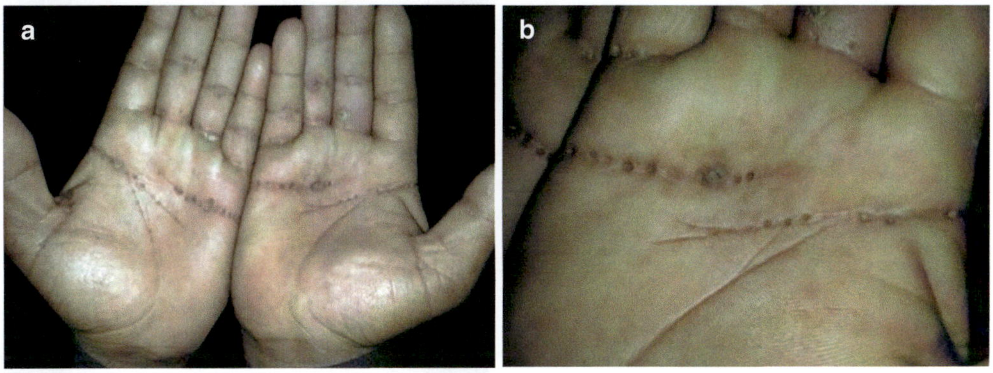

Fig. 2.9 Punctate keratosis of palmar crease. Depression filled with comedo-like keratin plug) (**a**, **b**)

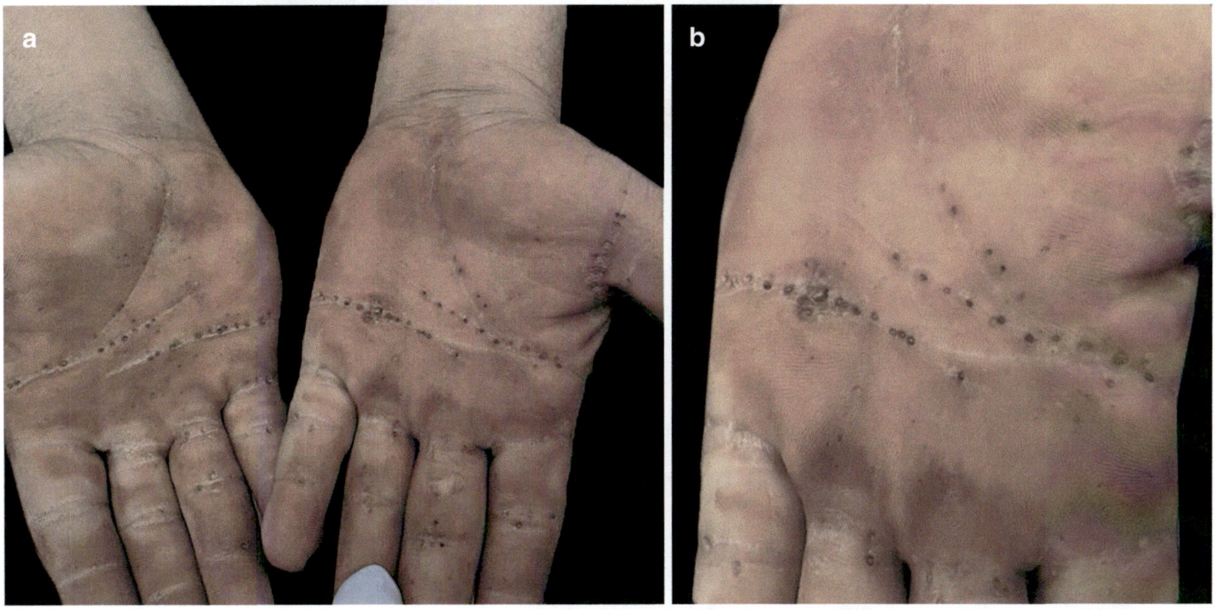

Fig. 2.10 Punctate keratosis of palmar crease. Depression filled with comedo-like keratin plug) (**a**, **b**)

Punctate Keratosis of Palmar Creases [5] (Figs. 2.9 and 2.10)

The lesions begin in adolescence or early adulthood with the formation of hyperkeratotic plugs on the palms, which break off, leaving characteristic pits.

Cole Disease (AD) [6] (Figs. 2.11 and 2.12)

- Defect in ectonucleotide pyrophosphatase/phosphodiesterase 1 (*ENPP1*) gene, which is responsible for the generation of inorganic pyrophosphate, a natural inhibitor of mineralization.

Fig. 2.11 Cole disease. Guttate hypopigmentation on hands, trunk (**a**–**c**) and Punctate palmoplantar keratoderma on the sole (**d**)

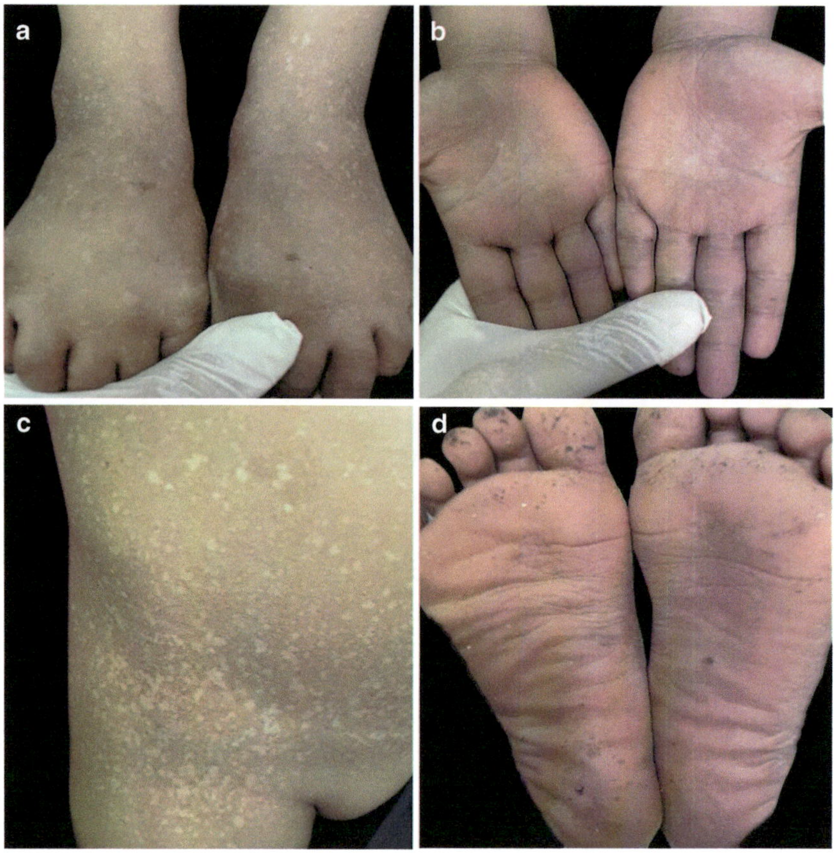

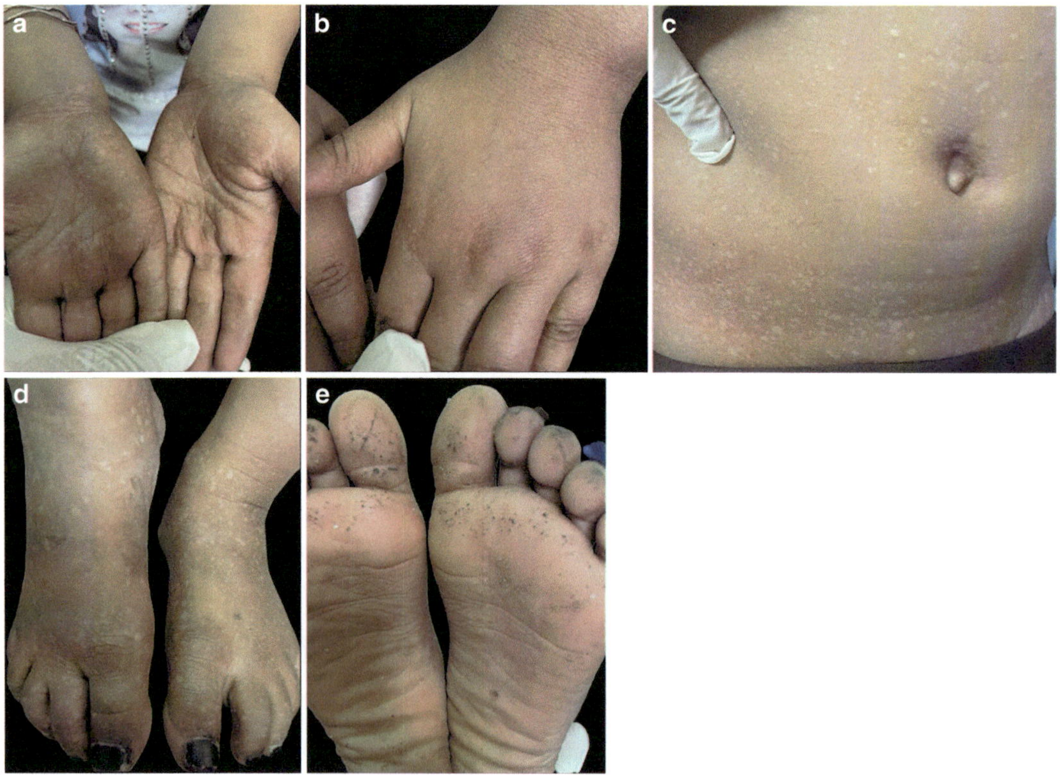

Fig. 2.12 Cole disease in the sister of the previous patient in Fig. 2.11. Guttate hypopigmentation on hands (**a**, **b**), abdomen (**c**), feet (**d**) and punctate palmoplantar keratoderma of the sole (**e**)

- Onset: at birth and develops during the first year of life.
- Clinical characteristics:
  - Punctate PPK.
  - Guttate hypopigmentation typically on arms and legs.
  - Cutaneous calcifications (uncommon).

PPK Striate (AD) [7] (Fig. 2.13)

- Defect in *DSG1*, *Desmoplakin,* and *KRT1* genes.
- Onset: early infancy.
- Clinical characteristics:
  - Areas of hyperkeratosis on the plantar aspect of the feet with no transgrediens.
  - Linear hyperkeratotic plaque on volar aspect of fingers and palms.
- May be associated with Carvajal syndrome (early during childhood, woolly hair, dilated left ventricular cardiomyopathy, and early heart failure).

PPK Areata (AD) [8] (Fig. 2.14)

- Defect in DSG1, Desmoplakin and KRT1 genes.
- Onset: childhood, increased severity with repetitive friction.
- Clinical characteristics:
  - Keratotic painful lesion on weight bearing area.
  - May be associated with Howel-Evans Syndrome, Richner-Hanhart Syndrome, pachyonychia congenita type 1.

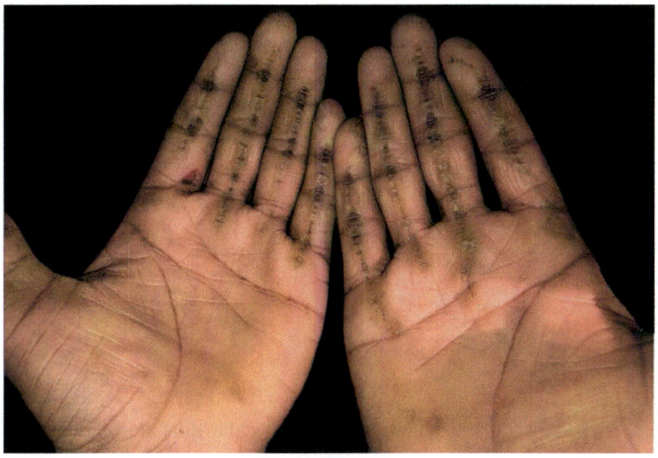

Fig. 2.13 Palmoplantar keratoderma striata. Linear hyperkeratotic plaque along the volar surfaces of fingers

Carvajal Syndrome (AD) (Cardio-Cutaneous Syndrome) [9] (Fig. 2.15)

- Defect in *Desmoplakin* gene.
- Clinical characteristics:
  - Focal non-transgredient PPK (during first year of life).
  - Woolly hair (at birth).
  - Left ventricular cardiomyopathy and early heart failure.

Howel-Evans Syndrome (AD) (Tylosis with Esophageal Cancer) [10] (Fig. 2.16)

- Defect in *RHBDF2* genes of rhomboid protease family, which result in abnormal regulation of epidermal growth factor receptor and inhibition of tumor necrosis factor.
- Onset: early infancy.
- Clinical characteristics:
  - Thick yellow waxy keratoderma and fissures mainly on pressure points, especially on the feet more than the palms.
  - May be associated with oral leukokeratosis or oral leukoplakia.
- There are two types of Howel-Evans Syndrome:
  - Type A Tylosis: It has a late-onset (5–15 years) and is mostly associated with esophageal cancer.
  - Type B Tylosis: It has an early onset (within the first 12 months) and has usually a benign course (association with esophageal cancer is less often seen).

Richner-Hanhart Syndrome (AR) (Tyrosinemia Type II) (Oculocutaneous Tyrosinemia) [11] (Fig. 2.17)

- Defect in tyrosine aminotransferase (*TAT*) gene. As a consequence of the TAT deficiency, there is an accumulation of tyrosine.
- Onset:
  - Ophthalmological features: They are often the earliest manifestations in the form of photophobia, scleral inflammation and pseudoherpetiform corneal ulcerations.
  - Cutaneous manifestations typically develop during the first 2 years of life and include painful, erythematous hyperkeratotic acral plaques. The keratoderma is usually symmetric and focal. Hair and teeth are unaffected. Intellectual disability is highly variable in severity. Patients have a normal life span.

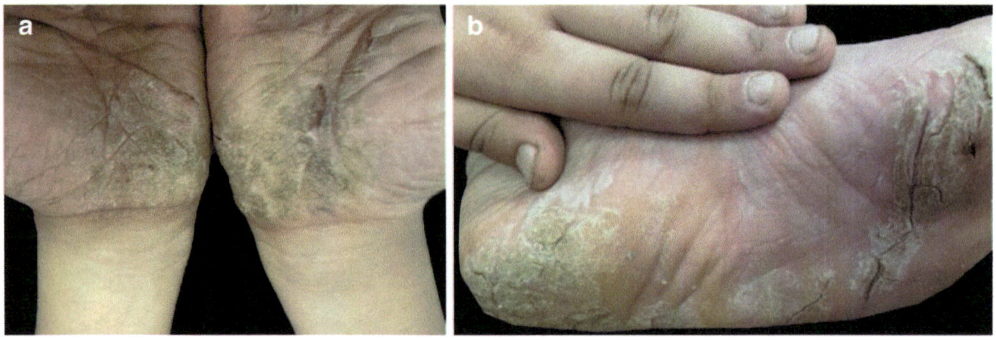

Fig. 2.14 Palmoplantar Keratoderma areata. Keratotic lesions on pressure areas (palms and soles) (**a**, **b**)

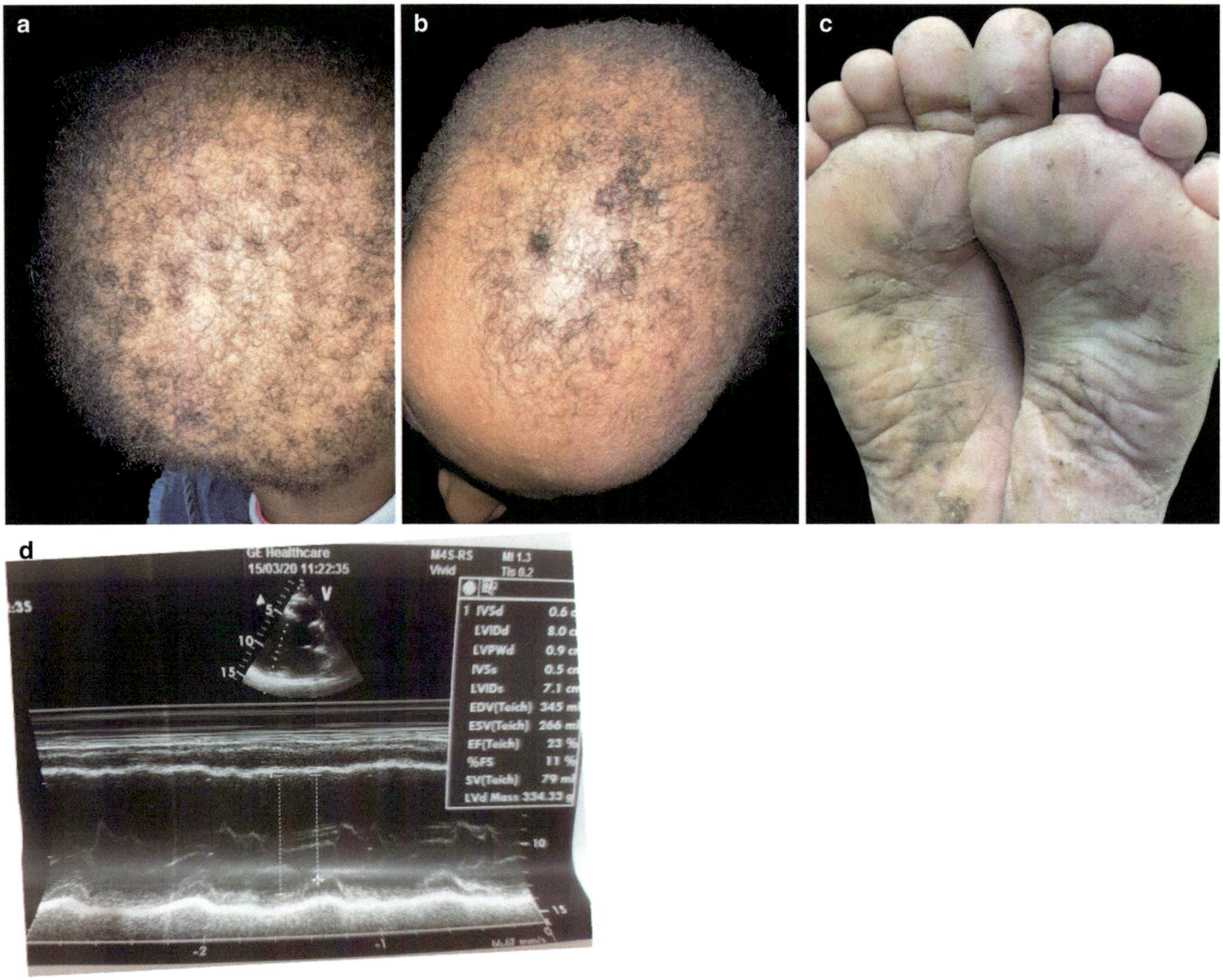

Fig. 2.15 Carvajal Syndrome. A child with wooly hair (**a**, **b**) with focal hyperkeratosis of the sole (**c**). Left ventricular dilatation with severe dysfunction (**d**)

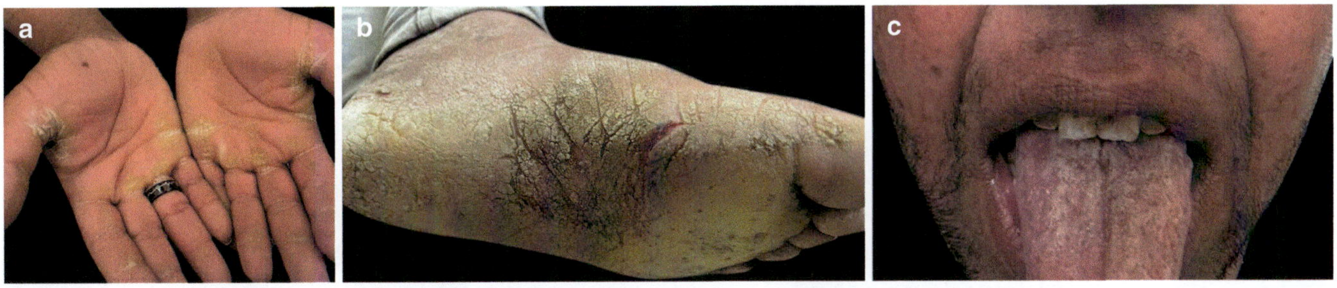

Fig. 2.16 Howel-Evans syndrome. Thick yellow wax keratoderma on palms and soles (**a**, **b**) and oral leukokeratosis (**c**)

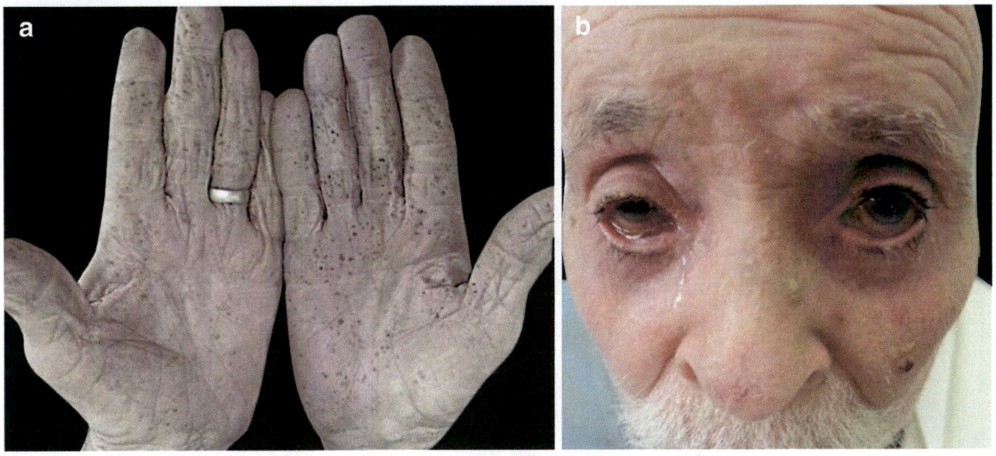

Fig. 2.17 Richner-Hanhart Syndrome. Palmar hyperkeratosis (**a**), Painful pseudo-herpetic dendritic keratitis (**b**)

Pachyonychia Congenita Type 1 (AD) [12] (Figs. 2.18, 2.19, 2.20, and 2.21)

- Mutation in keratin genes: *KRT6A* and *KRT16.*
- Clinical characteristics:
  - Hypertrophic nail dystrophy or pachyonychia with wedge shaped subungual hyperkeratosis.
  - Painful calluses and blisters mainly on the soles of the feet (focal plantar hyperkeratosis). Pain is one of the distinct characteristics. Calluses may also form on the palms (palmar hyperkeratosis).
  - Leukokeratosis.
  - Follicular hyperkeratosis at friction sites such as waist, hips, knees, elbows.
  - Deep itch under, around, or in the calluses.

Diffuse Palmoplantar Keratoderma (PPK)

Diffuse PPK involves most of the palms and soles. Some types are associated with abnormalities of internal organs "syndromic keratoderma." It may be either transgredient or non-transgredient keratoderma.

Transgredient keratodermas extend beyond the palms and soles onto the back of the hands and feet and in some cases up to the wrists and ankles. Skin around the mouth, eyes, nose, and over the elbows and knees may also be affected.

Non-transgredient keratodermas do not extend beyond the palms and soles. They may affect the knuckle pads and nails but do not involve the skin on the top of the feet or hands.

Transgredient and non-transgredient keratodermas are associated with several syndromes (Table 2.2).

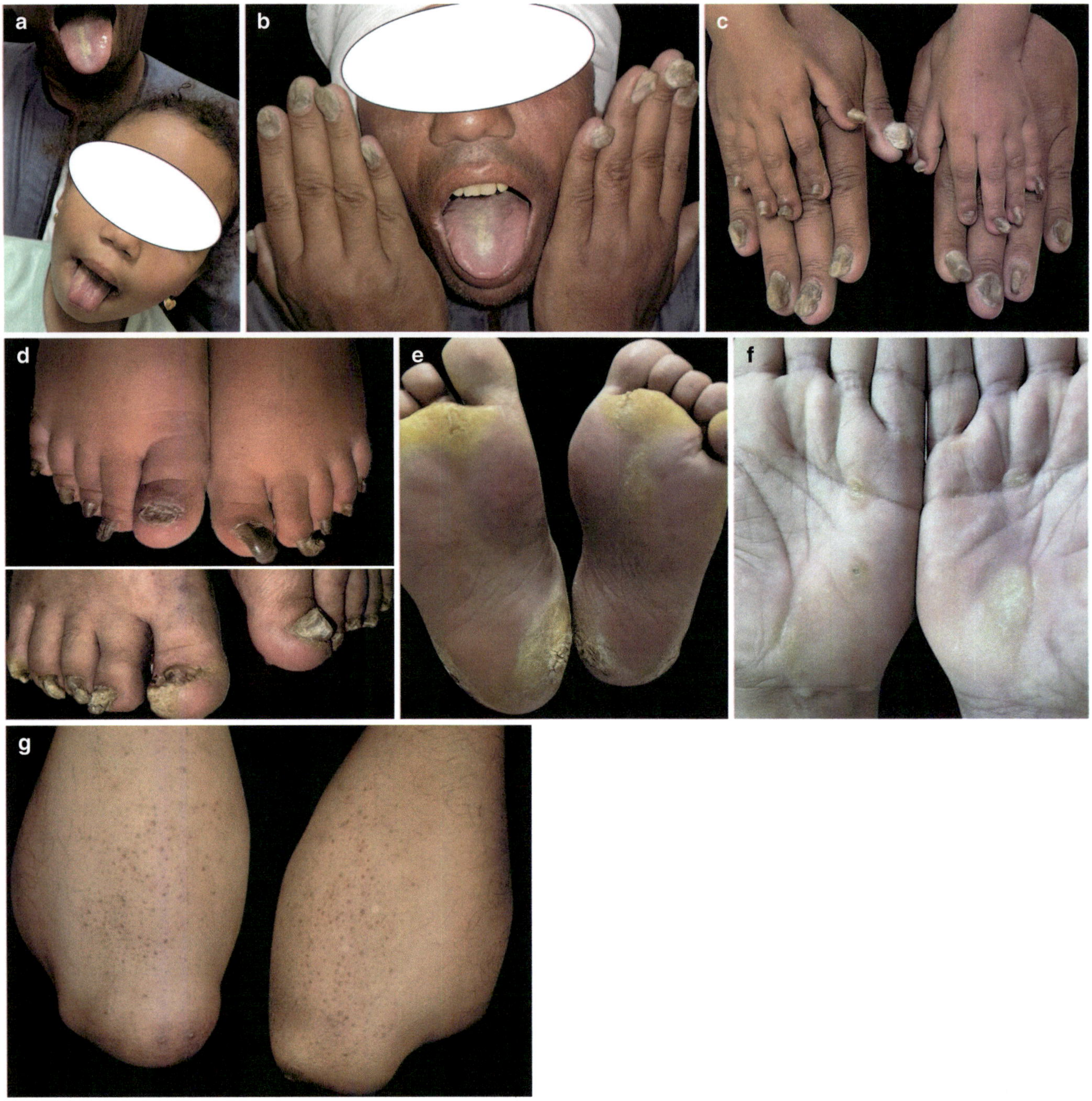

Fig. 2.18 Pachyonychia congenita. Father and his daughter having pachyonychia congenita. Oral leukokeratosis and angular cheilitis (**a**, **b**). Wedge shaped subungual hyperkeratosis with hypertrophic nail dystrophy of both hands and feet of the father and the daughter (**c**, **d**). Painful focal palmoplantar keratoderma (areata), yellow calluses (**e**, **f**) and follicular hyperkeratosis of elbows (**g**)

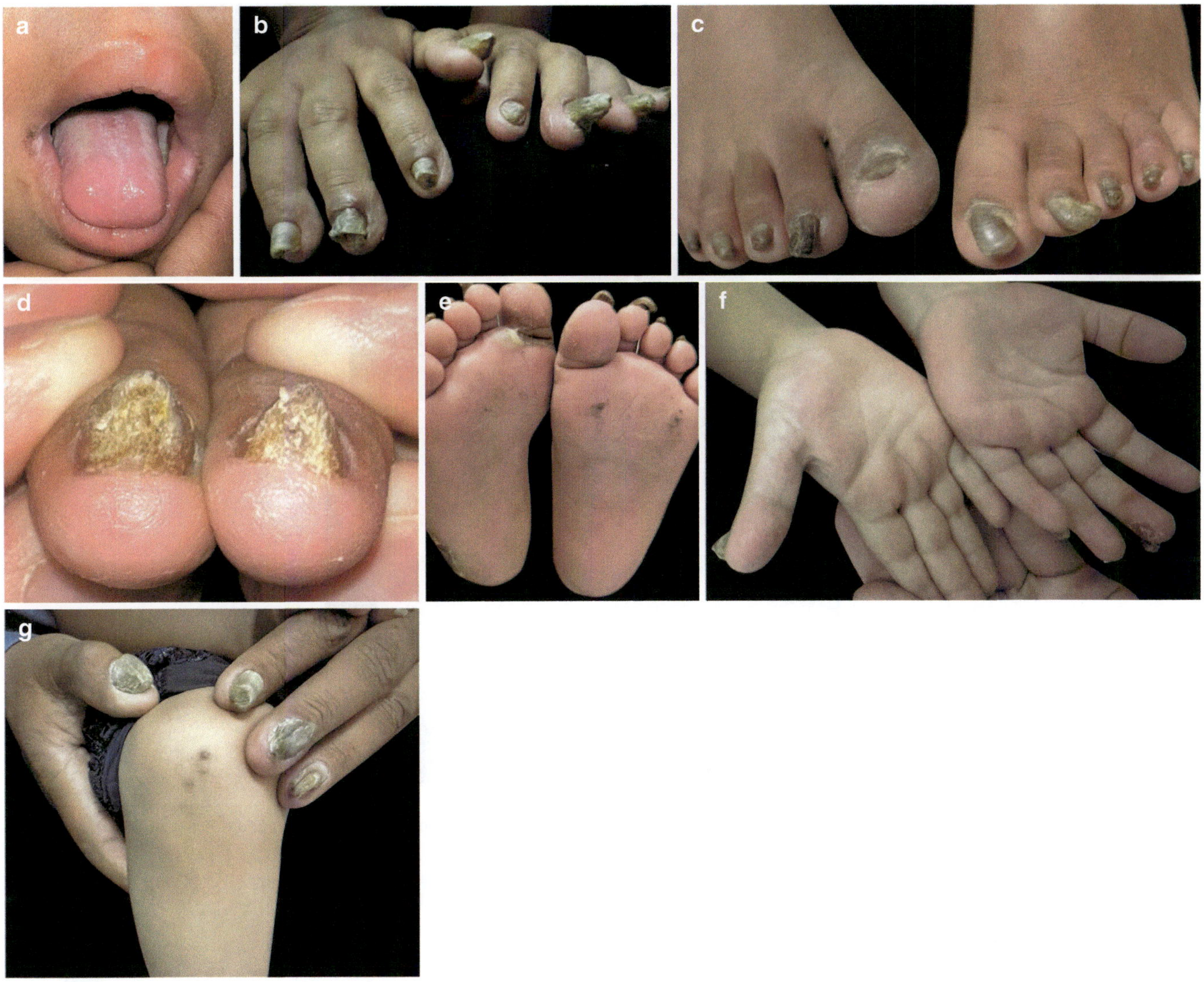

Fig. 2.19 Pachyonychia congenita. Oral leukokeratosis, angular cheilitis (**a**), wedge shaped subungual hyperkeratosis with hypertrophic nail dystrophy (**b**–**d**). Painful focal palmoplantar keratoderma (areata) (**e**, **f**) and follicular hyperkeratosis of knee (**g**)

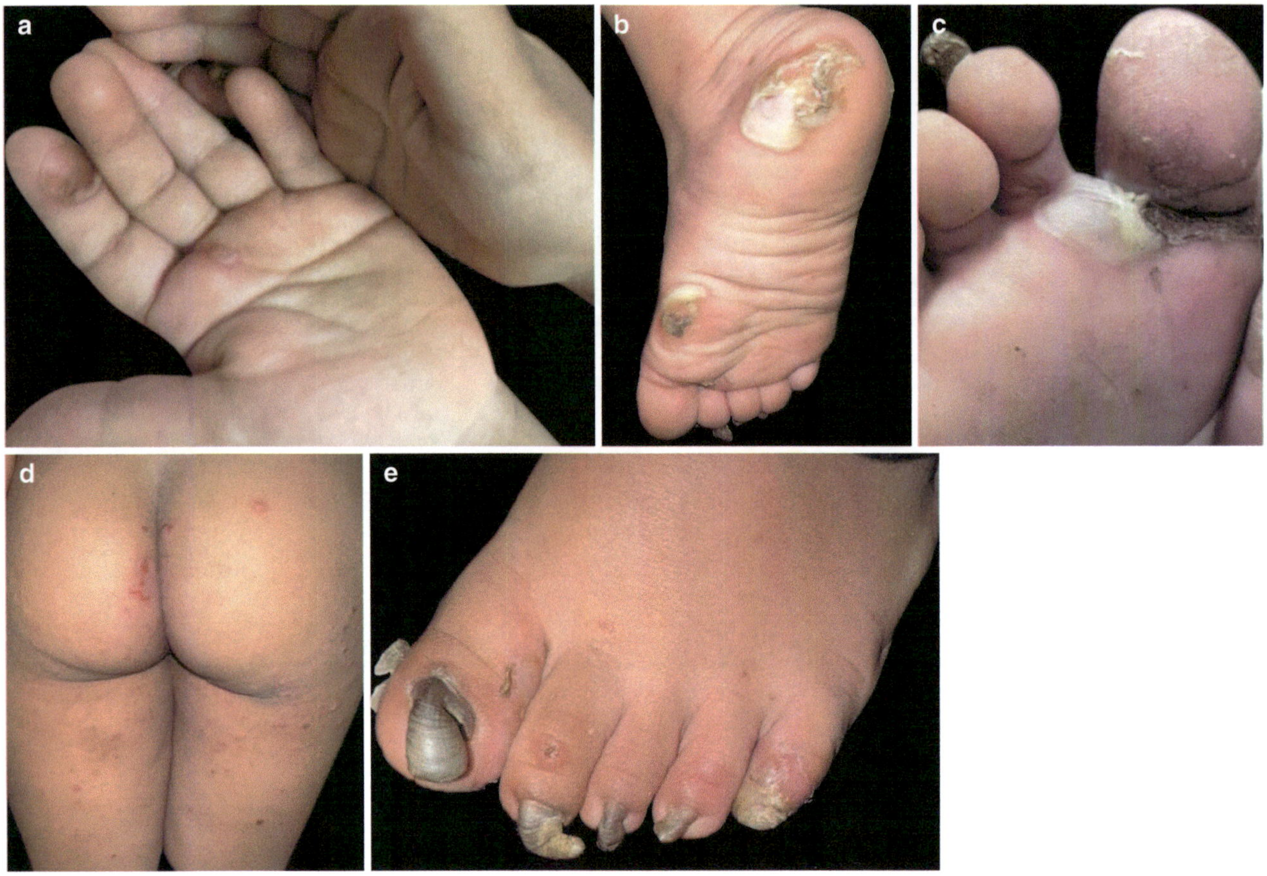

Fig. 2.20 Pachyonychia congenita. The same patient of Fig. 2.19 developed blistering on palms, soles, buttocks and dorsum of the foot (**a**–**e**)

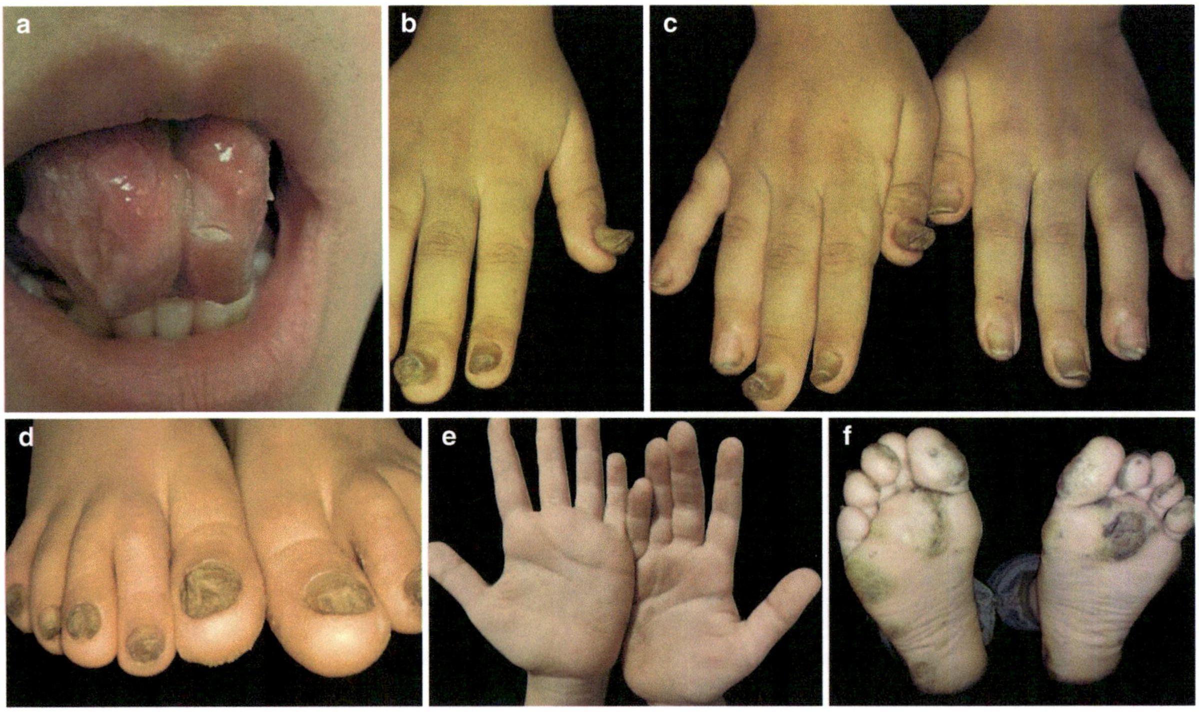

Fig. 2.21 Pachyonychia congenita. Oral leukokeratosis with angular cheilitis (**a**), wedge shaped subungual hyperkeratosis with hypertrophic nail dystrophy (**b**–**d**), painful focal palmoplantar keratoderma (areata) (**e**, **f**)

Table 2.2 Syndromes associated with diffuse palmoplantar keratoderma

Transgredient PPK	Non-transgredient PPK
• Mal de Meleda • Greither's disease • Papillon-Lefèvre syndrome • Vohwinkel syndrome • Bart-Pumphrey syndrome • Olmsted syndrome • Huriez syndrome	• Unna-Thost syndrome • Vorner syndrome • Naxos syndrome

Transgredient Keratodermas

Mal de Meleda PPK (AR) (Keratosis Extremitatum Hereditaria Trangrediens et Progrediens) [13, 14] (Figs. 2.22, 2.23, 2.24 , 2.25, and 2.26)

- Genetic *mutations in SLURP-1* gene which provides instructions for making a protein called secreted LY6/ uPAR-related protein-1.
- Onset: soon after birth.

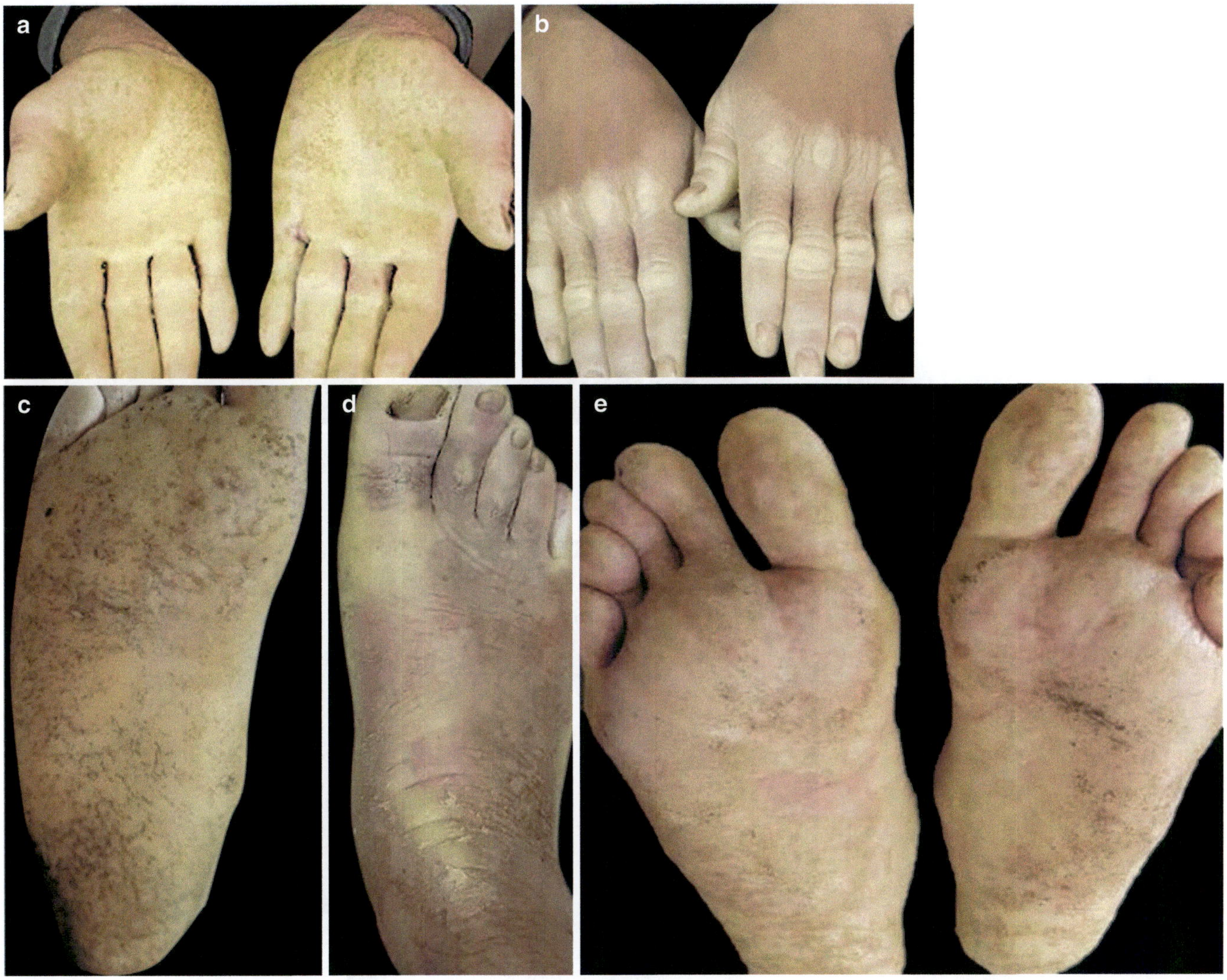

Fig. 2.22 Mal de Meleda. Adult patient with diffuse yellow transgredient palmoplantar keratoderma with macerated and well demarcated border (glove and stock) (**a**–**e**)

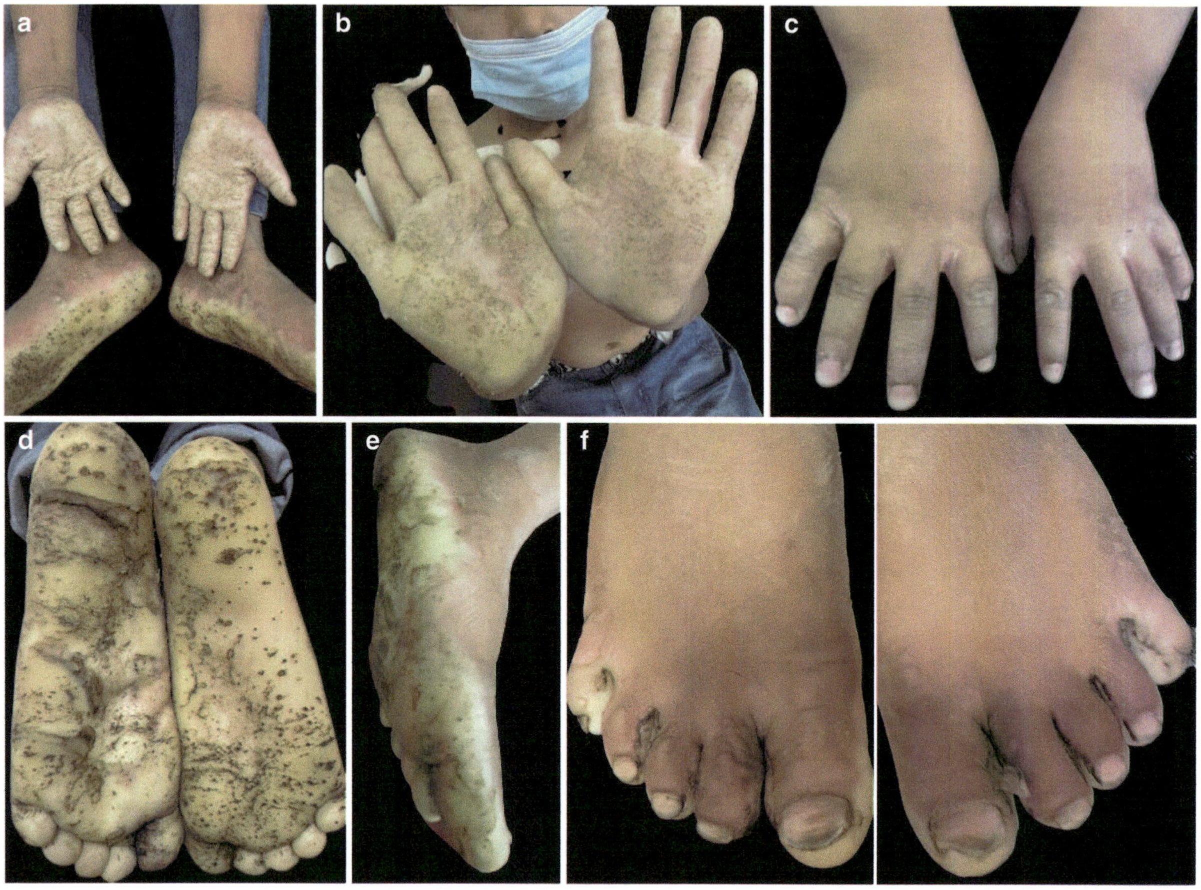

Fig. 2.23 Mal de Meleda. A child with diffuse transgredient macerated palmoplantar keratoderma (glove and stock) with maceration between toe webs (**a**–**f**). Conical tapering of finger tips (**c**). (*Courtesy, Samar Ashry*)

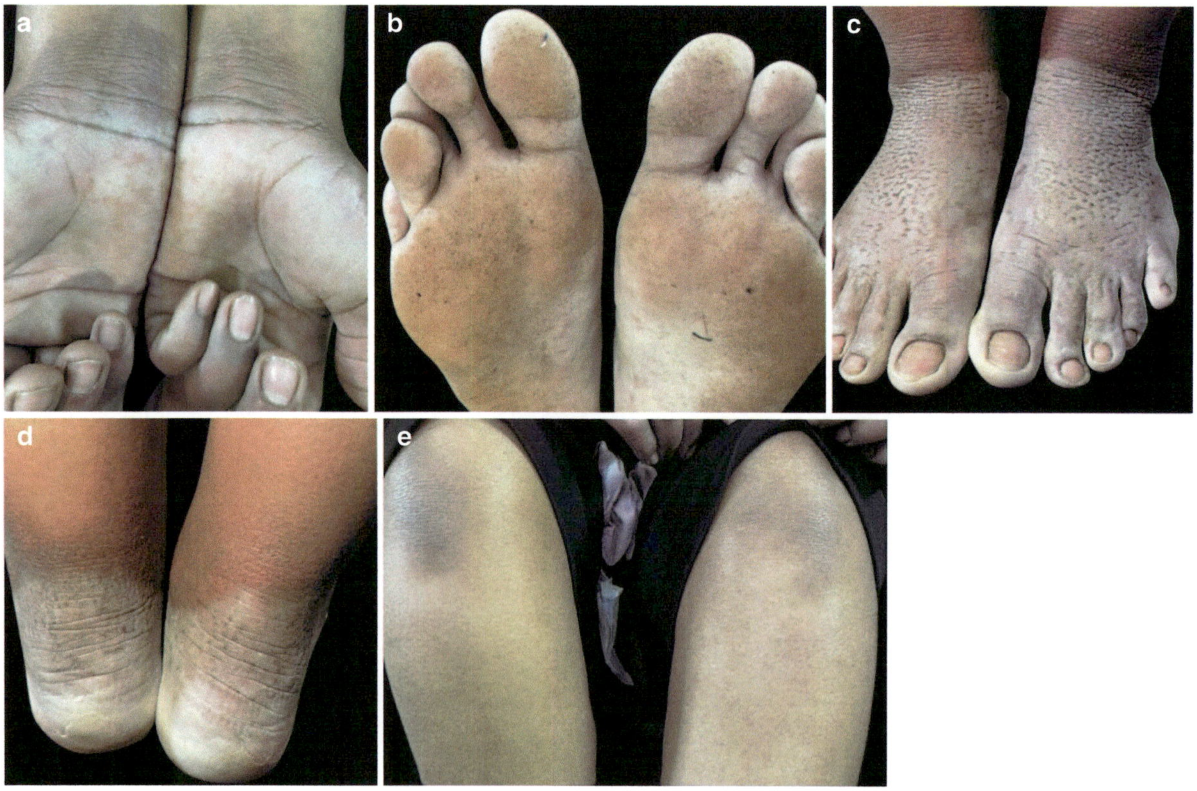

Fig. 2.24 Mal De Meleda. Diffuse transgredient palmoplantar keratoderma (glove and stock) (**a**–**d**) and hyperkeratosis on knees (**e**)

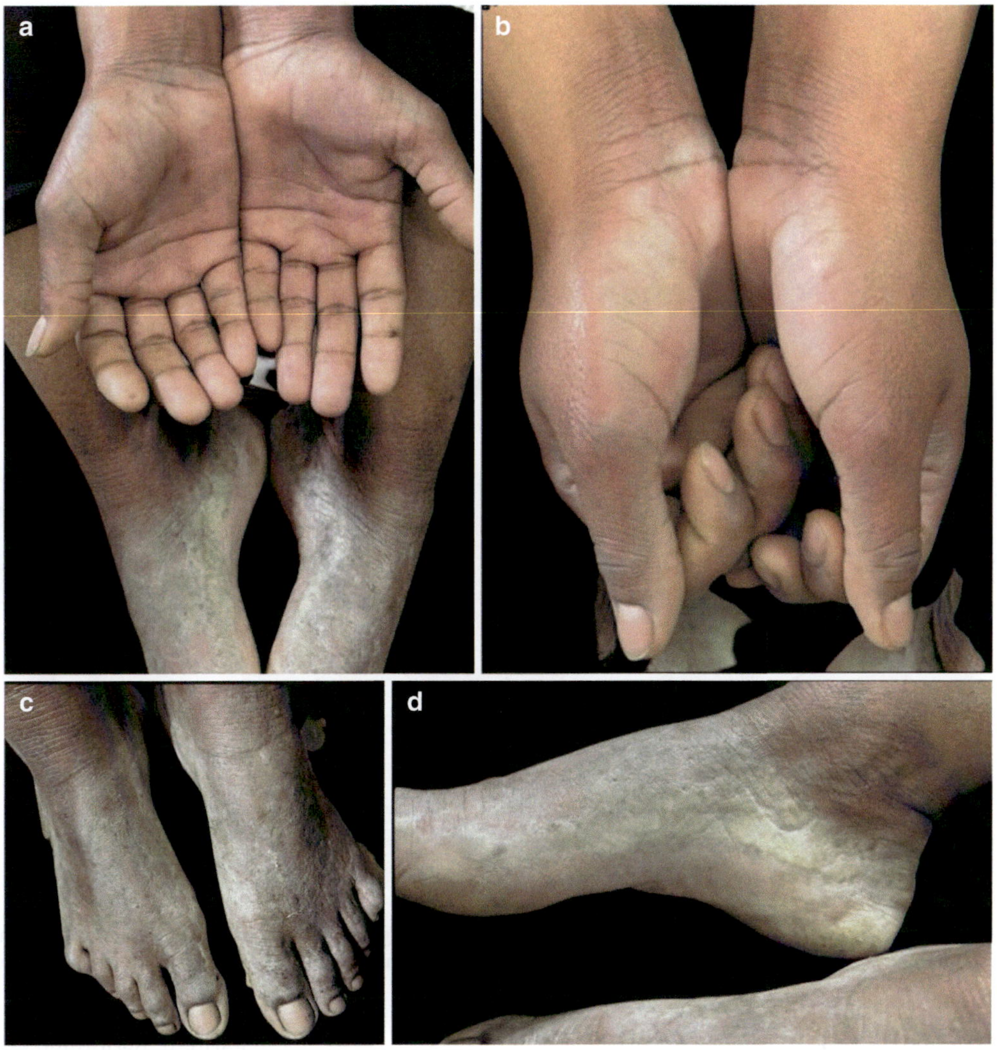

Fig. 2.25 Mal De Meleda (*the sister of patient in* Fig. 2.24) with diffuse transgredient macerated palmoplantar keratoderma (**a–d**)

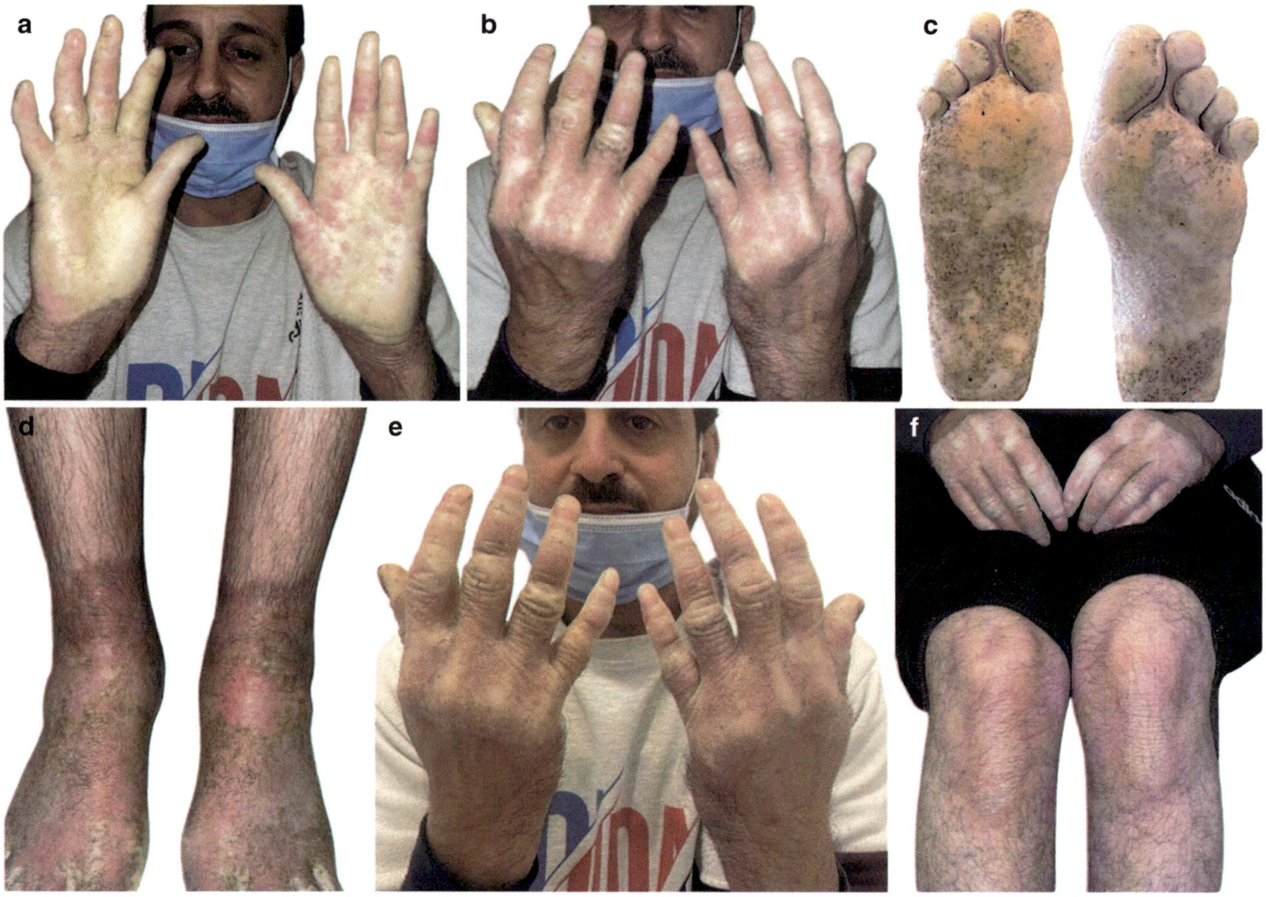

Fig. 2.26 Mal de Meleda. Adult patient with diffuse yellow transgredient palmoplantar keratoderma with macerated and well demarcated border (glove and stock) (**a**–**d**), Notice pseudoainhum constrictions on the digits (**e**) and psoriasiform lesions on the knees (**f**)

- Clinical characteristics:
  - It starts at birth as palmoplantar erythema, which progresses to develop thick lesions during the first 3–4 years of life and manifests clinically as bilateral thick yellow to brown PPK with prominent erythematous border.
  - The hyperkeratosis spreads to the dorsal aspects of hands and feet, like gloves and socks (transgrediens).
  - Hyperkeratosis progresses without a tendency to spontaneous resolution.
  - Keratoderma is most often complicated by hyperhidrosis, secondary bacterial and fungal infections, and is associated with foul smell.
  - Conical tapering of the fingertips may be seen.
  - The progressive form of disease presents with severe mutilation, constricting bands around digits, pseudoainhum, amputation of digits, and contractures.
- Associations:
  - Well-circumscribed psoriasis-like plaques may be present on the knees and the elbows.
  - Perioral, periorbital erythema, and hyperkeratosis.
  - Nail changes: koilonychia, subungual hyperkeratosis.
  - Syndactyly, hair on the palms and the soles, high-arched palate, and left-handedness.

Greither's Disease (AD) (Transgrediens et Progrediens PPK) [15] (Figs. 2.27 and 2.28)

- Missense mutation in *KRT1* gene.
- Usually presents after 2 years of age.
- Clinical characteristics:
  - Diffuse moderate to severe PPK with an erythematous border, extending to the dorsal aspects of the hands, feet, and/or wrists and involving the skin over the Achilles' tendon (transgrediens), gradually worsening with age (progrediens) to include patchy hyperkeratosis over the shins, knees, elbows, and, sometimes, skin flexures.
  - Hyperhidrosis is usually associated.

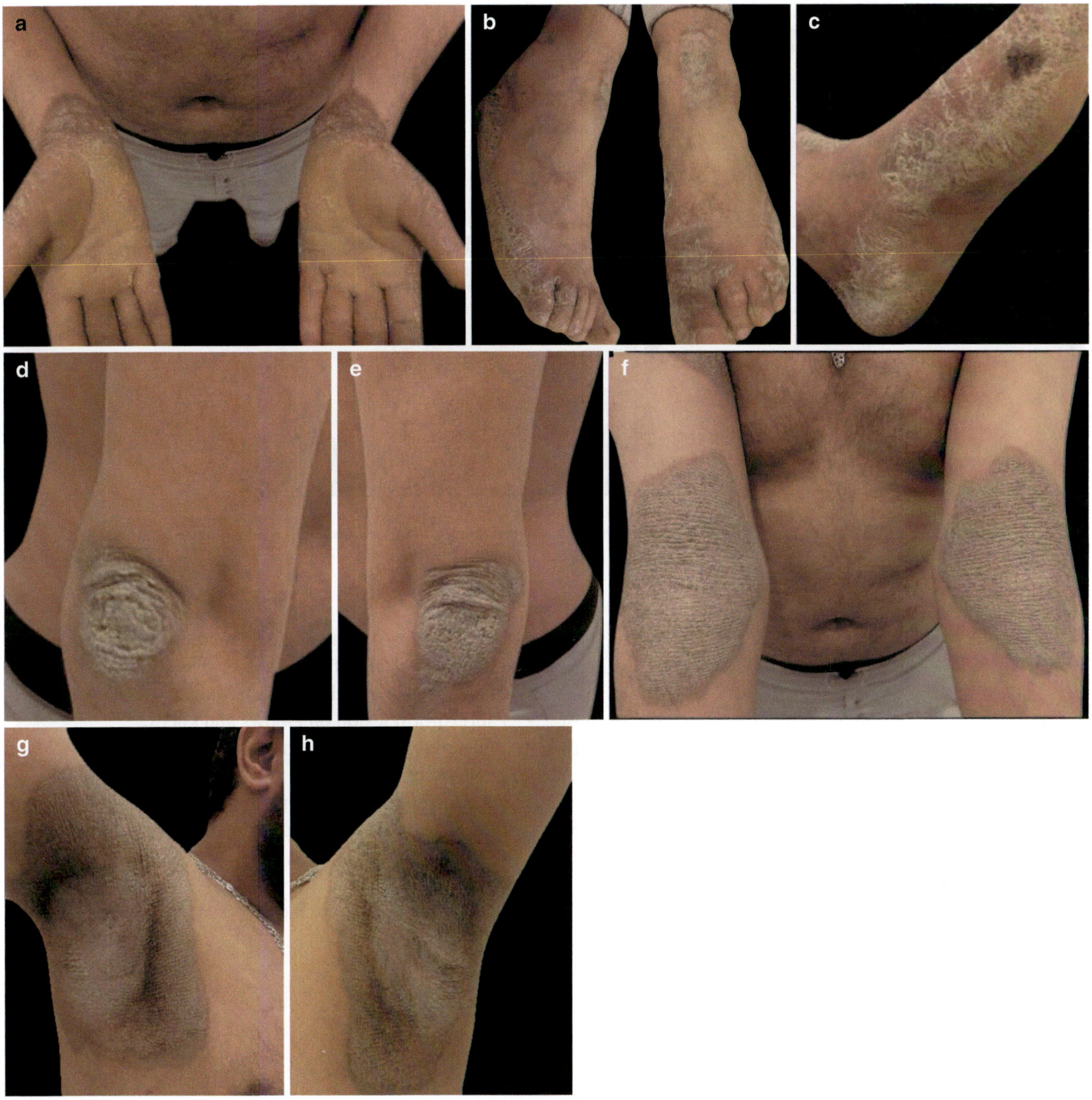

Fig. 2.27 Greither's Disease. Diffuse transgredient palmoplantar keratoderma with an erythematous border (**a**–**c**). Patchy hyperkeratotic plaques on elbows, flexures and axillae (**d**–**h**).

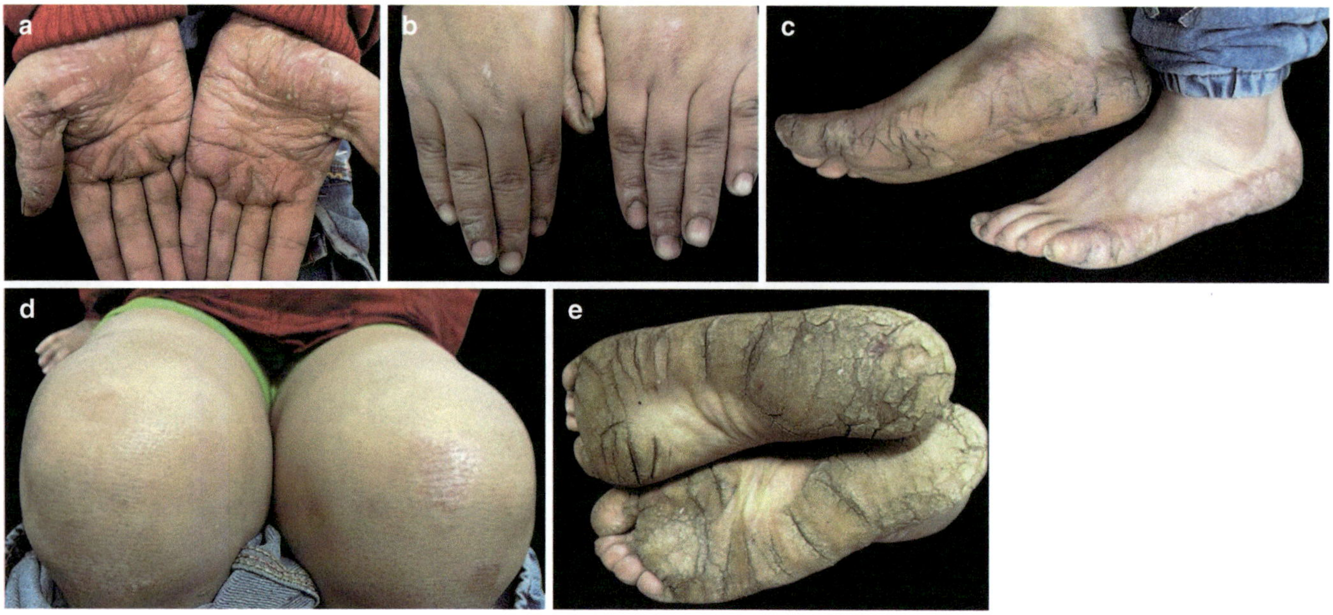

Fig 2.28 Greither's Disease. Diffuse transgredient palmoplantar with an erythematous border (**a–c**). Patchy mild hyperkeratosis of knees (**d**). Plantar keratoderma of the sole (**e**)

Papillon-Lefèvre Syndrome (AR) [16] (Figs. 2.29, 2.30, 2.31, 2.32, and 2.33)

- Mutation in *cathepsin C* gene, dysregulation of host immune response which in turn predisposes to cutaneous and systemic infections.
- Onset: at birth or early infancy.
- Characterized by the triad of symmetrical keratoderma with transgrediens, early onset severe periodontitis with loss of primary and permanent dentitions, and susceptibility to cutaneous and systemic infections.
- PPK: Diffuse transgredient mutilating (stocking and glove). Soles are affected more severely than palms and malodorous hyperhidrosis is frequent.
- Psoriasiform lesion on elbows and knees.
- Pyogenic bacterial infection: liver abscess and pyoderma.
- Pseudoainhum of distal phalanges, acral osteolysis, nail dystrophy, transverse groove of finger nails, and loss of alveolar bone may occur.
- Painful mastications.
- Blue sclera and bad oral odor.

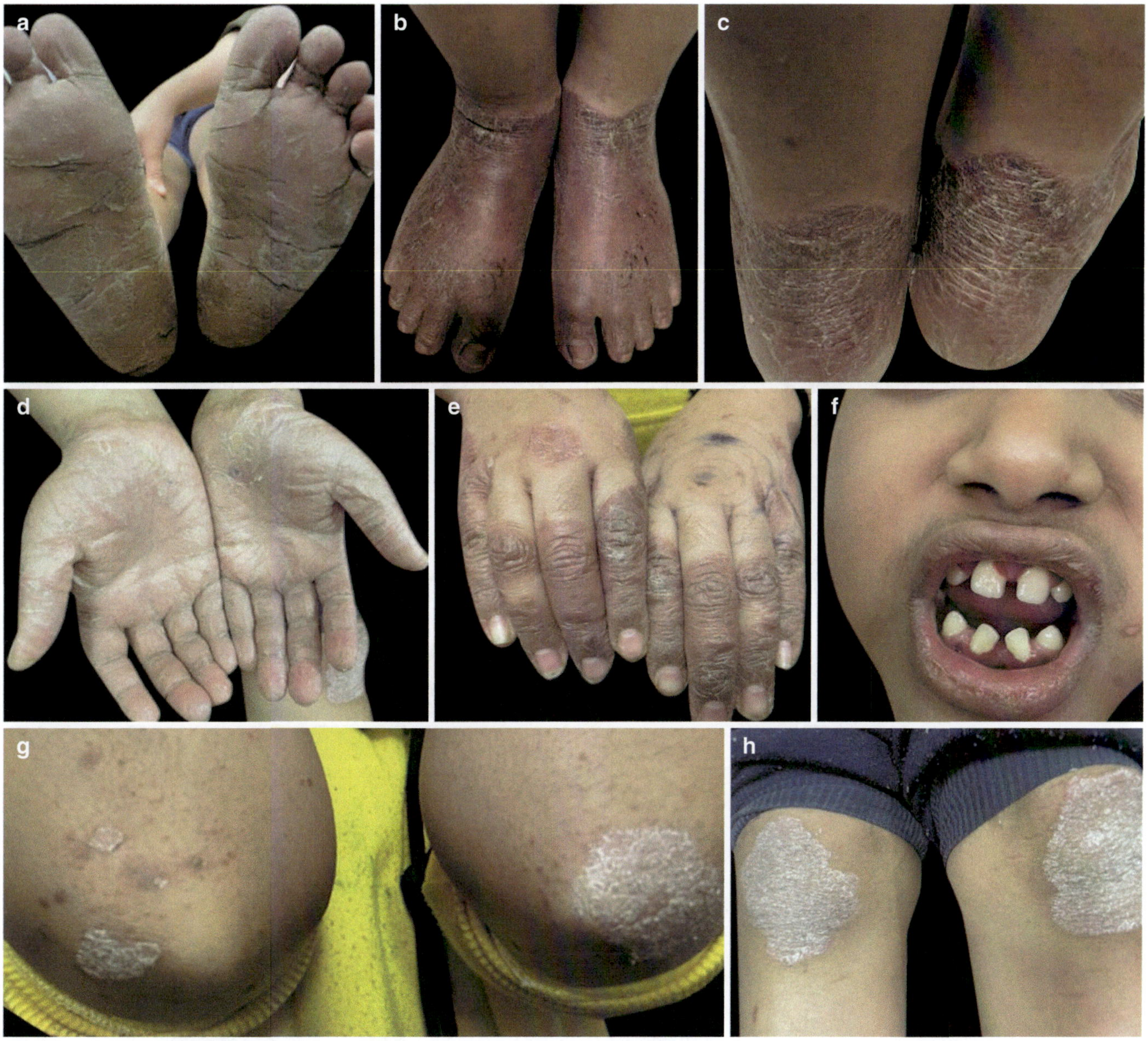

Fig 2.29 Papillon-Lefèvre Syndrome. Diffuse transgredient palmoplantar keratoderma (stocking and glove). Soles are affected more severely than palms (**a**–**e**). Periodontitis (**f**) and psoriasiform lesions on elbows and knees (**g**, **h**)

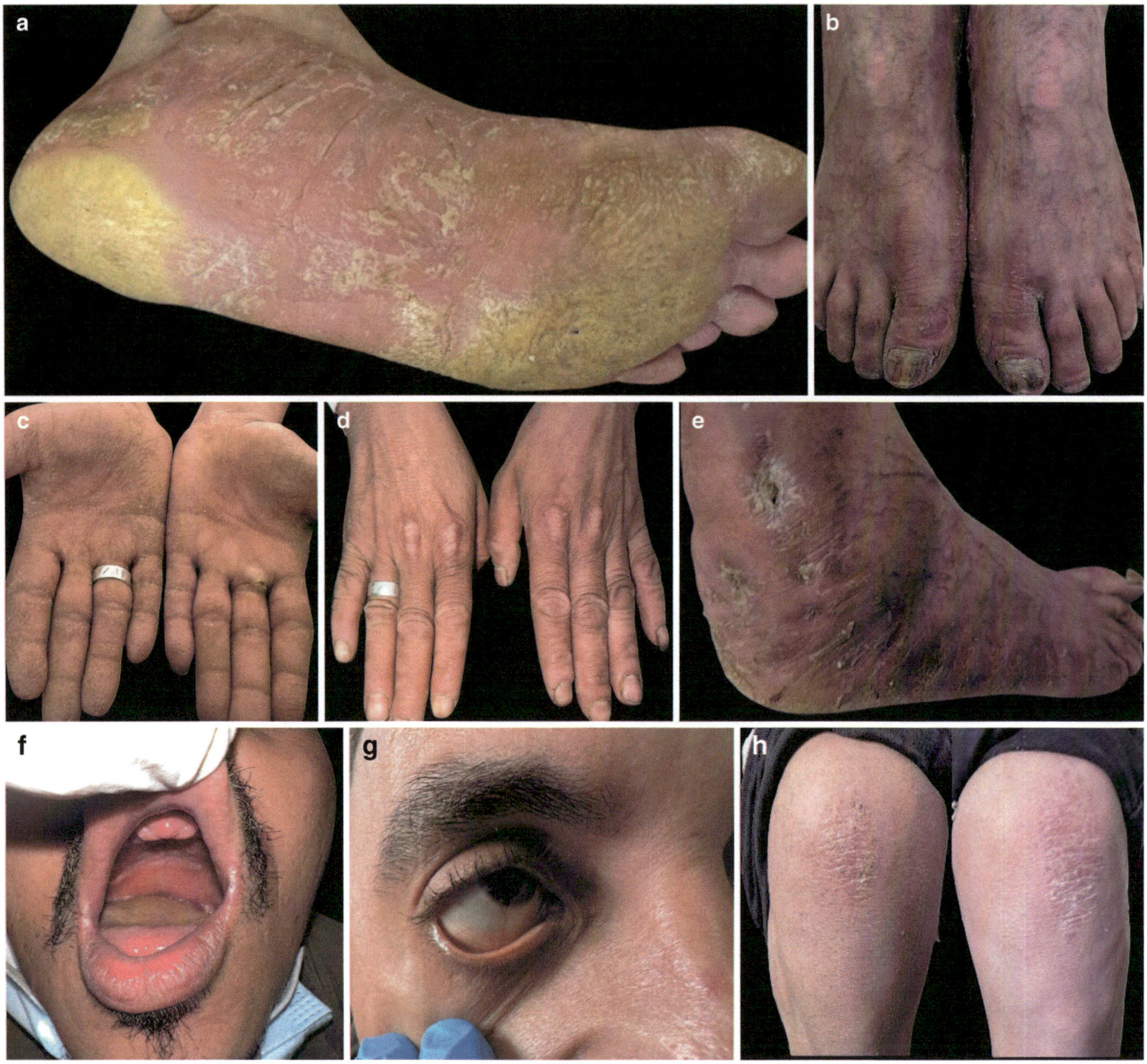

Fig. 2.30 Papillon-Lefèvre Syndrome. Diffuse transgredient PPK. Soles are affected more severely than palms with cutaneous infections in lower leg (**a**–**e**). Loss of teeth (**f**), blue sclera (**g**) and psoriasiform lesions on knees (**h**)

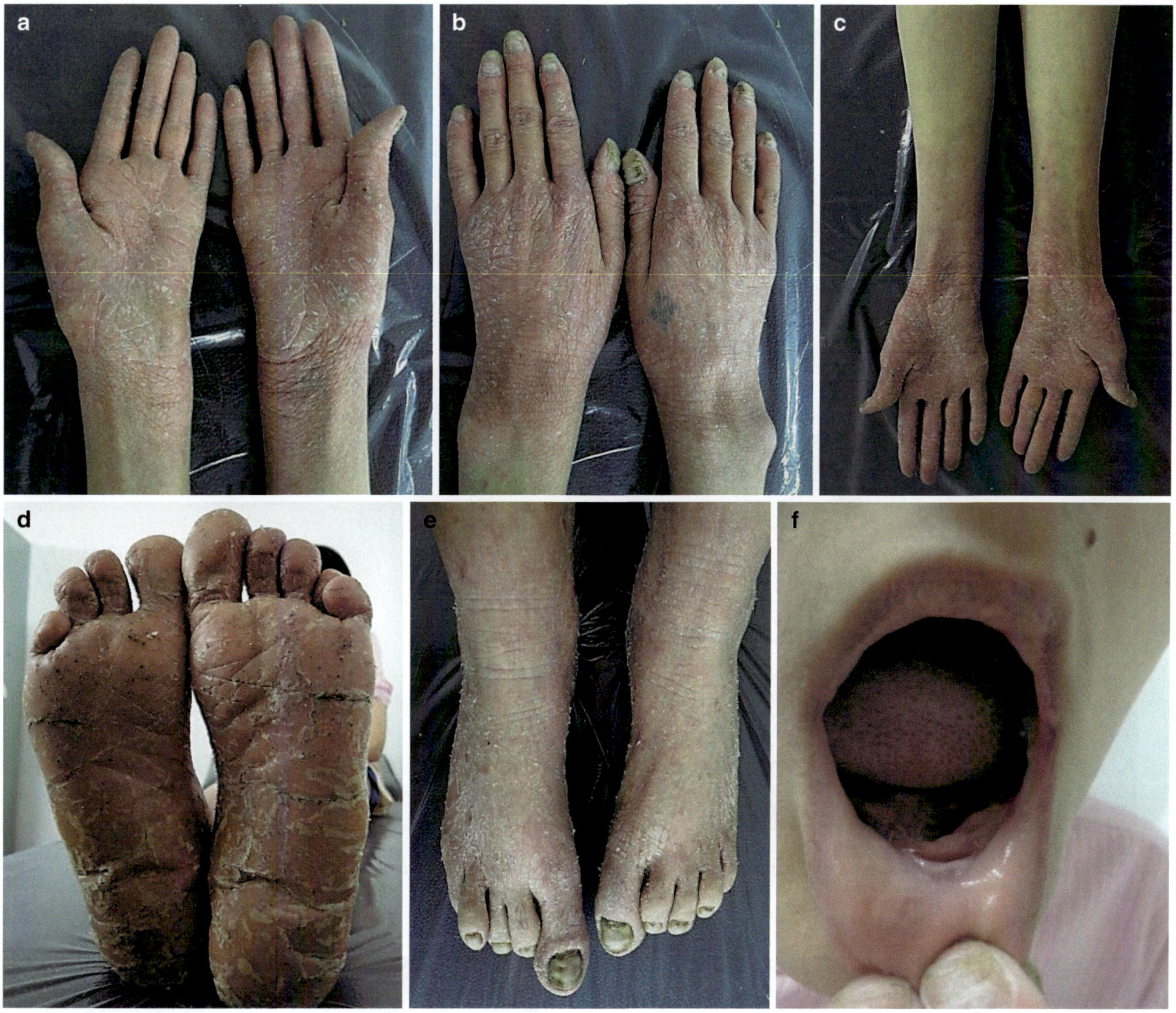

Fig. 2.31 Papillon-Lefèvre Syndrome. Diffuse transgredient PPK (stocking and glove) with nail dystrophy (**a**–**e**). Loss of teeth (**f**)

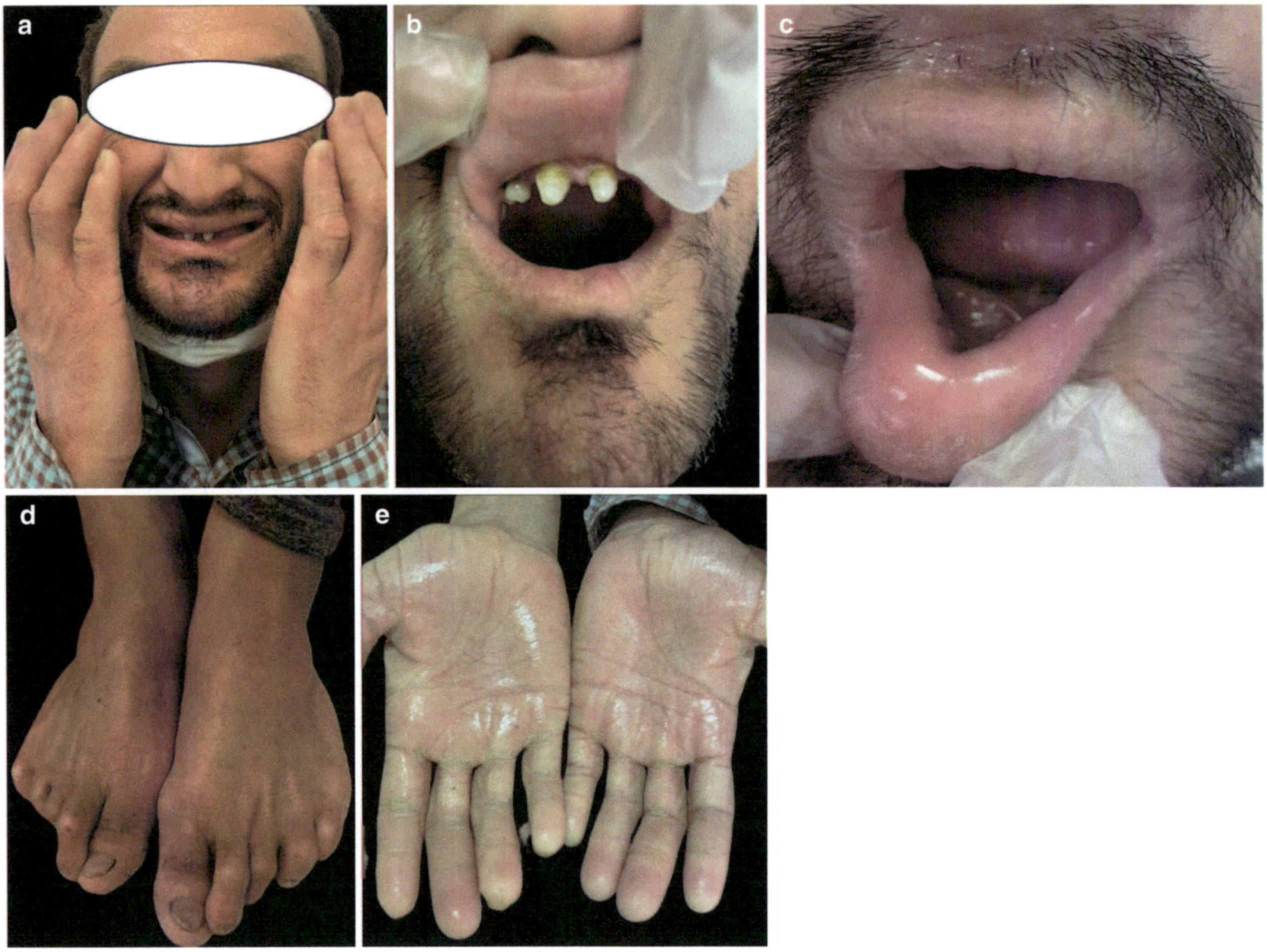

Fig. 2.32 Papillon-Lefèvre Syndrome. Periodontitis with loss of teeth (**a–c**). Diffuse hyperkeratosis of dorsum of hands and feet (**d**) with hyperhidrosis (**e**)

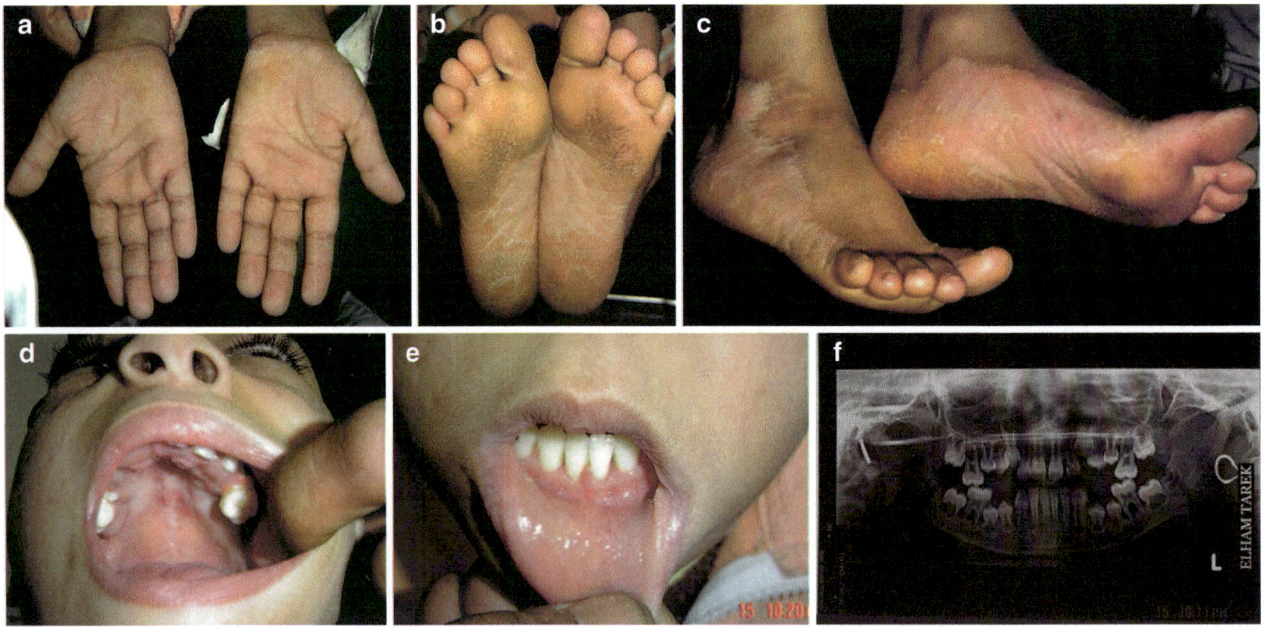

Fig. 2.33 Papillon-Lefèvre Syndrome. Diffuse transgredient PPK with well demarcated border (**a–c**). Periodontitis with loss of teeth (**d**, **e**). Panorama show loosely attached teeth (f). (*Courtesy, Hala Shawky*)

Vohwinkel Syndrome (AD) [17] (Keratoderma Hereditaria Mutilans) (PPK with Honeycomb Pattern) (Fig. 2.34)

- Defect in *GJB2* encoding Cx26.
- Onset: infancy or early childhood.
- The honeycomb appearance of PPK with a fine discernible superficial pattern replacing normal dermatoglyphics and starfish-shaped keratotic plaques over the knuckles, wrists, elbows, and knees are highly diagnostic.
- Over time, the affected children develop constricting fibrous bands and pseudoainhum and autoamputation of the toes and fingers particularly of the fifth digit.
- Other features include moderate to severe sensory neural deafness, myopathy, spastic paraplegia, mental retardation, acanthosis nigricans, ichthyosiform dermatitis, alopecia, and nail abnormalities.

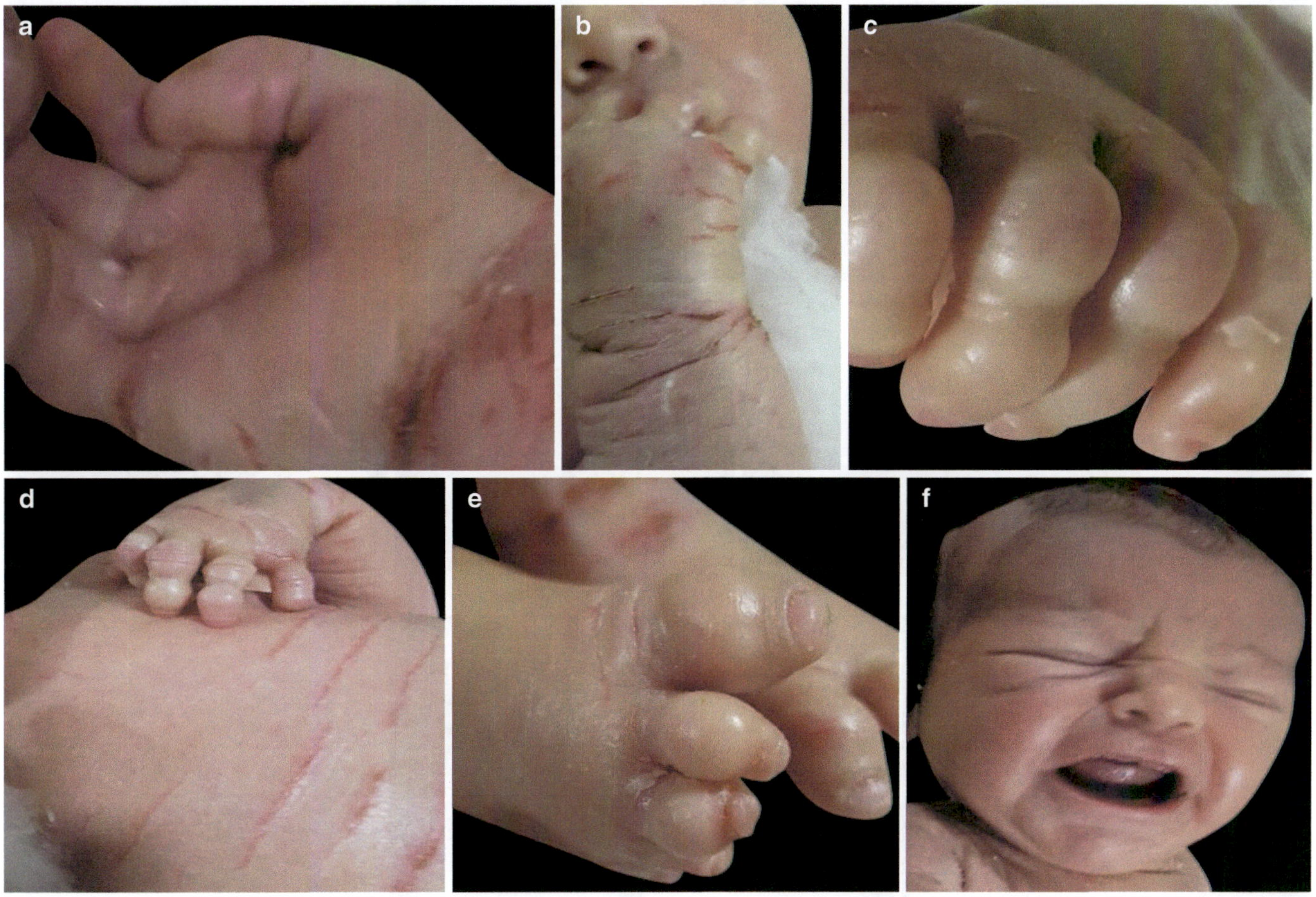

Fig. 2.34 Vohwinkel Syndrome. Palmar keratoderma with loss of dermatoglyphics (**a**), starfish-shaped keratotic plaques over the wrists (**b**). Constricting bands around fingers, wrist, toes (**c–e**) and alopecia (**f**)

Bart-Pumphrey Syndrome (AD) [18] (Fig. 2.35)

- Defect in *GJB2* encoding Cx26.
- Onset: infancy or early childhood.
- Clinical characteristics:
  - PPK: diffuse or striate with a granular surface. It is particularly evident along the skin creases.
  - Knuckle pads: hyperkeratosis on metacarpophalangeal, proximal, and distal interphalangeal joints.
  - Leukonychia which may improve with age.
  - Deafness.

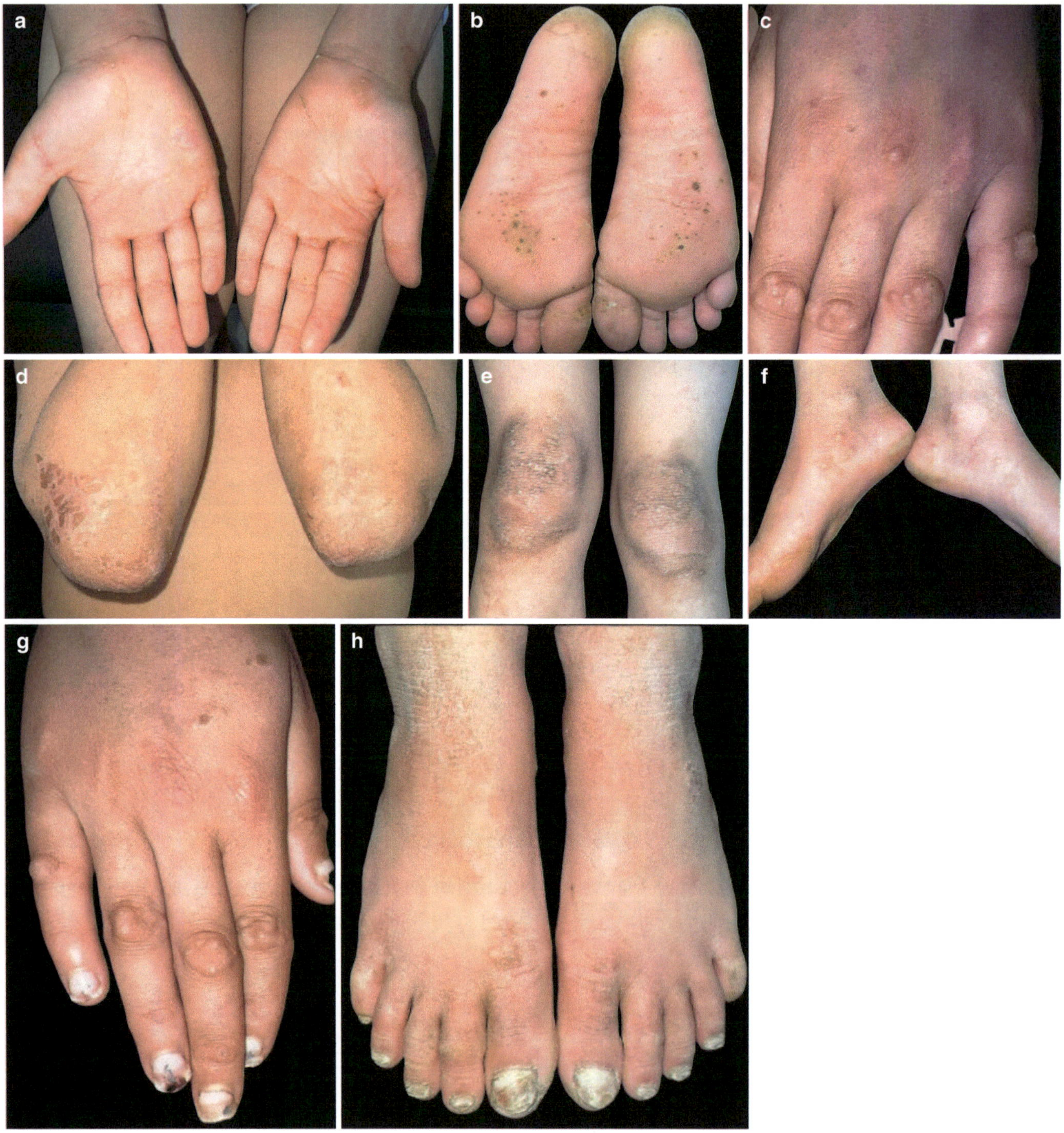

Fig. 2.35 Bart Pumphrey syndrome. Palmoplantar keratoderma (**a**, **b**), warty hyperkeratosis over the knuckles, interphalangeal joints, elbows, knees and feet (**c**–**f**)

Olmsted Syndrome (AD/R, XLR) (Diffuse Mutilating Keratoderma with Periorificial Plaques) [19] (Fig. 2.36)

- Mutations in transient receptor potential vanilloid-3 (*TRPV3*) gene in AD or AR forms. Mutations in membrane-bound transcription factor protease, site 2 (*MBTPS2*) gene in XLR form.
- Onset: at birth or early childhood.
- Clinical characteristics:
  - The disease has a slow, but progressive course.

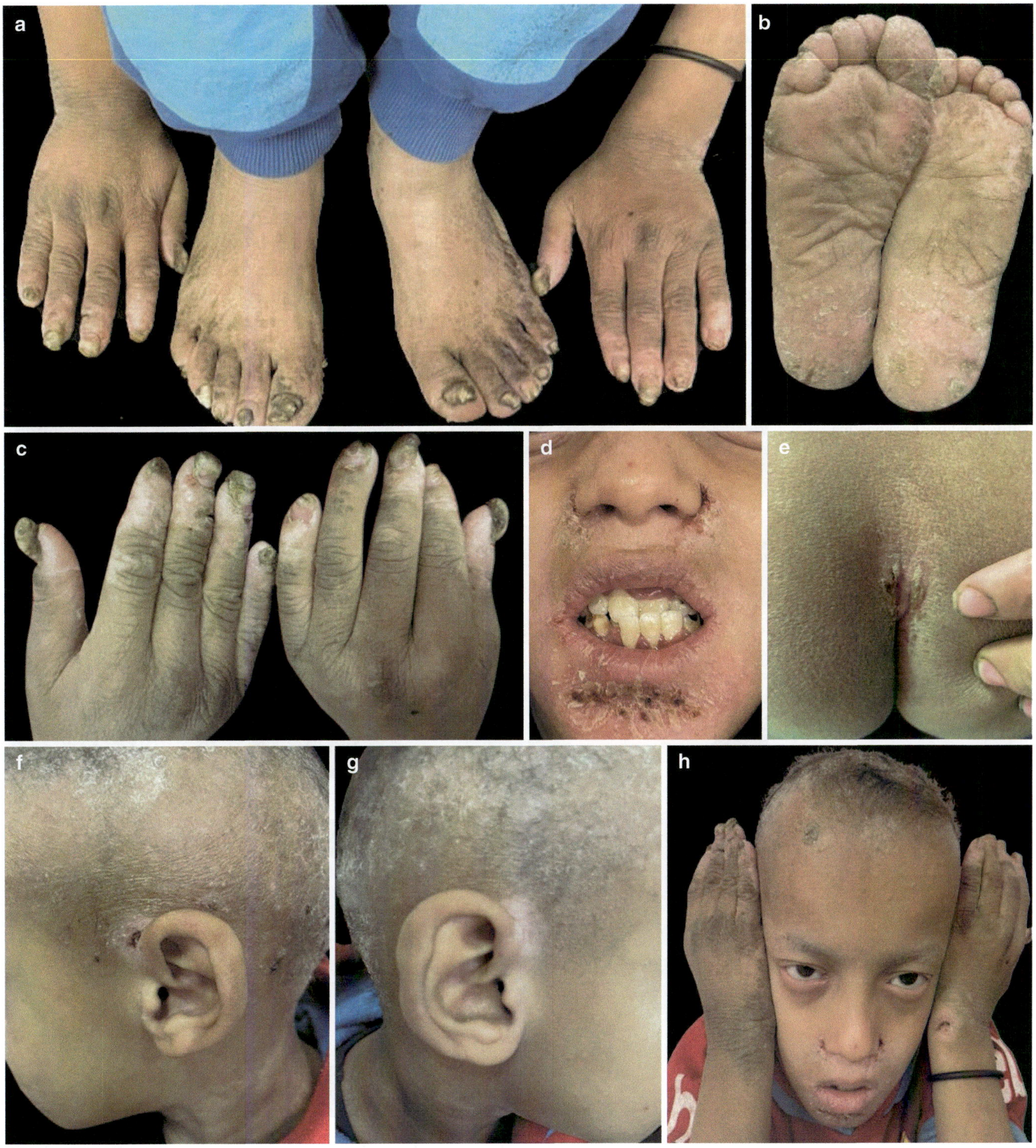

Fig. 2.36 Olmsted Syndrome. Diffuse transgredient palmoplantar keratoderma with nail dystrophy (**a**–**c**), periorificial and perianal hyperkeratotic plaques (**d**, **e**). Alopecia (**f**, **g**) and loss of eyebrows (**h**). (Courtesy of Samar Ashry)

- The two major cutaneous features of Olmsted syndrome are the symmetrical involvement of PPK with transgrediens, and the symmetrical hyperkeratotic plaques around the body orifices.
- Severe mutilation, contractures, constrictions, and autoamputation of digits occur over time.
- Severe itching.
- Corneal defects, alopecia universalis, keratosis pilaris, oral leukokeratosis, teeth abnormalities, and sensory neural deafness.

Huriez Syndrome (AD) (Sclerotylosis) [20] (Fig. 2.37)

- Onset: at birth.
- Characterized by the triad of congenital scleroatrophy of the distal extremities, PPK, and hypoplastic nails. The development of aggressive squamous cell carcinoma arising in the scleroatrophic area is also a distinctive feature of the syndrome.

Non-Transgredient Keratodermas

Unna-Thost and Vorner PPK are two clinically similar phenotypes PPK; non-epidermolytic (Unna-Thost) and epidermolytic (Vorner) and PPK. K9 is palmoplantar skin-specific keratin and its mutation results in keratoderma confined to palms and soles. However, K1 is expressed on palmoplantar and glabrous skin.

Unna-Thost Syndrome (AD) [21] (Figs. 2.38, 2.39, and 2.40)

- Mutation in *KRT1* gene.
- Onset: early infancy.
- Keratoderma begins in early infancy as patchy hyperkeratosis and is well developed by 3–4 years of age manifesting as symmetric, diffuse thick yellowish palmoplantar hyperkeratosis with a sharply demarcated erythematous lateral margins that is typically non-transgrediens.

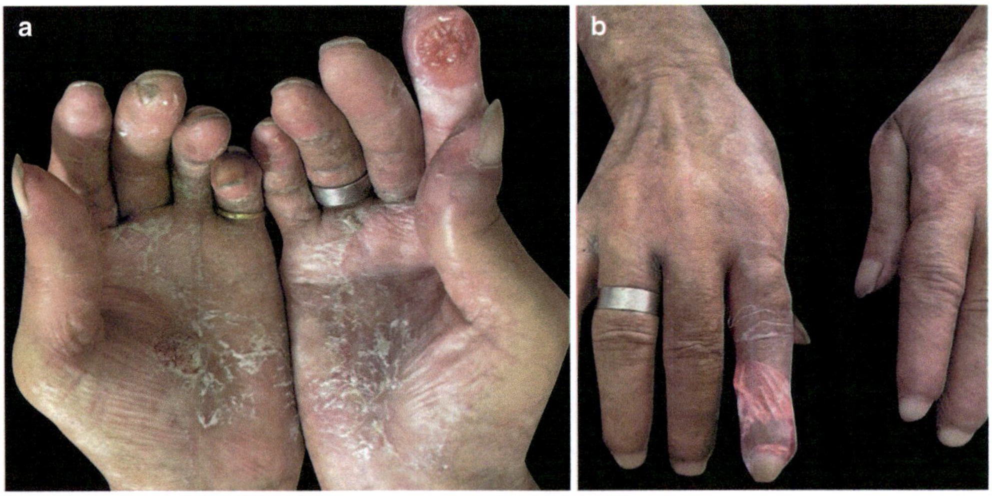

Fig. 2.37 Huriez Syndrome. Diffuse palmar keratoderma with scleroatrophy of the distal extremities developing squamous cell carcinoma diagnosed histopathologically (**a**) and hypoplastic nails (**b**)

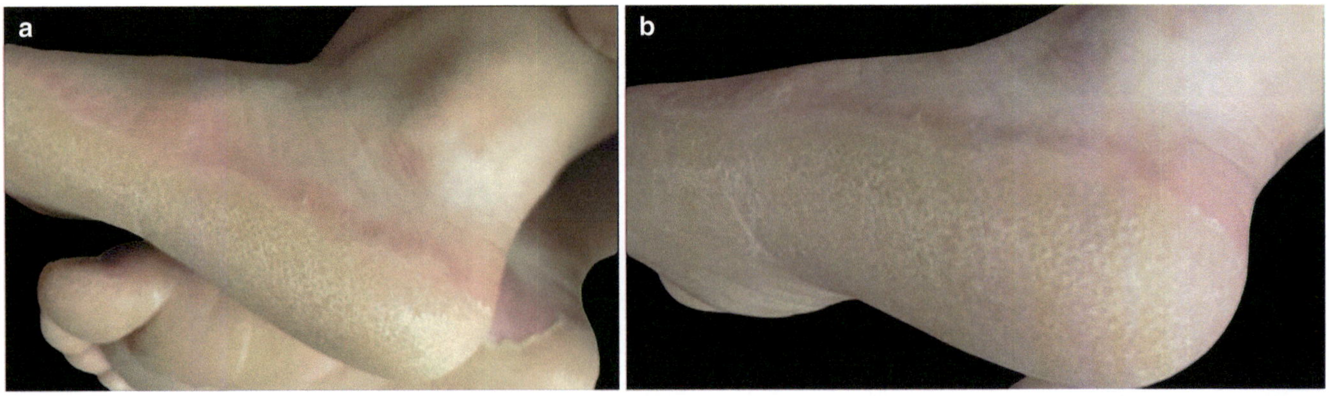

Fig 2.38 Unna-Thost Syndrome: Diffuse, yellowish non-transgredient plantar hyperkeratosis with a sharply demarcated erythematous lateral margins (**a**, **b**)

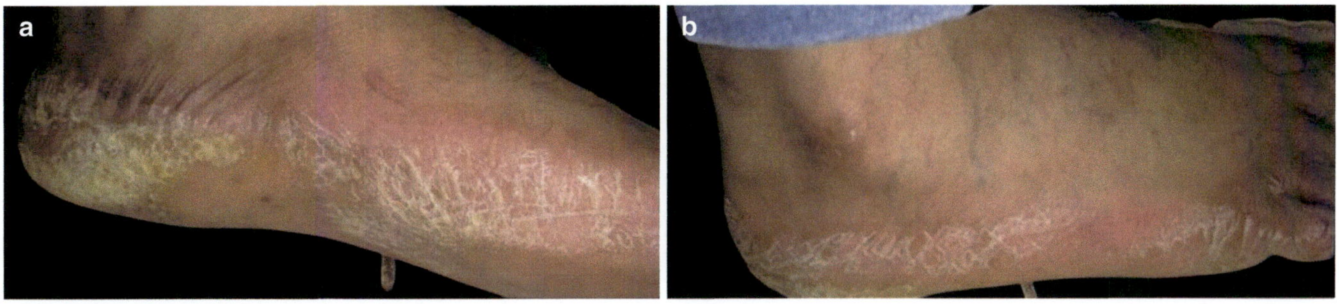

Fig. 2.39 Unna-Thost Syndrome. Diffuse, thick, yellowish non-transgredient plantar hyperkeratosis with a sharply demarcated erythematous lateral margins (**a**, **b**)

Fig. 2.40 Unna-Thost Syndrome: Diffuse, thick, yellowish non-transgredient PPK with a sharply demarcated erythematous lateral margins (**a**, **b**).

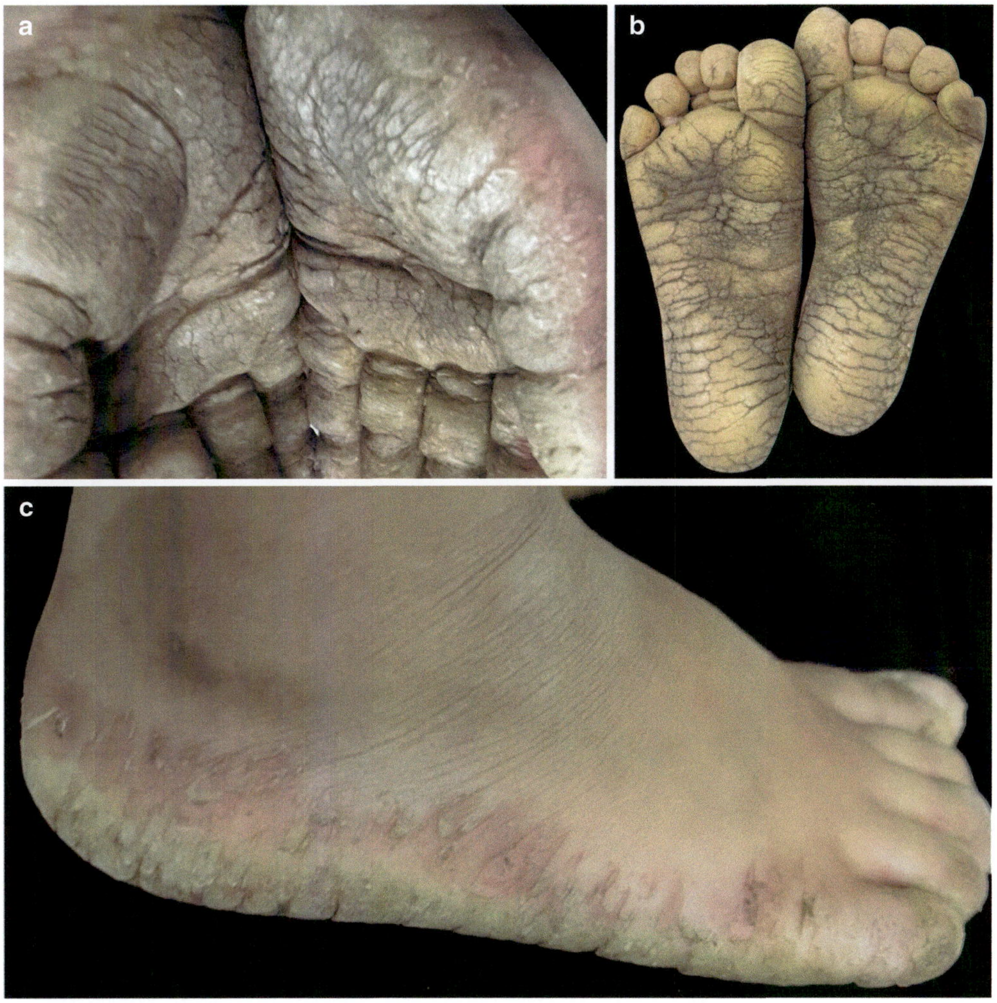

- Usually associated with hyperhidrosis, secondary dermatophyte infection, and pitted keratolysis associated with pruritus and malodor.
- Histopathology: non-epidermolytic hyperkeratosis.

Vorner Syndrome (AD) [22] (Fig. 2.41)

- Mutation in *KRT9* gene.
- Onset: early infancy.
- Diffuse non-transgredient isolated waxy yellowish PPK with well-demarcated erythematous border.
- Histopathology: epidermolytic hyperkeratosis.

Naxos Disease (AR) [23] (Fig. 2.42)

- Mutation in junction plakoglobin (*JUP*) gene.
- Diffuse PPK, woolly hair, right ventricular cardiomyopathy, arrhythmias in adolescence, alopecia.
- Woolly hair appears from birth, PPK develop during the first year of life and cardiomyopathy is clinically manifested by adolescence with 100% penetrance.

A syndrome with the same cutaneous phenotype and predominantly left ventricular involvement has been described in families from India and Ecuador (Carvajal syndrome, Fig. 2.15).

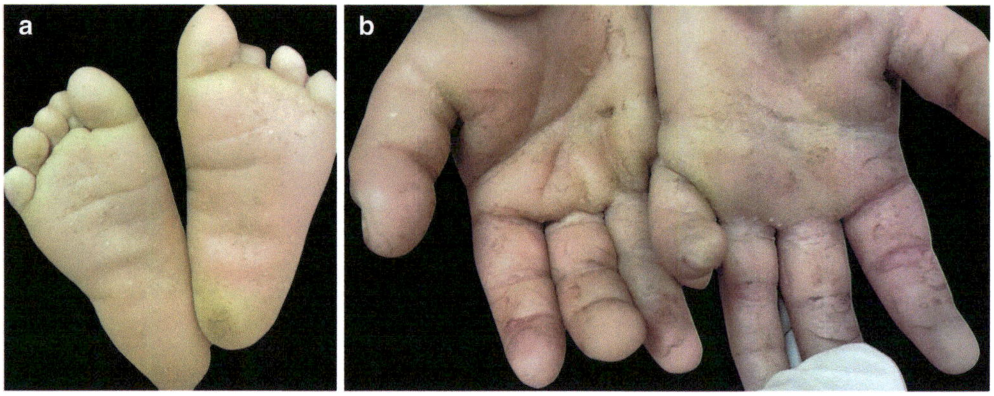

Fig. 2.41 Vorner Syndrome. Diffuse yellowish hyperkeratosis of palms and soles (**a**, **b**)

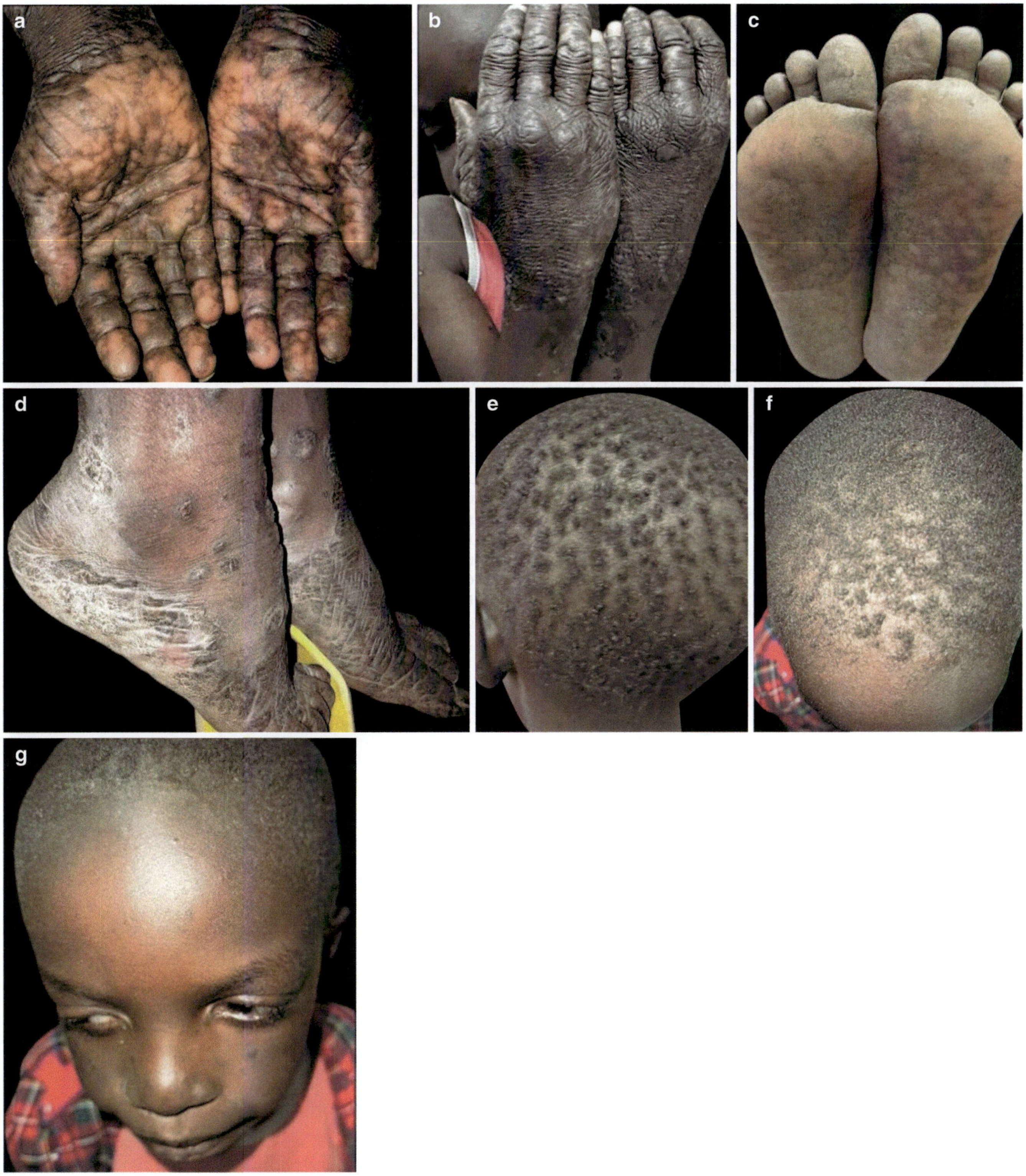

Fig. 2.42 Naxos Disease. Diffuse transgredient PPK (**a**–**d**), wooly hair (**e**, **f**) and alopecia (**g**)

References

1. Ishida-Yamamoto A. Erythrokeratodermia variabilis et progressiva. J Dermatol. 2016;43(3):280–5.
2. Tarikci N, Göncü EK, Yüksel T, et al. Progressive symmetrical erythrokeratoderma on the face: a rare condition and successful treatment with calcipotriol. JAAD Case Rep. 2016;2:70–1.
3. Zhang XJ, Li M, Gao TW, et al. Identification of a locus for punctate palmoplantar keratoderma at chromosome 8q24.13-8q24.21. J Invest Dermatol. 2004;122:1121–5.
4. Marques LP, Trope BM, Pina JC, et al. Inverse papular acrokeratosis of Oswaldo costa: a case report. Clin Aesthet Dermatol. 2010;3(6):51–3.
5. Mo HJ, Mo HJ, Kim TY, et al. A case of keratosis punctata of the palmar creases. Ann Dermatol. 2002;14(2):114–6.
6. Eytan O, Morice-Picard F, Sarig O, et al. Cole disease results from mutations in ENPP1. Am J Hum Genet. 2013;93(4):752–7.
7. Bragg J, Rizzo C, Mengden S. Striate palmoplantar keratoderma (Brunauer-Fohs-Siemens syndrome). Dermatol Online J. 2008;14(5):26.
8. Padial A, Morales V, Armario-Hita JC, et al. Keratoderma palmoplantaris varians (striata et areata), a form of chronic idiopathic acrokeratosis described by Degos. Actas Dermosifiliogr. 2008;99(2):134–7.
9. Srinivas SM, Kumar P, Basavaraja GV. Carvajal syndrome. Int J Trichology. 2016;8(1):53–5.
10. Sroa N, Witman P. Howel-Evans syndrome: a variant of ectodermal dysplasia. Cutis. 2010;85(4):183–5.
11. Čulic V, Betz RC, Refke M, et al. Tyrosinemia type II (Richner–Hanhart syndrome): a new mutation in the *TAT* gene. Eur J Med Genet. 2011;54(3):205–8.
12. Shah S, Boen M, Kenner-Bell B, et al. Pachyonychia congenita in pediatric patients: natural history, features, and impact. JAMA Dermatol. 2014;150(2):146–53.
13. Perez C, Khachemoune A. Mal de Meleda: a focused review. Am J Clin Dermatol. 2016;17(1):63–70.
14. Sethy M, Chatterjee S, Srinivas CR, et al. Mal De Meleda with flexural involvement. Indian Dermatol Online J. 2022;13(5):636–9.
15. Arif T, Adil M, Amin AA, et al. Transgrediens et progrediens palmoplantar keratoderma: a case of Greither's disease. Przegl Dermatol. 2017;104(1):66–7.
16. Sreeramulu B, Shyam ND, Ajay P, et al. Papillon-Lefèvre syndrome: clinical presentation and management options. Clin Cosmet Investig Dent. 2015;15(7):75–81.
17. Shuja Z, Li L, Gupta S, et al. Connexin26 mutations causing palmoplantar keratoderma and deafness interact with connexin 43, modifying gap junction and hemichannel properties. J Invest Dermatol. 2016;136:225–35.
18. Al-Hamdi KI, Qais Saadoon A, Abduljabbar NH. Bart-pumphrey syndrome. JAMA Dermatol. 2020;156(10):1126.
19. Duchatelet S, Hovanian A. Olmsted syndrome: clinical, molecular and therapeutic aspects. Orphanet J Rare Dis. 2015;10(33):1–10.
20. Çelik NS, Yaşar Ş, Aytekin S, et al. A rare syndrome resembling scleroderma: Huriez syndrome. Skin Appendage Disord. 2018;4(2):82–5.
21. Geetha M, Bhat R, Kiran B, et al. Unna thost syndrome: a case report. Int J Contemp Pediatr. 2019;6(4):1767–70.
22. Dev T, Mahajan VK, Sethuraman G. Hereditary palmoplantar keratoderma: a practical approach to the diagnosis. Indian Dermatol Online J. 2019;10(4):365–79.
23. Protonotarios N, Tsatsopoulou A. Naxos disease: cardiocutaneous syndrome due to cell adhesion defect. Orphanet J Rare Dis. 2006;1(4):1–5.

3 Epidermolysis Bullosa

Genetic skin fragility disorders, collectively designated epidermolysis bullosa (EB), manifest with trauma-induced blistering and erosions of the skin; the most severe forms also involve the mucous membranes. Residual manifestations of skin fragility comprise pigment anomalies, epidermal atrophy, or scarring. The appendages of the skin, nails, hair, and teeth, as well as other organs may also be affected. Severe EB subtypes evolve as systemic diseases with secondary multiorgan involvement and premature death.

Based on the level of skin cleavage, four EB types are distinguished: EB simplex, junctional EB, dystrophic EB, and Kindler syndrome. Disease-causing mutations in distinct genes lead to the defective mechanical stability of keratinocytes and reduced intraepidermal or dermal-epidermal adhesion (Tables 3.1 and 3.2).

Table 3.1 Epidermolysis bullosa: level of skin cleavage, major types, and subtypes [1]

Level of skin cleavage	Major EB type	Major EB subtypes
Intraepidermal	EBS	– Suprabasal EBS – Basal EBS
Intralamina lucida	JEB	– JEB, generalized – JEB, localized
Sublamina densa	DEB	– DDEB – RDEB
Mixed	Kindler EB	–

DDEB Dominant Dystrophic Epidermolysis Bullosa, *DEB* Dystrophic Epidermolysis Bullosa, *EB* Epidermolysis Bullosa, *EBS* Epidermolysis Bullosa Simplex, *JEB* Junctional Epidermolysis Bullosa, *RDEB* Recessive Dystrophic Epidermolysis Bullosa

N. Moftah et al., *Atlas of Common and Rare Genodermatoses*, https://doi.org/10.1007/978-3-031-60788-2_3

Table 3.2 Epidermolysis bullosa major types, subtypes, and targeted proteins [1–3]

EB Major Types	EB Subtypes		Targeted Protein
EBS	Suprabasal	Acral peeling skin syndrome[a]	Transglutaminase
		EBS superficialis[a]	Unknown
		Acantholytic EBS[a]	Desmoplakin, plakoglobin
		Skin fragility syndromes[a] – Desmoplakin deficiency (EBS-desmoplakin; skin fragility-woolly hair syndrome)[a] – Plakoglobin deficiency (EBS-plakoglobin; skin fragility-plakoglobin deficiency)[a] – Plakophilin deficiency (EBS-plakophilin; skin fragility-ectodermal dysplasia syndrome)[a]	– Desmoplakin – Plakoglobin – Plakophilin 1
	Basal	– EBS, localized – EBS, generalized intermediate – EBS, generalized severe – EBS with mottled pigmentation[a] – EBS, migratory circinate[a] – EBS, autosomal recessive K14[a] – EBS with muscular dystrophy – EBS with pyloric atresia[a] – EBS-Ogna[a] – EBS, autosomal recessive-BP230 deficiency[a]	– K5; K14 – K5; K14 – K5; K14 – K5 – K5 – K14 – Plectin – Plectin; a6β4 integrin – Plectin – Bullous pemphigoid antigen-230
JEB	Localized	JEB, localized	Collagen XVII Integrin a6β4 Laminin-332
		JEB, inversa[a]	Laminin-332
	Generalized	Severe (Herlitz)	Laminin 332
		Intermediate (non-Herlitz)	Laminin 332 Collagen XVII (BPAg2)
		With pyloric atresia[a]	α6β4 integrin
DEB	Autosomal recessive	– Severe (Hallopeau-Siemens) – Intermediate (non-Hallopeau-Siemens) – Inversa – Localized – Pruriginosa – Self-improving	Collagen VII
	Autosomal dominant	– Intermediate (Cockayne-Touraine) – Localized – Pruriginosa – Albopapuloid – Self-improving	
Kindler EB	Autosomal recessive		Kindlin-1

EB Epidermolysis bullosa, *EBS* Epidermolysis Bullosa Simplex, *JEB* Junctional Epidermolysis Bullosa, *DEB* Dystrophic Epidermolysis Bullosa
[a] Rare variants

Epidermolysis Bullosa Simplex (EBS) [1–5]

Epidermolysis Bullosa Simplex (EBS) encompasses all subtypes of EB having mechanical fragility and superficial blistering confined to the epidermis. EBS was separated into suprabasal and basal subgroups, based on the histopathologic site of cleavage within the epidermis.

When the classification system was last revised in 2019, peeling skin disorders, and other disorders with skin fragility, where blisters are only a minor part of the clinical picture or are not seen because skin cleavage is very superficial, are classified as separate categories although should be taken into account in the differential diagnosis of EB.

Acral Peeling Skin Syndrome (APPS) (AR) [6] (Figs. 3.1, 3.2, 3.3, and 3.4)

- Mutations in transglutaminase 5 (*TG5*) gene.
- APSS belongs to the group of peeling skin syndromes (PSS), rare autosomal recessive disorders which include localized acral form (APSS) and a diffuse form; non-inflammatory and inflammatory subtypes. APSS was first described as a specific entity in 1982 by Levy and Goldsmith.
- Although PSS was previously considered a subtype of epidermolysis bullosa simplex, it is now classified as a separate entity in the group of "other disorders with skin fragility."
- It presents at birth or in early childhood with the formation of flaccid blisters and superficial painless peeling limited to the hands and feet, leaving a painless residual erythema that heals without scarring and with no mucosal fragility.
- The manifestations are exacerbated by humidity and by physical factors such as trauma or friction.

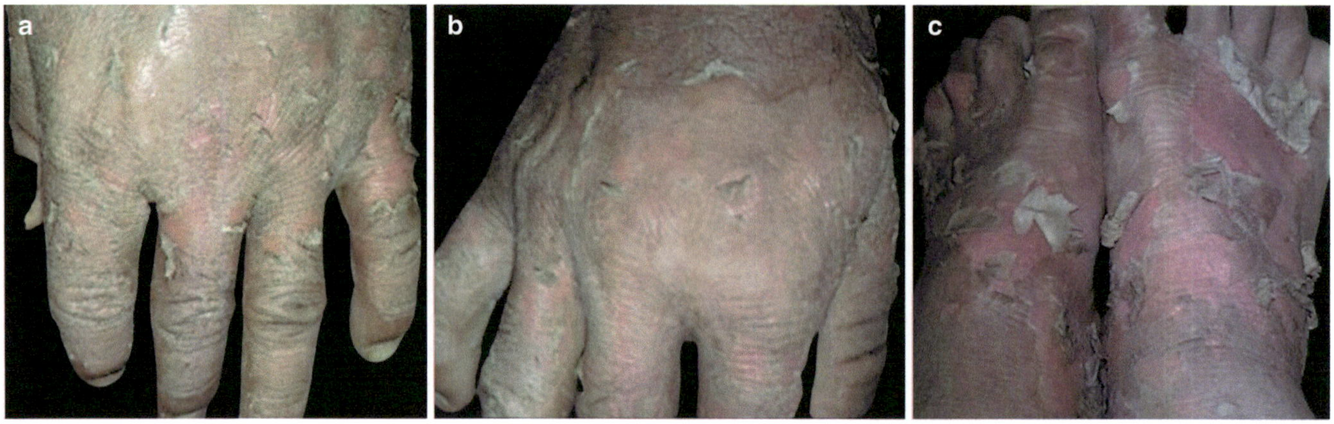

Fig. 3.1 Acral peeling skin syndrome. Superficial peeling of hands (**a**, **b**) and feet (**c**) with underlying erythema and no scar

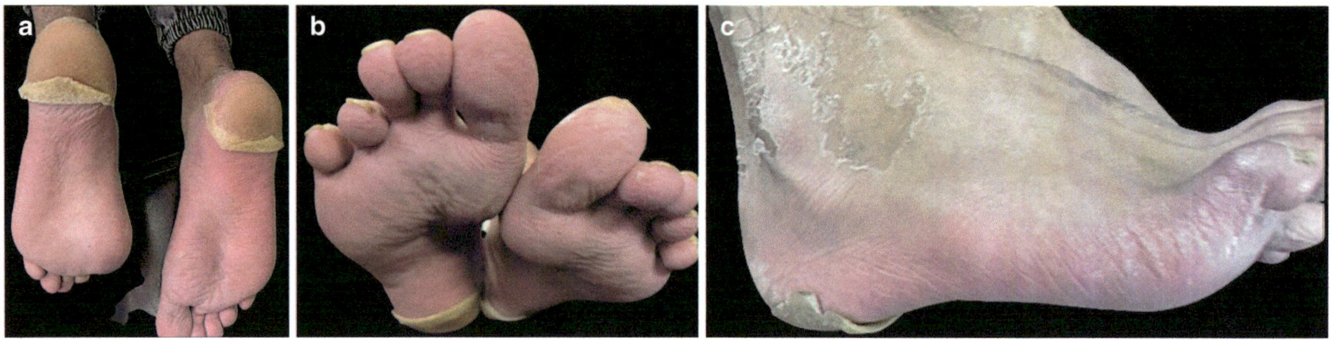

Fig. 3.2 Acral peeling skin syndrome. Superficial peeling of the feet (**a**–**c**) with underlying erythema and no scar

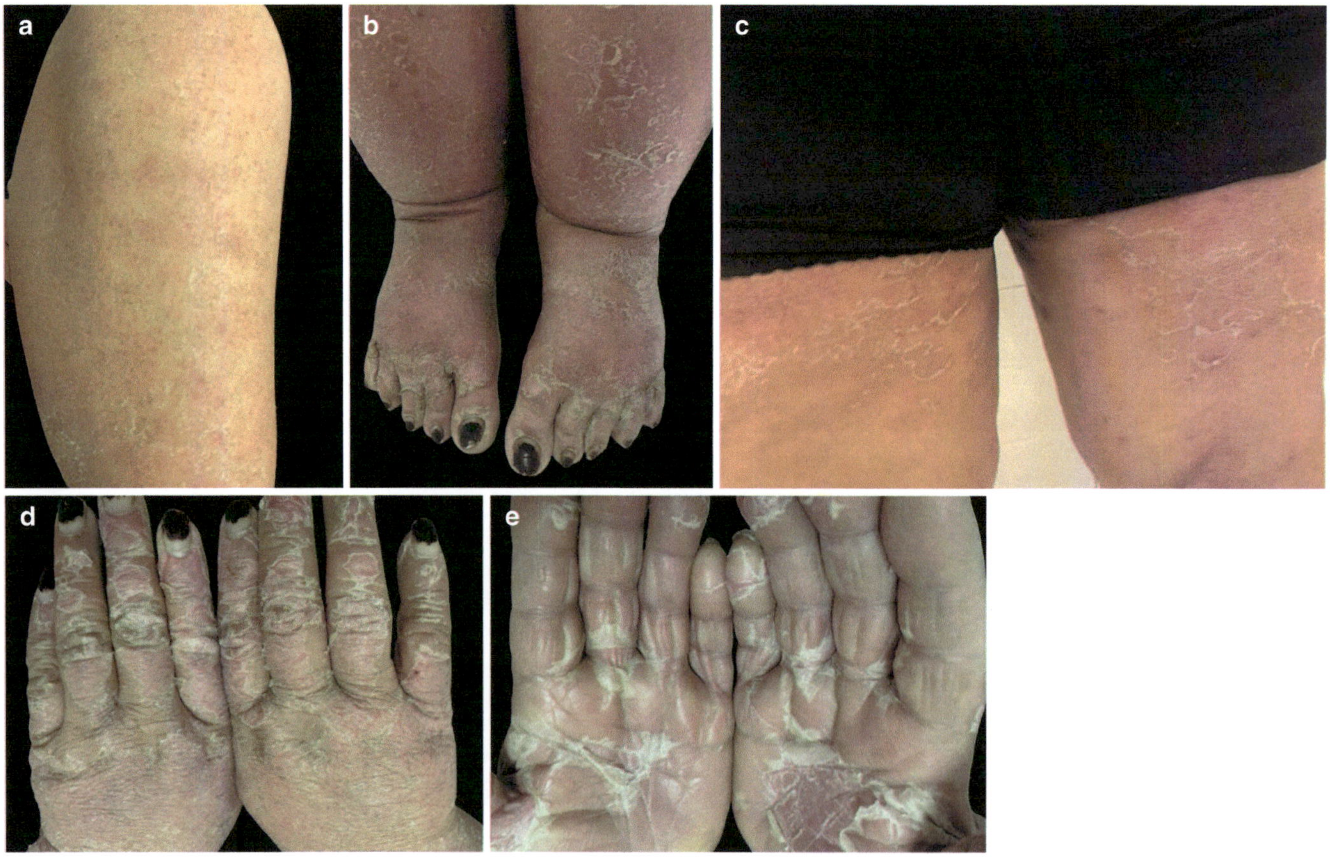

Fig. 3.3 Peeling skin syndrome, diffuse type. Generalized superficial skin peeling with underlying erythema (**a**–**e**)

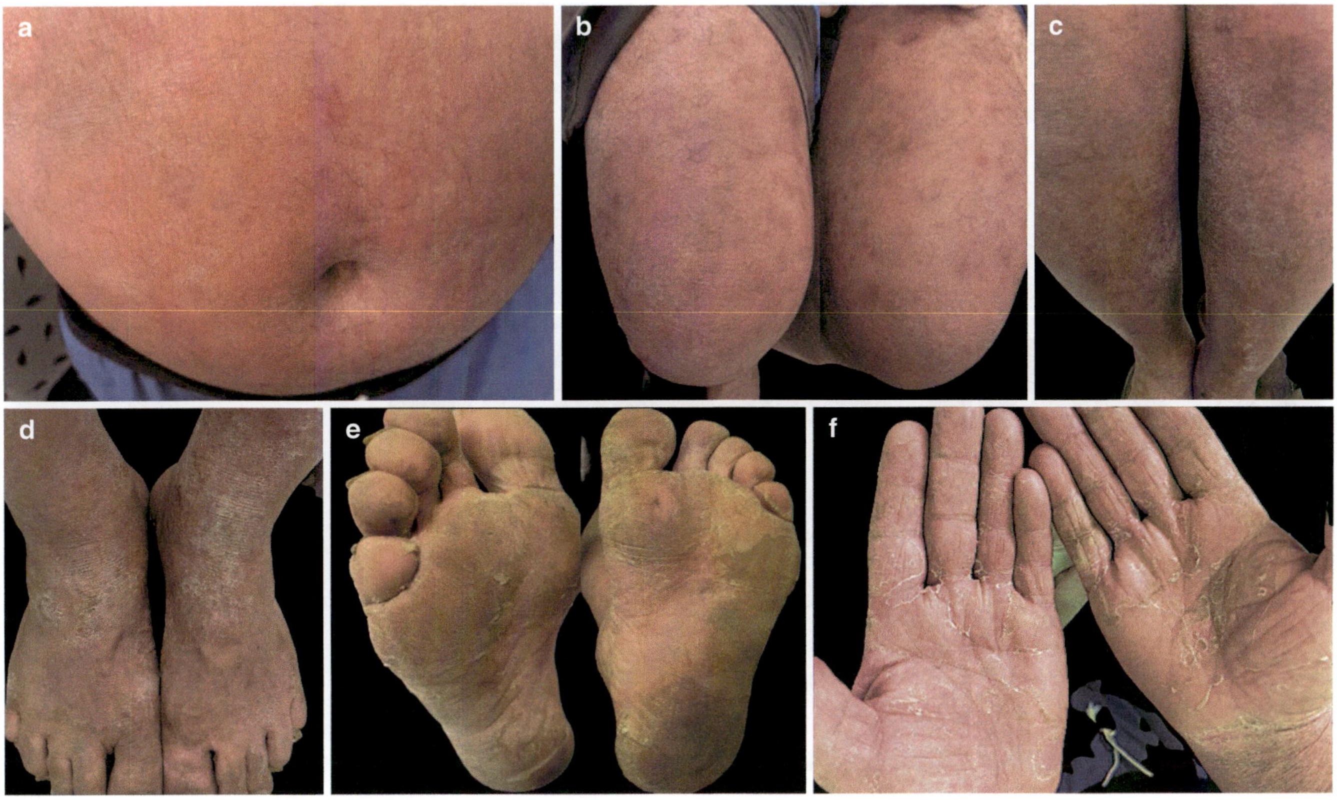

Fig. 3.4 Peeling skin syndrome, diffuse type. Generalized superficial skin peeling with underlying erythema (**a**–**f**)

Skin Fragility Syndrome [7] (Figs. 3.5 and 3.6)

- A rare cutaneous condition characterized by trauma-induced blisters and erosions due to mutations in *desmoplakin, plakoglobin, or plakophilin* genes.
- Skin fragility-woolly hair syndrome is a rare autosomal recessive genetic, ectodermal dysplasia syndrome characterized by persistent skin fragility caused by defective desmoplakin, an important desmosomal plaque protein. It is characterized by fragile skin with recurrent flaccid blisters and erosions dure to minor trauma, focal or diffuse palmoplantar keratoderma, woolly hair, varying degrees of alopecia, and dystrophic nails. Unlike other disorders associated with *desmoplakin* mutation, no cardiac symptoms are reported in this disease.

Epidermolysis Bullosa Simplex (EBS), Localized Subtype (AD) [5, 8] (Fig. 3.7)

- Formerly known as Weber-Cockayne.
- Most common subtype of EBS.
- Onset is usually in late infancy or early childhood.
- Defect in *KRT5* and *14* genes.
- Trauma-induced skin blisters, most frequently occur on the palms and soles exacerbated by warm weather and heal without scar.
- Hyperhidrosis can accompany this disorder.

Epidermolysis Bullosa Simplex (EBS), Generalized Subtype (AD) [5, 8] (Fig. 3.8)

- Generalized EBS is further subdivided into intermediate (previously known as generalized intermediate or Köebner) and severe (previously known as generalized severe or Dowling-Meara) subtypes.
- Defect in *KRT5* and *14* genes.
- Both forms typically present with a generalized onset of blisters that occurs at or shortly after birth.
- Hands, feet, and extremities are the most common sites of involvement.
- EBS, intermediate subtype is characterized by non-herpetiform blisters and erosions arising in particular at sites of friction.

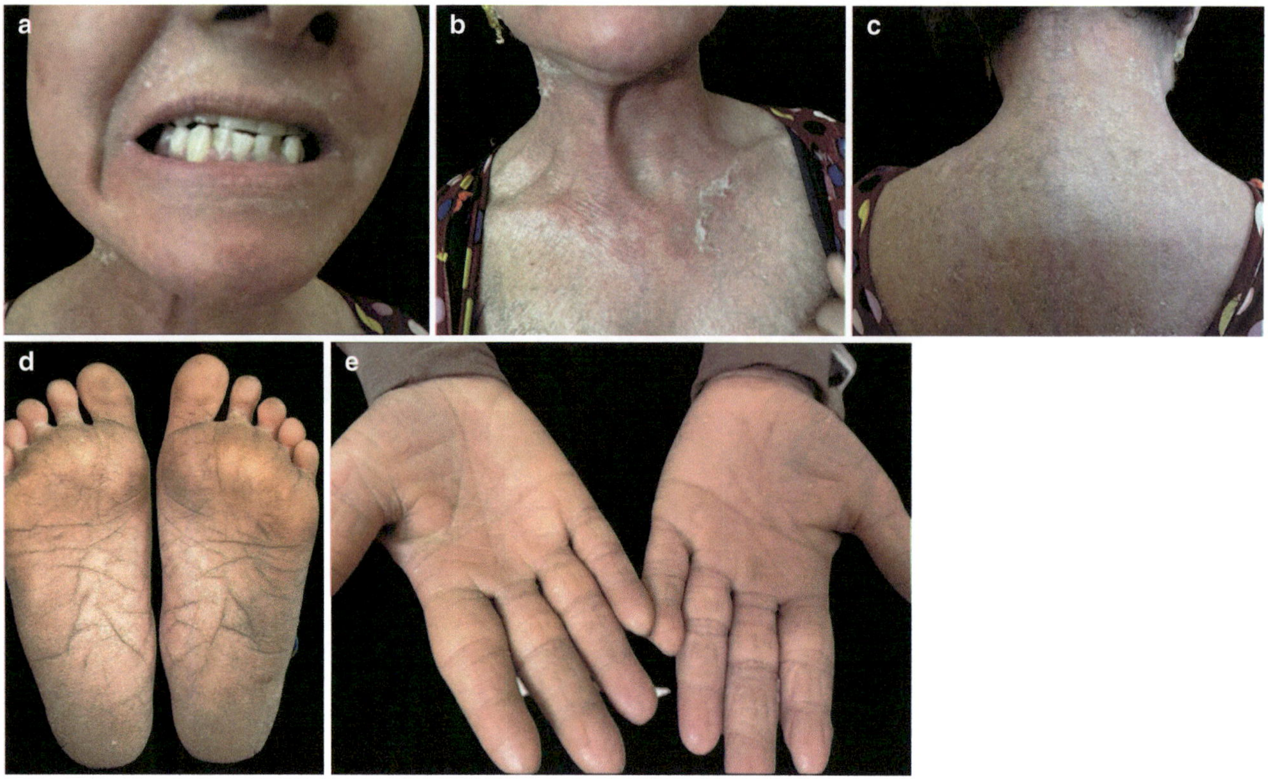

Fig. 3.5 Skin fragility syndrome. Persistent fragile skin with minor trauma on face (**a**), neck (**b**), and back (**c**) with diffuse palmoplantar keratoderma (**d**, **e**)

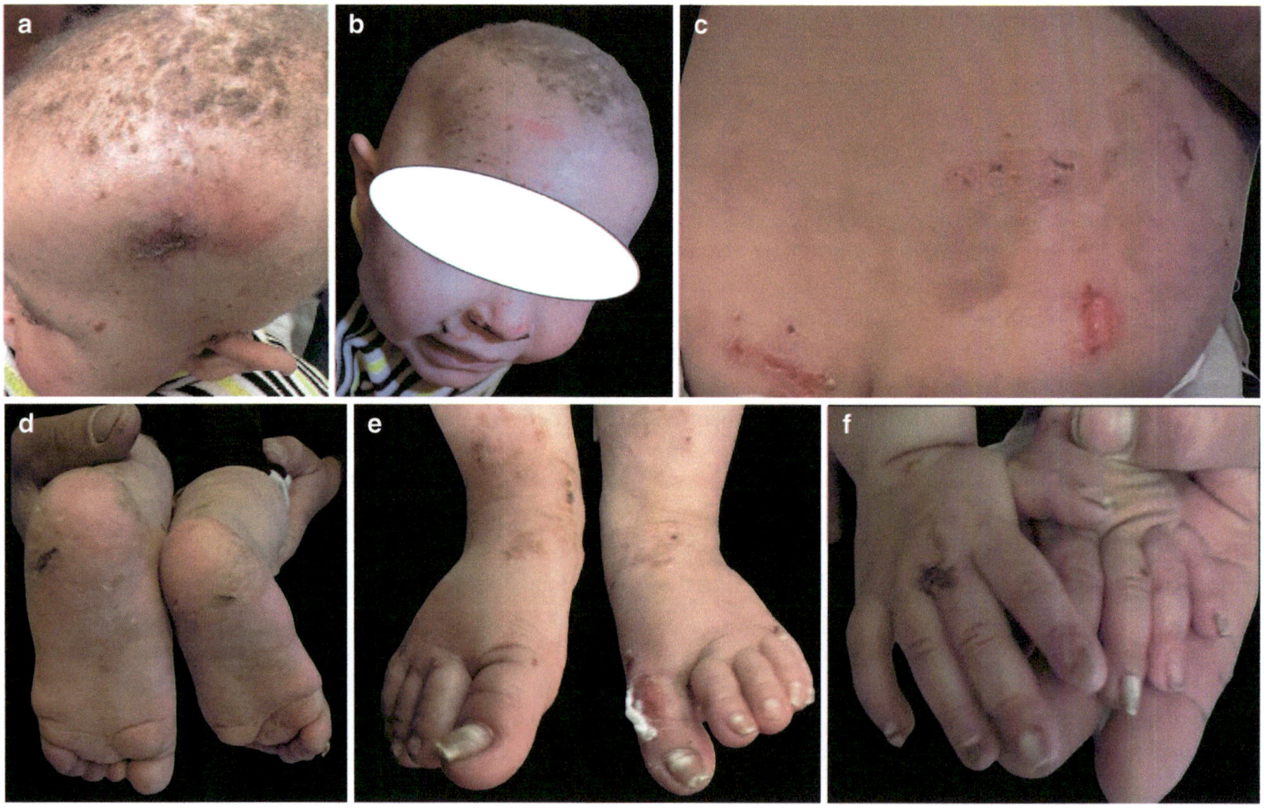

Fig. 3.6 Skin fragility with woolly hair syndrome. A child with woolly hair (**a**, **b**) and multiple minor trauma-induced blisters on back (**c**) and extremities with nail dystrophy (**d**–**f**)

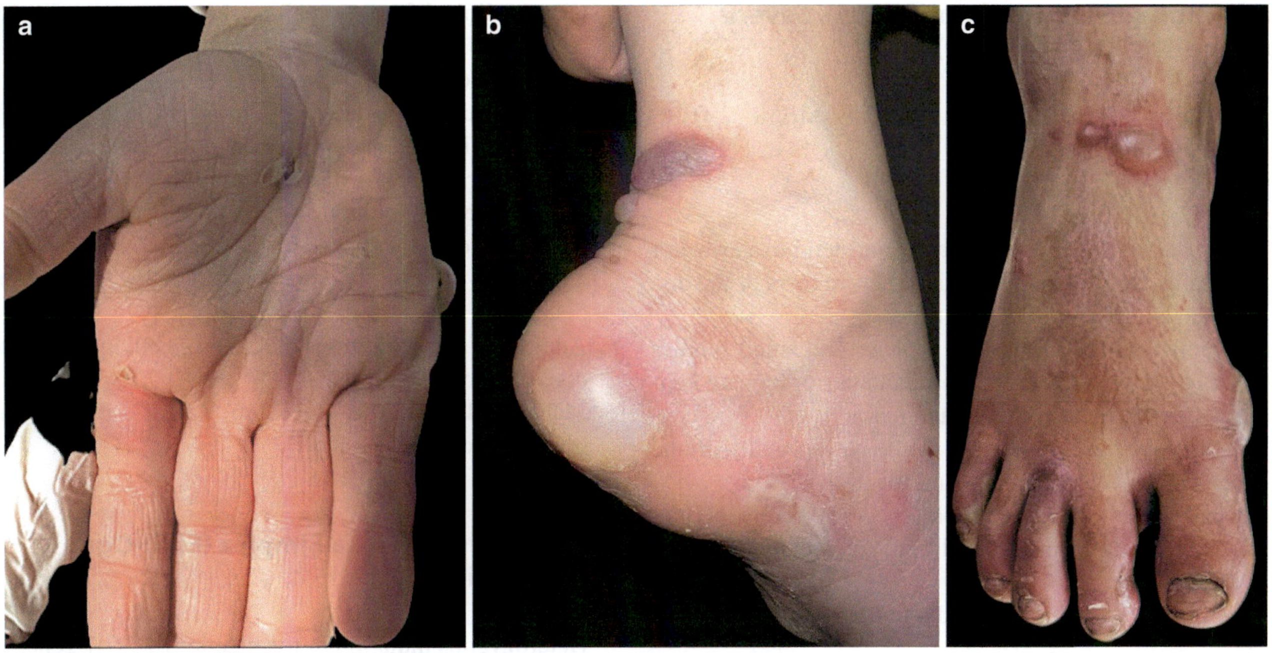

Fig. 3.7 Localized epidermolysis bullosa simplex (Weber-Cockyane). A child with multiple localized trauma-induced blisters on the palms (**a**) and feet (**b**, **c**) that heal without scar

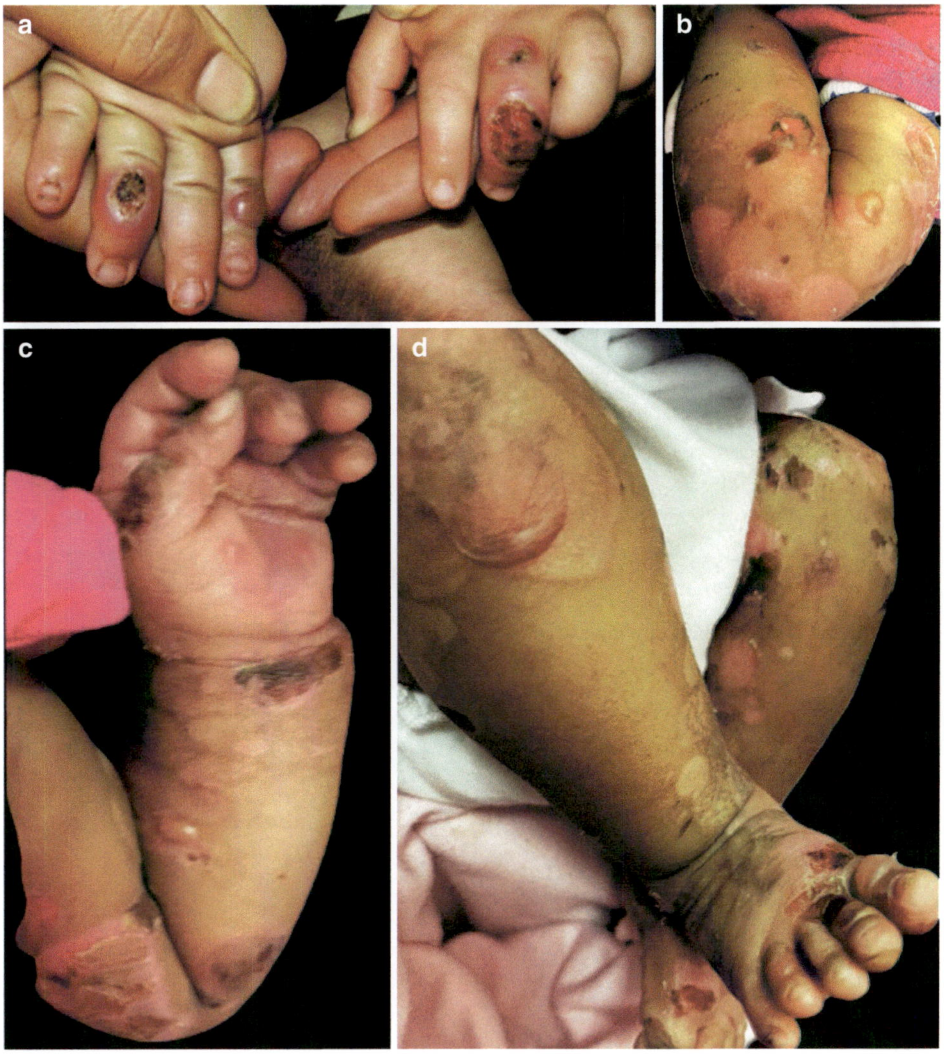

Fig. 3.8 Generalized epidermolysis bullosa simplex (Köebner). An infant with generalized trauma-induced blisters that heal without scar on hands (**a**), upper (**b**, **c**), and lower extremities (**d**)

Epidermolysis Bullosa Simplex (EBS), Severe Subtype (AD) [5, 8] (Fig. 3.9)

- Previously known as Dowling-Meara (EBS Herpetiformis).
- Most severe form of EBS.
- Defect in *KRT5* and *14*.
- Appear at birth and early infancy and tend to get better over time. However, infants with a severe form of the disease die within the first year of life.
- Characterized by generalized vesicles and small blisters arranged in grouped herpetiform annular or arcuate configuration that heal with scar and milia.
- Blisters may develop all over the body, especially on the face, hands, feet, arms, legs, and trunk.
- Laryngeal and esophageal (hoarseness) involvement, palmoplantar keratoderma, and nail dystrophy may be present.
- Electron microscopy: clumped tonofilaments.

Epidermolysis Bullosa Simplex (EBS) with Mottled Pigmentation (AD) [9] (Figs. 3.10 and 3.11)

- Rare form of EBS.
- Defect in *KRT5* gene.
- Classic clinical features include serous, non-scarring blisters on the distal part of the extremities and slowly progressing mottled skin pigmentation.
- Blisters usually appear at birth or in early infancy, tend to decrease with age, and only occasionally appear in adults, after minor trauma or friction.
- The mottled pigmented lesions appear later in infancy or childhood, not preceded by blisters, spread slowly, and tend to greatly lessen eventually but do not disappcar.
- Additional manifestations as photosensitivity and dental disorders may be present.
- Many adults also develop focal palmoplantar hyperkeratosis.

Epidermolysis Bullosa Simplex (EBS)-Ogna (AD) [10] (Fig. 3.12)

- Heterozygous mutation in the plectin (*PLEC*)1 gene.
- Onset typically at birth.
- Characterized by primarily acral blistering, easy bruisability, hemorrhagic blistering, and onychogryphosis.

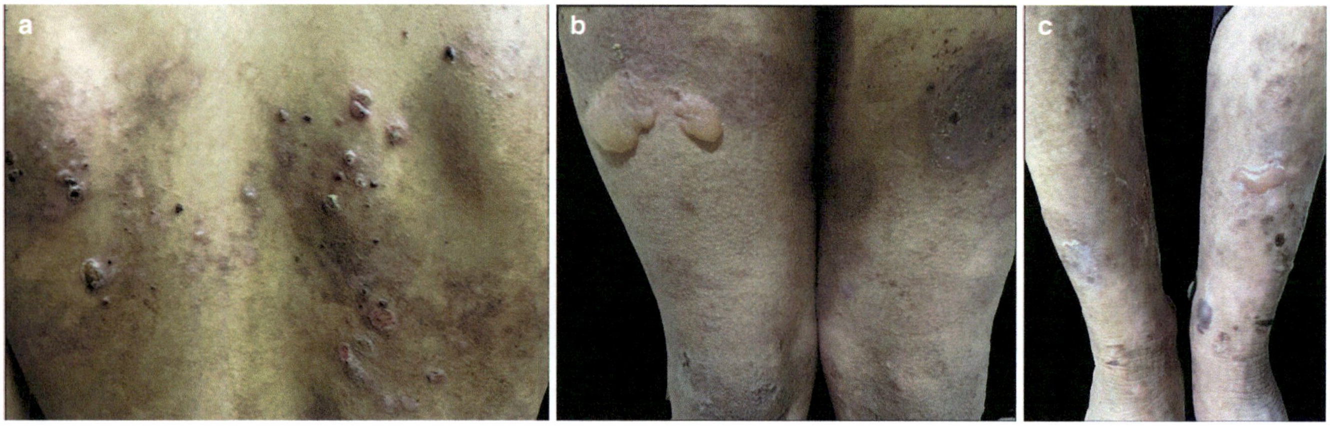

Fig. 3.9 Epidermolysis bullosa simplex (Dowling-Meara). A child with grouped flaccid blisters on back (**a**), and lower limbs (**b**, **c**), dating since early infancy

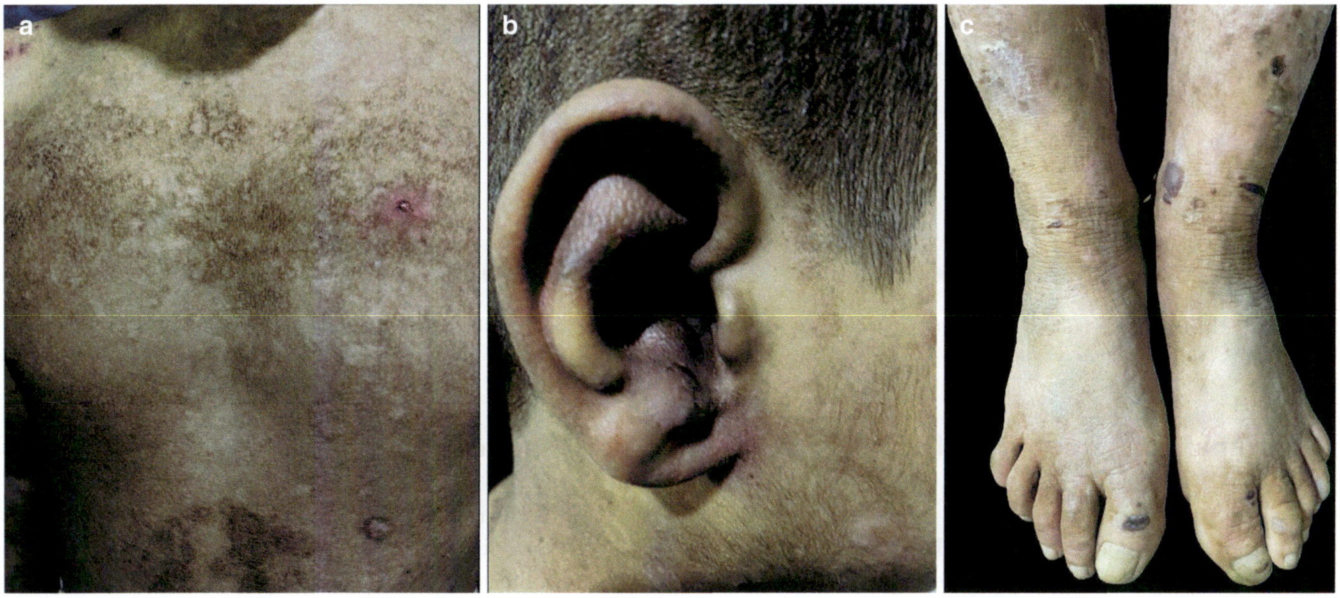

Fig. 3.10 Epidermolysis bullosa simplex with mottled pigmentation. Mottled appearance of the skin of the trunk (**a**) and the face (**b**) with acral blisters (**c**)

Fig. 3.11 Epidermolysis bullosa simplex with mottled pigmentation. A child (sister of patient in Fig. 3.10) with mottled pigmentation on trunk (**a**) upper extremities (**b**), acral blisters (**c**), and dental disorders (**d**)

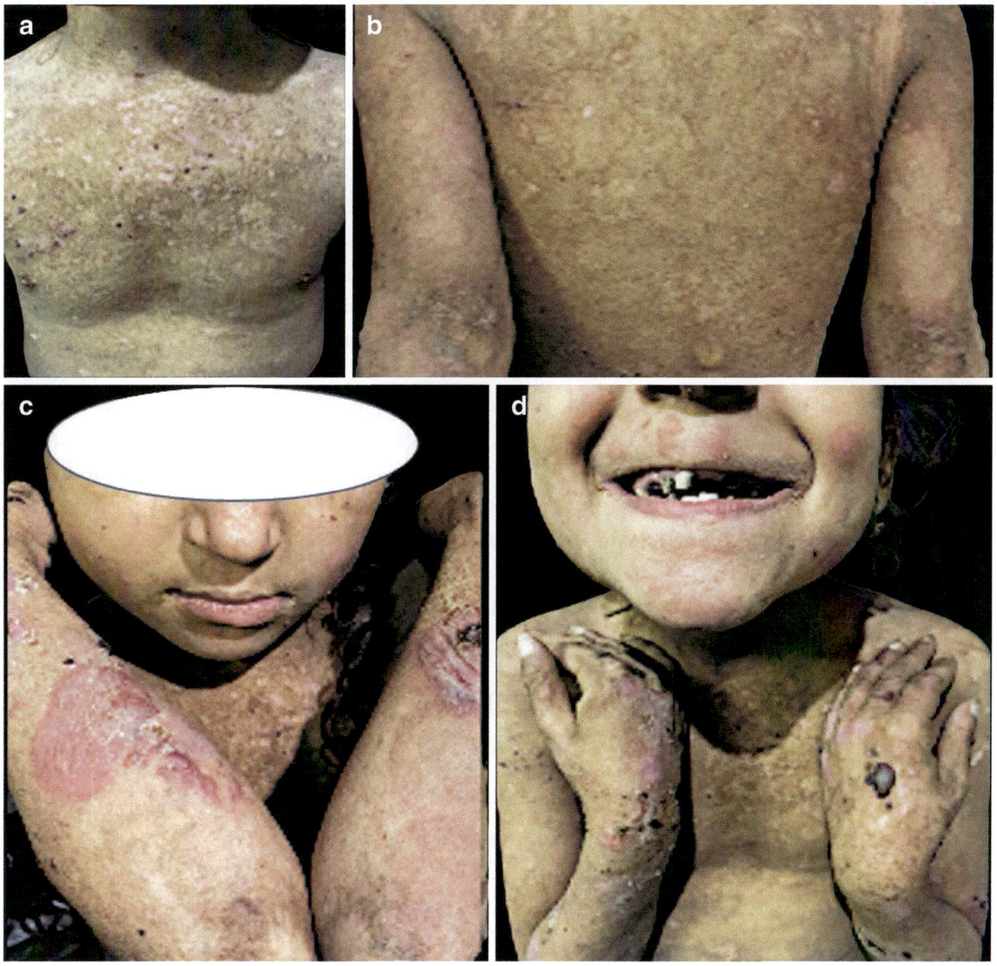

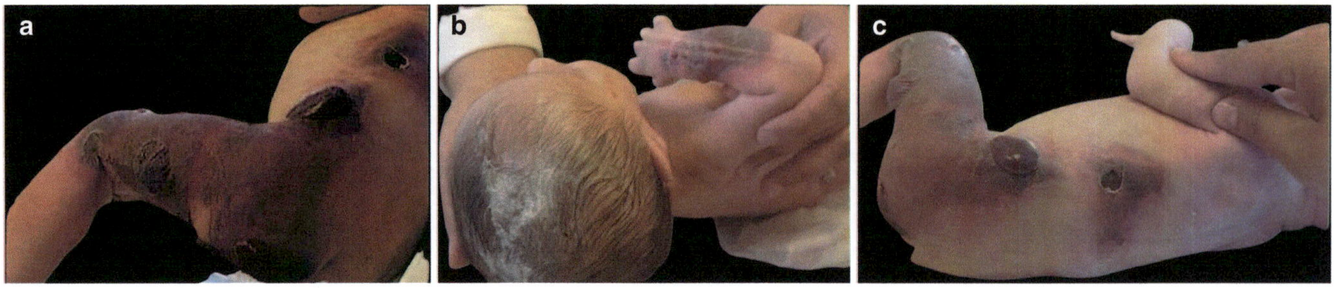

Fig. 3.12 Epidermolysis bullosa simplex (Ogna type). An infant at birth with hemorrhagic blisters and bruises on the extremities (**a**, **b**) and the trunk (**c**). (*Courtesy, Ghada Raslan*)

Junctional Epidermolysis Bullosa (JEB) [5, 11, 12]

Junctional epidermolysis bullosa (JEB) is characterized by skin fragility, manifested by blistering with little or no trauma. The two major subtypes of JEB are severe JEB (previously known as JEB generalized severe, Herlitz or letalis JEB) and intermediate JEB (previously known as JEB generalized intermediate, non-Herlitz JEB).

Junctional Epidermolysis Bullosa (JEB)-Severe Subtype (AR) [3, 11] (Figs. 3.13 and 3.14)

- Formerly termed JEB Herlitz or letalis.
- Due to mutation in *laminin 332*.
- Onset at birth or early infancy.
- Characterized by fragility of skin and mucous membranes with little or no trauma, with generalized blistering at birth, significant internal involvement, and a poor prognosis.
- Periorificial blisters, erosions and granulation tissues around the mouth, eyes, and nares, fingers, and toes, and internally around the upper airway.
- Patients are at increased risk for death from sepsis or other complications secondary to the profound epithelial disadhesion.
- Early lethality in the first 6–24 months of life.

Junctional Epidermolysis Bullosa (JEB)-Intermediate Subtype (AR) [5, 11, 12] (Fig. 3.15)

- Generalized JEB; either with significant mucosal involvement and early lethality (loss of laminin 332) or without (loss of BPAg2/collagen XVII).
- Clinical characteristics of patients with loss of *laminin 332*:
  - Mucosal involvement, patients may develop the same periorificial erosive hypergranulation tissue as those with the severe variant.
  - They can also show significant oropharyngeal, esophageal, and urogenital erosions and scarring.
  - Enamel hypoplasia, and nail dystrophy or loss of nails can occur.
  - Even though this group of patients with significant mucosal involvement survives infancy, life expectancy is often reduced.
- Clinical characteristics of patients with loss of BPAg2/collagen XVII:
  - Formerly known as generalized atrophic benign epidermolysis bullosa (GABEB).
  - Characterized by generalized cutaneous blistering presenting at birth, worsened by increased ambient temperature and heal with a distinctive atrophic appearance.
  - Extracutaneous involvement is rare, except for teeth, with hypoplastic enamel formation resulting in significant tooth decay. Nail dystrophy and a non-scarring alopecia are other common clinical manifestations.
  - Affected patients have the potential to bear children and to have a typical life expectancy.
  - This subtype has been shown to display phenotypic reversion, a correction of blistering occurring in localized regions, most often on the arms and other subexposed regions.

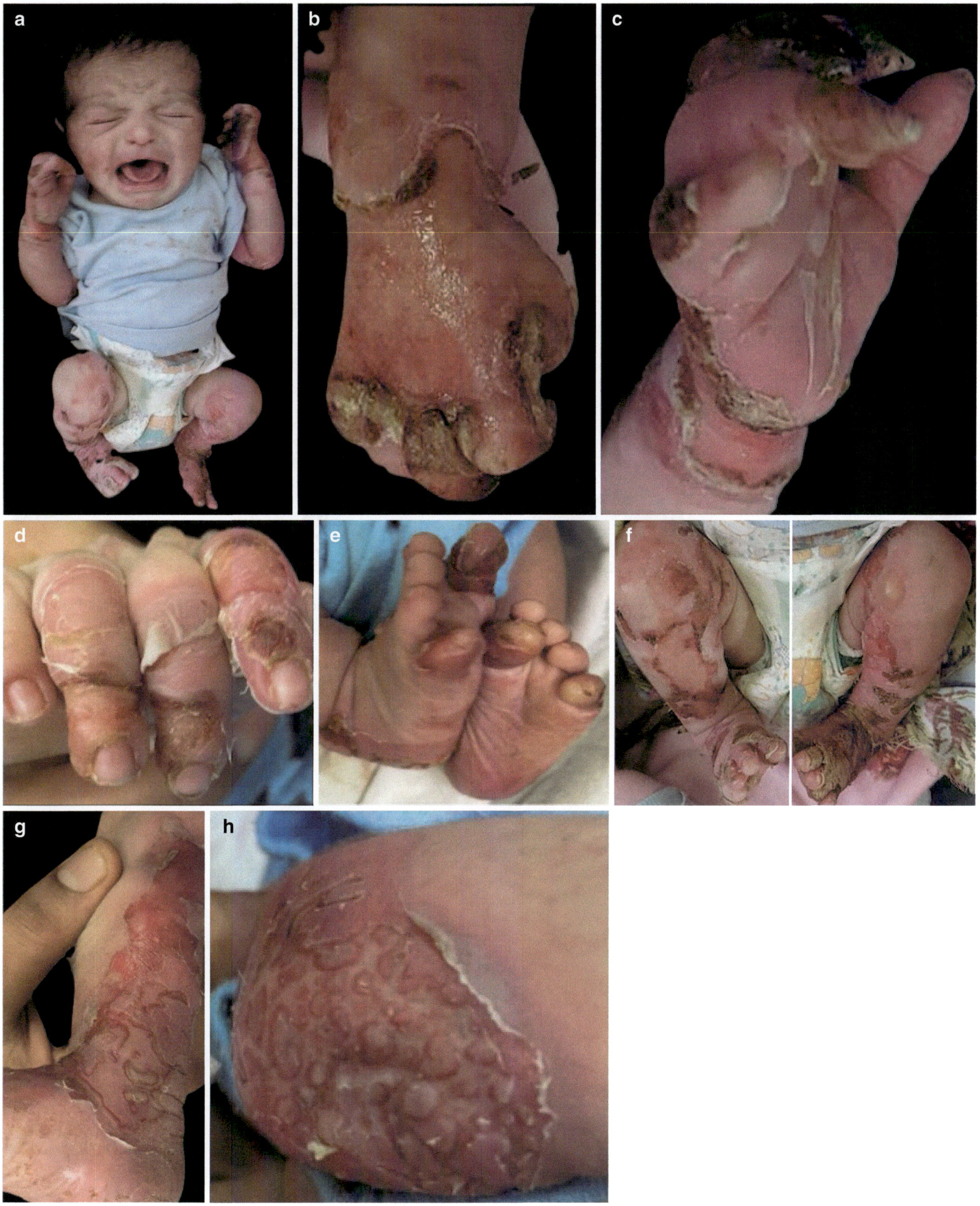

Fig. 3.13 Junctional epidermolysis bullosa, severe subtype (Herlitz). An infant with extensive blistering, large areas of denuded skin of extremities (**a**–**f**), non-healing exuberant granulation tissue on leg and buttock (**g**, **h**)

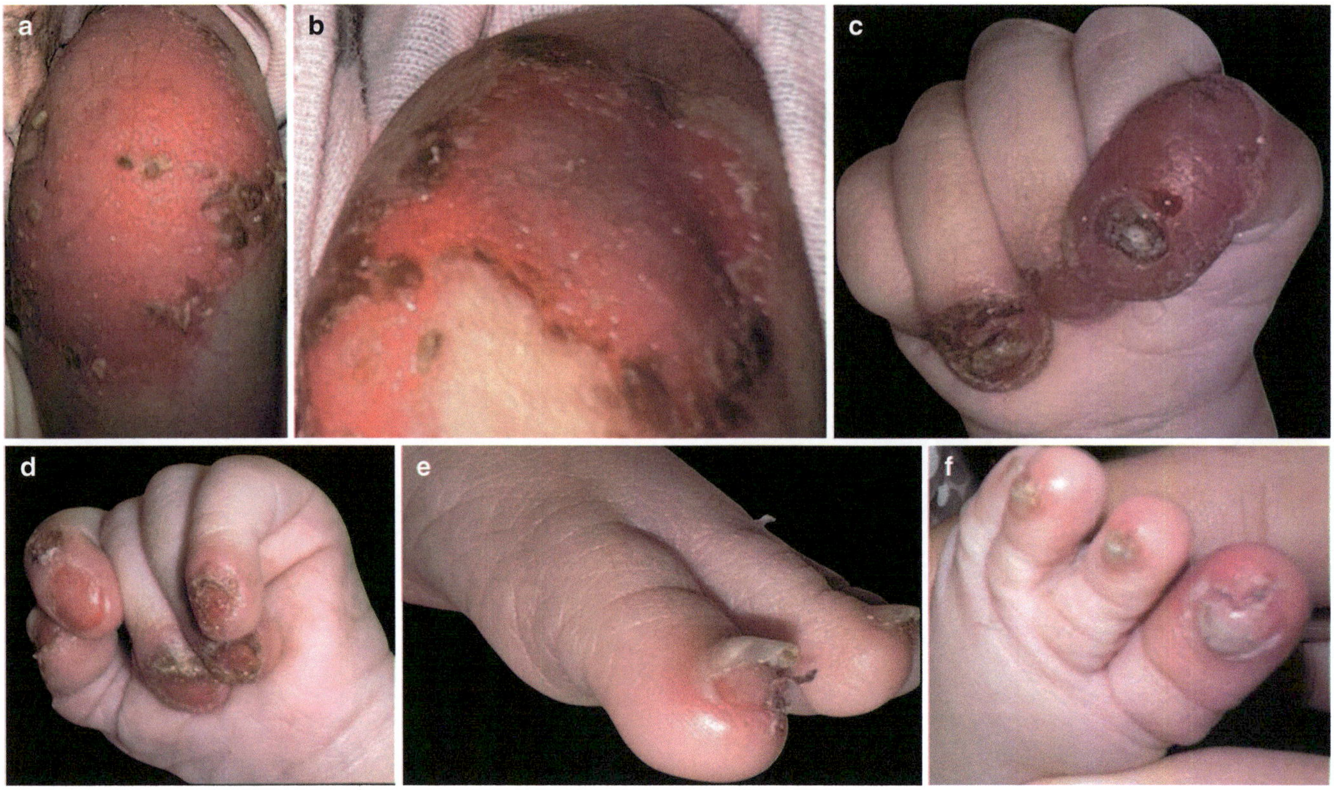

Fig. 3.14 Junctional epidermolysis bullosa, severe subtype (Herlitz). An infant with large area of non-healing denuded skin and granulation tissue on extremities (**a**, **b**), fingers (**c**, **d**), and toes (**e**, **f**)

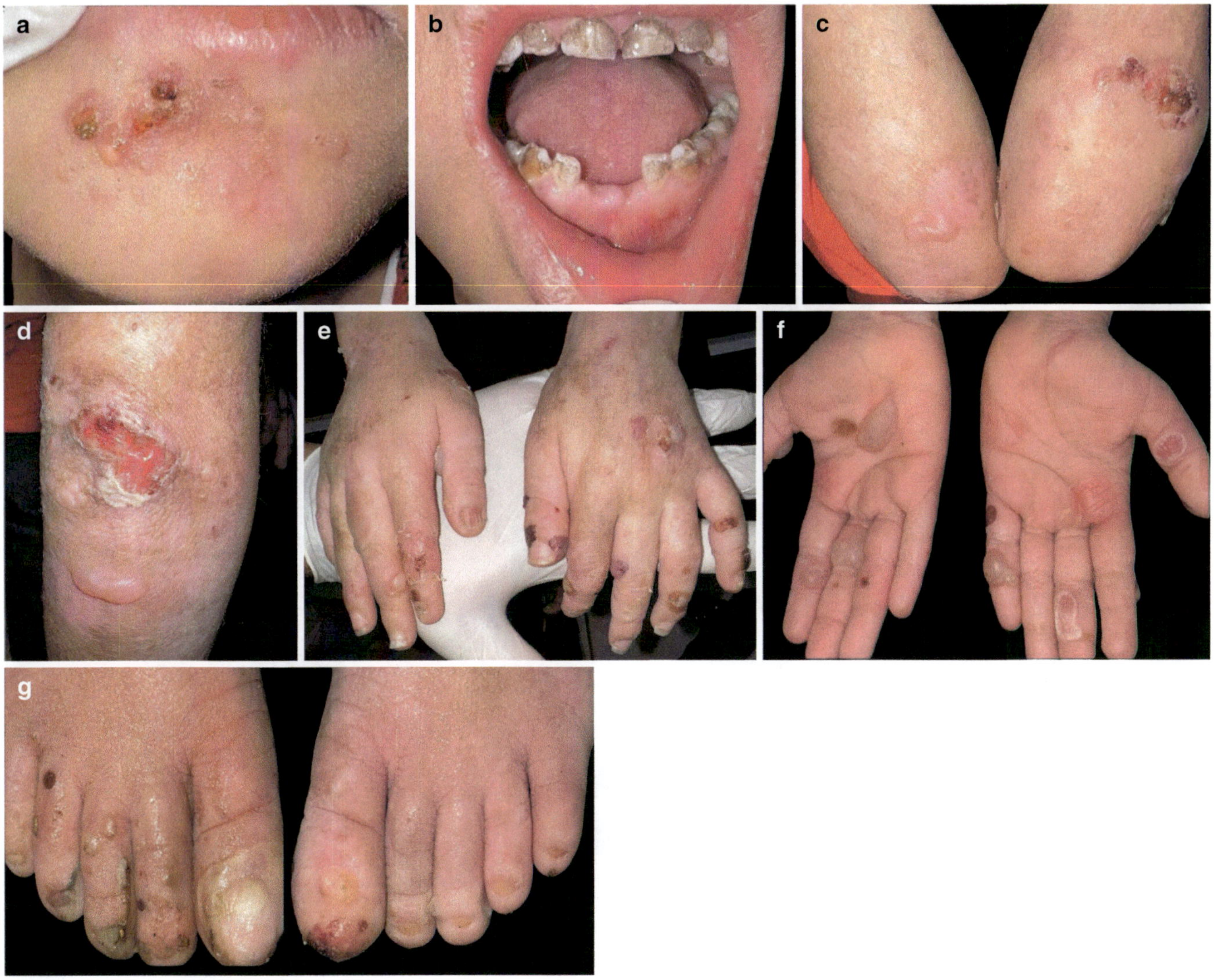

Fig. 3.15 Junctional epidermolysis bullosa (Non-Herlitz). A child with periorificial non-healing erosions (**a**), dental enamel hypoplasia and dental caries (**b**), blisters and hemorrhagic bullae and erosions on forearms, elbow (**c**, **d**), hands (**e**, **f**), and feet with nail dystrophy (**g**)

Dystrophic Epidermolysis Bullosa (DEB) [5]

Dystrophic Epidermolysis Bullosa (DEB) may be inherited as a dominant (DDEB) or recessive trait (RDEB) Generally, RDEB is more severe than dominant disease; however, there is considerable phenotypic overlap between types. DEB results from defect in type VII collagen.

The hallmark of DEB is that of scarring following blistering, both in the skin and in a variety of mucosae. Milia are also a specific finding in areas of healed blistering in DEB. Secondary extracutaneous complications are common in the more severe forms of RDEB.

Major subtypes of DEB include localized DDEB (previously encompassing nails only, pretibial and acral DDEB), intermediate DDEB (previously known as generalized DDEB), intermediate RDEB (previously known as RDEB generalized intermediate, non-Hallopeau-Siemens RDEB), and severe RDEB (previously RDEB generalized severe, Hallopeau-Siemens RDEB).

Recessive Dystrophic Epidermolysis Bullosa (RDEB), Severe Subtype [5, 13] (Figs. 3.16 and 3.17)

- Formerly known as RDEB of Hallopeau-Siemens.
- Characterized by the presence of blistering and erosions affecting the whole body (most prominent on the acral surfaces) in the neonatal period.

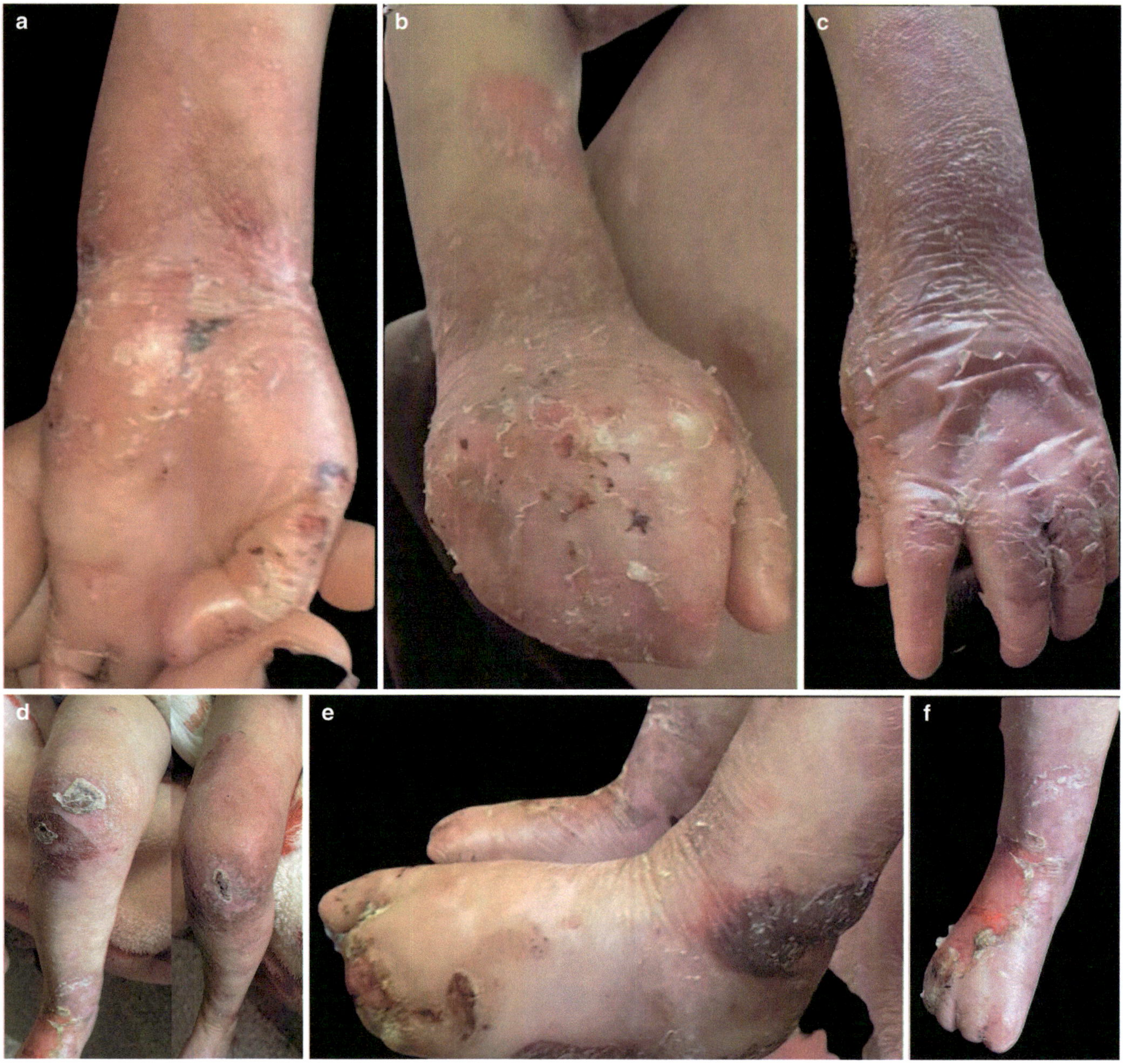

Fig. 3.16 Recessive dystrophic epidermolysis bullosa (Hallopeau-Siemens). An 8-year-old female patient with multiple recurrent blistering that heal with atrophic scars (**a**–**f**), pseudosyndactyly (**e**, **f**), absent fingernails (**c**), and toenails (**e**, **f**). (*Courtesy, Shaimaa Farook*)

- Hand deformities: pseudosyndactyly, flexion contractures and, in advanced stages, as a mitten-like deformity. This results in the complete loss of function of the hands and consequently to severe psychosocial problems for the young patients.
- Oral involvement may lead to mouth blistering, fusion of the tongue to the floor of the mouth, and progressive diminution of the size of the oral cavity.
- Esophageal erosions can lead to webs and strictures that can cause severe dysphagia. Consequently, malnutrition and vitamin and mineral deficiency may lead to growth restriction in young children.
- Urethral and anal erosions and stenosis may be also present.
- Eyes: corneal erosions can lead to scarring and loss of vision.
- Nails and teeth may be also affected.
- Patients who survive to childhood are at significant risk of developing aggressive SCC in areas of chronic erosions.

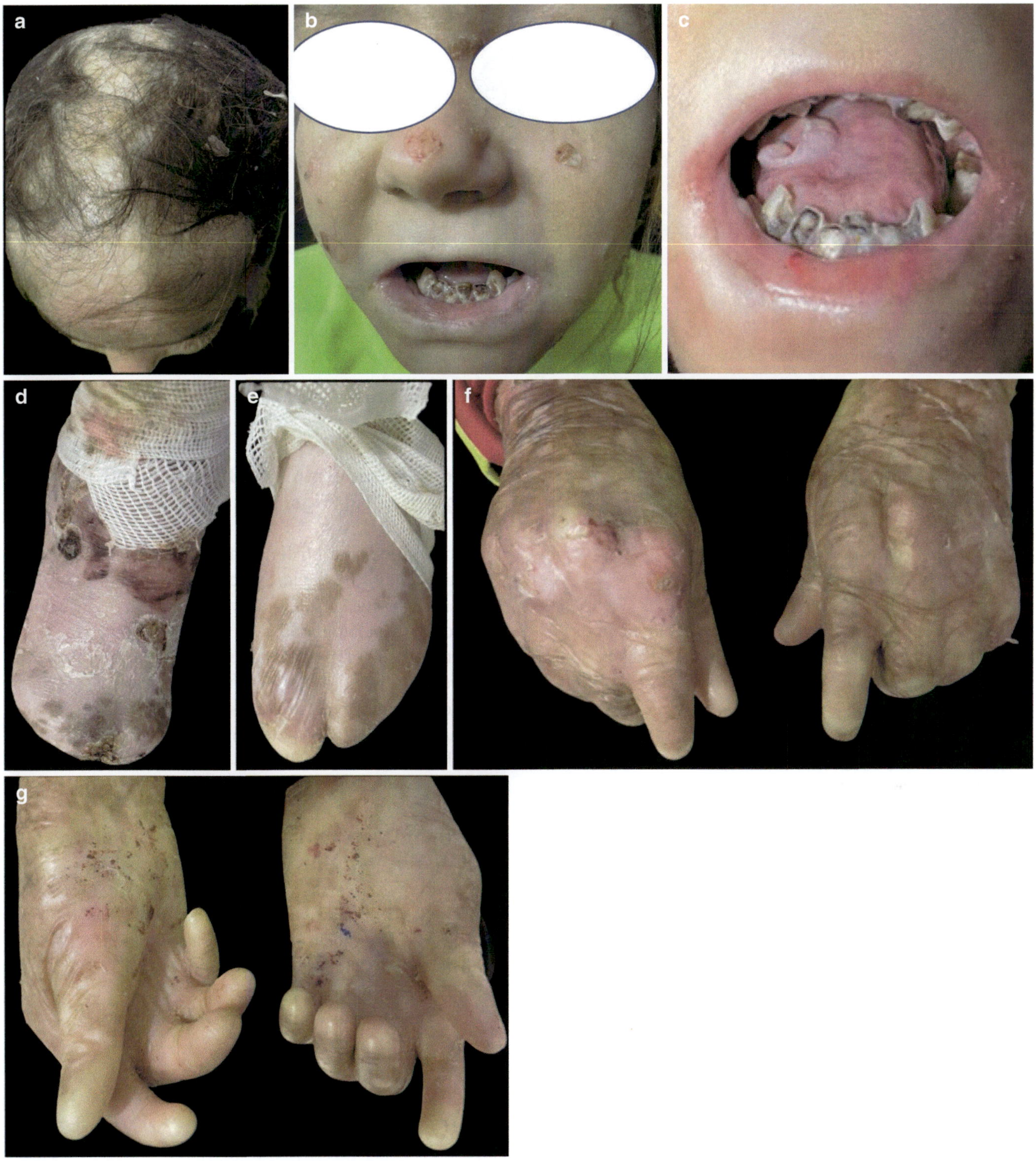

Fig. 3.17 Recessive dystrophic epidermolysis bullosa (Hallopeau-Siemens). A 12-year-old female patient with scalp cicatricial alopecia following blistering (**a**), erosions and atrophic scars on the face (**b**), teeth crowding, dental caries, and traumatic lingual ulcer (proven by biopsy) with loss of papillae (**b**, **c**), atrophic scars on hands and feet, pseudosyndactyly with absent toenails and fingernails (**d**–**g**)

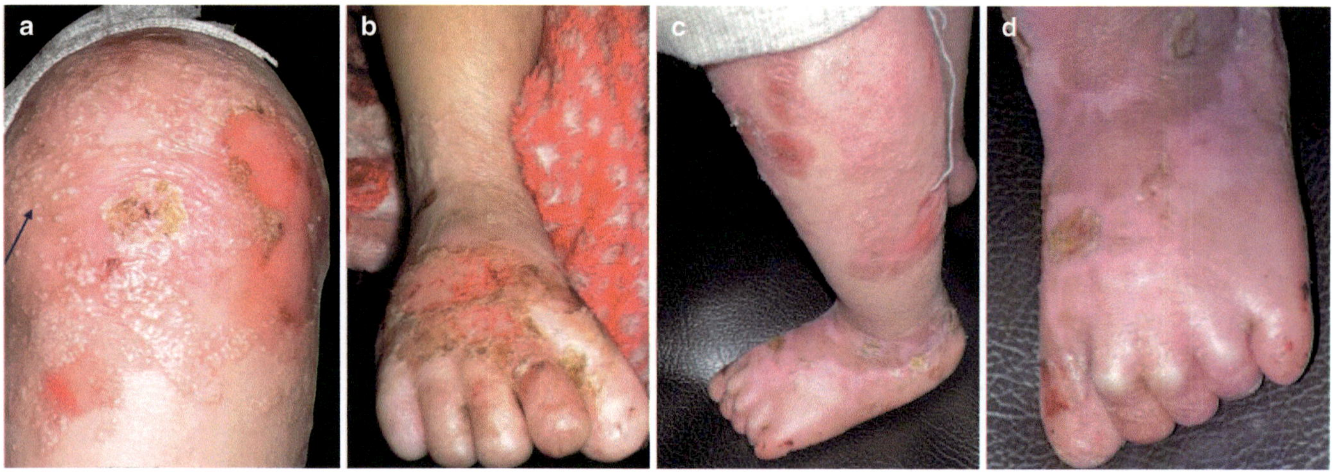

Fig. 3.18 Autosomal dominant dystrophic epidermolysis bullosa (Cockayne-Touraine). An infant with multiple blisters, erosions, and crusts on lower extremities which heal with milia (arrow) (**a**) and atrophic scars with absent nails (**b–d**)

Dominant Dystrophic Epidermolysis Bullosa (DDEB), Intermediate Subtype [5, 14, 15] (Fig. 3.18)

- Previously known as generalized DDEB, Cockayne-Touraine type.
- It usually manifests at birth with the development of blisters, primarily affecting the limbs. Blisters heal by numerous milia and scars particularly visible on the elbows, knees, and hands.
- Nail dystrophy, always present, can lead to loss of nail plates. Usually, fingers and toes are not affected by major cicatricial retractions.
- Blisters can develop in the mucosa, mainly in the oral cavity and, less commonly, in the esophagus, where they can cause strictures, often in sharp contrast with the scarce cutaneous involvement.
- Dental caries are relatively frequent.
- Corneal and genitourinary tract involvement, anemia, and growth delay are rare.

Dystrophic Epidermolysis Bullosa (DDEB) Pruriginosa [16] (Figs. 3.19 and 3.20)

- Skin fragility and blistering lesions usually manifest in infancy and heal with atrophic scarring and milia.
- Intense pruritus is frequently delayed until the adolescence or even adulthood.
- At the onset of pruritus, the clinical picture generally worsens with the development of papules, nodules, lichenoid, and hypertrophic lesions in a linear distribution, preferentially on extensor surfaces of the limbs.
- Nail dystrophy is usually present.

Dominant Dystrophic Epidermolysis Bullosa (DDEB) Albopapuloid (AD) [17] (Fig. 3.21)

- White perifollicular papules (flesh colored scar like papules) mainly on the trunk (lumbosacral region) with small blisters (spontaneous or trauma induced).
- Nail dystrophy.
- Hardly any mucosa or tooth damage can be seen.

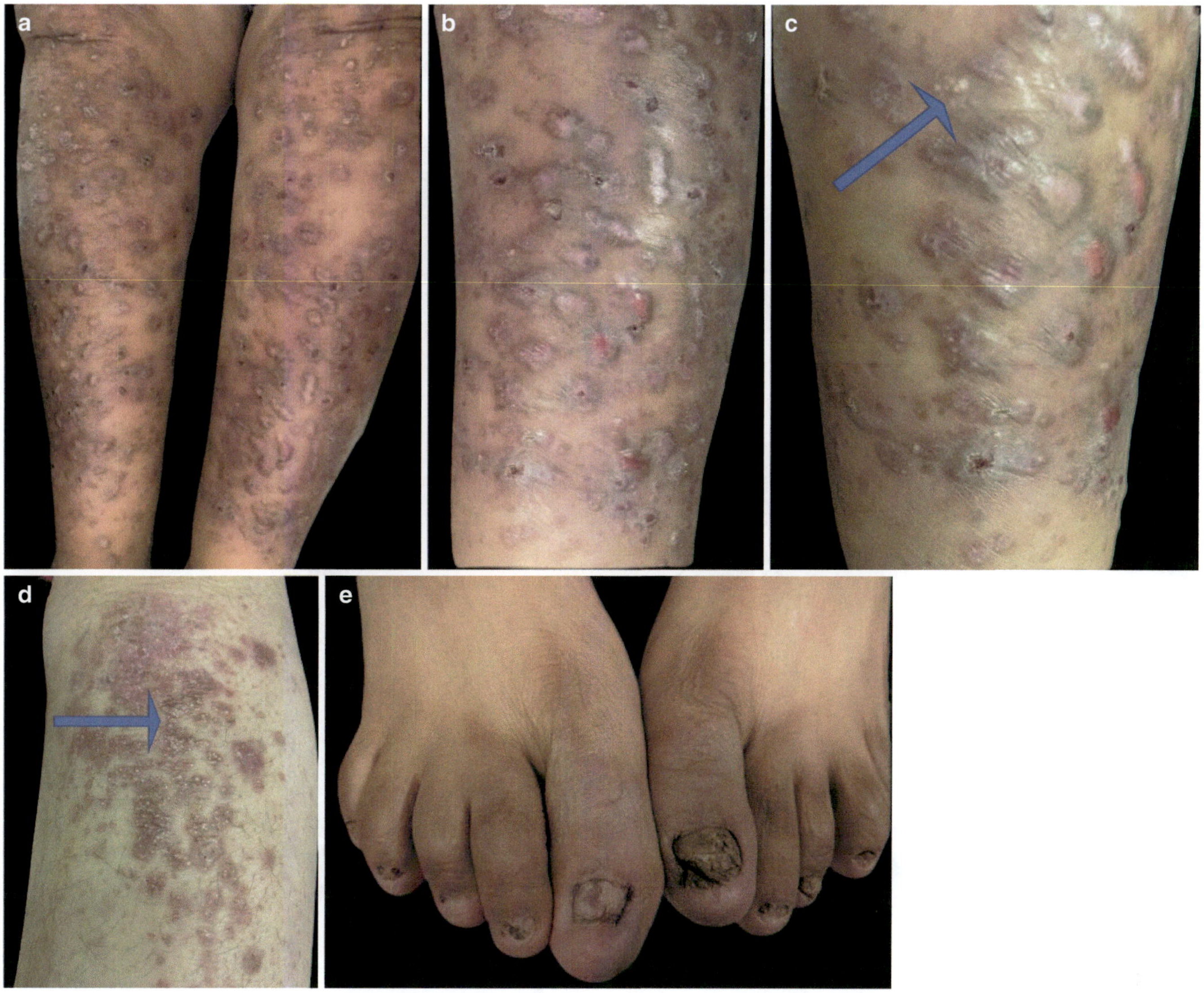

Fig. 3.19 Dystrophic epidermolysis bullosa pruriginosa. An adult patient with severe pruritus, lichenified prurigo like nodules coalescing to form linear plaques (**a**, **b**), multiple blisters, erosions, crusts, and prurigo like nodules on lower extremities (shin of tibia) which heal with milia (blue arrow) and scars (**c**, **d**) with nail dystrophy (**e**)

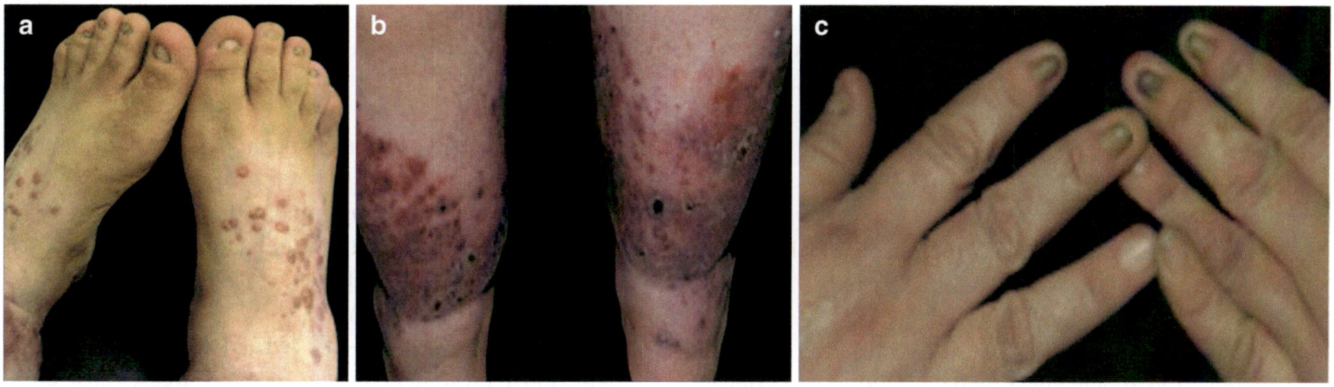

Fig. 3.20 Dystrophic epidermolysis bullosa pruriginosa. An adult with severe pruritus, prurigo like nodules on dorsa of feet (**a**), multiple blisters, erosions and crusts on lower extremities with hemorrhagic bullae (**b**) and nail dystrophy (**a**, **c**)

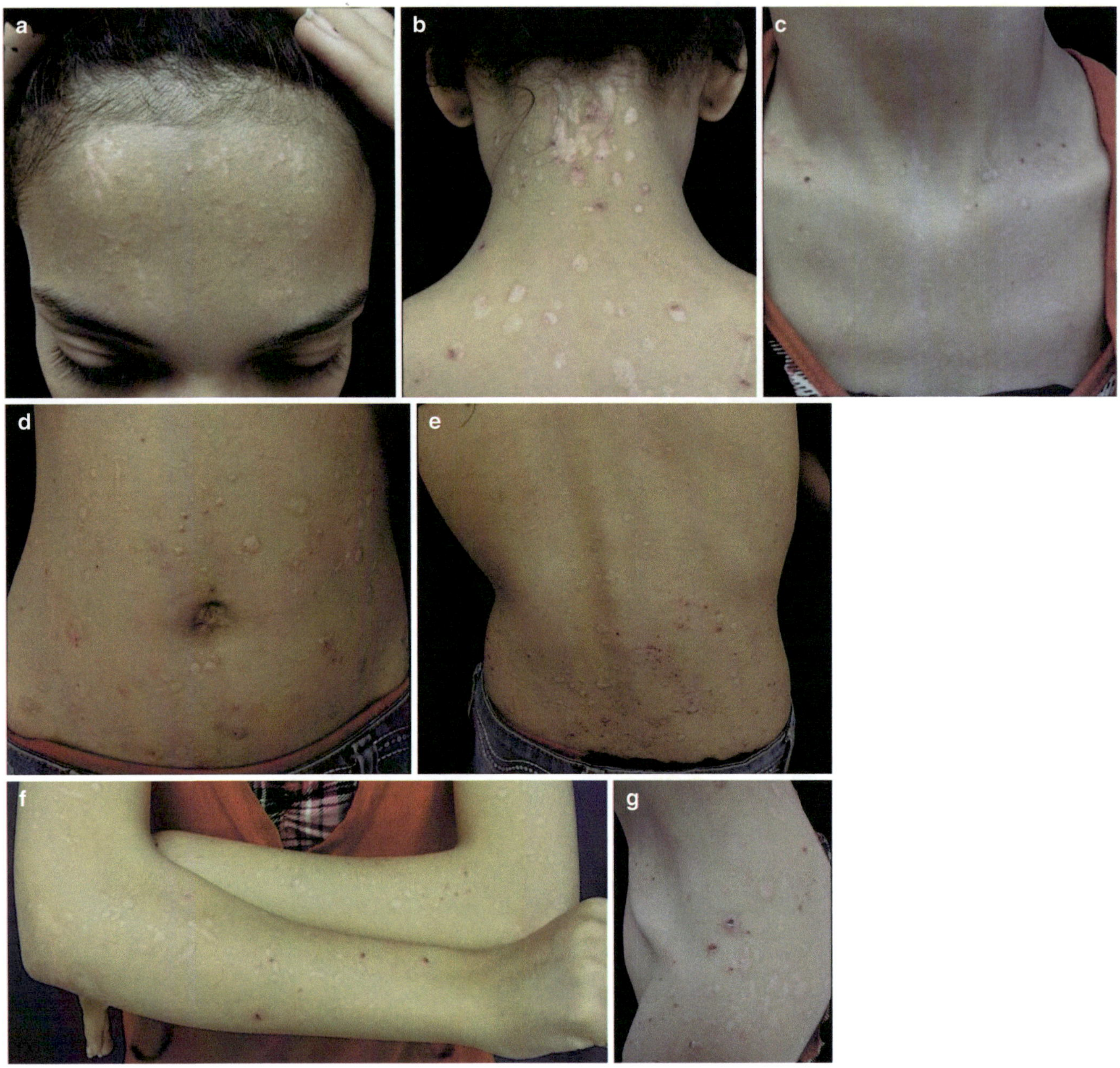

Fig. 3.21 Dystrophic epidermolysis bullosa albopapuloid. An adult patient with small eroded blisters and white perifollicular papules (flesh colored scar like papules) on face (**a**), neck (**b**), chest (**c**), abdomen (**d**), back (**e**), upper (**f**), and lower extremities (**g**)

Kindler Epidermolysis Bullosa (AR) [18, 19] (Figs. 3.22, 3.23, 3.24, 3.25 and 3.26)

- Previously known as Kindler syndrome and bullous acrokeratotic poikiloderma of Kindler and Weary.
- Defect in *FERMT1* gene (*Kindlin-1*).
- A combination of features of inherited blistering skin disorders (e.g., dystrophic epidermolysis bullosa) and congenital poikilodermas (e.g., Rothmund-Thomson syndrome).
- Characterized by *congenital* blistering associated with mild photosensitivity and progressive *poikiloderma.*
- Acral blisters and erosions at birth, induced by trauma or sun exposure.
- Photosensitivity, most prominent during childhood and usually decreases over time, coinciding with decreased blister formation by 10–12 years of age.
- Diffuse cutaneous atrophy.
- Atrophic cigarette paper-like (wrinkled, thin, and fragile) skin, most prominent in sun-exposed areas, most commonly on the dorsal surfaces of the hands and feet.
- Poikiloderma and atrophy, often progressive, with discrete skip areas.

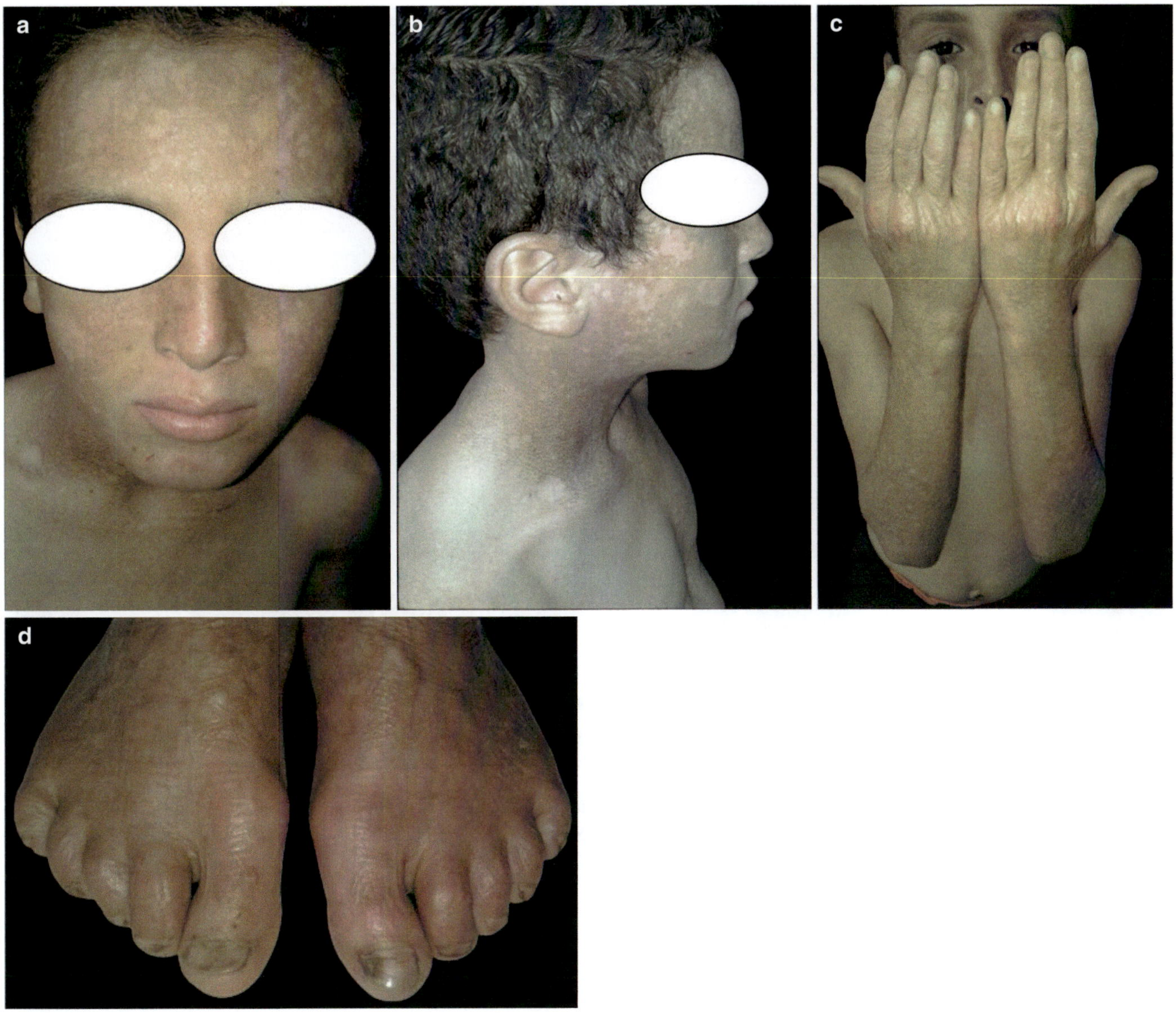

Fig. 3.22 Kindler syndrome. Poikiloderma of the face (**a**) and the neck with "skip areas" (**b**), wrinkled atrophic skin (cigarette paper-like) of dorsum of hands (**c**) and feet with toenails dystrophy (**d**)

- Mucous membrane: erosive gingivitis, gingival hyperplasia, periodontitis, poor dentition, loss of teeth, orogenital leukokeratosis, strictures of esophagus, urethra, anus, and vagina.
- Eye: ectropion, corneal ulcer, recurrent keratoconjunctivitis (symblepharon).
- Nail dystrophy.
- Palmoplantar keratoderma with a common glassy palmar appearance, obscuring the dermatoglyphics.
- Pseudosyndactly, mild webbing of fingers and toes and pseudoanihum may occur.
- Early development of actinic keratoses.
- Increased risk of developing squamous cell carcinoma (Figs. 3.22, 3.23, 3.24, 3.25 and 3.26).

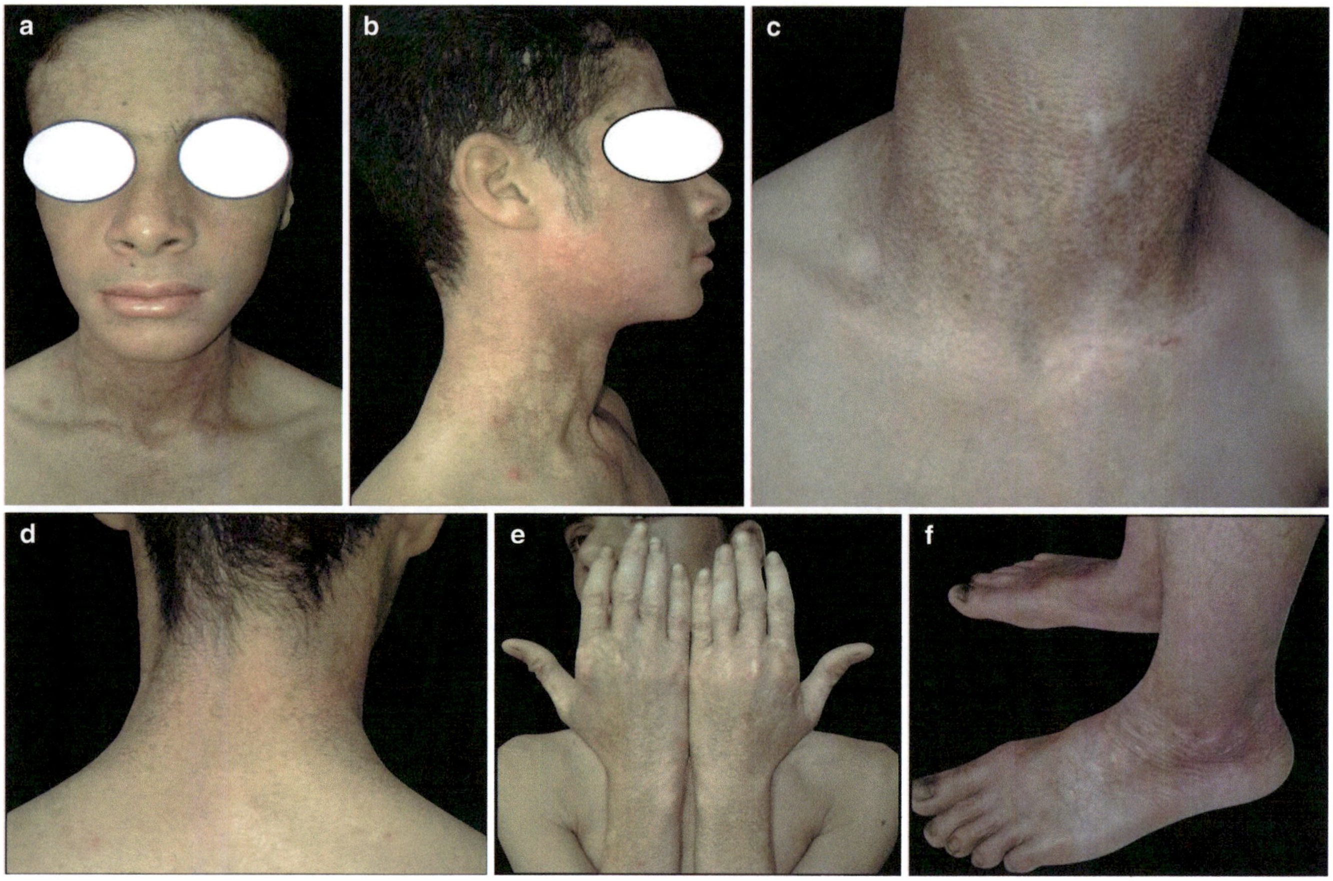

Fig. 3.23 Kindler syndrome (brother of the patient of Fig. 3.22). Poikiloderma of the face and the neck with "skip areas" (**a**–**d**), wrinkled atrophic skin (cigarette paper-like) of dorsum of hands and feet with nail dystrophy (**e**, **f**)

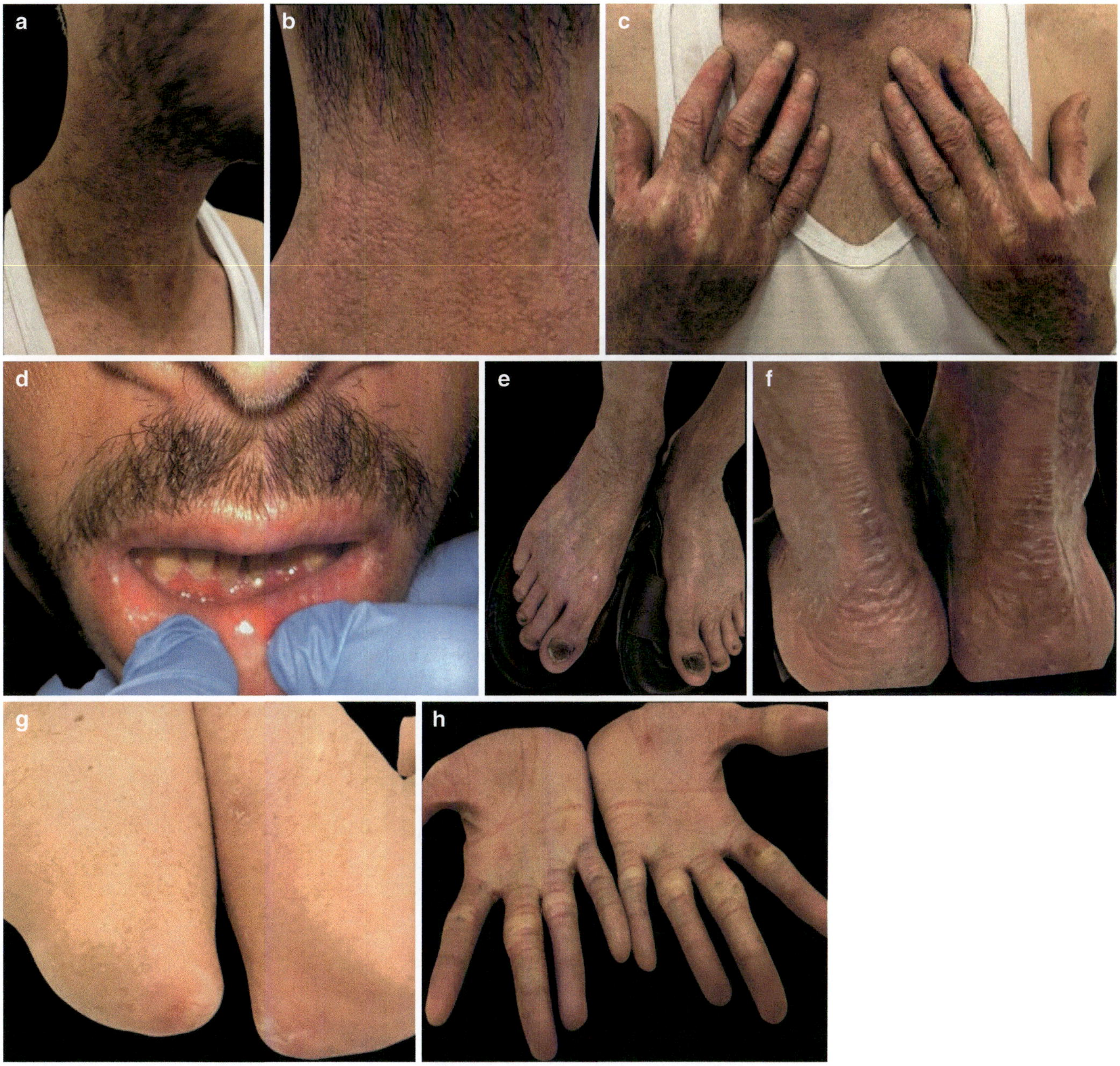

Fig. 3.24 The same patient of Kindler syndrome (Fig. 3.23) at age of 24 years. Poikiloderma of face, neck and upper chest (with "skip areas" (**a**–**c**), gingivitis (**d**), erythema, wrinkle and atrophy (cigarette paper-like) of the skin of the dorsum of hands and feet and nail dystrophy (**c**–**f**), hyperkeratosis of elbows (**g**) with mild webbing between fingers and palmar hyperkeratosis (**h**)

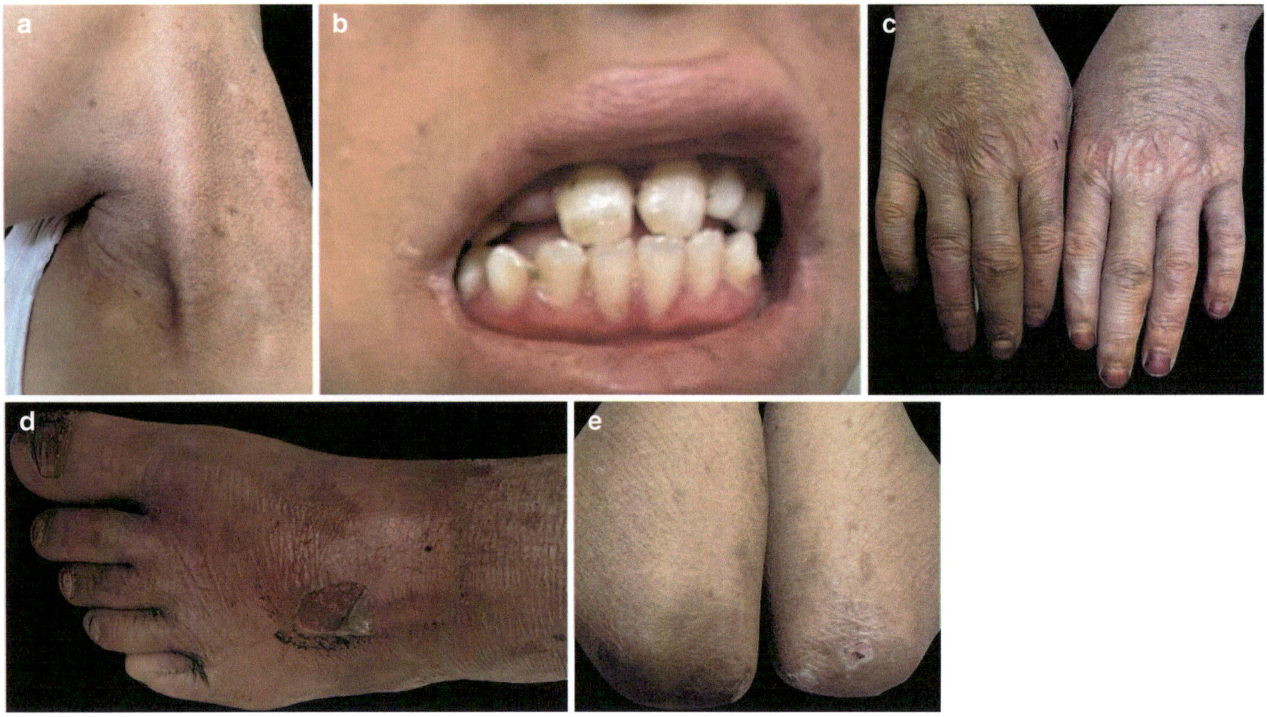

Fig. 3.25 Kindler syndrome. Poikiloderma of the neck with "skip areas" (**a**), gingivitis and angular stomatitis (**b**), wrinkled atrophic skin (cigarette paper-like) of dorsum of hands and feet (**c**, **d**), large erosion on foot (**d**), and hyperkeratosis of the elbows (**e**). Courtesy of Samar Ashry

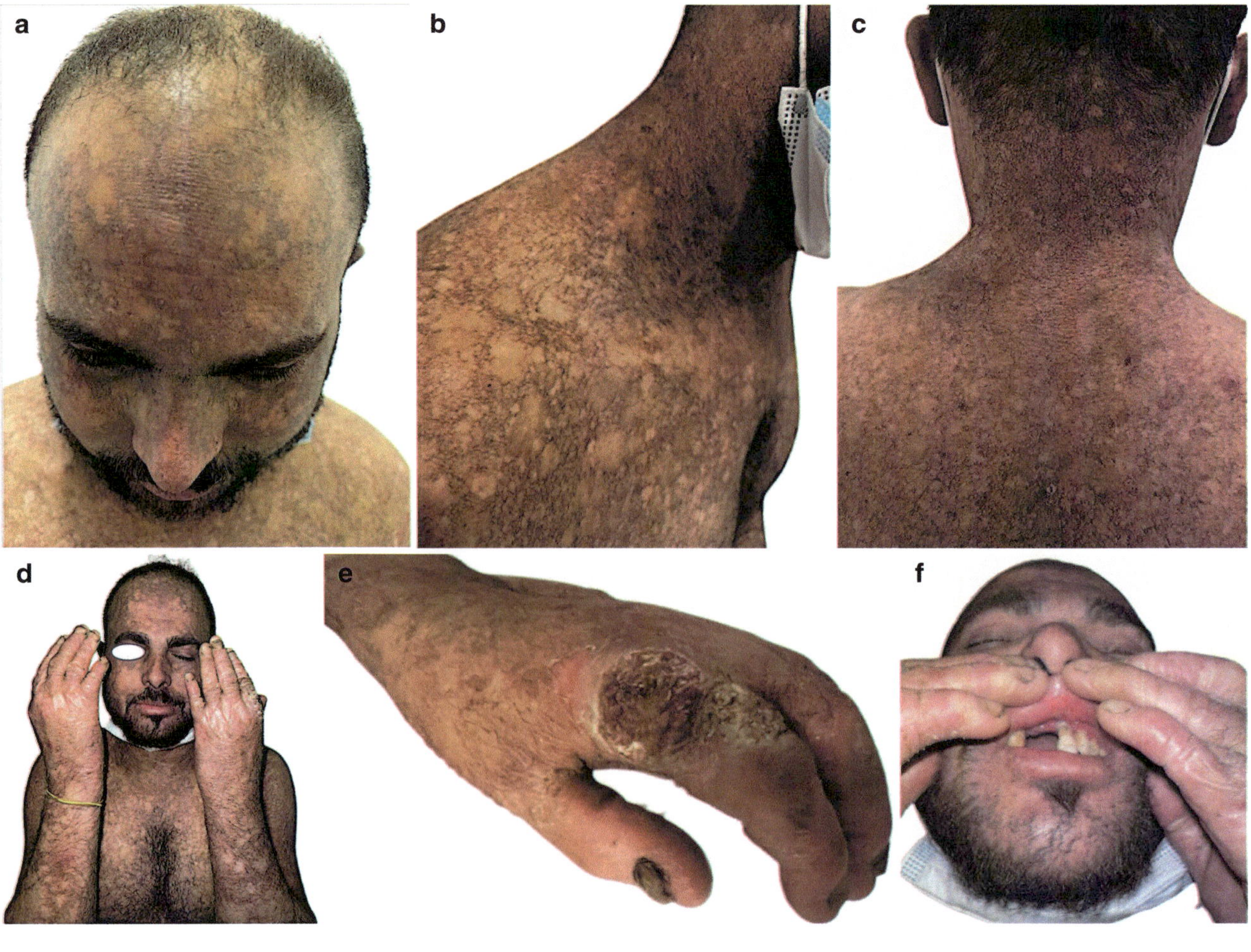

Fig. 3.26 Kindler syndrome. Poikiloderma of face, neck, and upper back with "skip areas" (**a–c**), wrinkled atrophic skin (cigarette paper-like) of the dorsum of hands showing sclerodactyly and squamous cell carcinoma (**d**, **e**). Gingival hypertrophy with loss of teeth is seen (**f**)

References

1. Fine JD, Bruckner-Tuderman L, Eady RAJ, et al. Inherited epidermolysis bullosa: updated recommendations on diagnosis and classification. J Am Acad Dermatol. 2014;70(6):1103–26.
2. Bardhan A, Bruckner-Tuderman L, Chapple ILC, et al. Epidermolysis bullosa. Nat Rev Dis Primers. 2020;6(1):78.
3. Fine JD, Eady RAJ, Bauer JA, et al. The classification of inherited epidermolysis bullosa (EB): report of the third international consensus meeting on diagnosis and classification of EB. J Am Acad Dermatol. 2008;58:931–50.
4. Harvey N, Youssefian L, Saeidian AH, et al. Pathomechanisms of epidermolysis bullosa: beyond structural proteins. Matrix Biol. 2022;110:91–105.
5. Has C, Bauer JW, Bodemer C, et al. Consensus reclassification of inherited epidermolysis bullosa and other disorders with skin fragility. Br J Dermatol. 2020;183:614–27.
6. Riveroa JR, Domingueza MC, Blancob VP, et al. Acral peeling skin syndrome: a case report and literature review. Actas Dermosifiliogr. 2016;107(8):702–4.
7. Whittock NV, Wan H, Eady RAJ, et al. Compound heterozygosity for non-sense and Mis-sense mutations in Desmoplakin underlies skin fragility/woolly hair syndrome. J Invest Dermatol. 2002;118(2):232–8.
8. Horn HM, Tidman MJ. The clinical spectrum of epidermolysis bullosa simplex. Br J Dermatol. 2000;142(3):468–72.
9. Echeverria-Garci B, Vicente A, Hernandez A, et al. Epidermolysis bullosa simplex with mottled pigmentation: a family report and review. Pediatr Dermatol. 2013;30(6):125–31.
10. Kiritsi D, Pigors M, Tantcheva-Poor I, et al. Epidermolysis bullosa simplex Ogna revisited. J Invest Dermatol. 2013;133(1):270–3.
11. Kao CH, Chen SJ, Hwang B, et al. Junctional epidermolysis bullosa. J Chin Med Assoc. 2006;69(10):503–6.
12. Bhinder MA, Arshad MW, Zahoor MY, et al. Junctional epidermolysis bullosa (non-Herlitz type). J Coll Physicians Surg Pak. 2017;27(5):308–10.
13. Gurevich I, Agarwal P, Zhang P, et al. In vivo topical gene therapy for recessive dystrophic epidermolysis bullosa: a phase 1 and 2 trial. Nat Med. 2022;28(4):780–8.
14. Intong LR, Murrell DF. Inherited epidermolysis bullosa: new diagnostic criteria and classification. Clin Dermatol. 2012;30(1):70–7.
15. Das BB, Sahoo S. Dystrophic epidermolysis bullosa. J Perinatol. 2004;24(1):41–7.
16. Pai VV, Sori T, Naveen KN, et al. Epidermolysis bullosa pruriginosa: a report of two cases. Indian Dermatol Online J. 2014;5(1):44–7.
17. Nomura K, Umeki K, Sawamura D, et al. Dominant dystrophic epidermolysis bullosa albopapuloidea Pasini—ultrastructural observations of albopapuloid lesions and a type VII collagen DNA polymorphism study of a family. Acta Derm Venereol. 1997;77(4):277–80.
18. Ashton GH. Kindler syndrome. Clin Exp Dermatol. 2004;29(2):116–21.
19. D'Souza MA, Kimble RM, McMillan JR. Kindler syndrome pathogenesis and fermitin family homologue 1 (kindlin-1) function. Dermatol Clin. 2010;28(1):115–8.

Pigmentary Genodermatoses

4

This chapter includes both hypomelanosis and hypermelanosis genodermatoses. Hypomelanosis may be related to a defect of embryological development of melanocytes, a defect of biogenesis of melanosomes, or a defect of melanosomes transport. Hypermelanosis may be in the form of diffuse linear hyperpigmentation, reticular hyperpigmentation, non-figurate hyperpigmentation, genodermatoses associated with café-au-lait macules and associated with lentiginosis.

Hypomelanosis

1. Piebaldism
2. Waardenburg syndrome
3. Ziprkowski–Margolis syndrome/Woolf syndrome
4. Hermansky–Pudlak syndrome
5. Griscelli–Prunieras syndrome
6. Vogt–Koyanagi–Harada syndrome
7. Alezzandrini syndrome
8. Hypomelanosis of Ito (incontinentia pigmenti achromians)

Hypomelanosis [1]

Hypomelanosis Related to a Defect of Embryological Development of Melanocytes

Piebaldism (AD) [1, 2] (Figs. 4.1, 4.2, 4.3, and 4.4)

- It is a very rare congenital hypomelanosis.
- Autosomal dominant inheritance, with mutation of *KIT* proto-oncogene.
- It is due to defect of embryological development of melanocytes.
- Age of onset: at birth.
- Clinical characteristics:
  - Leukoderma affects the anterior midline trunk, extremities and forehead, but spares the posterior midline, hands, feet, and shoulders.
  - Occasional normal pigmented and hyperpigmented macules and patches, ranging from few millimeters to several centimeters in diameter, may be identified within the white patches. Hyperpigmented patches may occur within normal skin.
  - White forelock of hairs (midline in location, triangular or diamond-shaped) with involvement of eyebrows and eyelashes in 80%–90% of cases.
- D.D: contrary to vitiligo, these patches are sparing hands, feet, and periorificial areas, stable with time and do not repigment.
- Histopathology: total absence of melanocytes within hair bulb and epidermis. The hyperpigmented macules are characterized by abundance of melanosomes in melanocytes and keratinocytes.

Waardenburg Syndrome (AD/AR) [1, 2] (Figs. 4.5, 4.6, and 4.7)

- Waardenburg syndrome (WS) is a rare hypomelanosis, with sensorineural deafness.
- Age of onset: at birth.
- There are four types of WS: autosomal dominant (WS 1, WS2, and WS 3) or less frequently autosomal recessive disorder (WS 4). Mutation occurs in certain genes including; *PAX3*, microphthalmia-associated transcription factor (*MITF)*, endothelin-B receptor (*EDNRB*), endothelin-3 (*EDN3),* and *SOX10.*
- Clinical characteristics:
  - WS 1 (classic form):
    The white forelock, as in piebaldism, is the most frequent manifestation (20–60% of cases).
    Hypopigmented patches in about 1/3 of cases.
    Ocular manifestations in about 1/3 of cases [heterochromia iridis and dystopia canthorum (movement of the internal canthus to external without any change of the external canthus)].
    Facial dysmorphia [broad nasal root and synophrys (confluent eyebrows)] in about 2/3 of cases.

N. Moftah et al., *Atlas of Common and Rare Genodermatoses*, https://doi.org/10.1007/978-3-031-60788-2_4

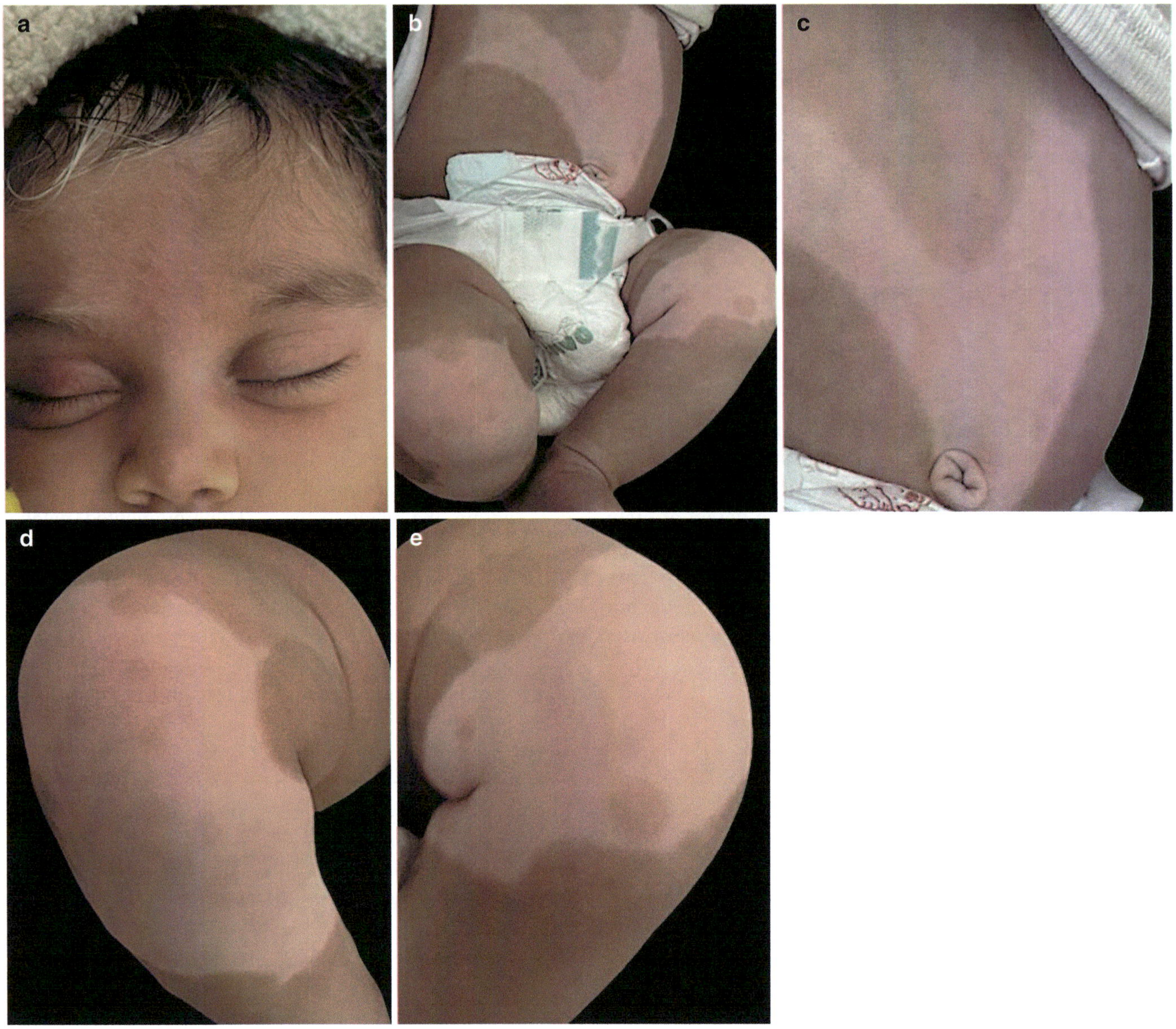

Fig. 4.1 Piebaldism. White forelock (**a**) and characteristic depigmented patches on the mid forehead (**a**), central anterior trunk and mid extremities (**b–e**). Hyperpigmented patches within the leukoderma (**e**)

Sensorineural deafness in one or both sides in 1/3 to 1/5 of cases.
- WS2:
  As WS1 without dystopia canthorum, however, congenital deafness is more frequent.
- WS 3:
  As WS1 with upper limb abnormalities (hypoplasia, syndactyly, and flexor contractures).
- WS 4:
  As WS 1 with Hirschsprung's disease (neonatal intestinal obstruction, megacolon) and deafness.

- Histopathology; melanocytes are absent in depigmented patches. In normal pigmented skin, melanocytes are normal or presented with short dendrites and abnormal melanosomes.

Hypomelanosis Related to a Defect of Melanogenesis

Albinism (AR/XLR) [1, 3]

- Albinism can affect eyes [ocular albinism (OA)] or eyes and skin [oculocutaneous albinism (OCL)]
- Albinism has many clinical types.
- Autosomal recessive inheritance, with mutations in tyrosinase (*TYR*) gene, *P* protein gene, tyrosinase related protein (*TYRP*)-1 gene and membrane-associated transporter protein (*32* gene in OCA type 1, OCA type 2, OCA type 3, and OCA type 4, respectively. Mutations in protein unknown (4q24), in membrane-associated transport protein (SLC24A5) and protein unknown (10q22.2-3) in OCA type 5, 6, and 7, respectively. However, OA 1 is an

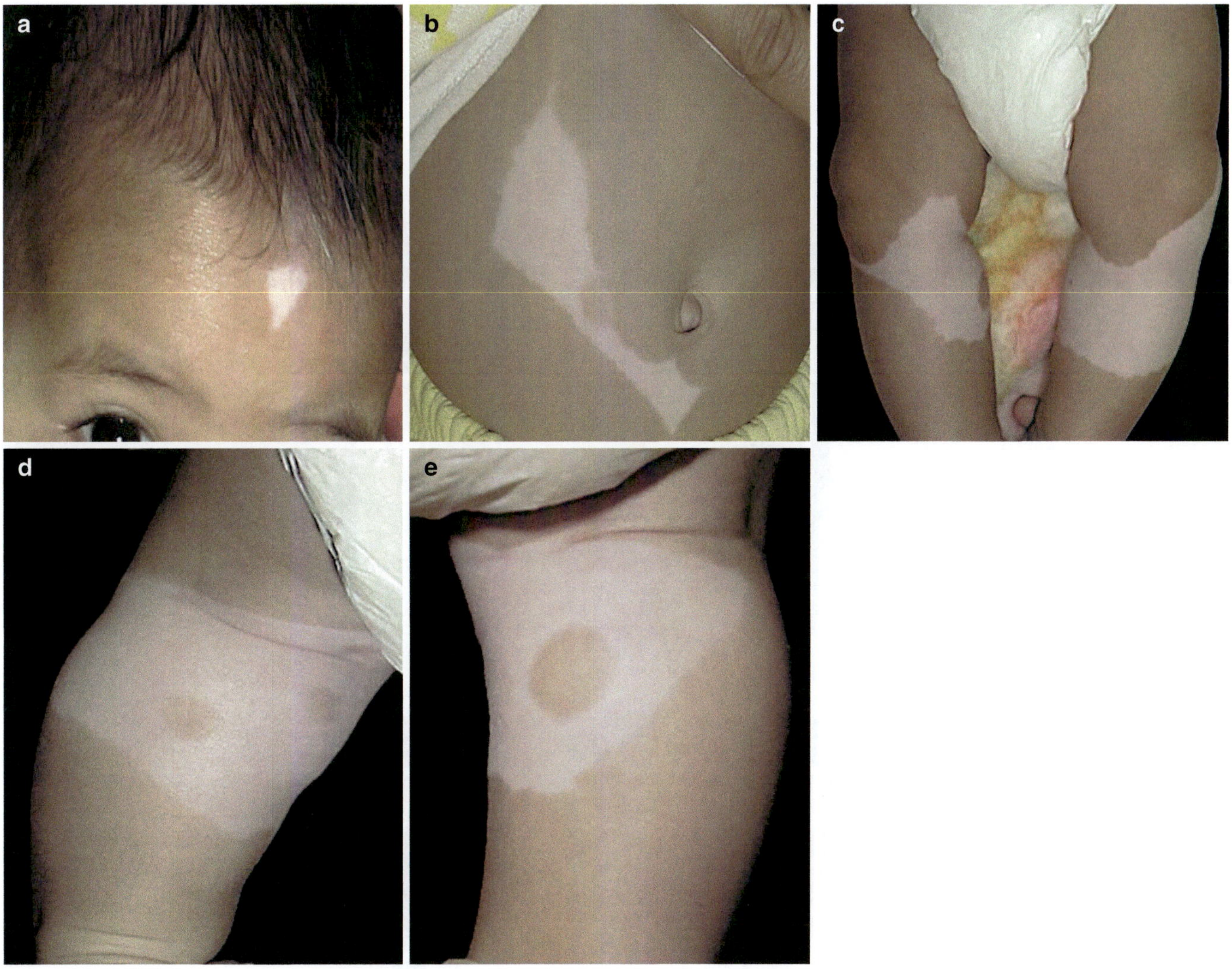

Fig. 4.2 Piebaldism. White forelock and characteristic depigmented patches on the mid forehead (**a**), central anterior trunk and mid extremities (**b–d**). Hyperpigmented patches within the leukoderma (**b–e**)

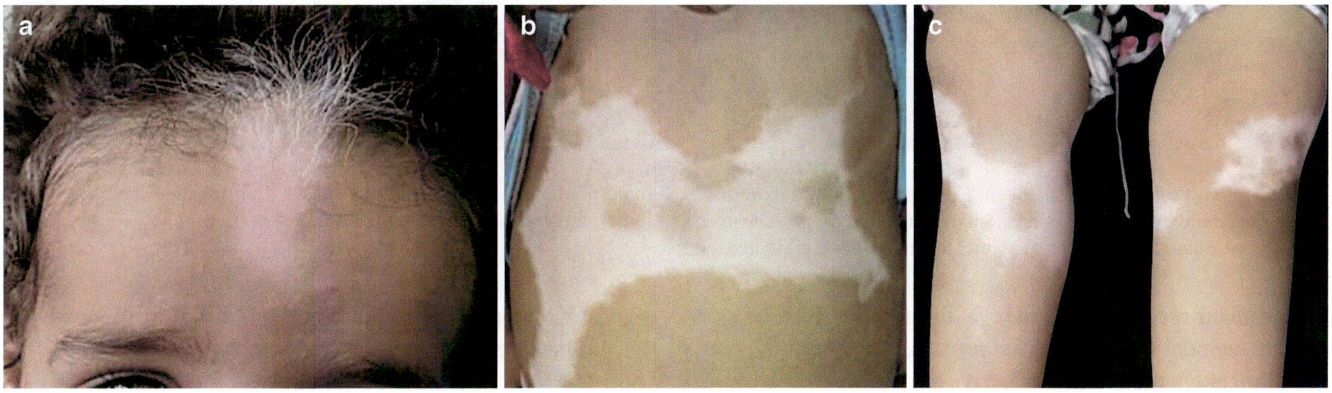

Fig. 4.3 Piebaldism: White forelock and characteristic depigmented patches on the mid forehead (**a**), central anterior trunk and mid extremities (**b**, **c**). Hyperpigmented patches within the leukoderma (**b**, **c**)

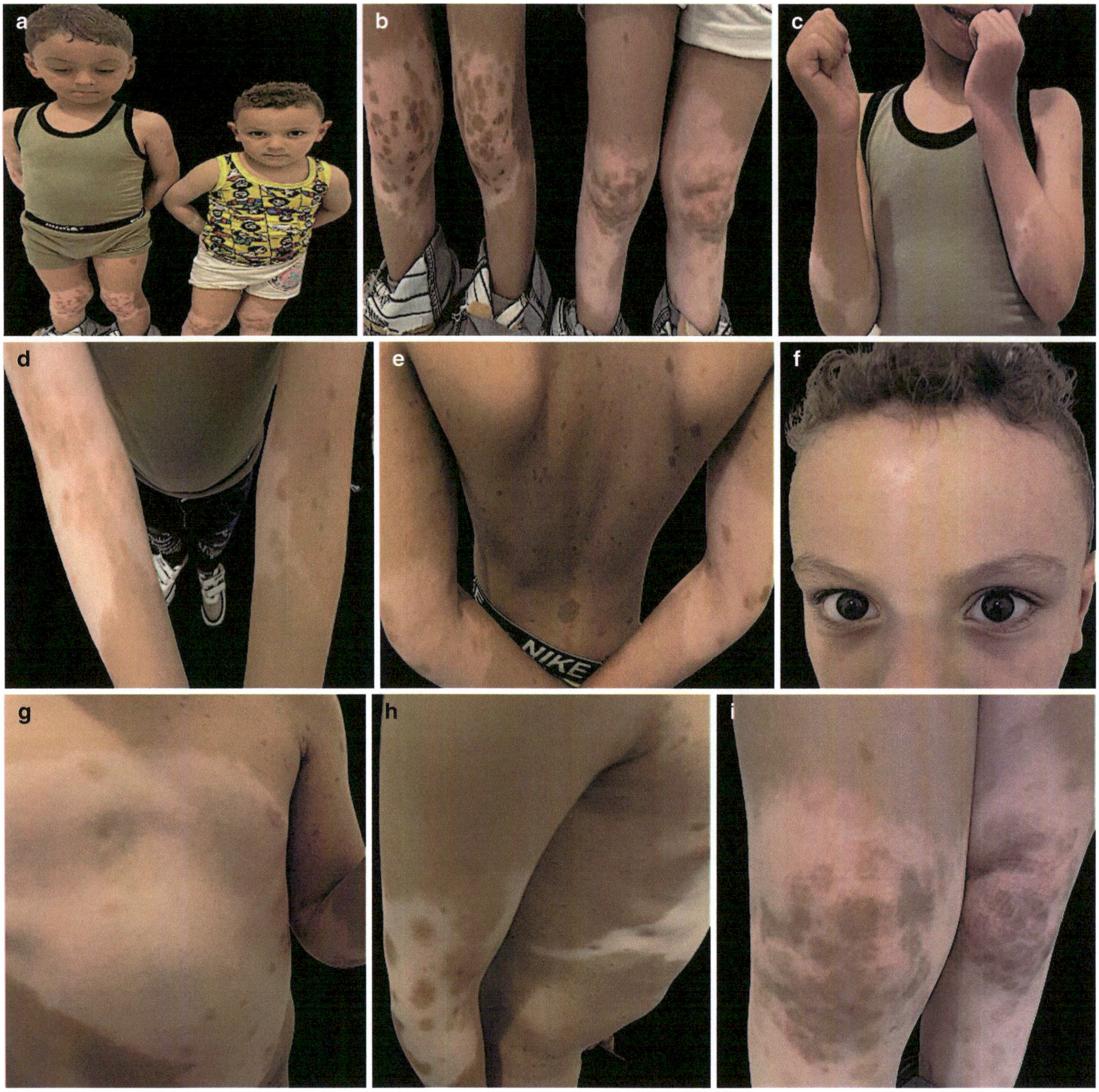

Fig. 4.4 Two brothers of piebaldism. Leukoderma in mid-extremities (**a–i**). The youngest showing amelanotic patch on the mid forehead and the central anterior trunk (**f**, **g**). Note the normally pigmented and hyperpigmented macules and patches within leukodermas (**b–i**), with hyperpigmented patches on the normal skin (**e**, **g**, **i**)

X-linked recessive disorder, with mutation in *OA1* gene that encodes a melanosomal protein.

- Clinical characteristics:
  - OCA type 1: the first most common form;

    These persons are white, with fair skin (skin type I), blond hair and blue eyes.

    Sunburn is common on unprotected skin.

    Ocular manifestations include severe nystagmus, photophobia, and reduced visual acuity.
  - OCA type 2: the second most common form, mostly in black people.

    During childhood, phenotype is similar to OCA1; however, progressively little amount of pigment is accumulated into skin and eyes.

    With time, lentigos, pigmented nevi and freckles can be seen in photo-exposed areas.

    Ocular manifestations are less severe, and nystagmus and visual acuity tend to get better with time.

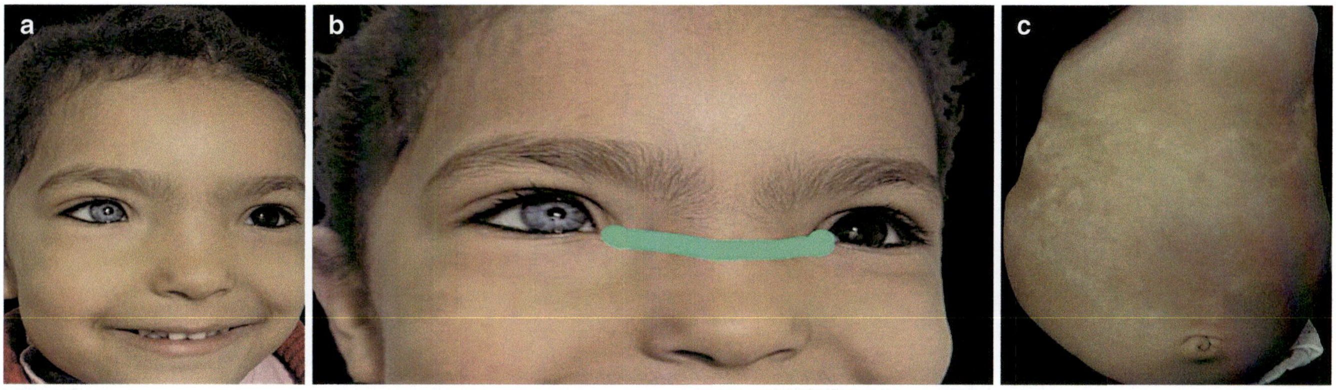

Fig. 4.5 Waardenburg syndrome with deafness. Heterochromia irides associated with dystopia canthorum (**a**, **b**), and leukoderma in mid trunk (**c**). (*Courtesy, Aya A. Abu Oun*)

Fig. 4.6 Waardenburg syndrome with deafness. Depigmented patches on the face, broad nasal root, white hair in medial part of the eyebrows, dystopia canthorum (**a**, **b**), and leukoderma in the trunk and upper limb (**c**, **d**)

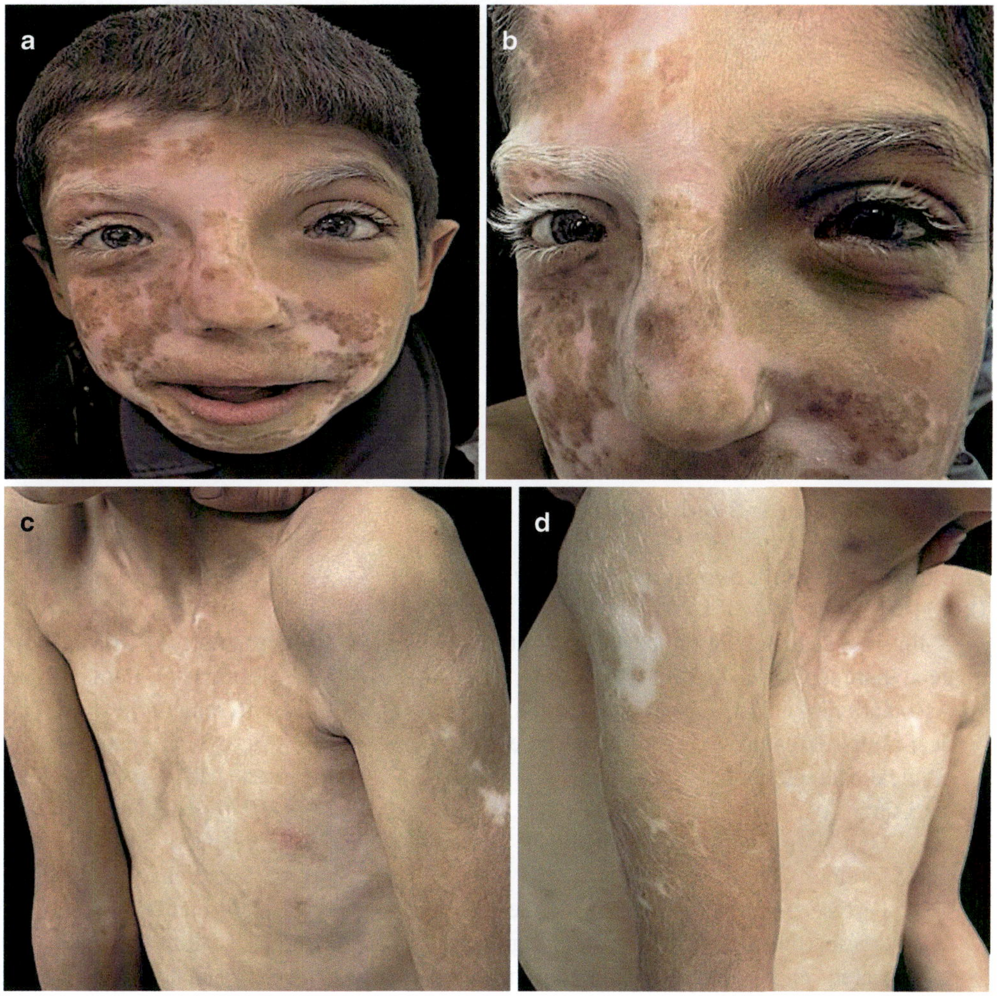

– OCA type 3: It is most commonly seen in African people.

  At birth, skin and hairs are light brown and iris is gray or light brown; however, hairs and iris can become darker with time.

  Ocular manifestations are present but are usually less severe. Nystagmus is constant.

– OCA type 4, 5, 6, and 7: rare forms of OCA.

  Phenotype is similar to OCA2.

– OA: It is a rare form of albinism

  Limited to the eyes. In fact, hypopigmentation in the skin is light but most easily seen in black people.

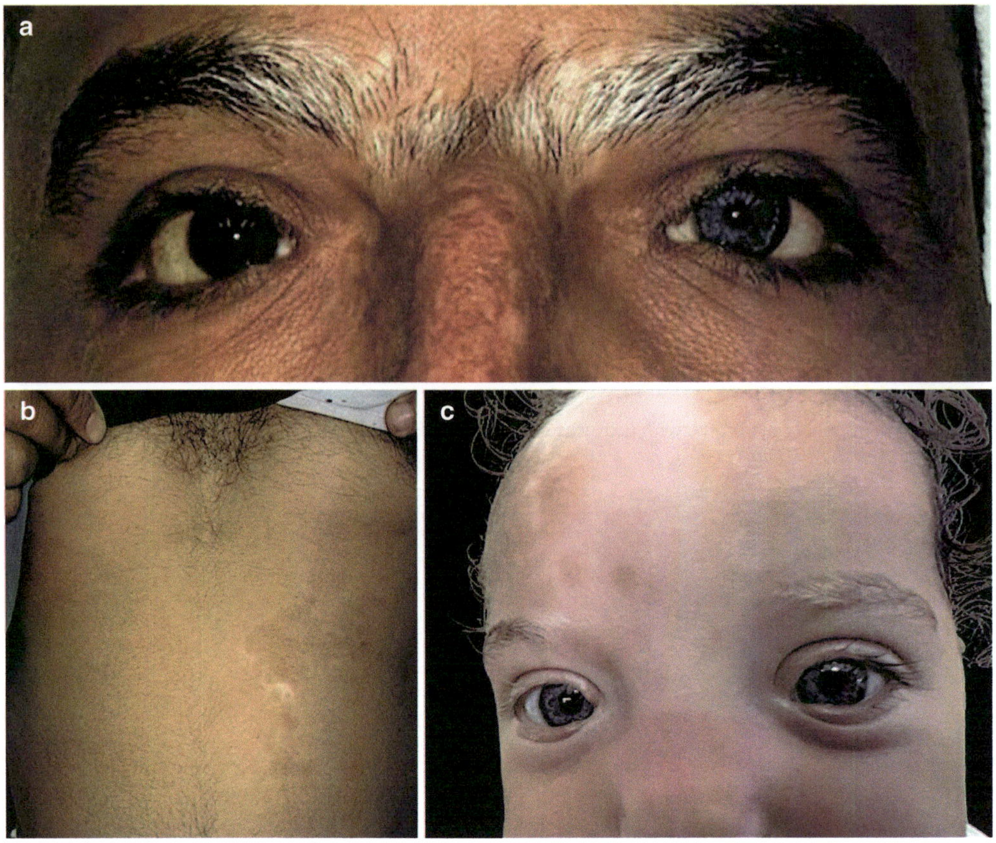

Fig. 4.7 Waardenburg syndorme in an elderly male and in an infant. The elderly male is showing heterochromia irides and white hairs in medial eyebrows with dystopia canthorum, confluent eyebrows (**a**) and leukoderma in central trunk (**b**). The infant is showing same color of the iris in both eyes (**c**)

Ocular abnormalities of albinism are present (including photophobia and nystagmus).

Albinism–Deafness Syndrome

Ziprkowski–Margolis Syndrome/Woolf Syndrome (XLR) [4] (Fig. 4.8)

- X-linked recessive inheritance, with mutation of unknown gene that mapped to Xq26.3-q27.
- Association of albinismus circumscriptus (without OA) + deaf mutism (features of Woolf syndrome).
- Clinical characteristics:
  - Skin:

    Hypopigmentation of piebaldism pattern (white forelock), but more diffuse.

    Diffuse pigmentary dilution of the hair and skin, sparing the buttocks and genital region.

    Later, multiple hyperpigmented macules appear, giving the skin a leopard-like appearance.
  - Ears: congenital sensorineural deafness.
  - Eyes: heterochromia iridis.
- Associations: Addison's and systemic sclerosis.

Hypomelanosis Related to a Defect of Biogenesis of Melanosomes

Phenotypically, extrapigmentary abnormalities are associated with OCA due to the involvement of lysosome-related organelles besides melanosomes.

Hermansky–Pudlak Syndrome (AR) [1, 5] (Fig. 4.9)

- Hermansky–Pudlak syndrome (HPS) is a rare disorder, with many types.
- Autosomal recessive disorder, with mutation in *HPS1* gene, *AP3B1* gene, *HPS3* gene, *HPS4* gene, *HPS5* gene, *HPS6* gene, and *DTNBP1* gene in HPS1, 2, 3, 4, 5, 6, and 7, respectively.
- Clinical characteristics:
  - Pigment dilution [OCA (tyrosinase +ve)]:

    Skin: the light color of skin is associated with pigmented nevi, granulomatous plaques, and "knife-cut" ulcers of vulva, intertriginous areas, and peristomal skin similar to cutaneous Crohn's disease.

    Hair: creamy colored hair.

    Ocular manifestations of albinism (nystagmus, reduced visual acuity, and photophobia).

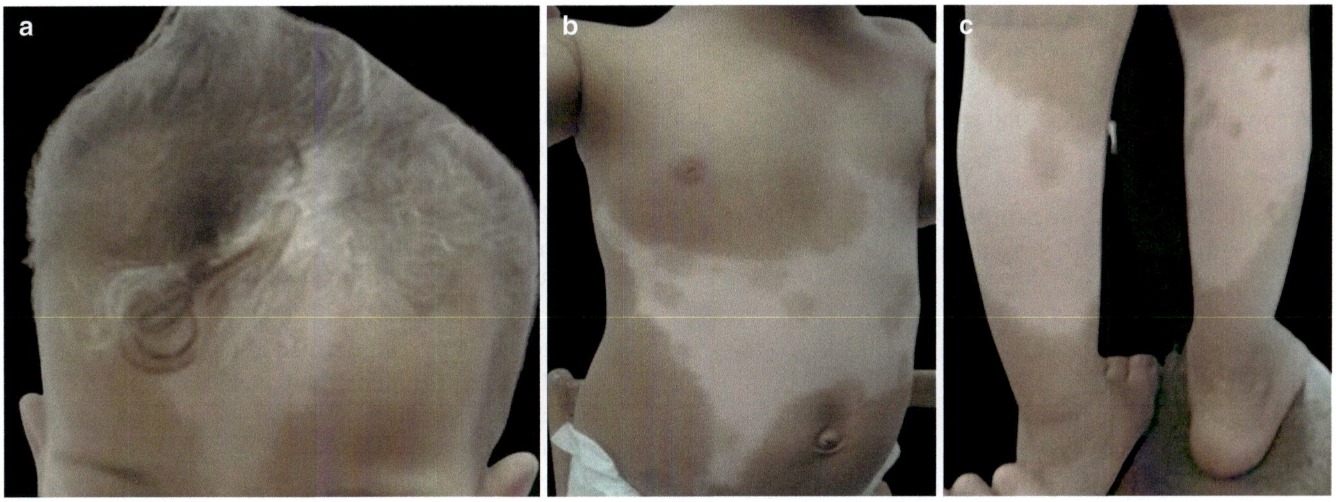

Fig. 4.8 Albinism–deafness syndrome (Ziprkowski–Margolis syndrome/Woolf syndrome). A piebaldism pattern (hypopigmentation on the trunk associated with white forelock) (**a–c**). The child is deaf

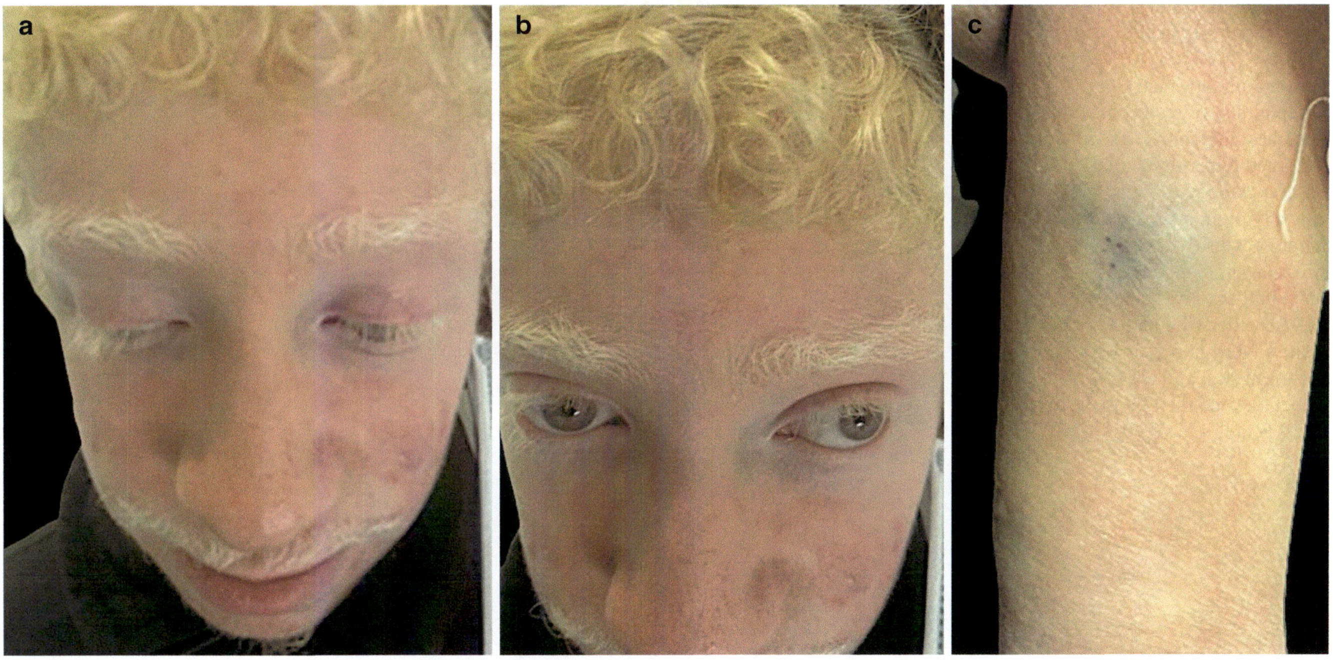

Fig. 4.9 Hermansky-Pudlack syndrome (OCA). Pigmentary dilution of skin, hair, and eye (**a**, **b**) with ecchymotic patch on upper limb (**c**). The patient complains of frequent epistaxis

- Systemic affection:
  Bleeding manifestations (epistaxis, gingival and genital bleeding, bloody diarrhea, petechial purpura).
  Deposition of ceroid-like material (degradation of lipids and glycoproteins) in lysosomes of:
    GIT: granulomatous colitis
    Lung: pulmonary fibrosis
    Heart: cardiomyopathy
    Renal: renal failure
    CNS: neurodevelopmental delay and seizures.

• Investigations:
  - Blood film: platelet count is normal, bleeding time and platelet function analyzer (PFA)-100 time are prolonged
  - Electron microscopy: Macromelanosomes as well as stage I– III and rarely stage IV melanosomes are seen within melanocytes and adjacent keratinocytes.
    Absence of dense bodies within platelets.
    Ceroid deposits are found within lysosomes in affected internal organs.

Hypomelanosis Related to a Defect of Melanosomes Transport

Phenotypically, pigmentary and extrapigmentary manifestations are observed.

Griscelli–Prunieras Syndrome (AR) [1, 6] (Fig. 4.10)

- Griscelli–Prunieras (GS) syndrome is a very rare disorder, with many types.
- Autosomal recessive disorder, with mutation in *MYO5A* gene, *RAB27A* gene, and *MLPH* gene in GS1, 2, and 3, respectively.
- Clinical characteristics:
  - Pigment dilution of:

    Skin: pigmentary dilution of skin due to pigment clumping within melanocytes.

    Hair: silver gray, monotonously white (due to large irregular melanin clumps in hair near medulla).
- Types.:
  - GS1: dilution of skin and hair with neurological impairment (developmental delay, hypotonia, and mental retardation)
  - GS2 (the most common): dilution of skin and hair with immune abnormalities and hemophagocytic syndrome.
  - GS3: dilution of skin and hair only.
- Investigations:
  - Histopathology: large irregular clumps of melanin in the hair near medulla. Enlarged hyperpigmented basal melanocytes with sparsely pigmented adjacent keratinocytes.
  - Electron microscopy: accumulation of melanosomes in melanocytes.

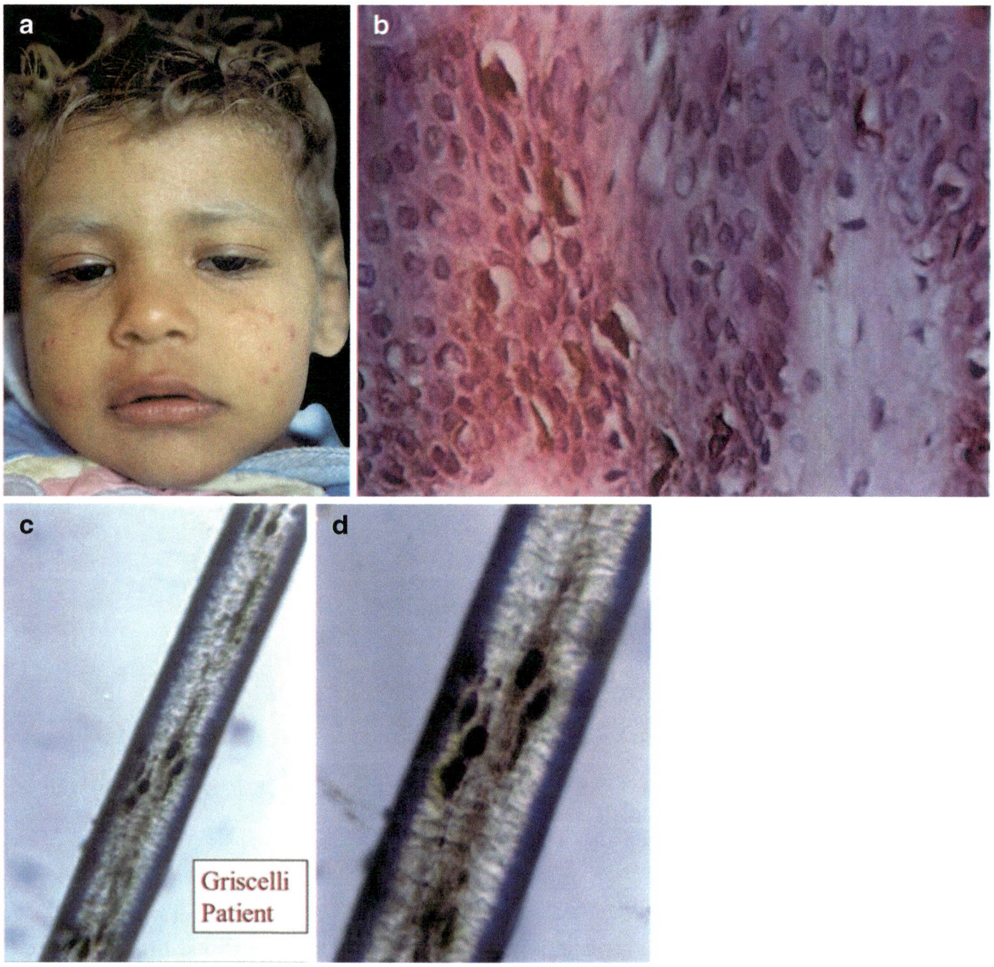

Fig. 4.10 Griscelli syndrome. Female child 3 years old having pigmentary dilution of skin and silvery-gray hairs of scalp and eyebrows born to a consanguineous marriage complaining of recurrent skin and chest infections (**a**). (**a**) Enlarged hyperpigmented basal melanocytes with sparsely pigmented adjacent keratinocytes (**b**), large irregular pigment clumps in hair shaft (**c**, **d**). She had an elder brother who had the same silvery gray hair with recurrent skin and chest infections and died by the age of 10 years

Other Hypomelanoses

Vogt–Koyanagi Harada Syndrome (Sporadic, AR) [1, 7, 8] (Figs. 4.11 and 4.12)

- Vogt–Koyanagi syndrome (VKH), a multisystem disease, results from T-cell mediated autoimmune reaction against melanin-pigmented antigens (*TYR, TRP-1, and S-100* protein).
- Inheritance: sporadic or autosomal recessive; an association with defect in *HLA-DR4*, *HLA-DRB1*, and *HLA-DQA1*.
- Clinical characteristics:
  - Aseptic meningitis
  - Bilateral, diffuse uveitis
  - Deafness, tinnitus, and vertigo
  - Vitiligo that appears after extracutaneous involvement, especially of face or sacral region.
  - Alopecia areata
  - Poliosis.
- Four stages of VKH are recognized including; prodromal stage, uveitic stage, convalescent stage, and chronic recurrent stage.
  - Prodromal stage;

    No symptoms, may mimic a non-specific viral infection or marked by flu-like symptoms.

    Meningismus.

    Ear; dysacusia (discomfort caused by loud noises or distortion in quality of heard sounds), tinnitus, and/or vertigo.

    Eye; orbital pain, photophobia, and tearing.

    Skin and hair may be sensitive to touch.

    Cranial nerve palsies and optic neuritis are uncommon.
  - Acute uveitic phase occurs few days later and typically lasts for several weeks;

    Bilateral panuveitis causing blurring of vision.
  - Convalescent phase;

    Gradual skin depigmentation with poliosis,

    Sometimes with nummular depigmented scars

    Alopecia.

    Eye; diffuse fundus depigmentation [classic orange-red discoloration "sunset glow fundus" and retinal pigment epithelium clumping and/or migration]. Sugiura's sign (perilimbal vitiligo) is the earliest depigmentation to occur.
  - Chronic recurrent phase;

    Repeated bouts of low-grade or subclinical uveitis leading to granulomatous anterior inflammation, cataracts, glaucoma, and ocular hypertension.

    Dysacusia.
- Investigations:
  - Cerebrospinal fluid pleocytosis in prodromal phase up to 8 weeks even if chronic uveitis persists.
  - Electroretinogram and visual field testing.
  - Imaging tests such as retinography, fluorescein or indocyanine green angiography, optical coherence tomography, and ultrasound.
- DD: Alezzandrini syndrome, sarcoidosis, tuberculosis, syphilis, sympathetic ophthalmia, primary intraocular B-cell lymphoma, and posterior scleritis.

Alezzandrini Syndrome [9] (Fig. 4.13)

- Alezzandrini syndrome is an autoimmune disorder of unilateral melanocyte destruction in skin, hair, eye (retina, uvea), and ear (cochlea and vestibular labyrinth) from an unknown origin, however, viral or autoimmune processes may lead to this melanocyte destruction.
- Defect in *HLA-DQA1* and *HLA-DRB1* genes.
- Clinical characteristics:
  - Aseptic meningitis followed by:
  - Skin: ipsilateral facial vitiligo
  - Hair: ipsilateral poliosis (white scalp hair, eyebrows, eyelashes)
  - Eye: ipsilatera degenerative retinitis
  - Ear: ipsilateral deafness.
- D.D.: VKH share similar cutaneous and ocular signs, however, Alezzandrini syndrome is unilateral in addition to neurological involvement typical of VKH syndrome (cranial nerve damage, sterile meningitis) is not reported in Alezzandrini syndrome.
- Investigations: regular ophthalmological assessment (fundus examination, visual acuity, fundus autofluorescence, and optical coherence tomography) and audiometry.

Hypomelanosis of Ito [1, 10] (Figs. 4.14 and 4.15)

Incontinenia Pigmenti Achromians

- It is due to chromosomal mosaicism and sporadic mutations.
- It is not an inherited disorder as the chromosomal defect occurs after conception.
- The specific gene(s) is most likely a balanced translocation of Xp21.2.
- Constitutional autosomal or X autosome translocations are reported.
- Onset: apparent at birth or usually appear in the first year of life.
- Clinical characteristics:

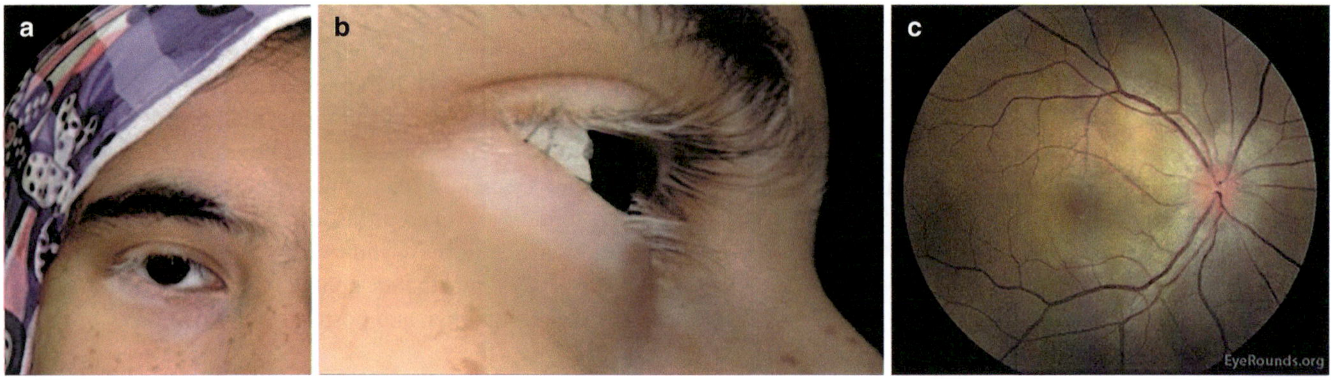

Fig. 4.11 Vogt-Koyanagi-Harada syndrome. Vitiligo around eye associated with poliosis (**a**, **b**). Non-inflammatory depigmented lesions of ocular fundus (**c**)

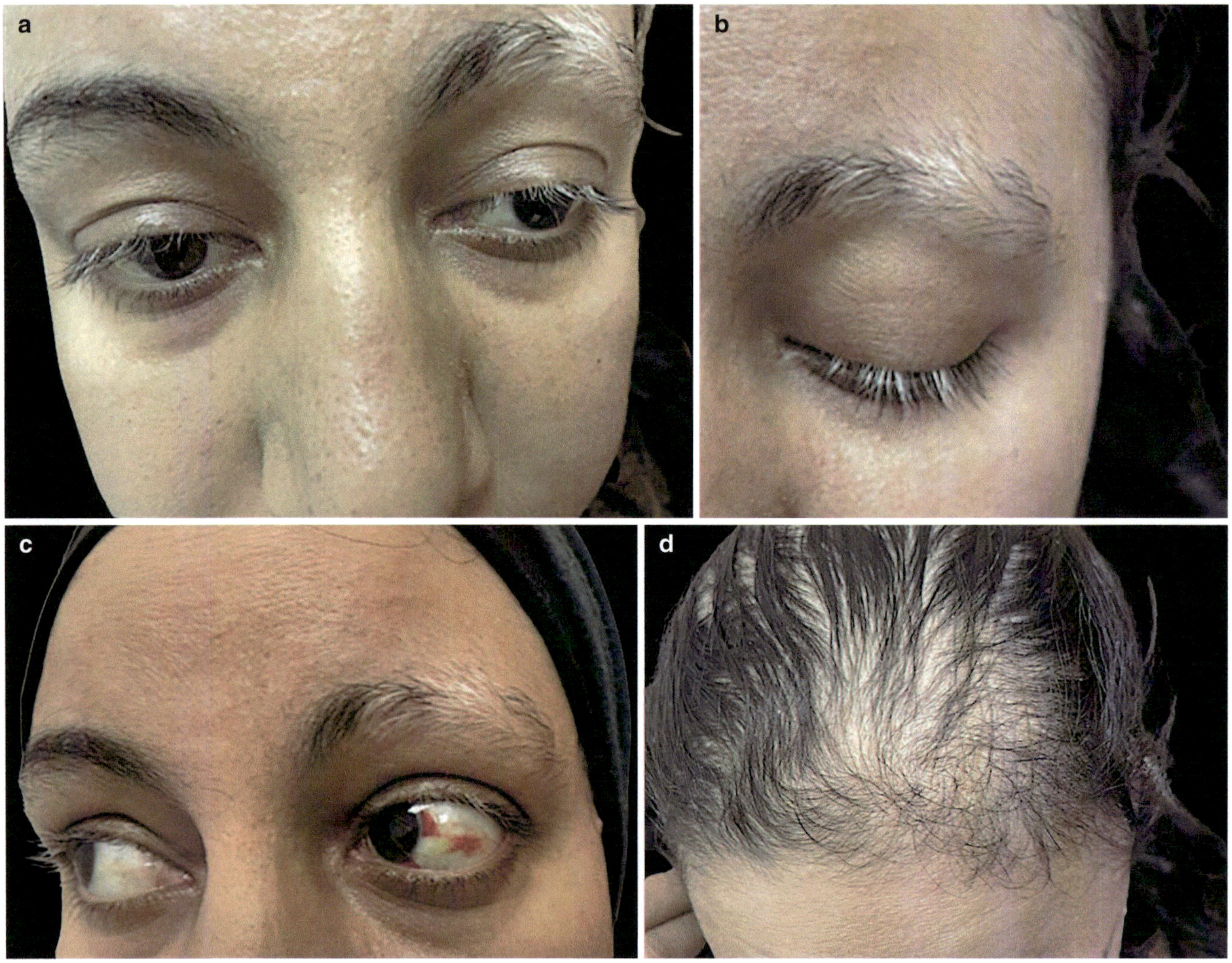

Fig. 4.12 Vogt-Koyanagi-Harada syndrome. Vitiligo in the upper eyelid associated with poliosis (**a**, **b**), subconjunctival hemorrhage (**c**), and diffuse alopecia areata (**d**). The patient is suffering from optic neuritis

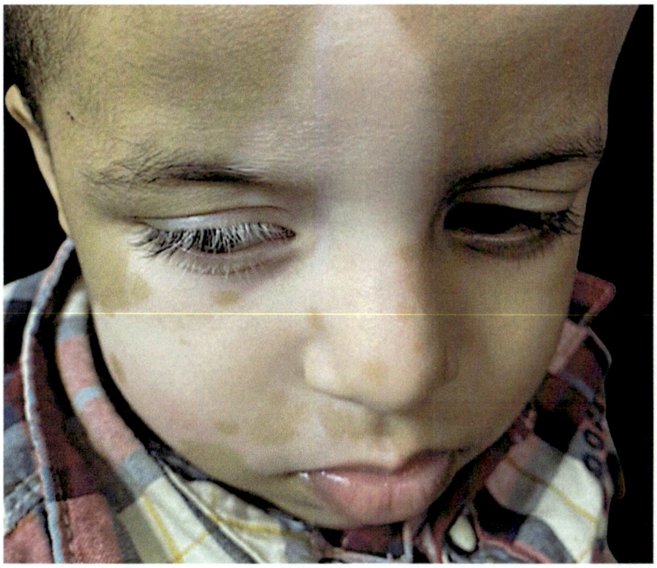

Fig. 4.13 Alezzandrini syndrome. A 7-year-old boy presenting with unilateral gradual loss of vision and degenerative retina followed by Ipsilateral facial vitiligo with Ipsilateral poliosis

  - Skin: unusual unilateral or bilateral streaks, whorls, and swirls of hypopigmentation along the lines of Blaschko. Superimposed lentigines, hypertrichosis, and alopecia are occasionally observed.
  - CNS: mental retardation and seizures may be found.
  - Orthopedic, hearing, and visual problems may be encountered.
- Light and electron microscopy show few melanocytes and melanosomes.

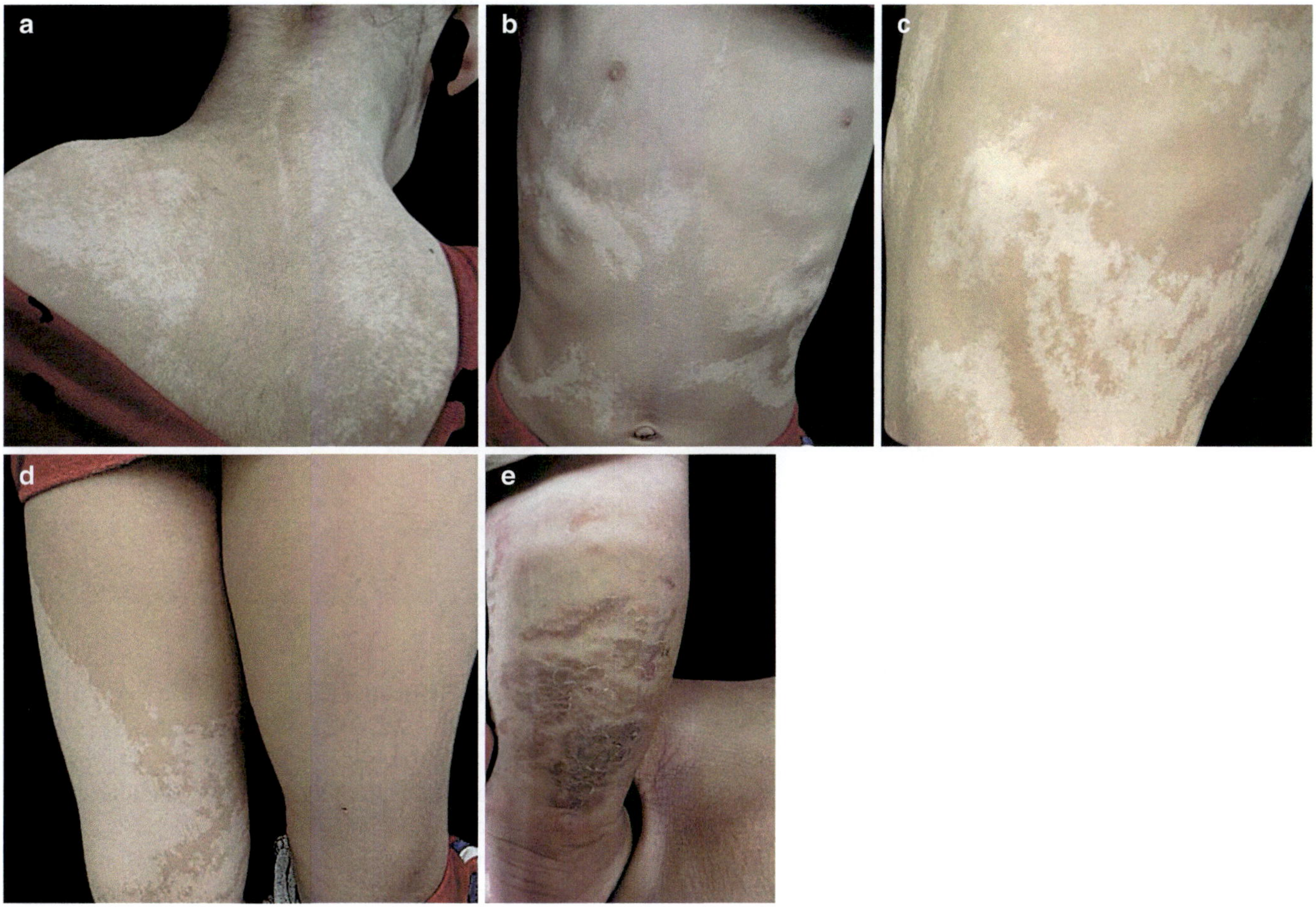

Fig. 4.14 Hypomelanosis of Ito. Patches and swirls of hypopigmentation along the Blaschko lines on the neck (**a**), trunk (**b**, **c**), and lower extremities (**d**, **e**)

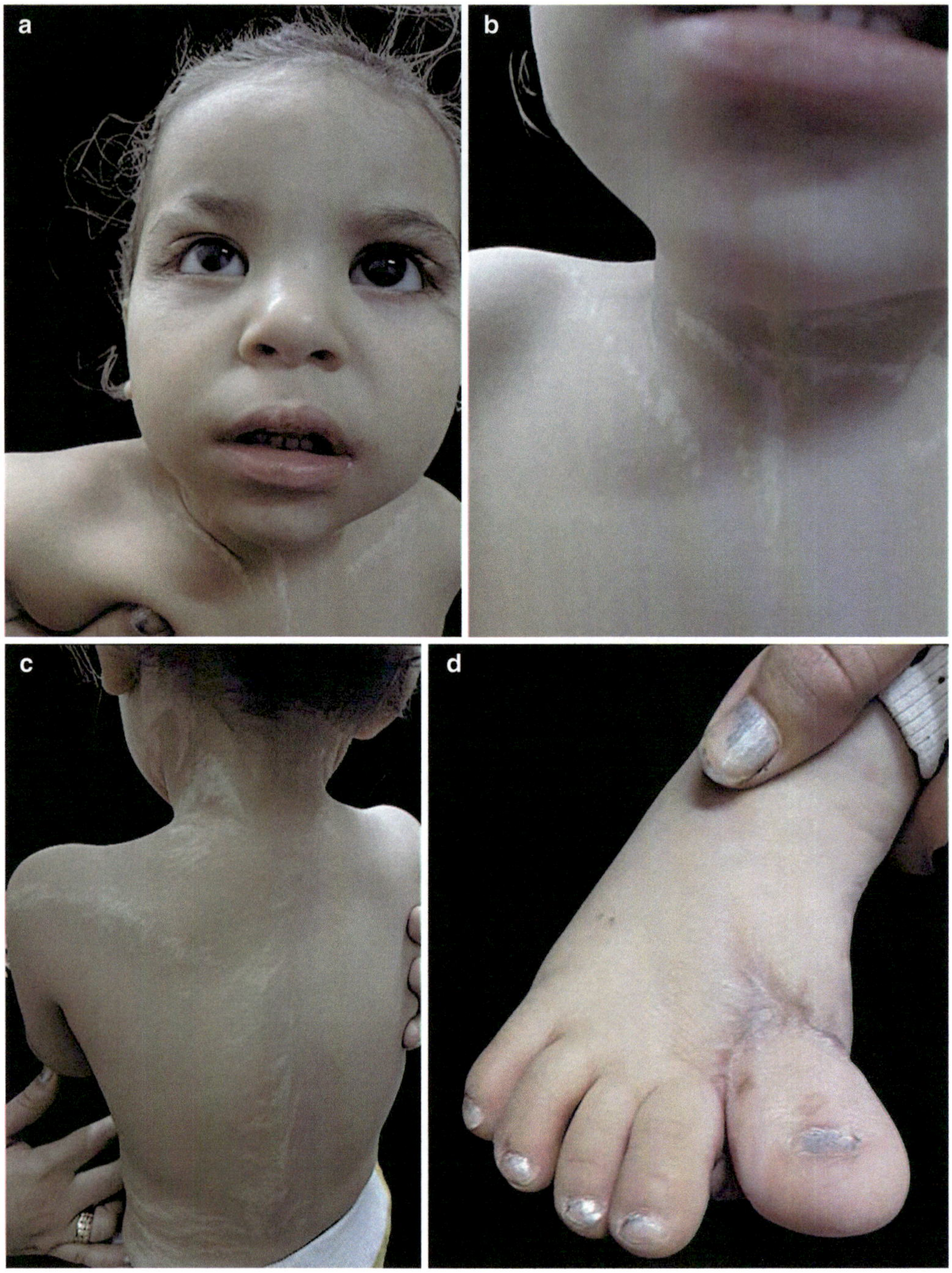

Fig. 4.15 Hypomelanosis of Ito. Streaks of hypopigmentation along the Blaschko lines on the neck and trunk (**a**–**c**) with previous orthopedic operation of skeletal anomalies of the right foot (**d**)

Hypermelanosis

1. Incontinentia pigmenti
2. Linear and whorled nevoid hypermelanosis
3. Dowling–Degos disease
4. Reticulate acropigmentation of Kitamura
5. Reticulate acropigmentation of Dohi
6. Dyschromatosis universalis hereditaria
7. Naegeli–Franceschetti–Jadassohn syndrome
8. Familial gigantic melanocytosis
9. McCune–Albright syndrome
10. Peutz–Jeghers syndrome.
11. Laugier–Hunziker syndrome

Incontinentia Pigmenti (XLD) [11] (Figs. 4.16, 4.17, 4.18, 4.19, 4.20, 4.21, 4.22, and 4.23)

- It is a rare condition affecting ectodermal structures (skin, teeth, eyes, and nails) and CNS.
- X-linked dominant inheritance, with mutation of *IKBKG* (*NEMO*) gene.
- Onset: first few weeks to months of life.
- Incidence: almost only observed in females as being lethal in males before birth.
- Clinical characteristics:

- Skin: lesions follow Balshcko lines.
  First stage (inflammatory) (2 weeks after birth): linear vesicles on scalp and limbs, most prominent on lower extremities, and rare on face.
  Second stage (verrucous) (2–6 weeks after birth): linear verrucous lesions on extremities, and it disappears later in infancy.
  Third stage (hyperpigmentation) (childhood): streaks and swirls of reticulate grayish-brown hyperpigmentation (Chinese letters) on trunk and intertriginous areas. Keratotic nodules (including subungual lesions) occasionally arise after puberty.
  Forth stage (hypopigmentation) (third decade): linear hypopigmented bands lacking hair and sweat glands, especially on calves and may be the only stigmata of the disease during adulthood.
- Hair (30–40% of patients): alopecia (linear absence of hair)
- Nails (10–20% of patients): dystrophy and trachyonychia.
- Teeth (40–50% of patients): Cone-shaped, agenesis and pegged teeth.
- Eye (20–40% of patients): retinal vascular affection, strabismus, cataracts, microphthalmia, and optic atrophy.
- CNS (<30% of patients): microcephaly, seizure, hemorrhagic stroke, motor and intellectual delay.
- Skeletal defects (uncommon): skull anomalies and scoliosis.
- Lung (uncommon): pulmonary hypertension.

• DD: Bullous lesions in infancy: bullous impetigo, candidiasis, and linear immunoglobulin A (IgA) bullous disease of childhood and epidermolysis bullosa.
• Investigations:
  - CBC: eosinophilia.
  - Histopathology: an intraepidermal vesicle filled with eosinophils (biopsy from intact blister).

Linear and Whorled Nevoid Hypermelanosis (LWNH) [12] (Fig. 4.24)

• Linear and whorled nevoid hypermelanosis (LWNH) is a rare sporadic pigmentary anomaly.
• Genetic studies: different chromosomal abnormalities (trisomy 7, 14, 18, 20, X-chromosome mosaicism).
• Onset: within a few weeks of age, with no preceding inflammation or palpable lesion.
• Clinical characteristics:
  - Skin:
    Reticulate hyperpigmented macules coalescing to form streaks and whorled areas over trunk, extremities, and neck following the lines of Blaschko, and do not cross the midline. The pigmented streaks display V-shaped pattern over spine, S-shaped or whorled pattern over anterior and lateral aspects of trunk, and linear arrangement over extremities and genitalia.
    Sparing of the face, palms and soles, eyes and mucous membranes.
  - Extracutaneous features:
    Skeletal, neurological, and ocular abnormalities.
    CNS diseases; microcephaly, arhinencephaly, and epilepsy
    Cardiac defects; ventricular septal defect and tetralogy of Fallot.
    Developmental retardation, facial and body asymmetry, and brachydactyly.
    Deafness.
• Investigations:
  - Dermatoscopic features; "net like" pattern of pigmentation along lines of Blaschko in both linear and whorled parts.
  - Histopathology; diffuse moderate hyperpigmentation in the basal layer and prominence or vacuolization of melanocytes. Pigmentary incontinence is usually, but not always absent.
• DD: incontinentia pigmenti, hypomelanosis of Ito and epidermal verrucous nevus.

Dowling-Degos Disease (DDD) (AD) [13] (Figs. 4.25 and 4.26)

• Dowling-Degos disease (DDD) is a rare disorder.
• Autosomal dominant inheritance, with genetic mutation of keratin 5 (KRT5), protein O-glucosyltransferase 1 (*POGLUT1*), protein O-fucosyltransferase 1 (*POFUT1*) or presenilin enhancer protein 2 gene (*PSENEN*).
• Onset: after puberty (the third to fourth decade of life).
• Clinical characteristics:
  - Acquired reticulated hyperpigmentation (lentigo-like brown macules) at flexural sites, face, neck, and upper chest.
  - Perioral pitted facial scars (concomitant acne-like scar) and acne form-like eruption.
  - Comedone-like lesions on back and neck.
  - Small brown papules with variable hyperkeratosis, hidradenitis suppurativa-like lesion, and cystic lesions (epidermoid cyst).
• Histopathology: filiform elongation of rete ridges involving the follicular infundibulum and melanocyte proliferation without melanin incontinence.

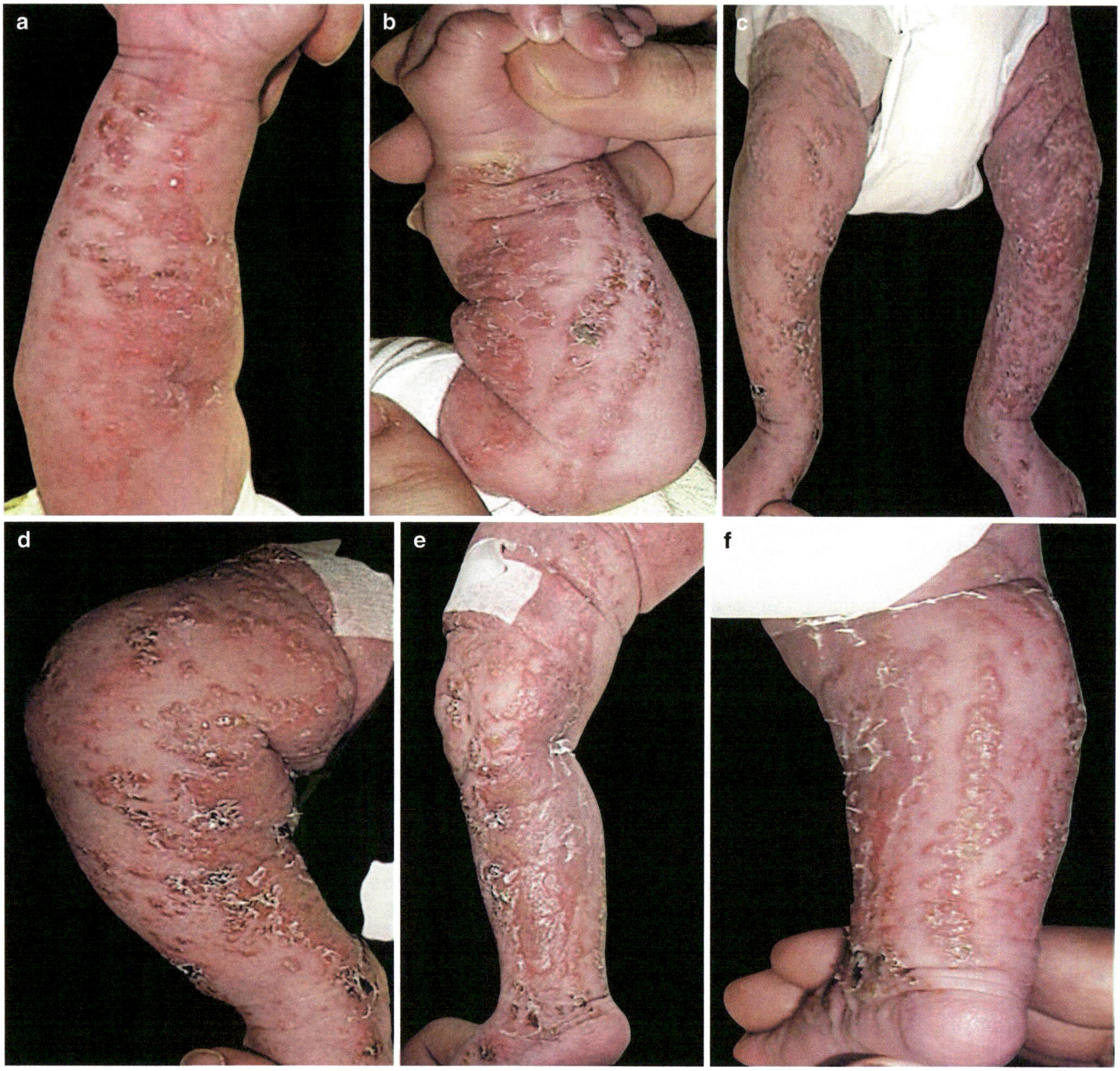

Fig. 4.16 Incontinentia pigmenti. Linear inflammatory vesicles and verrucous plaques on the limbs following Blaschko lines (**a**–**f**)

- D.D.: Reticulate acropigmentation of Kitamura (RAK), acanthosis nigricans, neurofibromatosis type 1
- Prognosis: there is no significant mortality associated with DDD.

Reticulate Acropigmentation of Kitamura (RAK) (AD) [14] (Fig. 4.27)

- RAK is a rare genodermatosis.
- Autosomal dominant inheritance, with mutation in *ADAM10* gene.
- Onset: childhood or adolescence.
- Clinical characteristics:
  - Lentiginous, hyperpigmented atrophic macules in a reticular pattern on the dorsal aspect of the hands and feet (no hypopigmentation).
  - Palmoplantar pits
  - Discontinuity of the fingerprint lines (break of dermatoglyphics)
  - Epidermoid cysts.
- Histopathology: the pigmented macules show epidermal atrophy and an increased number of basal melanocytes.

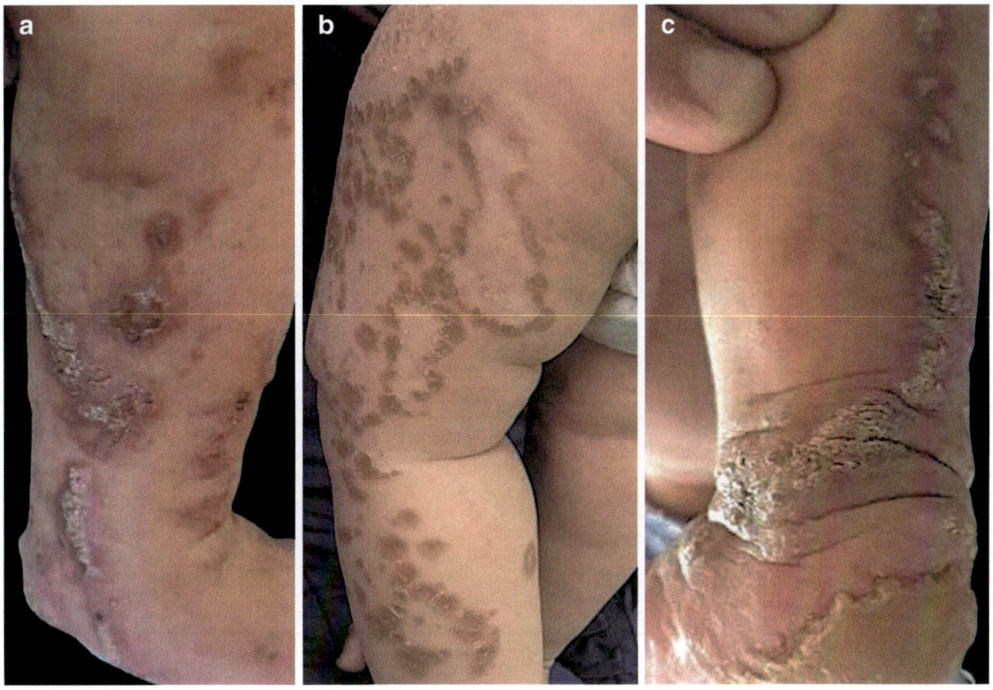

Fig. 4.17 Incontinentia pigmenti. Linear verrucous plaques on lower limbs following Blaschko lines (**a–c**)

Reticulate Acropigmentation of Dohi (RAD) (AD) [15] (Fig. 4.28)

- Reticulate acropigmentation of Dohi (RAD) is a rare dyschromic genodermatosis.
- Autosomal dominant inheritance, with mutation of Adenosine Deaminase gene
- Onset: Infancy or early childhood
- Clinical characteristics:
  - Reticulate hyperpigmented and hypopigmented pinpoint to pea-sized flat macules over dorsa of hands and feet without affection of palms and hands.
  - There were no palmar pits or breaks of fingerprint lines
  - Freckle-like macules on face.
- Histopathology: hyperpigmented and hypopigmented macules show basal melanosis and hypomelanosis, respectively.
- D.D.: DDD, RAK, dyschromatosis universalis hereditaria (DUH), xeroderma pigmentosum.

Dyschromatosis Universalis Hereditaria (DUH) (AD/AR) [16] (Figs. 4.29, 4.30, and 4.31)

- A spectrum of dyschromatoses disorders includes DUH, dyschromatosis symmetrica hereditaria (DSH) or RAD, and a segmental form called unilateral dermatomal pigmentary dermatosis.
- Autosomal dominant or autosomal recessive patterns of inheritance, with mutation of *ABCB6* gene
- Onset: Infancy or early childhood
- Clinical characteristics:
  - Generalized hypo- and hyperpigmented macules in reticulate pattern in trunk and extremities, spreading to the face, hands, and feet.
  - It usually spares palms and soles.
  - Hair, teeth, and nails may be involved.
- Histopathology: focal increase or decrease in melanin content of the basal layer (depending on the type of the lesion biopsied) and occasionally pigmentary incontinence.

Naegeli–Franceschetti–Adassohn Syndrome (NFJS) (AD) [17] (Fig. 4.32)

- Naegeli–Franceschetti–Jadassohn Syndrome (NFJS) is a rare form of ectodermal dysplasia that affects skin, sweat glands, nails, and teeth.
- Autosomal dominant inheritance, with mutation of *KRT14* gene.
- Onset: during infancy
- Clinical characteristics:
  - Reticulated hyperpigmentation on neck, chest and abdomen, and fading by puberty.
  - Palmoplantar keratoderma, brittle toenails, and absent dermatoglyphs.
  - Mucosal pigmentation.
  - Sparse scalp hair
  - Abnormal sweating and heat intolerance
  - Dental abnormalities (Defective dentures with yellow spots on the enamel)

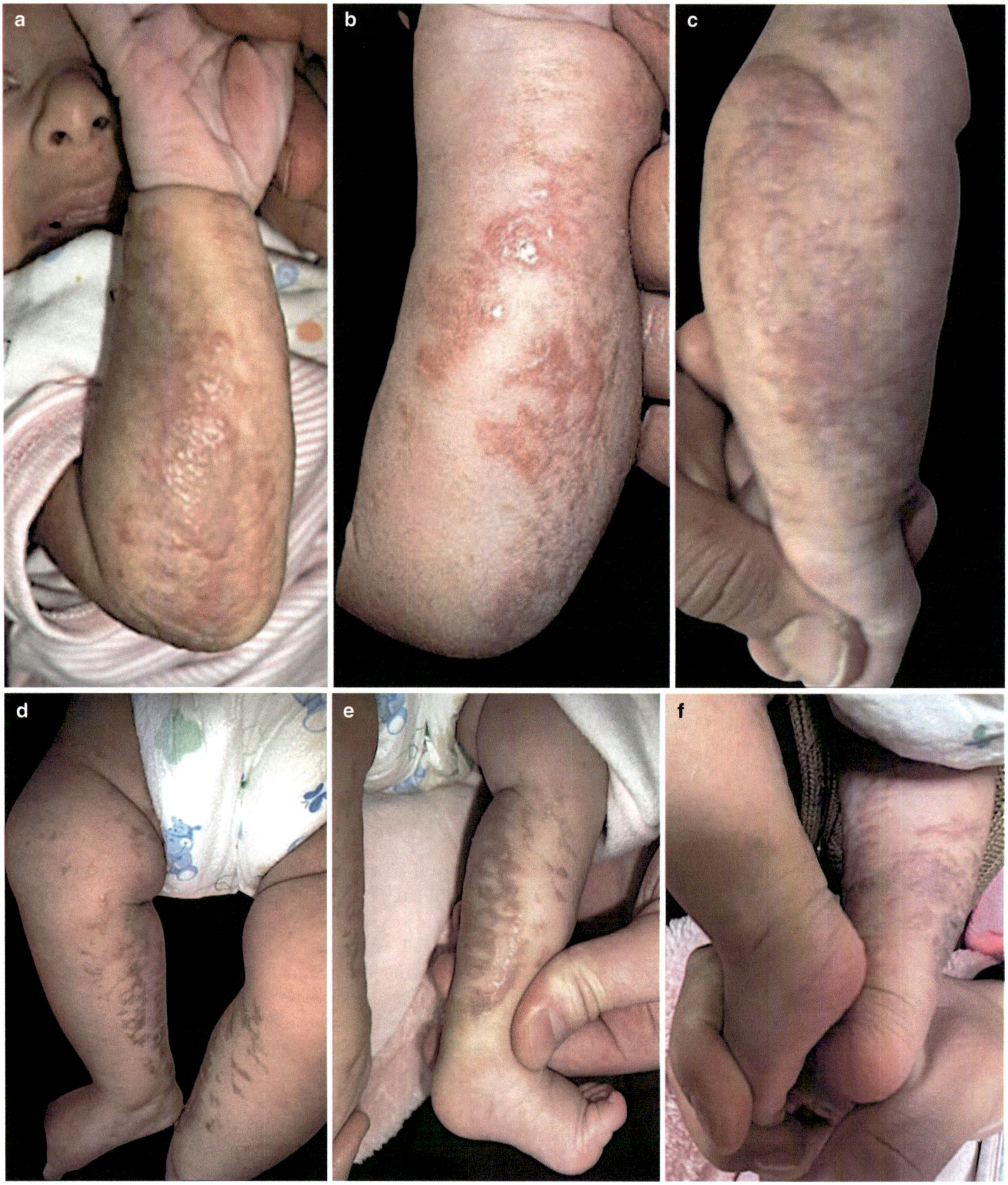

Fig. 4.18 Incontinentia pigmenti. An infant with linear verrucous erythematous plaques on the upper and lower limbs following Balshcko lines (**a**–**f**)

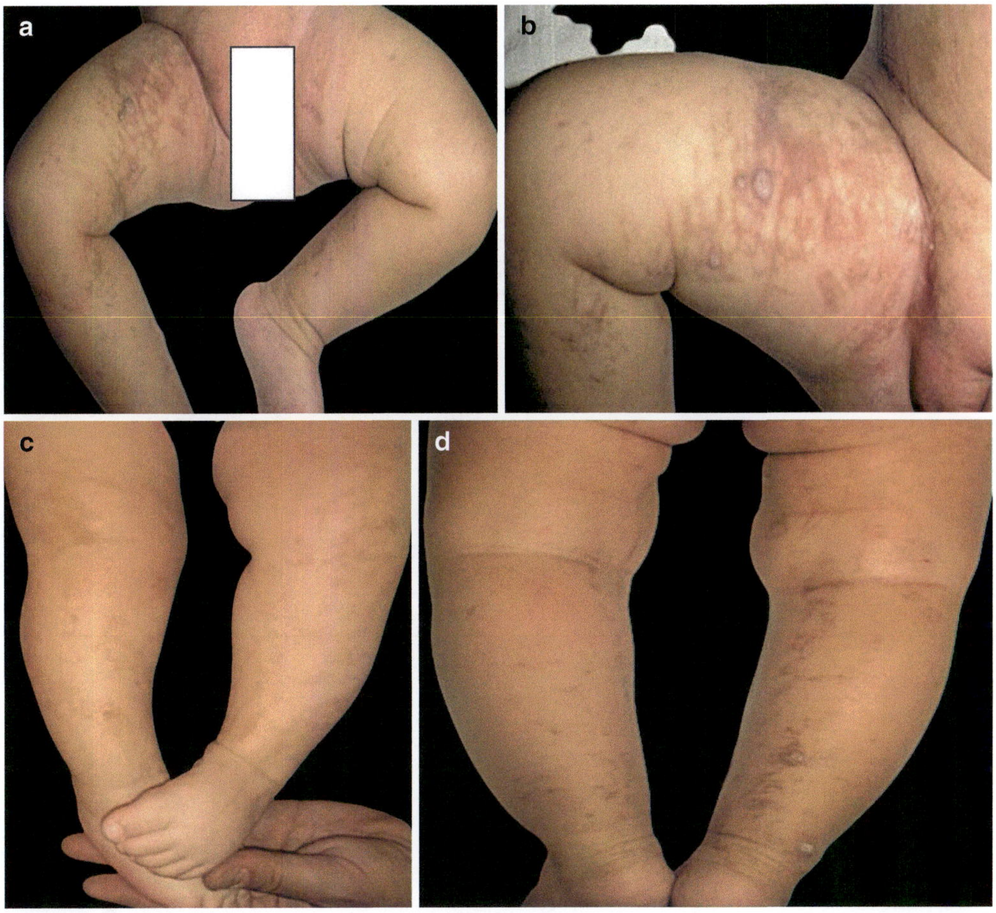

Fig. 4.19 Incontinentia pigmenti. Verrucous plaques and hyperpigmentation following Blaschko lines on the intertriginous areas and lower limbs (**a**–**d**)

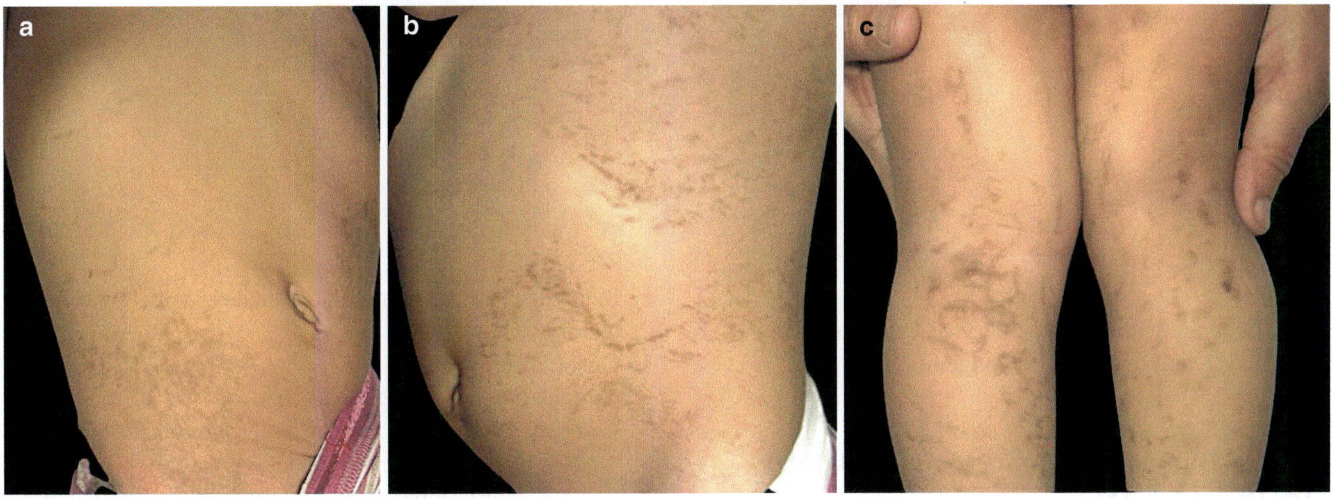

Fig. 4.20 Incontinentia pigmenti. Hyperpigmentation following Blaschko lines on the trunk and lower limbs (**a**–**c**)

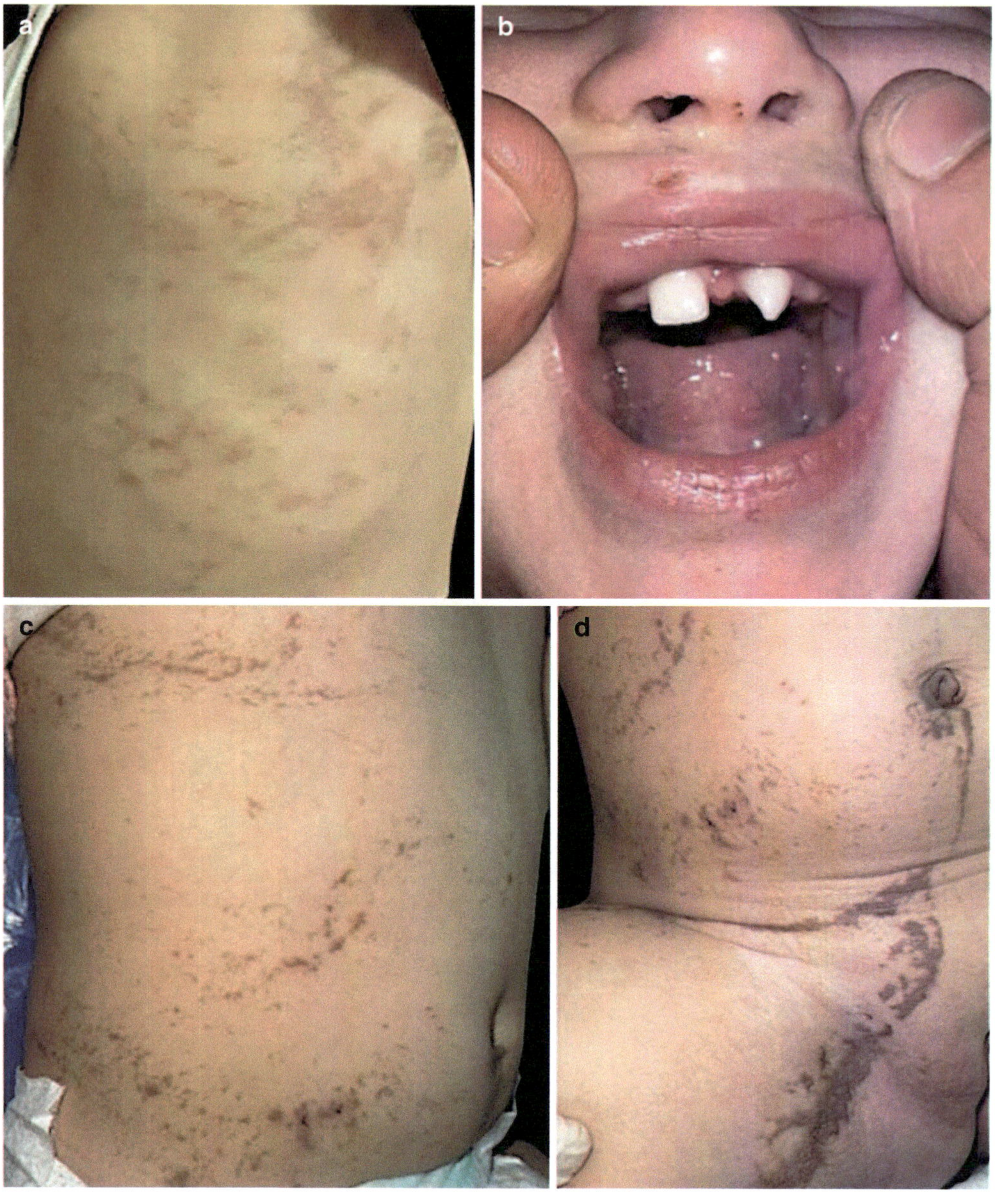

Fig. 4.21 Incontinentia pigmenti. Cone-shaped and agenesis of teeth (**a**, **b**), linear verrucous plaques on the trunk and intertriginous areas follow Blaschko lines (**c**, **d**)

- D.D.
  - Other reticulate pigmentary diseases as DDD, RAK, RAD, and dyskeratosis congenita.

Familial Gigantic Melanocytosis (FGM) (AD) [18, 19] (Fig. 4.33)

- Familial gigantic melanocytosis (FGM) is a rare disorder first described by El-Darouti et al. in 1984 and termed "familial melanopathy with gigantic melanocytes" (FMGM).
- Autosomal dominant inheritance.
- The cause of the disorder remains unknown, however, melanocytes in both hyper- and hypopigmented skin seem to be unable to deliver melanin to the surrounding keratinocytes.
- Incidence: more common in males, with +ve family history.
- Onset: after birth.
- Clinical characteristics:
  - There is a diffuse brown hyperpigmentation studded with raindrop hypopigmentation that affects the face, neck, chest, upper arms, and the trunk but with a lesser extent.
  - Affected skin is of normal texture and shows no redness, scaling, or atrophy. Photosensitivity is absent.
  - Sparse axillary and pubic hair
  - Light-colored scalp and body hair.
- Histopathology: presence of abnormally large melanocytes laden with melanin and moderately hypopigmented keratinocytes, particularly in the hypopigmented areas and the walls of the hair follicles.

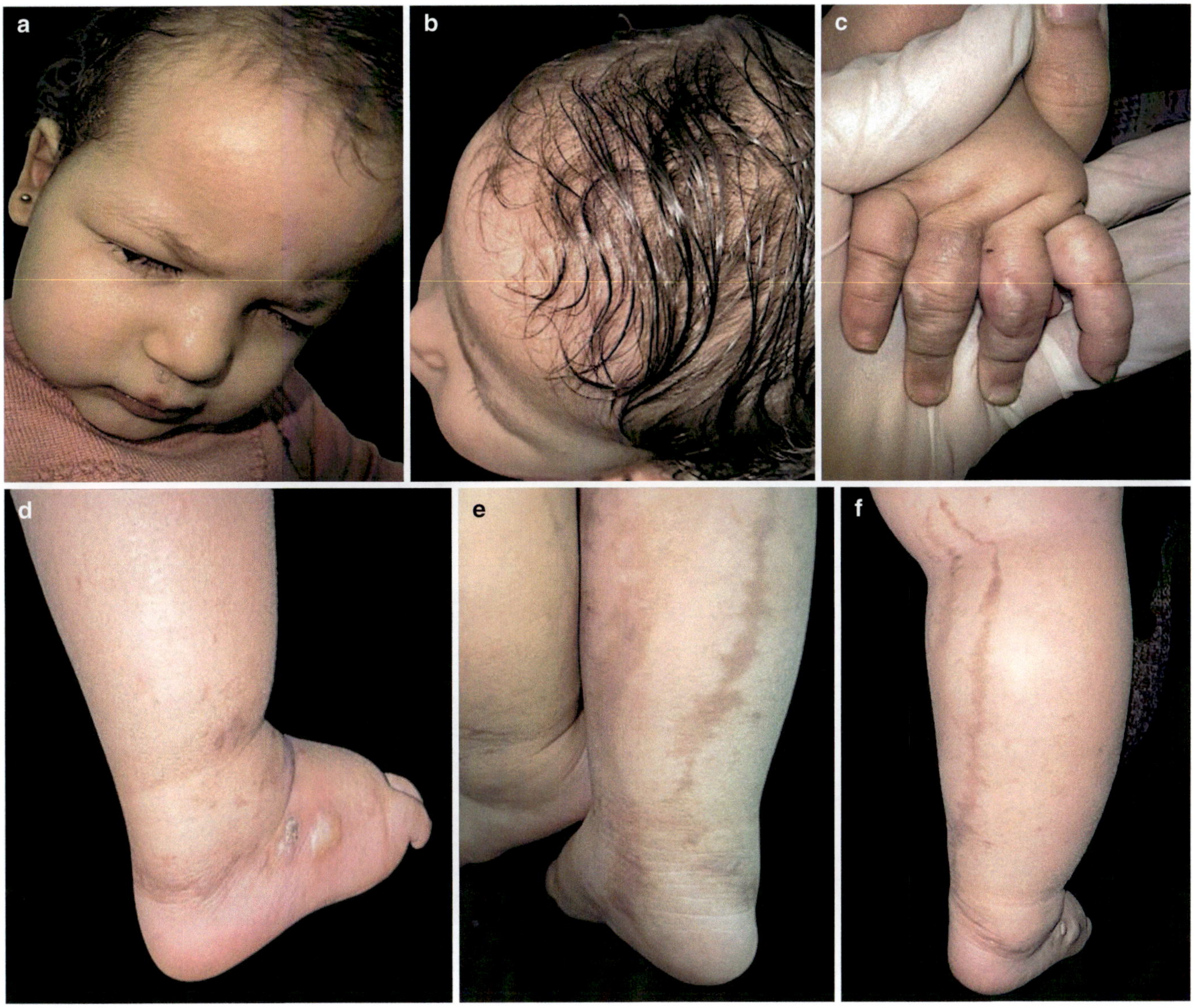

Fig. 4.22 Incontinentia pigmenti. A 9-months-old female infant with photophobia, diffuse hair loss (**a**, **b**), multiple erythematous vesicles on hand and feet (**c**, **d**), hyperpigmentation follow Blaschko lines on the lower limbs (**e**, **f**)

McCune–Albright Syndrome (MAS) [20] (Figs. 4.34 and 4.35)

- McCune–Albright syndrome (MAS) a sporadic disease affecting three areas: skeleton, skin, and endocrine system.
- Defect in *GNAS* gene, not inherited.
- Clinical characteristics:
  - Skin: Unilateral large café-au-lait hyperpigmented patches not crossing the midline with irregular geograpphic borders (coast of Maine). These spots must be differentiated from those characteristic of NF (NF = coast of California).
  - Bones: multiple pathologic fractures, scoliosis, unilateral polyostotic fibrous dysplasia.
  - Endocrinal:

    Precocious puberty (typically gonadotropin-independent). This includes breast development, genital maturation (with or without pubic hair growth), increased height velocity, and macroorchidism.

    Hypogonadotropic hypogonadism, particularly in the setting of hyperprolactinemia.

    Ovarian cysts.

    Hyperthyroidism; tachycardia, arrhythmias (mostly supraventricular), hypertension, hyperthermia, tremor, sleeplessness, weight loss, or failure to thrive (in infants).

    Cushing syndrome.

    Acromegaly from growth hormone excess.

    Pituitary tumors

    Hypophosphatemia (hypophosphatemic rickets).

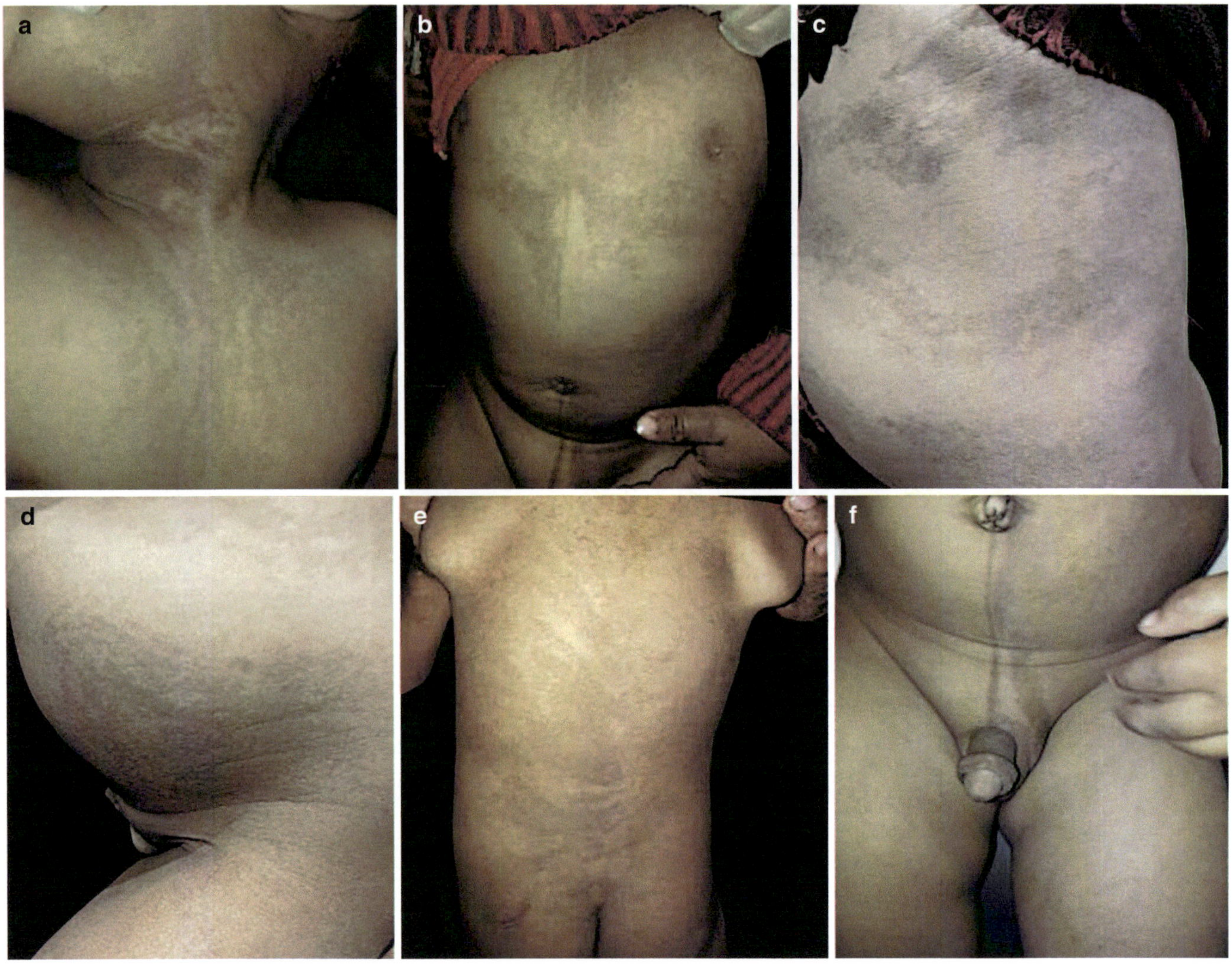

Fig. 4.23 Incontinentia pigmenti. Hyperpigmentations follow Balshcko lines on the neck, trunk, and intertriginous areas (**a**–**f**)

- Investigations:
  - Laboratory studies:
    Blood and urinary chemistries.
    Thyroid testing (thyroid-stimulating hormone [TSH], thyroxine [T4], antithyroid antibodies)
    Gonadotropin (luteinizing hormone [LH], follicle-stimulating hormone [FSH]), and sex hormone levels
    Adrenocorticotropic hormone (ACTH) levels
    Serum prolactin (PRL)
    Growth hormone (GH) and insulin-like growth factor 1 (IGF-1) levels
    Dexamethasone suppression testing (standard or low-dose/high-dose)
    Urine collection assayed for free cortisol (urinary free cortisol [UFC])
    Polymerase chain reaction (PCR) assay
  - Diagnostic imaging modalities:
    Plain radiography [mainly skull and mandibles (craniofacial survey), pelvis; as clinically indicated].
    Ultrasonography (neck and thyroid, ovarias and pelvis; as clinically indicated)
    Computed tomography (CT); as clinically pertinent.
    Magnetic resonance imaging (MRI); as clinically pertinent.
    Radionuclide bone scanning.
  - Others:
    Arterial blood gas determination (for suspected acidosis)
    Electrocardiography (ECG); for suspected arrhythmia.
    Gastrointestinal (GI) endoscopy to evaluate polyposis.
    Biopsy (bone, muscle, soft tissue, thyroid); as clinically pertinent.

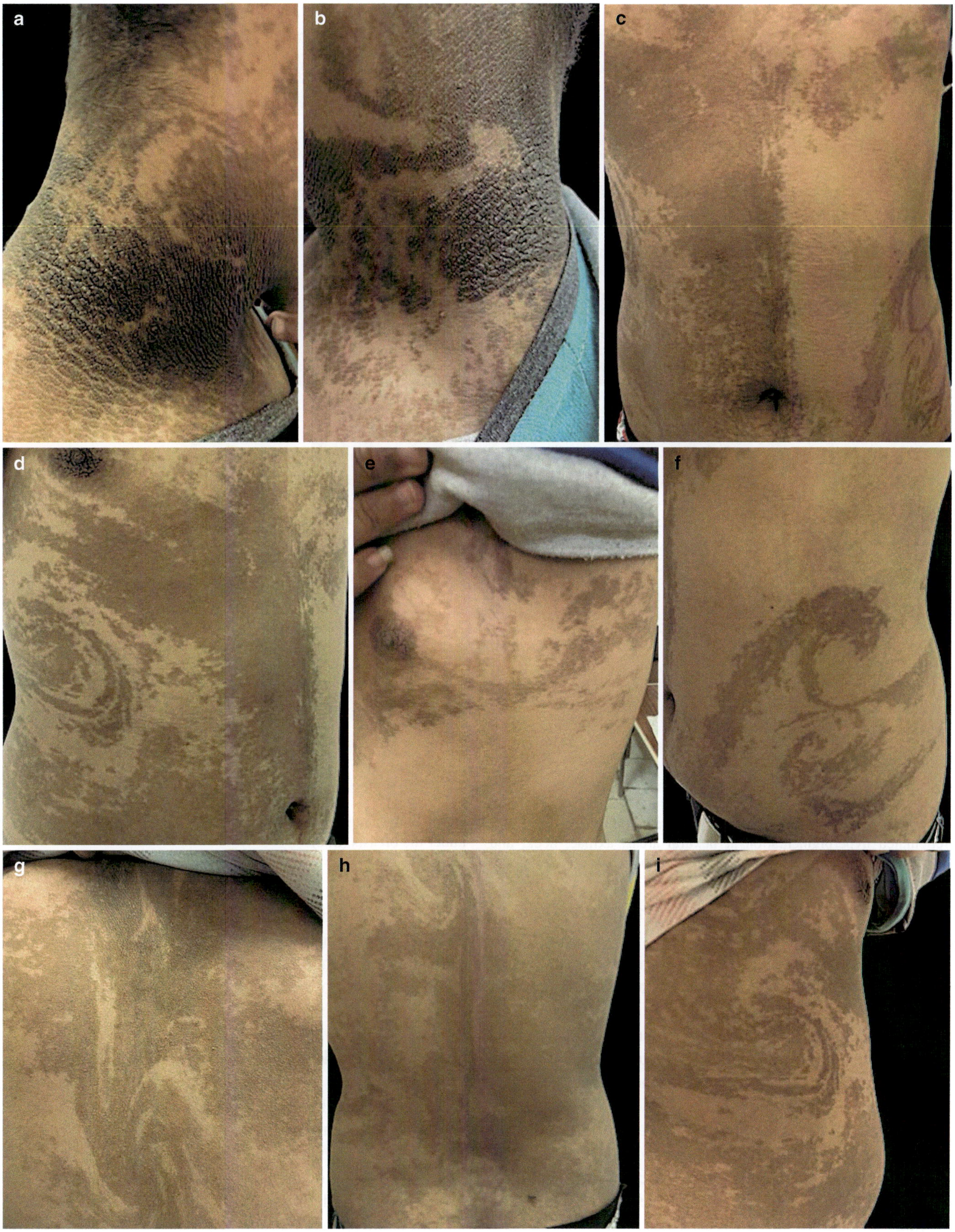

Fig. 4.24 Linear and whorled nevoid hypermelanosis. Streaks and swirls of hyperpigmentation along the Blaschko lines on the neck and trunk (**a**–**i**) with no preceding inflammation

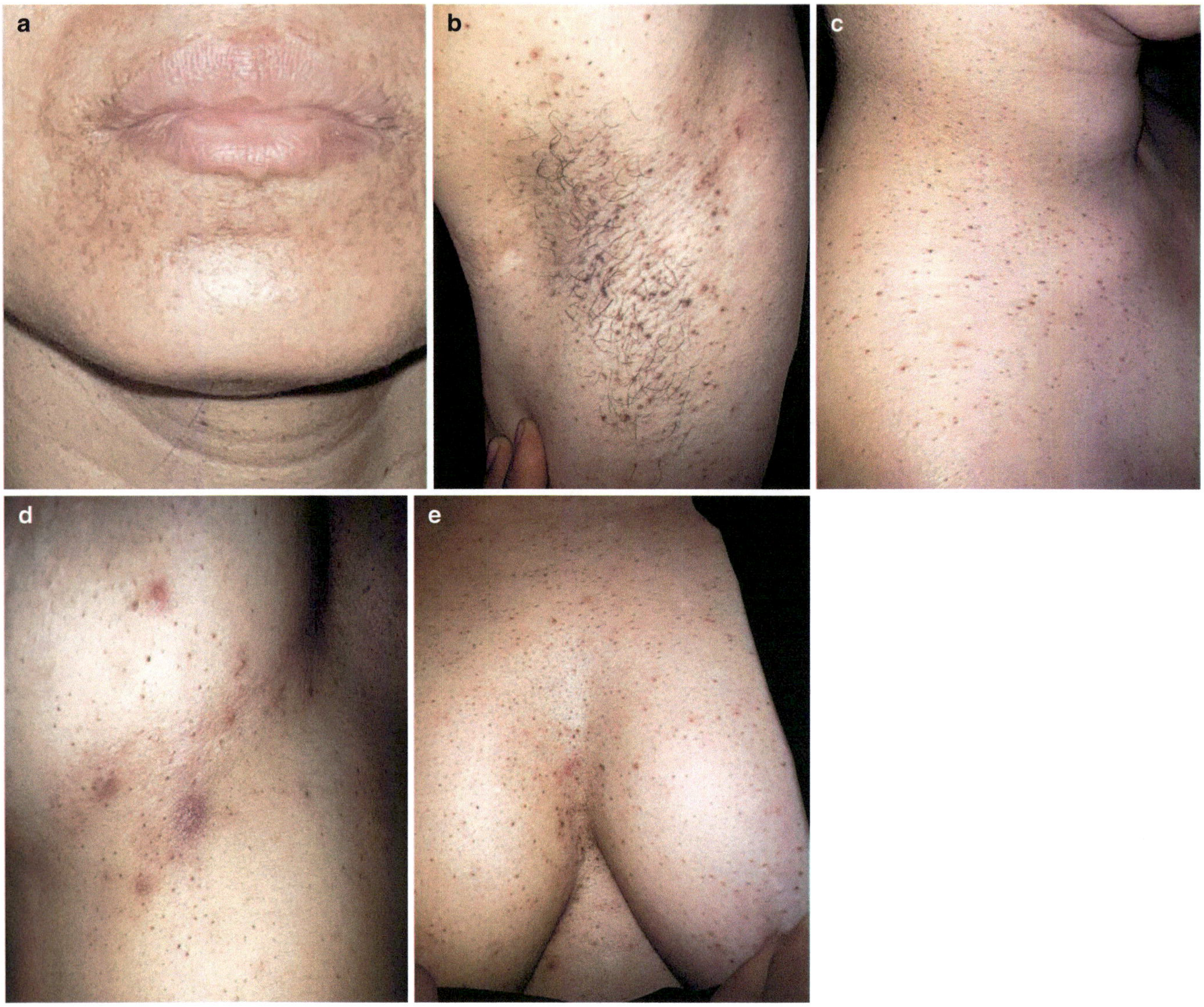

Fig. 4.25 Dowling–Degos disease. Perioral pitted facial scars (**a**), reticulated hyperpigmentation at flexural areas, axillae, neck, and upper chest (**b**–**e**), comedone-like lesions on neck, axillae, and upper chest (**b**–**e**), and hidradenitis suppurativa-like lesions inbetween and under the breasts (**d**, **e**)

Peutz–Jeghers Syndrome (AD) [21] (Fig. 4.36)

- The disease is caused by mutations in a tumor suppressor gene, *STK11* or *LKB1*, that is located on chromosome 19p13.3 ***se***
- There is pigmented or melanotic macules on the lips or in the mouth and polyps in the gastrointestinal tract.
- There is also a high risk of malignancy, particularly gastrointestinal cancer.
- The small bowel is the most common site for hamartomatous polyps followed by the colon and stomach.
- Polyps are also the most common cause for symptoms including obstructive symptoms, bleeding, anemia, and intussusception. The characteristics of polyps that are more likely to evolve into cancer is still unknown
- Polyps can also occur in other organs such as the lungs, renal pelvis, urinary bladder, and nasopharynx.
- There is a higher-than-expected risk in pancreas, lungs, breast, uterus, ovaries, and testes.

Laugier–Hunziker Syndrome [22] (Fig. 4.37)

- Laugier–Hunziker syndrome is a rare acquired macular hyperpigmentation of oral mucosa and lips frequently associated with longitudinal pigmentation of the nails usually beginning in the third to fifth decade of life with a female preponderance
- The pathogenesis is unknown, but no systemic involvement or malignant predisposition has been described.

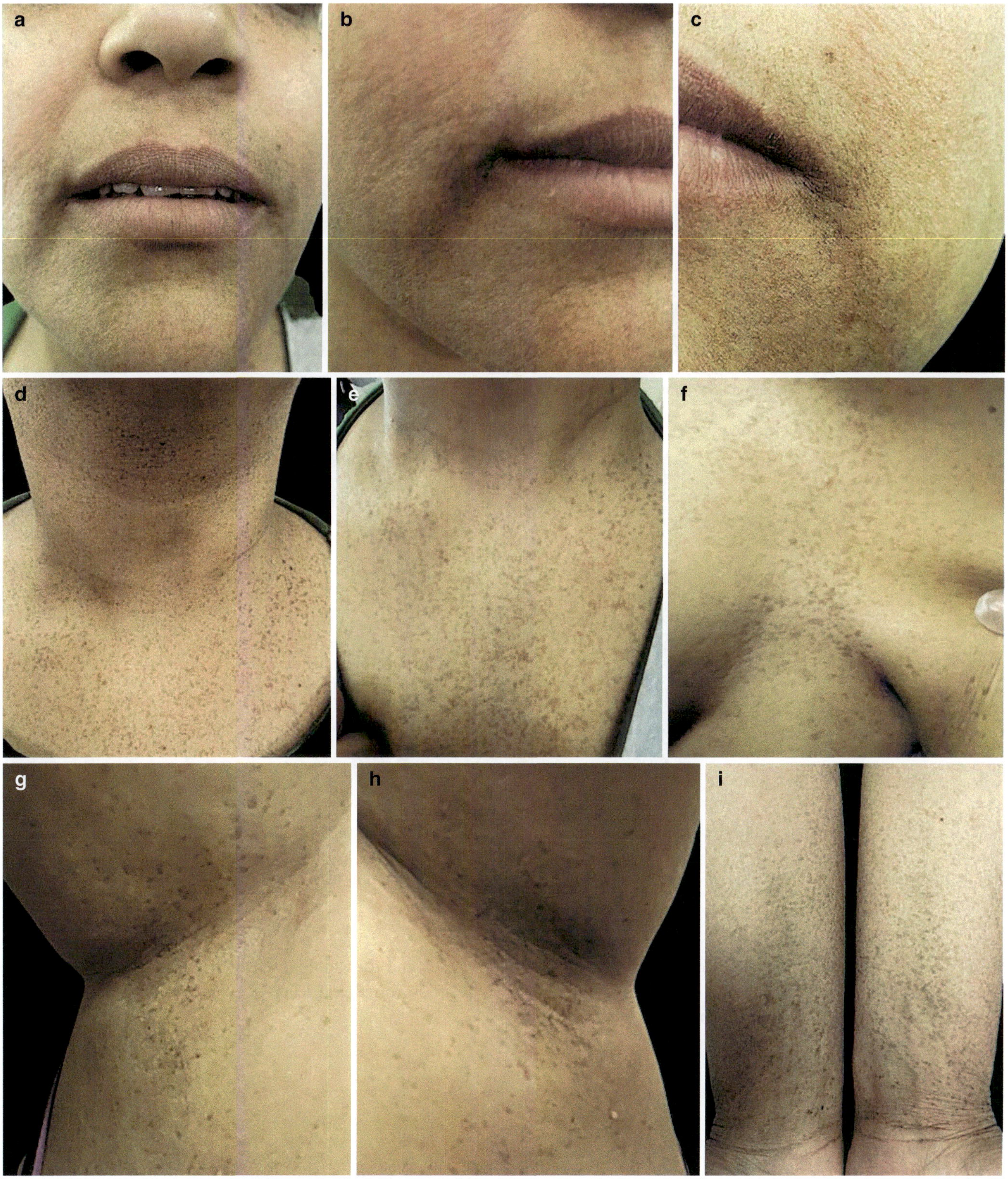

Fig. 4.26 Dowling-Degos disease. Perioral pitted facial scars (**a**–**c**), reticulated hyperpigmentation at neck, upper chest, axillae and popliteal fossae (**d**–**i**)

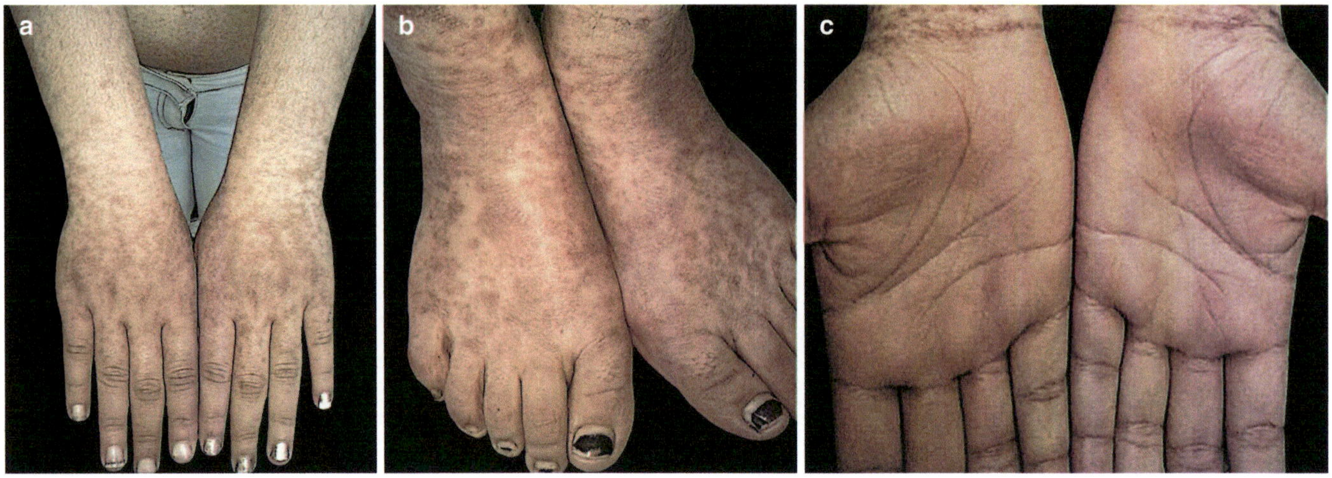

Fig. 4.27 Reticulate acropigmentation of Kitamura. Reticulate atrophic hyperpigmented macules (lentigo-like) on the dorsum of the hands and feet (**a**, **b**) and palmar pits (**c**)

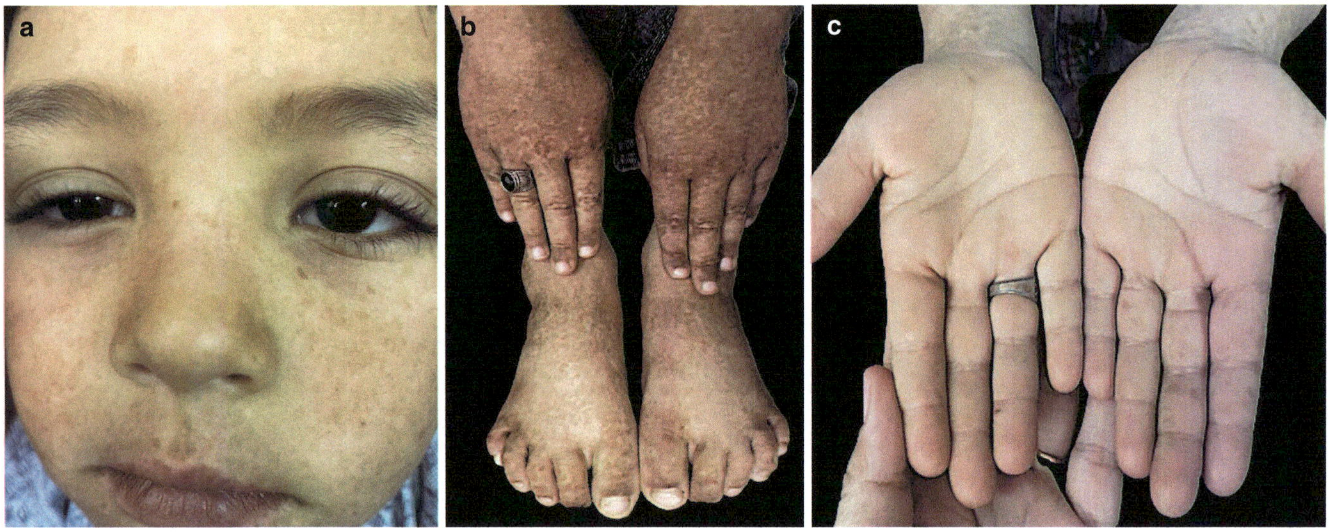

Fig. 4.28 Reticulate acropigmentation of Dohi. Reticulate hypo- and hyperpigmentation on the face, dorsum of the hands, and spare palms (**a**–**c**)

- The syndrome must be included in the differential diagnosis of diffuse oral pigmentation to exclude other conditions with systemic implications as Peutz–Jeghers syndrome or adrenal insufficiency, Carney complex, Carney complex, LEOPARD syndrome.

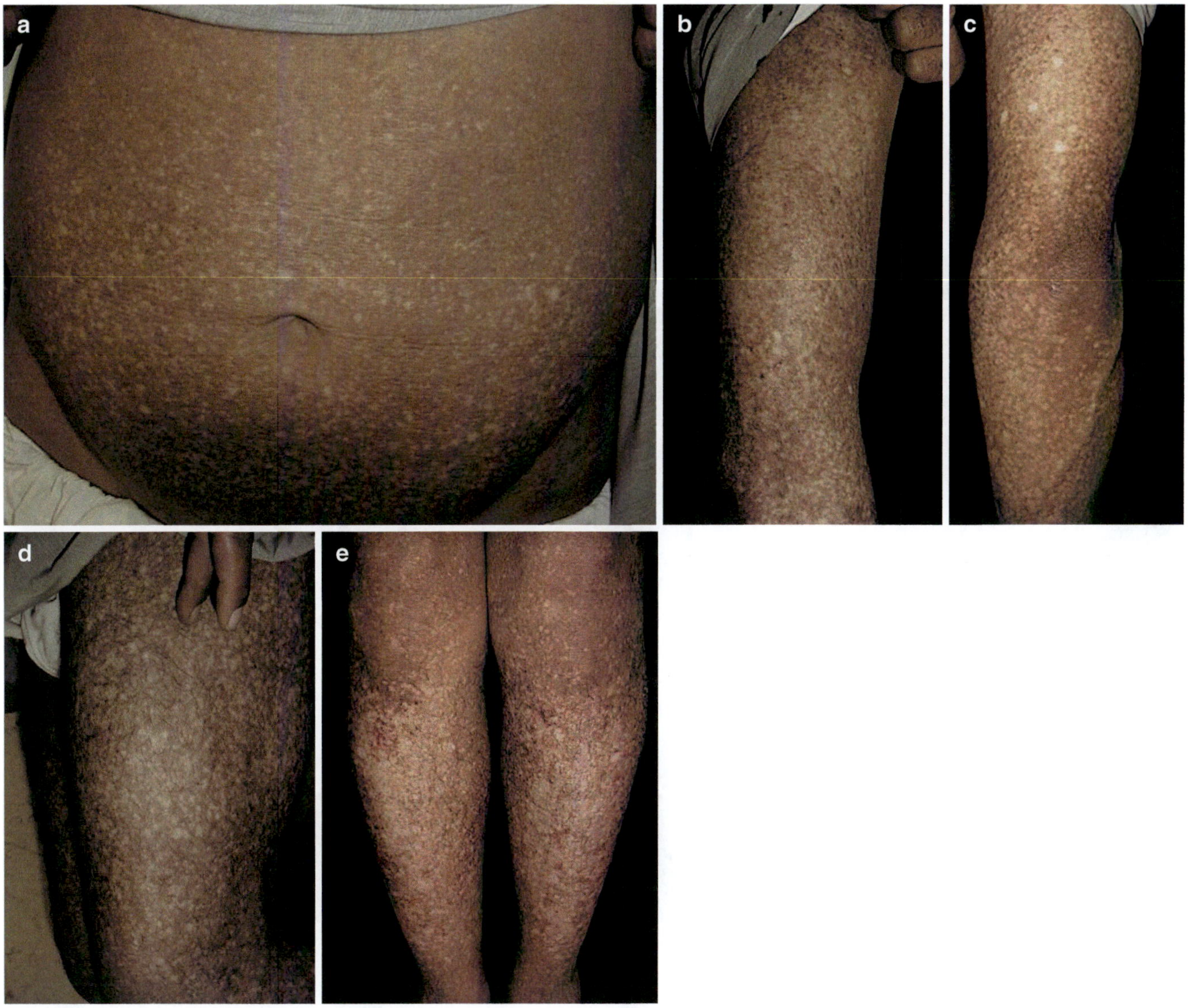

Fig. 4.29 Dyschromatosis universalis hereditaria. Generalized hypo- and hyperpigmented macules in reticulate pattern (**a**–**e**)

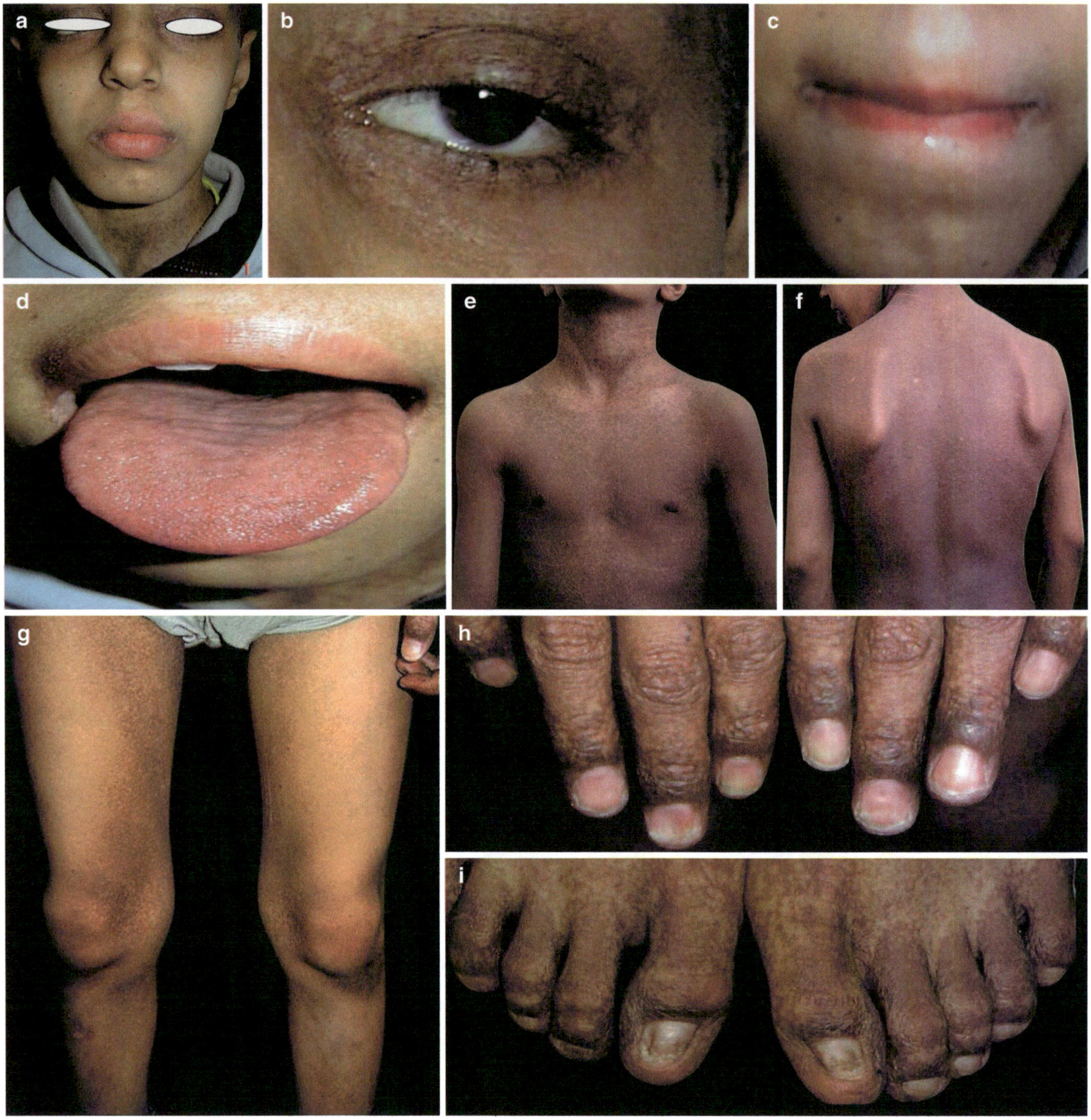

Fig. 4.30 Dyschromatosis universalis hereditaria. Generalized hypo- and hyperpigmented macules in reticulate pattern around eyes, neck, at angles of mouth (**a**–**d**), trunk, lower limbs and periungual and nails (**e**–**i**). (*Courtesy, Fatma Abdel Salam*)

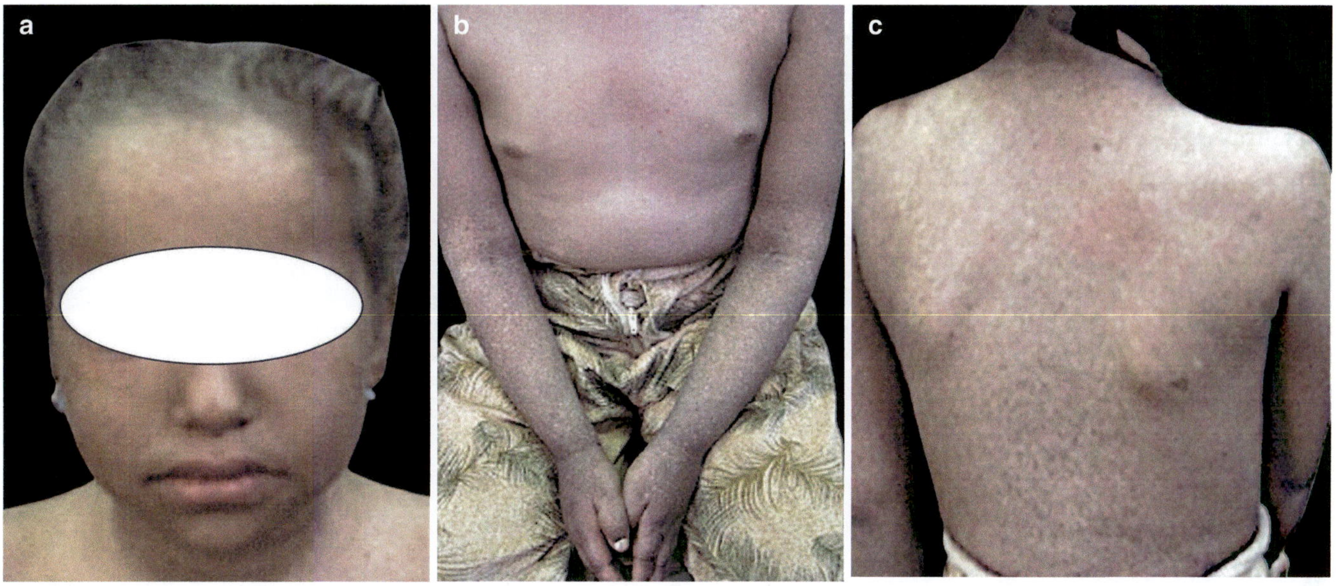

Fig. 4.31 Dyschromatosis universalis hereditaria. Generalized hypo- and hyperpigmented macules in reticulate pattern affecting the face, trunk, and limbs (**a**–**c**)

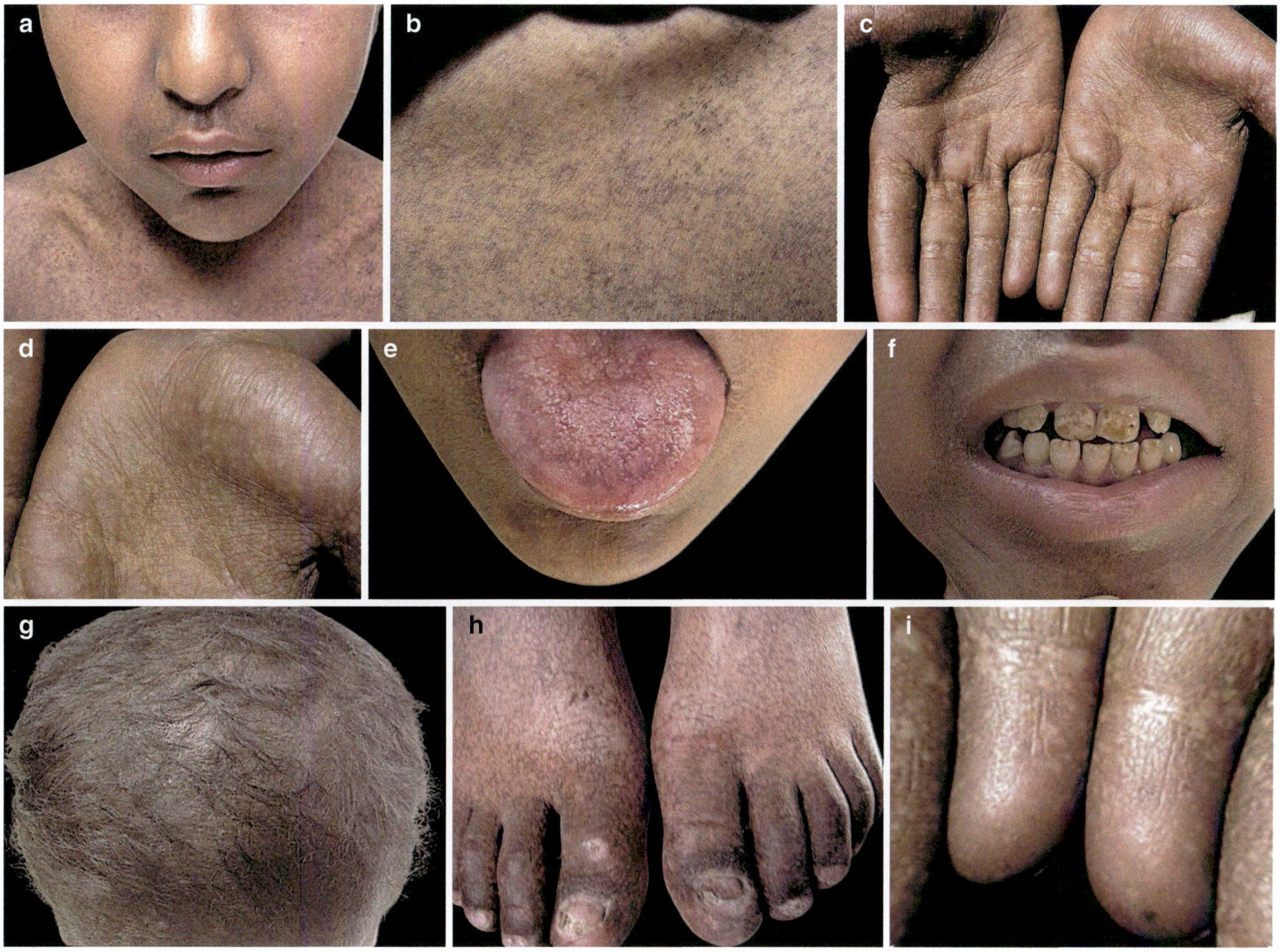

Fig. 4.32 Naegeli–Franceschetti–Jadassohn Syndrome (**a**–**d**): Reticulated hyperpigmentation during infancy peri-orally (**a**), and on chest (**b**) and hands (**c**, **d**). Mucosal pigmentation in tongue (**e**), yellow spots on the enamel (**f**), sparse scalp hair (**g**), periungual hyperpigmentation (**h**), and brittle toenails with absent dermatoglyphics (**i**)

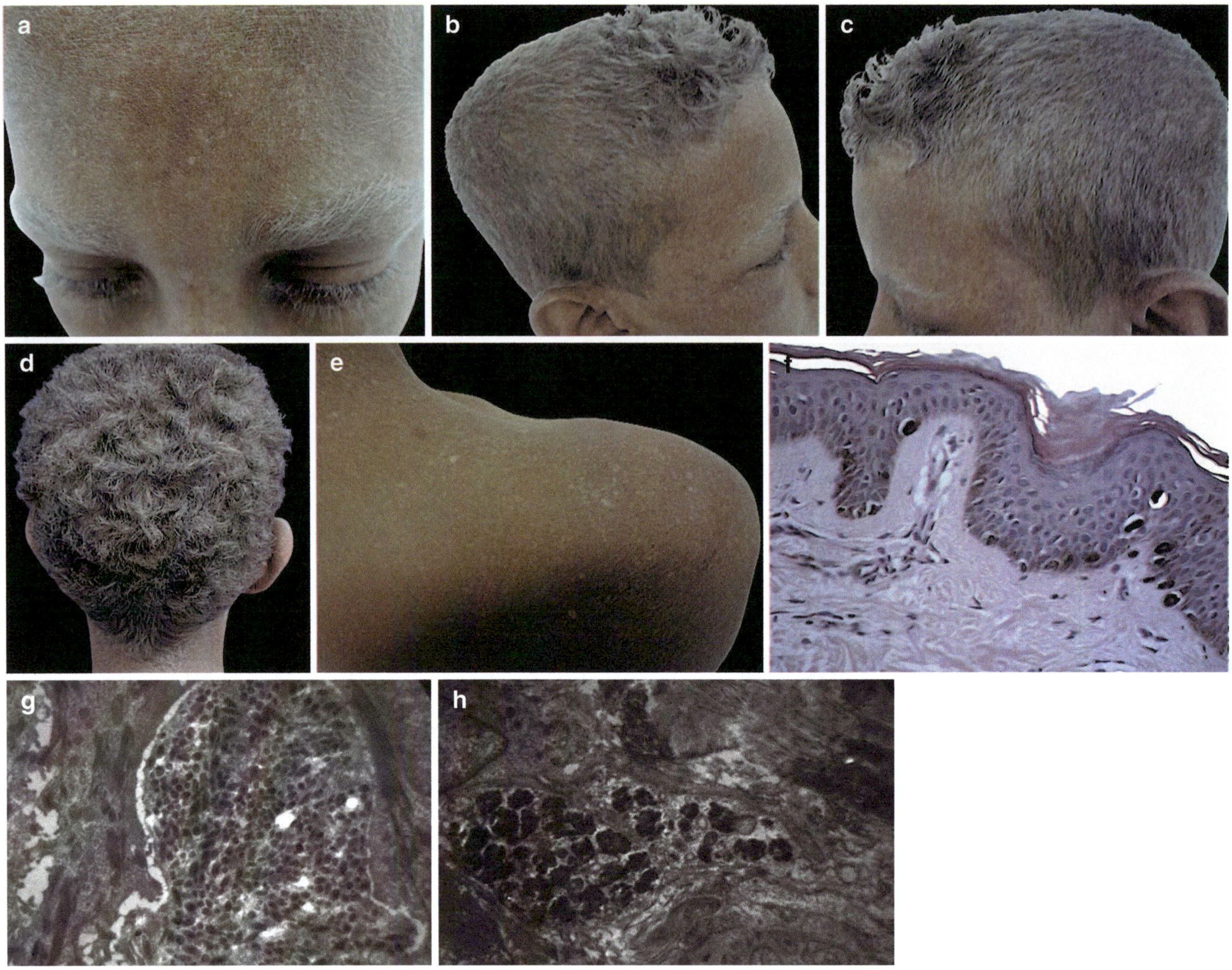

Fig. 4.33 Familial gigantic melanocytosis. Light colored scalp hairs (**a**–**e**), raindrop like hypopigmented macules (**a**–**c**, **f**), giant melanocytes (**g**), pericellular halos (**f**), large melanosomes by transmission electron microscopy (**g**, **h**)

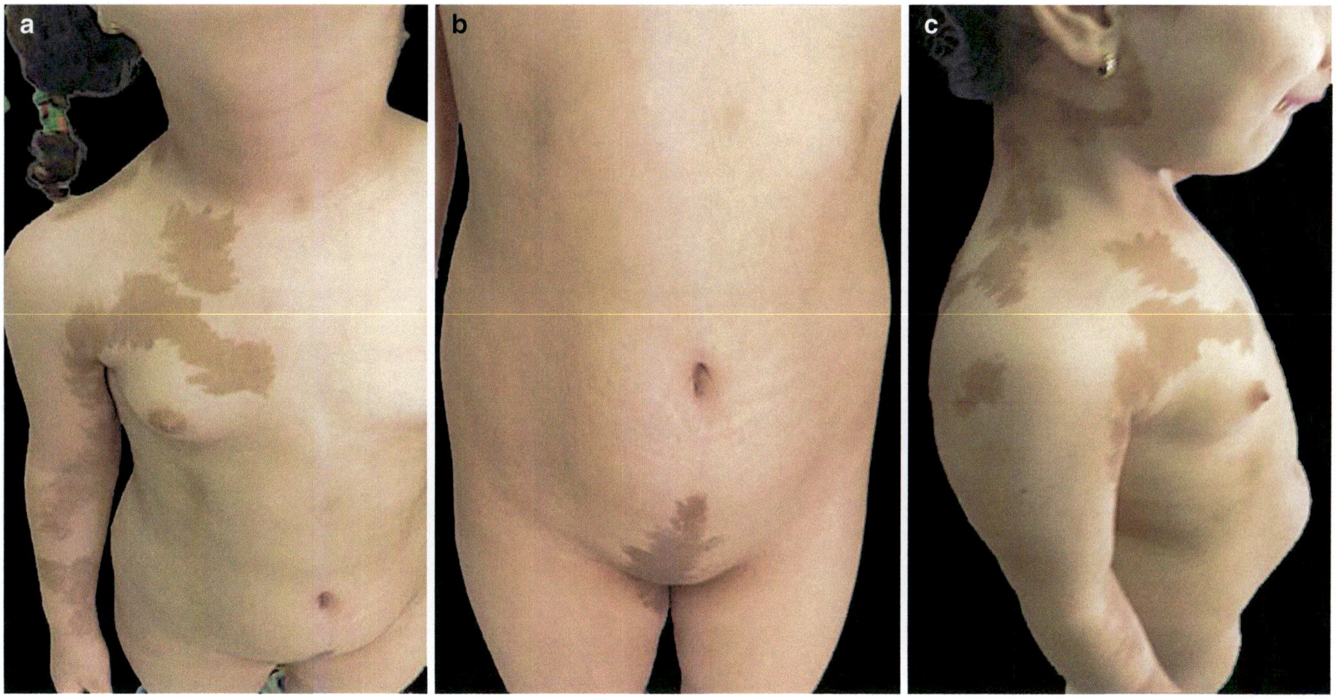

Fig. 4.34 McCune-Albright syndrome. Unilateral large café-au-lait patches not crossing the midline with irregular geographic borders (coast of Maine) (**a–c**). (*Courtesy, Ghada Raslan*)

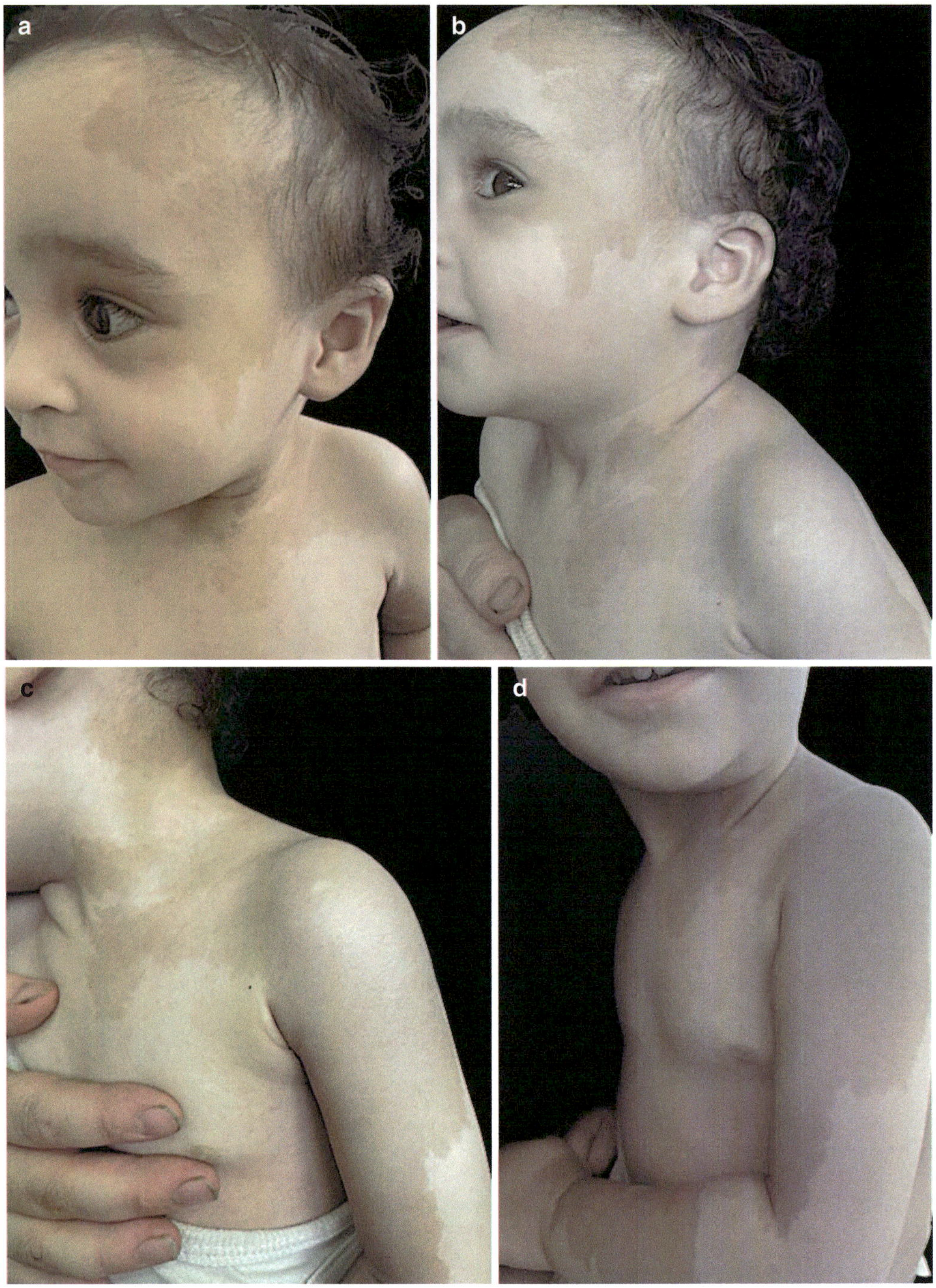

Fig. 4.35 McCune-Albright Syndrome. Unilateral large café-au-lait patches not crossing the midline with irregular geographic borders (coast of Maine) (**a–d**). (*Courtesy, Ghada Raslan*)

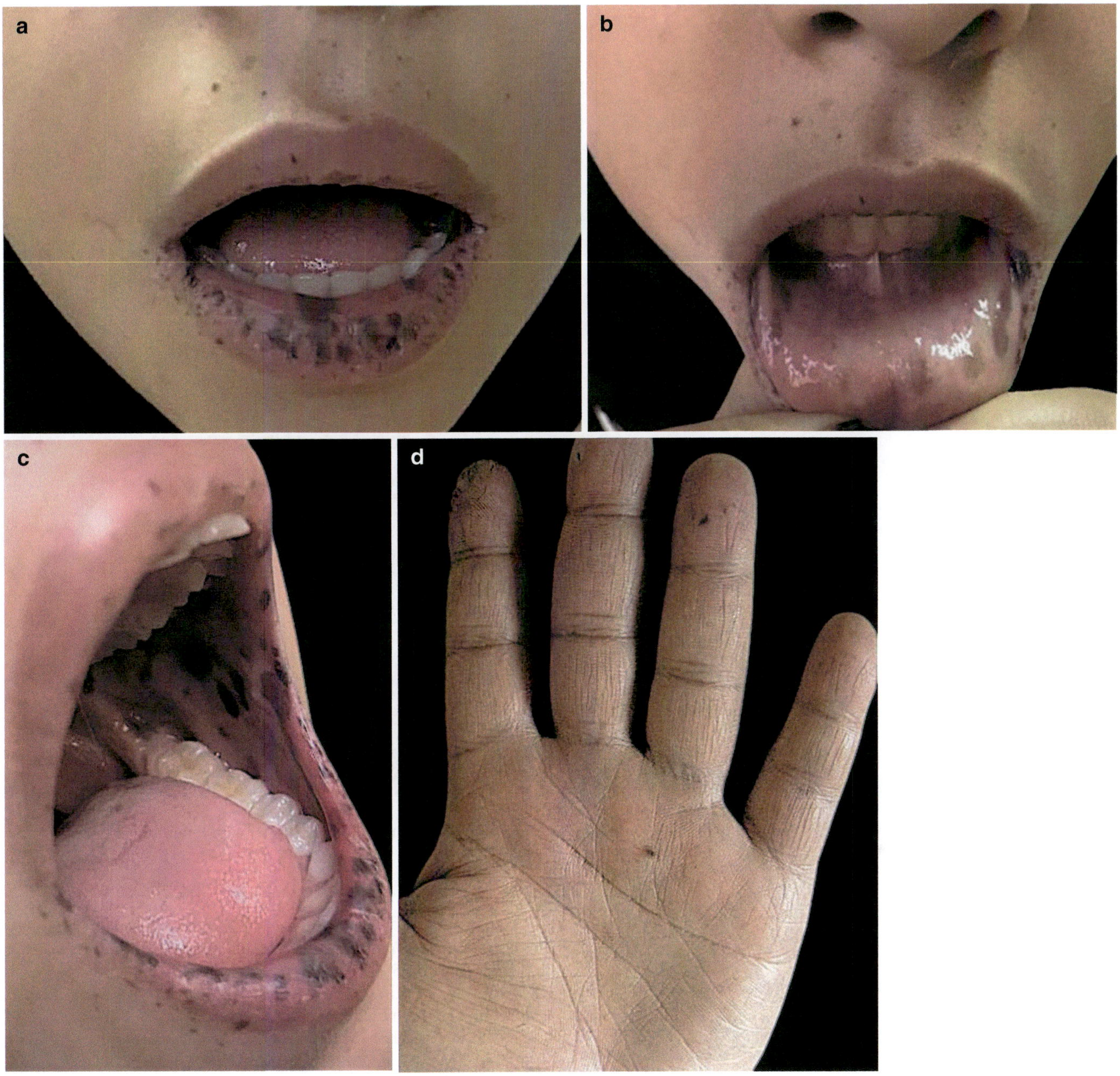

Fig. 4.36 Peutz Jegher syndrome. Dark brown mucocutaneous lentigines perioral, on mucocutaneous junction, the lips, buccal mucosa (**a**–**c**), and palm (**d**)

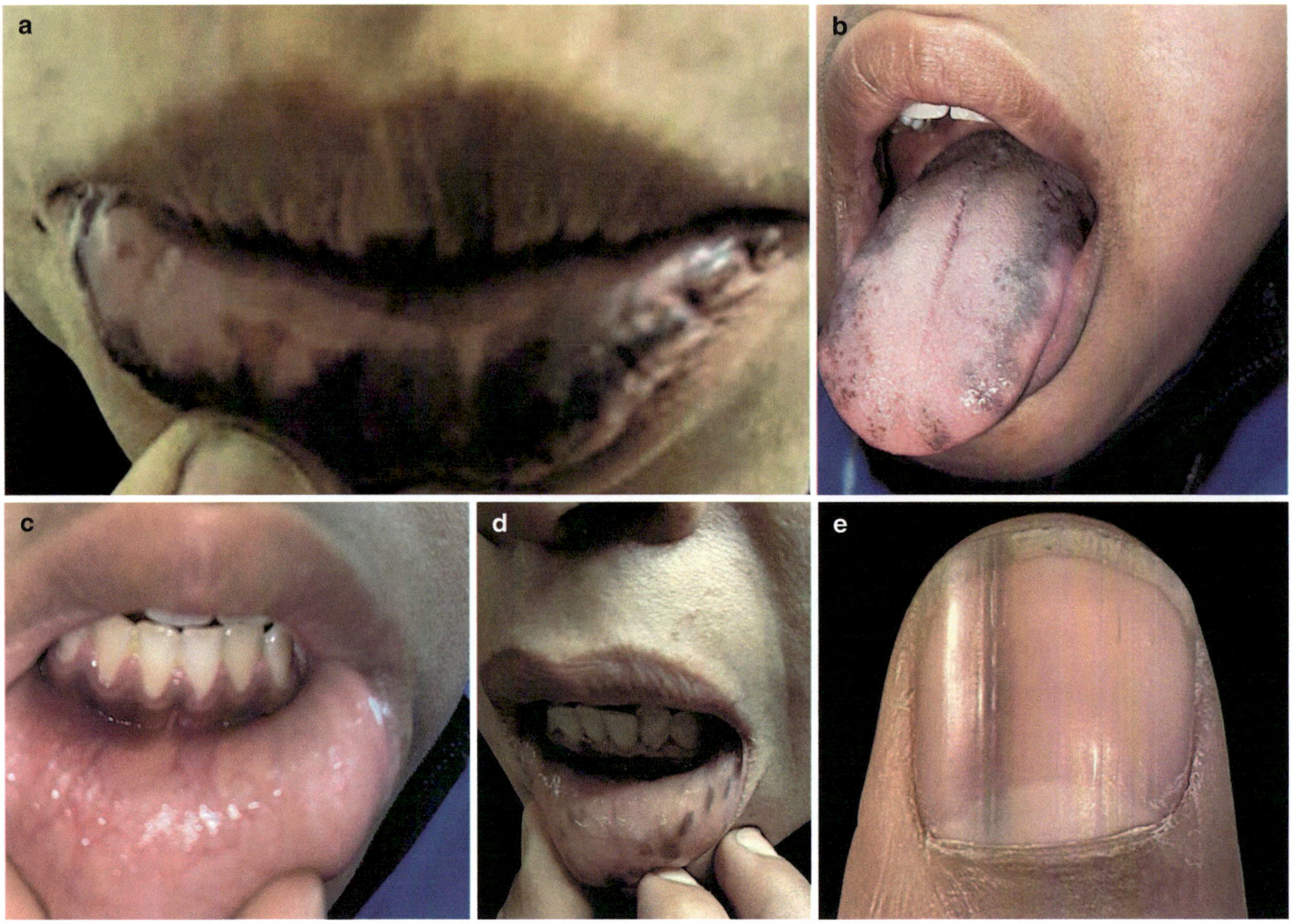

Fig. 4.37 Laugier-Hunziker syndrome. Pigmentation on lower lip, tongue, gum (**a–c**), lentigines on lower lip (**d**) with longitudinal melanonychia (**e**)

References

1. Passeron T, Mantoux F, Ortonne JP. Genetic disorders of pigmentation. Clin Dermatol. 2005;23:56–67.
2. Saleem MD. Biology of human melanocyte development, Piebaldism, and Waardenburg syndrome. Pediatr Dermatol. 2019;36:72–84.
3. Oetting WS, King RA. Molecular basis of albinism: mutations and polymorphisms of pigmentation genes associated with albinism. Hum Mutat. 1999;13:99–115.
4. Zlotogora J. X-linked albinism-deafness syndrome and Waardenburg syndrome type II: a hypothesis. Am J Med Genet. 1995;59:386–7.
5. Li W, Zhang Q, Oiso N, et al. Hermansky-Pudlak syndrome type 7 (HPS-7) results from mutant dysbindin, a member of the biogenesis of lysosome-related organelles complex 1 (BLOC-1). Nat Genet. 2003;35:84–9.
6. Menasche G, Ho CH, Sanal O, et al. Griscelli syndrome restricted to hypopigmentation results from a melanophilin defect (GS3) or a MYO5A F-exon deletion (GS1). J Clin Invest. 2003;112: 450–6.
7. Sakata VM, da Silva FT, Hirata CE, et al. Diagnosis and classification of Vogt-Koyanagi-Harada disease. Autoimmun Rev. 2014;13(4-5):550–5.
8. Damico FM, Kiss S, Young LH. Vogt-Koyanagi-Harada disease. Semin Ophthalmol. 2005;20:183–90.
9. Andrade A, Pithon M. Alezzandrini syndrome: report of a sixth clinical case. Dermatology. 2011;222:8–9.
10. Kuster W, Konig A. Hypomelanosis of Ito: no entity, but a cutaneous sign of mosaicism. Am J Med Genet. 1999;85:346–50.
11. Hand JL. What's new with common genetic skin disorders? Curr Opin Pediatr. 2015;27:460–5.
12. Sinha P, Chatterjee M, Singh KK, et al. Linear and whorled nevoid hypermelanosis with depigmentation. Indian Dermatol Online J. 2017;8:131–3.
13. Stephan C, Kurban M, Abbas O. Dowling-Degos disease: a review. Int J Dermatol. 2021;60:944–50.
14. Tang JC, Escandon J, Shiman M, et al. Presentation of reticulate acropigmentation of Kitamura and Dowling-Degos disease overlap. J Clin Aesthet Dermatol. 2012;5:41–3.
15. Mohana D, Verma U, Amar AJ, et al. Reticulate acropigmentation of Dohi: a case report with insight into genodermatoses with mottled pigmentation. Indian J Dermatol. 2012;57:42–4.

16. Sethuraman G, Srinivas CR, D'Souza M, et al. Dyschromatosis universalis hereditaria. Clin Exp Dermatol. 2002;27:477–9.
17. Shah BJ, Gupta NP, Dhamale SS. Naegeli–Franceschetti–Jadassohn syndrome: aa rare case. Indian Dermatol Online J. 2015;6:403–6.
18. El-Darouti MA. Familial melanopathy with gigantic melanocytes. Am J Dermatopathol. 1984;6(suppl):31–4.
19. El-Darouti MA, Fawzi SA, Marzook SA, et al. Familial gigantic melanocytosis. Int J Dermatol. 2005;44:1010–5.
20. Brillante B, Guthrie L, Van Ryzin C. McCune-Albright syndrome: an overview of clinical features. J Pediatr Nurs. 2015;30:815–7.
21. Tacheci I, Kopacova M, Bures J. Peutz-Jeghers syndrome. Curr Opin Gastroenterol. 2021;37:245–54.
22. Moore RT, Chae KAM, Rhodes AR. Laugier and Hunziker pigmentation: a lentiginous proliferation of melanocytes. J Am Acad Dermatol. 2004;50:S70–4.

5 Genodermatoses with Malignant Potential

Disease-associated malignancy may occur in several inherited conditions with dermatologic manifestations [1–3]. These genodermatoses include the following:

1. Tuberous sclerosis
2. Neurofibromatosis
3. Birt-Hogg-Dubé Syndrome
4. Cowden's disease
5. Gorlin Syndrome
6. Bazex-Dupré-Christol Syndrome
7. Rombo syndrome
8. Reed syndrome
9. Brooke-Spiegler Syndrome

Tuberous Sclerosis (AD) [3–6] (Figs. 5.1, 5.2, 5.3, 5.4, 5.5, 5.6, 5.7, and 5.8)

- Autosomal dominant syndrome with variable expression.
- Mutations in a tumor suppressor gene either *TSC1* or *TSC2*.
- Manifested by hamartomatous tumors in multiple organs, including brain, eyes, heart, kidneys, lungs, and skin.
- Typically shows three clinical features, the Vogt triad which consists of mental retardation, epilepsy, and facial angiofibroma; however, approximately half of the patients have normal intelligence and a quarter do not have seizures.
- Skin lesions occur in nearly all individuals and are important for diagnosis.
- Skin lesions include hypomelanotic macules, confetti skin lesions, facial angiofibromas, fibrous facial plaque, shagreen patch, and periungual fibromas.
- Hypomelanotic macules "Ash leaf spots": appear at birth or shortly after and are most useful in early diagnosis.
- Facial angiofibroma: erythematous lesions located on the cheeks, nose, nasolabial folds, and chin, often sparing the upper lip.
- Shagreen patch (characteristic truncal lesion): is a connective tissue hamartoma located in the lower back region. A shagreen patch has an orange peel or leathery texture and often presents in children aged 2–6 years but may not appear until puberty.
- Fibroma: multiple flesh-colored non-traumatic subungual or periungual fibroma (Koenen tumor) in toenail more than fingers.
- Other features include molluscum fibrosum pendulum; commonly seen on the neck, groin, axillae, and near flexures of extremities, especially in adults and café-au-lait macules.
- Associations:
  - CNS: low intelligence, seizures, infantile spasm, cortical tubers (hamartoma), cognitive impairment, behavioral problems, and autism.
  - Eyes: retinal phakomata, achromic retinal patch, retinal astrocytoma, retinal gliomas.
  - Cardiac: cardiac rhabdomyomas (earliest finding in the first 3 years of life).
  - Pulmonary: lymphangioleiomyomatosis, pulmonary cyst (pneumothorax).
  - Dental: enamel hypoplasia (pitted enamel common).
  - Renal: angiomyolipoma, multiple bilateral renal cysts, carcinoma, renal failure.
  - Endocrinal: precocious puberty and hypothyroidism.
- Definite diagnostic criteria for tuberous sclerosis include two major (excluding lymphangioleiomyomatosis and renal angiomyolipoma alone) or one major and two minor criteria and possible diagnosis include either one major feature or ≥two minor features (Table 5.1).

N. Moftah et al., *Atlas of Common and Rare Genodermatoses*, https://doi.org/10.1007/978-3-031-60788-2_5

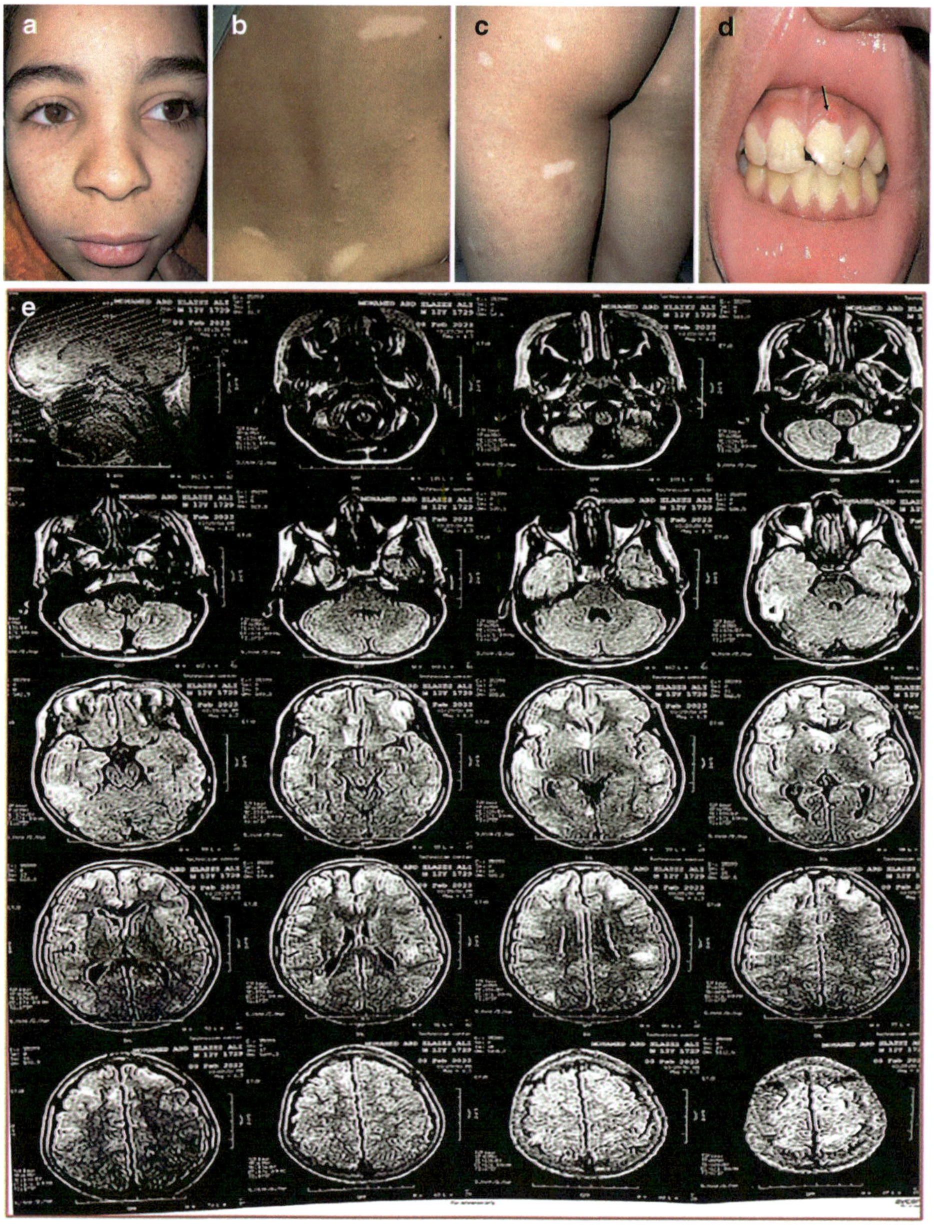

Fig. 5.1 Tuberous sclerosis. Facial angiofibroma (**a**), shagreen patches on the back (**b**), ash leaf hypopigmented patches on back, buttocks, and thighs (**b**, **c**), and angiofibroma of the gingiva (black arrow) (**d**). MRI showing multiple high signal foci in supra-tentorial cerebrum and intraventricular in frontal horn of the right lateral ventricle (**e**)

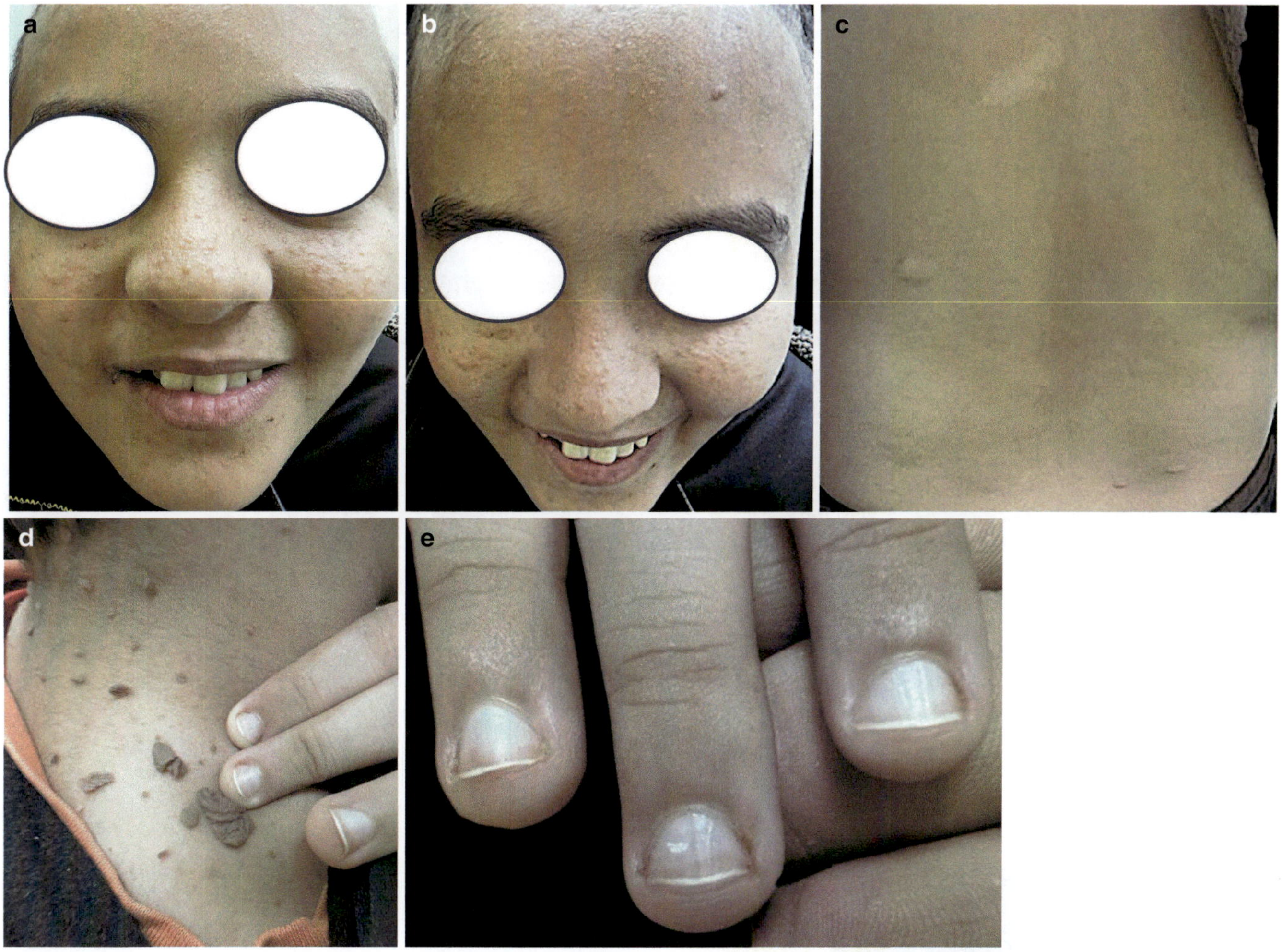

Fig. 5.2 Tuberous sclerosis. Facial angiofibroma with fibrous cephalic plaque of forehead (**a**, **b**), ash leaf hypopigmented patch, and shagreen patch on the back (**c**). Multiple skin tags like lesions on the neck (**d**). Nails show leukonychia (**e**). History of infantile spasm at age of 3 months. The patient is blind. MRI showed bilateral ventricular hyperdense subependymal nodules with marginal calcification

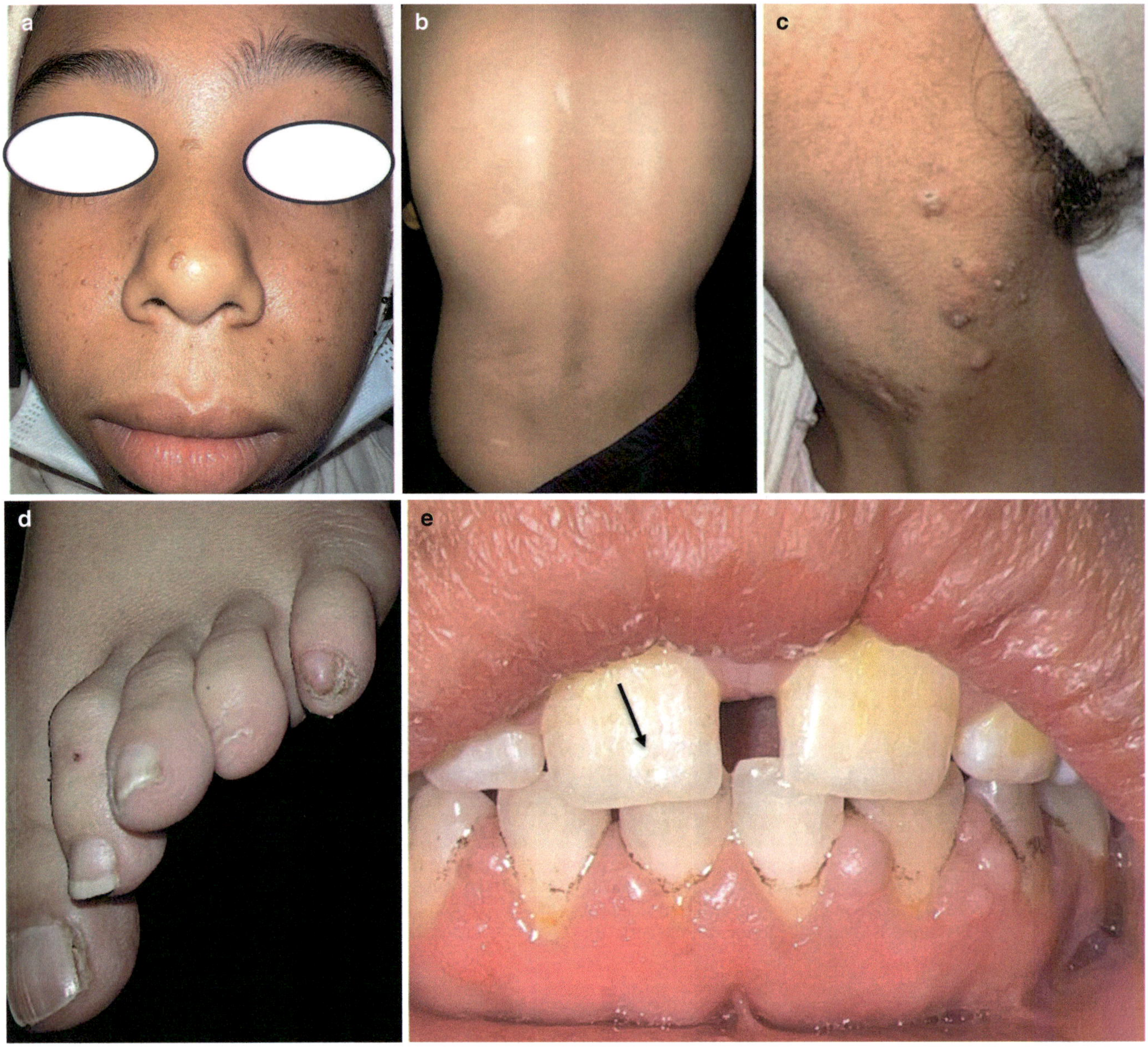

Fig. 5.3 Tuberous sclerosis. Facial angiofibroma (**a**), ash leaf patches on the back (**b**), shagreen patch on the neck (**c**), periungual (**d**), and gingival fibroma, dental enamel pits (black arrow) (**e**). History of repeated attack of seizures. MRI showed periventricular and subcortical calcifications (subependymal giant cell astrocytoma) (**f**)

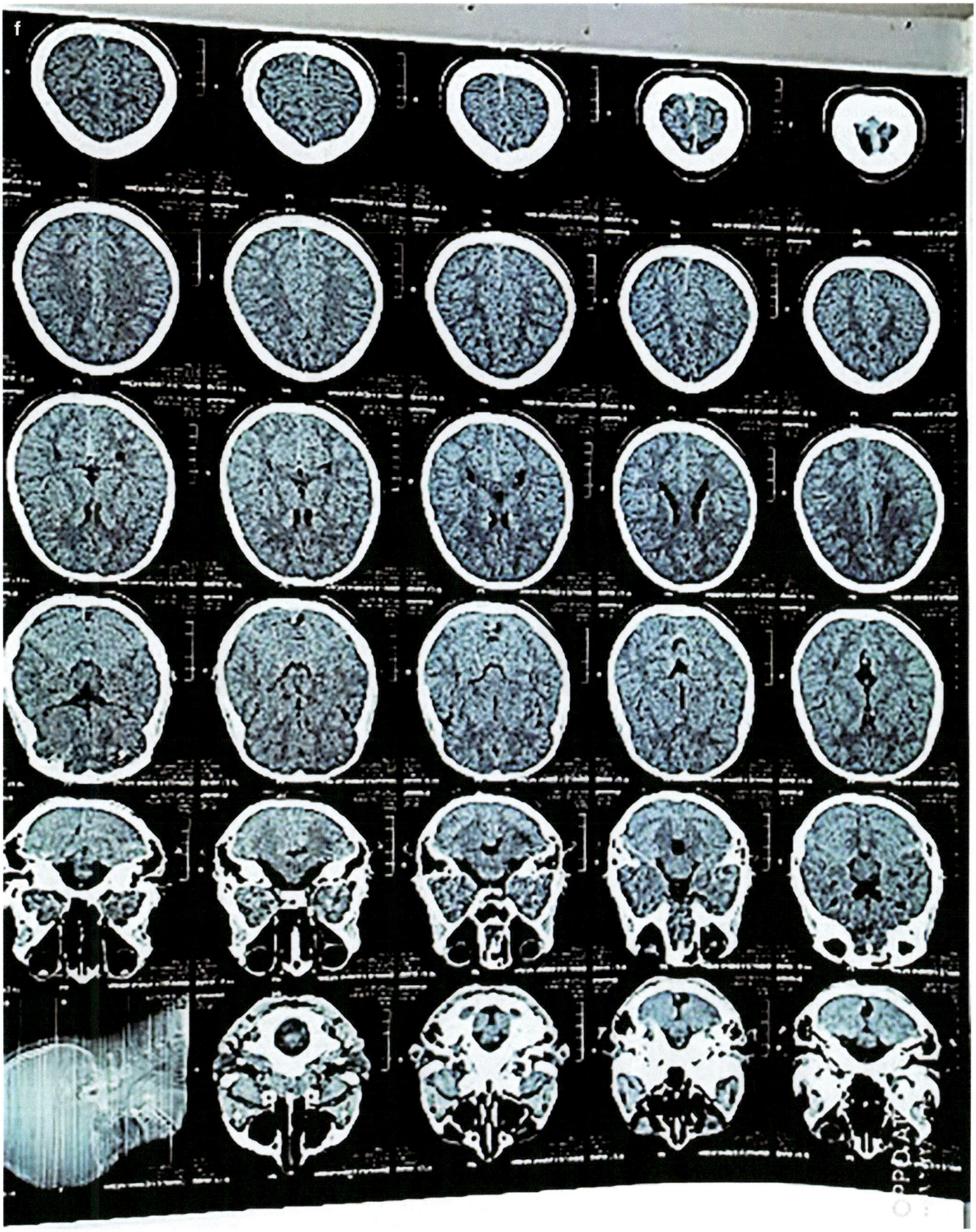

Fig. 5.3 (continued)

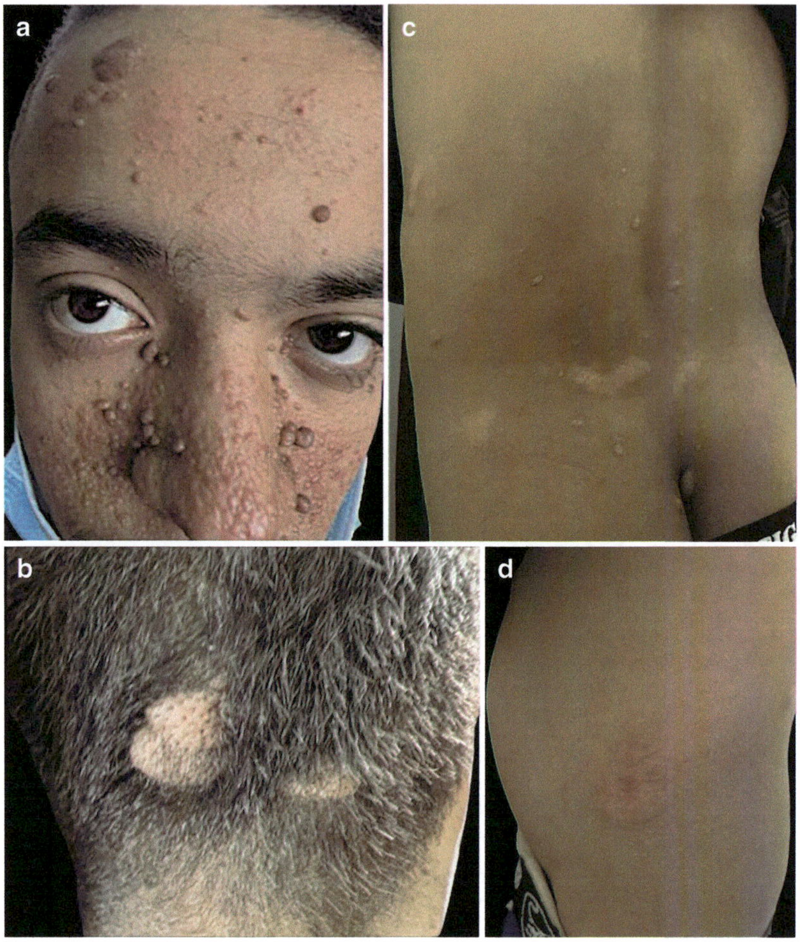

Fig. 5.4 Tuberous sclerosis. Facial angiofibroma with fibrous cephalic plaque of forehead and scalp (**a**, **b**), Ash leaf patches on back (**c**), shagreen patch on buttock (**d**). (*Courtesy, Doaa Atef*)

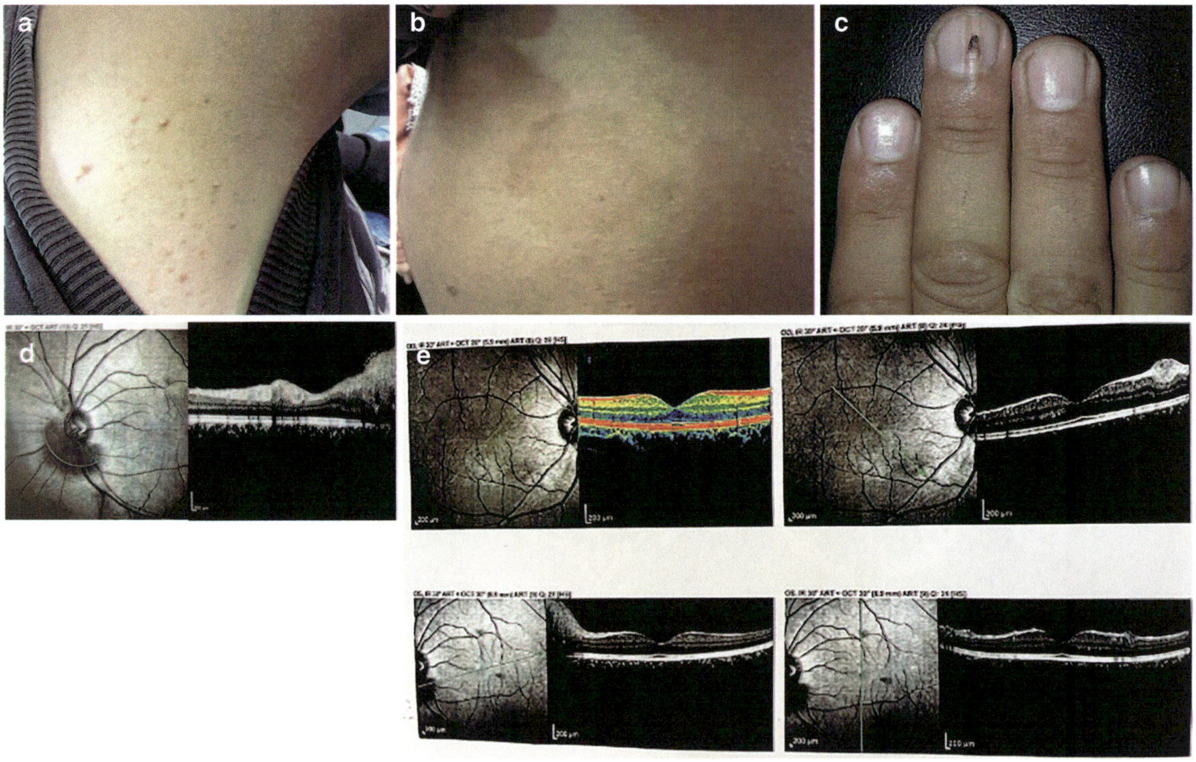

Fig. 5.5 Tuberous sclerosis. Skin tags like lesions on the neck (**a**), café-au-lait macules (CALM) on abdomen (**b**), and ungual fibroma (**c**). Fundus examination showed bilateral retinal hamartoma confirmed by ocular computerized tomography (**d**, **e**). MRI showed cortical and subependymal tuberous sclerosis (not shown)

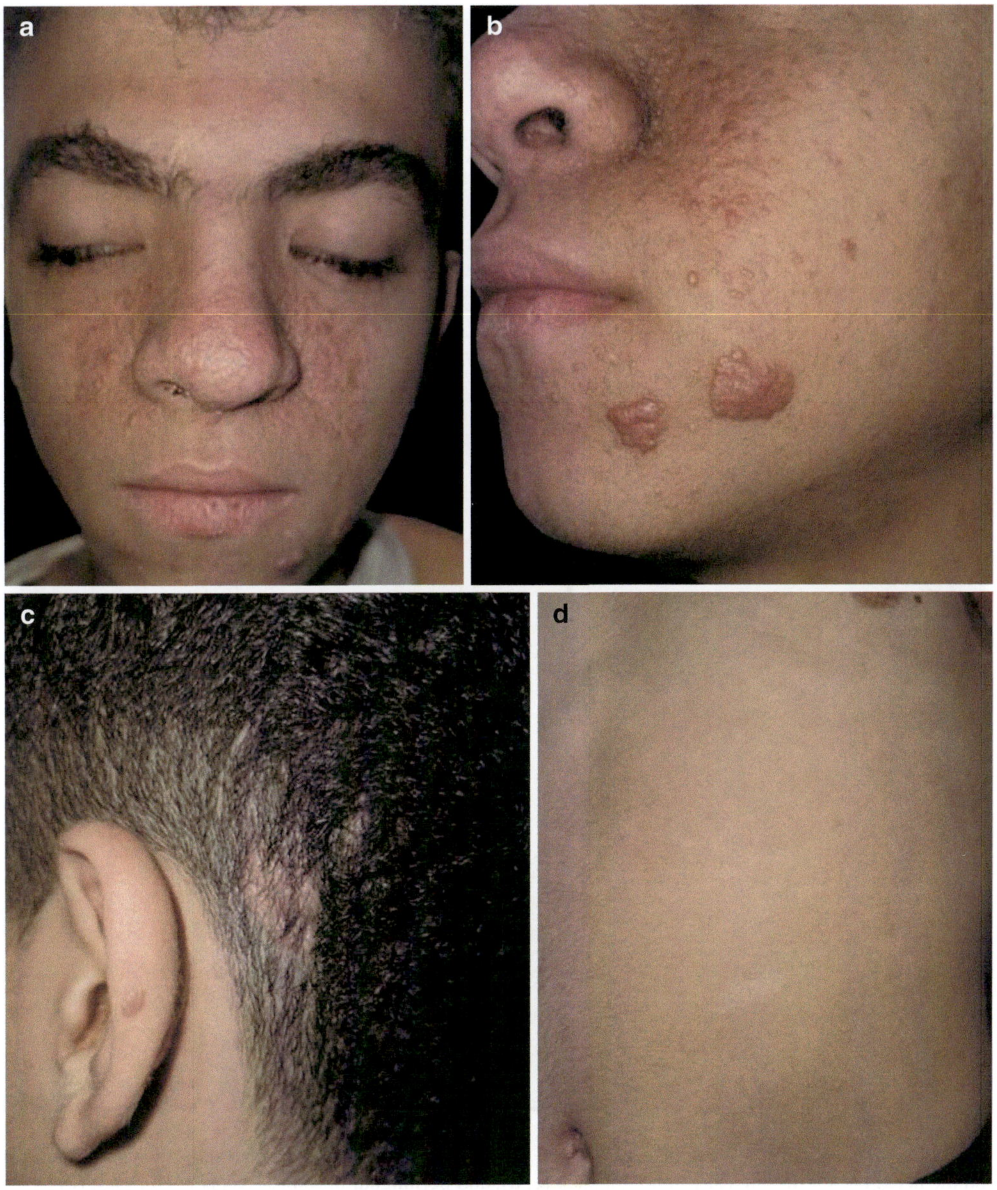

Fig. 5.6 Tuberous sclerosis. Facial angiofibroma (**a**, **b**), fibrous cephalic plaque (**b**) shagreen patch on scalp (**c**) and ash leaf patch on the abdomen (**d**)

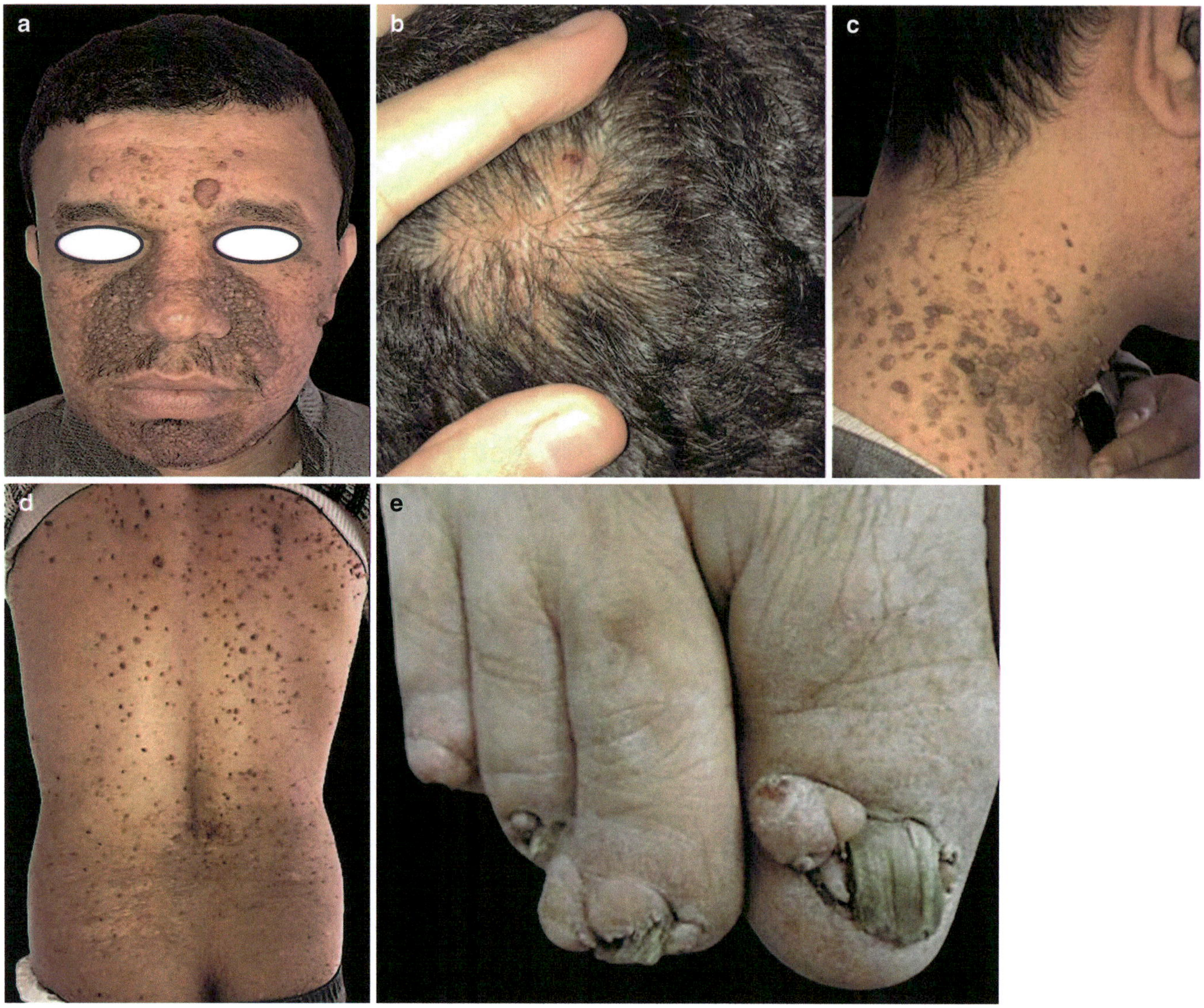

Fig. 5.7 Tuberous sclerosis. Facial angiofibroma with fibrous cephalic plaque of forehead (**a**), shagreen patch on scalp (**b**), skin tags like lesions on the neck, back with ash leaf patches on back (**c**, **d**), and periungual fibromas (Koenen's tumors) (**e**)

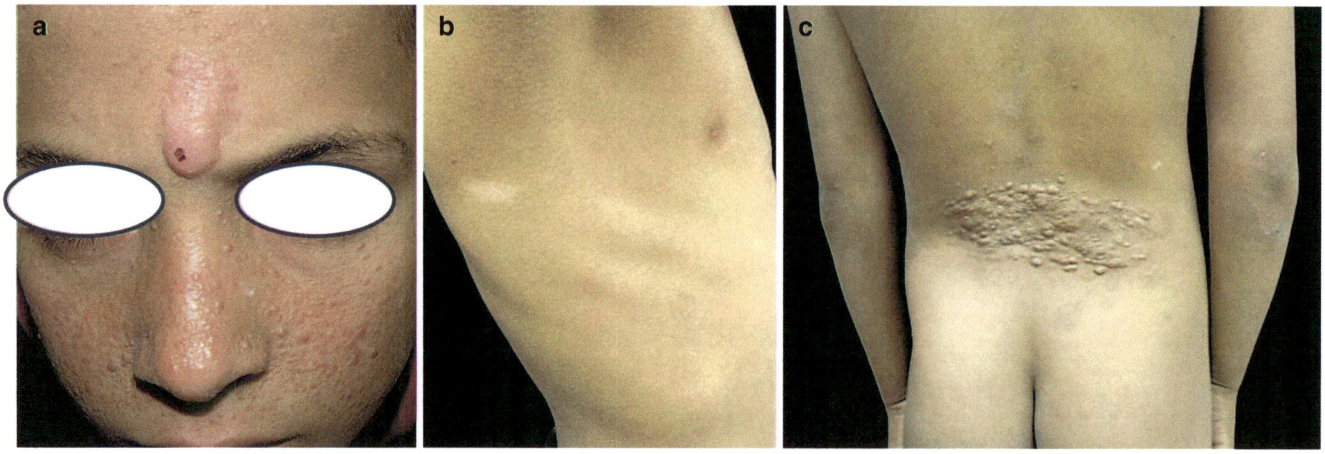

Fig. 5.8 Tuberous sclerosis. Facial angiofibroma, fibrous plaque on forehead (**a**), ash leaf patch (**b**), and shagreen patch on the back (**c**)

Table 5.1 Major and minor criteria for diagnosis of tuberous sclerosis [5]

Major criteria	Minor criteria
Hypomelanotic macules (≥3; at least 5 mm diameter)	"Confetti" skin lesions
Angiofibroma (≥3) or fibrous cephalic plaque	Dental enamel pits (≥3)
Ungual fibromas (≥2)	Intraoral fibromas (≥2)
Shagreen patch	Retinal achromic patch
Multiple retinal hamartomas	Multiple renal cysts
Multiple cortical tubers and/or radial migration lines	Nonrenal hamartomas
Subependymal nodule (≥2)	Sclerotic bone lesions
Subependymal giant cell astrocytoma	
Cardiac rhabdomyoma	
Lymphangioleiomyomatosis	
Renal angiomyolipomas (≥2)	

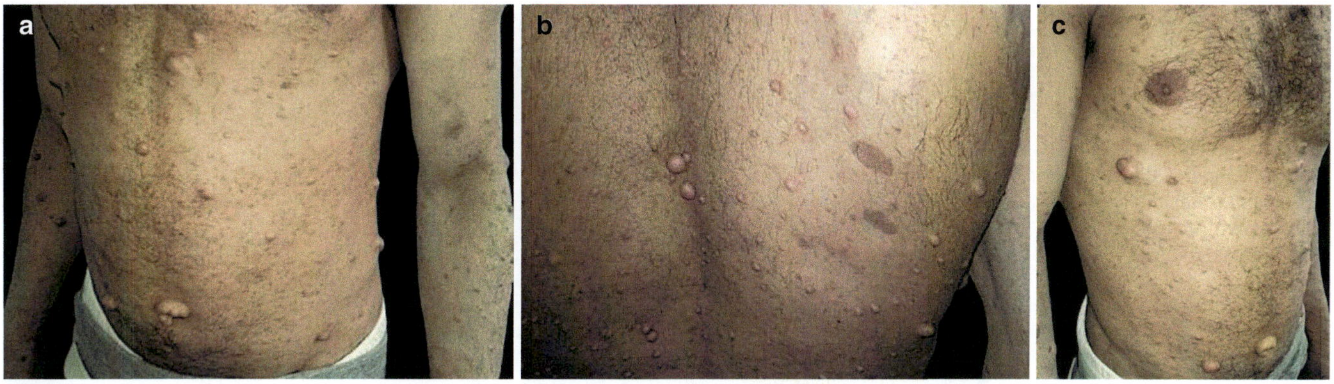

Fig. 5.9 Neurofibromatosis. Multiple neurofibroma and café-au-lait macules and patches on the trunk (**a**–**c**).

Neurofibromatosis (NF) (AD) [7–10] (Figs. 5.9, 5.10, 5.11, 5.12, 5.13, 5.14, 5.15, 5.16, 5.17, 5.18, 5.19, 5.20, 5.21, and 5.22)

Von Recklinghausen Syndrome

- The term neurofibromatosis (NF) is used for a group of genetic disorders that primarily affect the cell growth of neural tissues. Neurofibromatosis type 1 (NF1) is the most common type of NF and accounts for about 96% of all cases, while NF2 (bilateral acoustic neurofibroma) accounts for 3% and Schwannomatosis for <1%.
- Defect in the tumor suppressor *NF-1* gene in NF1.
- The diagnostic criteria for NF1 were updated by international consensus in 2021. In the absence of a parent with NF1, the criteria for clinical diagnosis includes two or more of the following:
  - Six or more café-au-lait (CAL) macules greater than 5 mm in diameter in prepubertal children and greater than 15 mm postpubertal.
  - Axillary or inguinal freckles (>2 freckles) (if only CAL and freckling are present, one of these two cutaneous manifestations should be bilateral, and Legius syndrome should be considered, though the diagnosis is still likely NF1).
  - Two or more typical neurofibromas or one plexiform neurofibroma.
  - Optic pathway glioma.
  - Two or more iris hamartomas (Lisch nodules), often identified only through slit-lamp examination by an ophthalmologist; or two or more choroidal abnormalities (bright, patchy nodules imaged by optical adherence tomography/near infrared reflectance imaging).
  - Sphenoid dysplasia or typical long-bone abnormalities such as pseudarthrosis (exception is sphenoid dysplasia does not count as a separate criterion in the case of ipsilateral orbital plexiform neurofibroma).
  - Heterozygous pathogenic NF1 variant with a variant allele fraction of 50% in apparently normal tissue.
- In the presence of a parent with NF1, the criteria for clinical diagnosis include one of the above criteria.
- Other cutaneous manifestations include nevus anemicus, juvenile xanthogranuloma, glomus tumors, Patrick-Yesudian sign: palmar melanotic macules (palmar freckling) and melanoma.
- Children with NF1 and juvenile xanthogranulomas have a 20–32-fold higher risk for juvenile chronic myeloid leukemia than do patients with NF1 who do not have juvenile xanthogranulomas (Fig. 5.19).

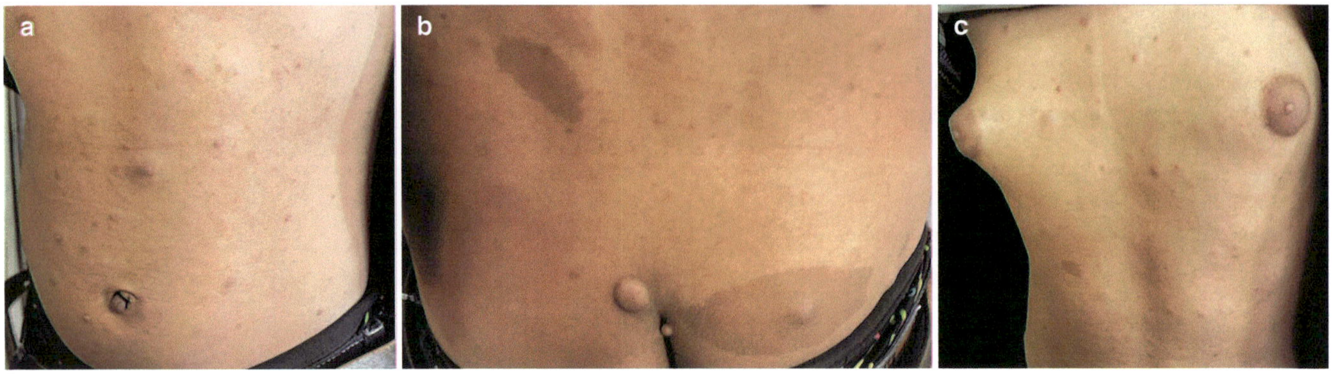

Fig. 5.10 Neurofibromatosis. Café-au-lait, freckles, neurofibromas, gynecomastia (**a**–**c**)

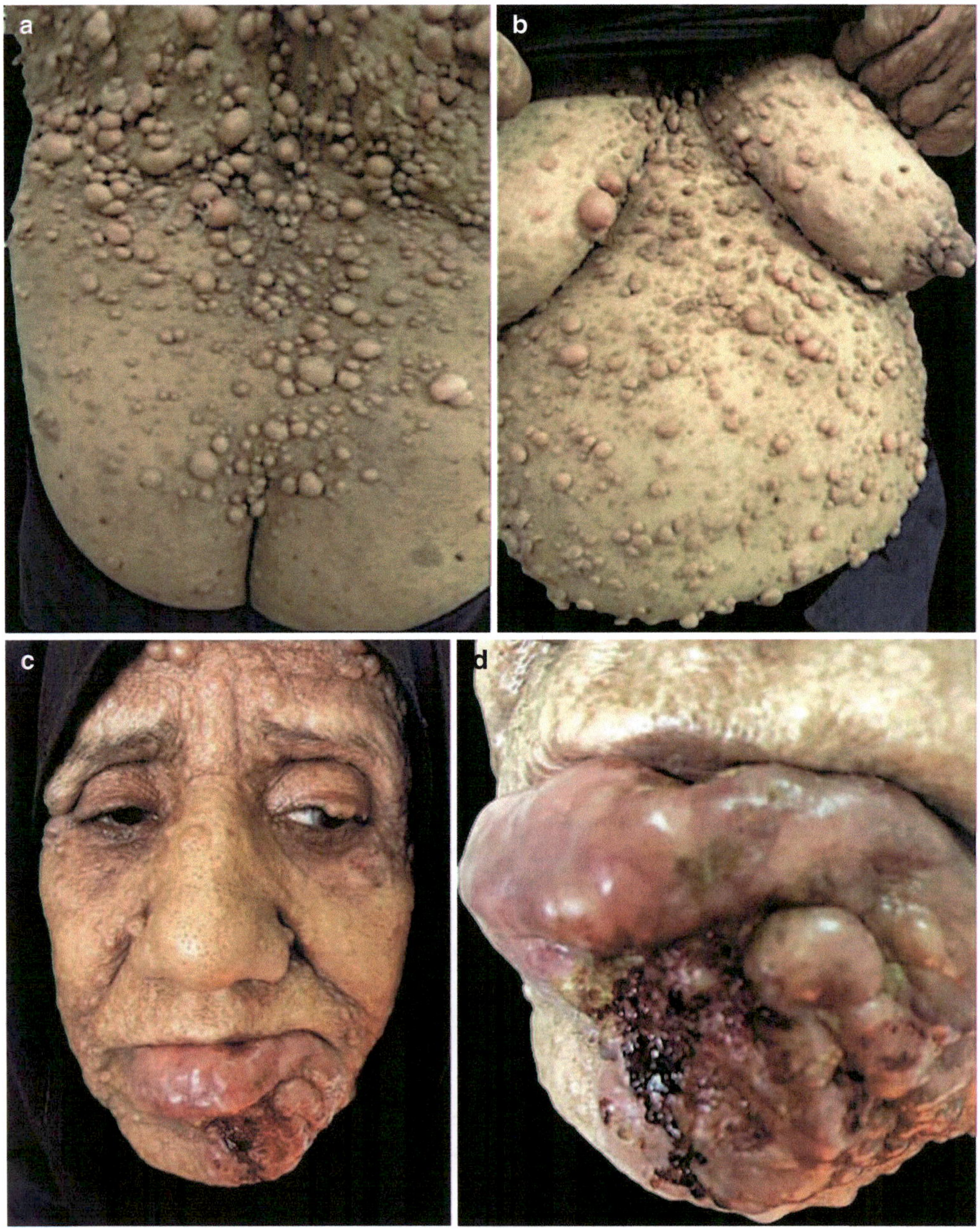

Fig. 5.11 Neurofibromatosis. Multiple neurofibromas on the trunk (**a**, **b**) and the face (**c**), some of them show ulcerative indurated lobulated mass on the chin and lip suggestive of neurofibrosarcoma (**d**)

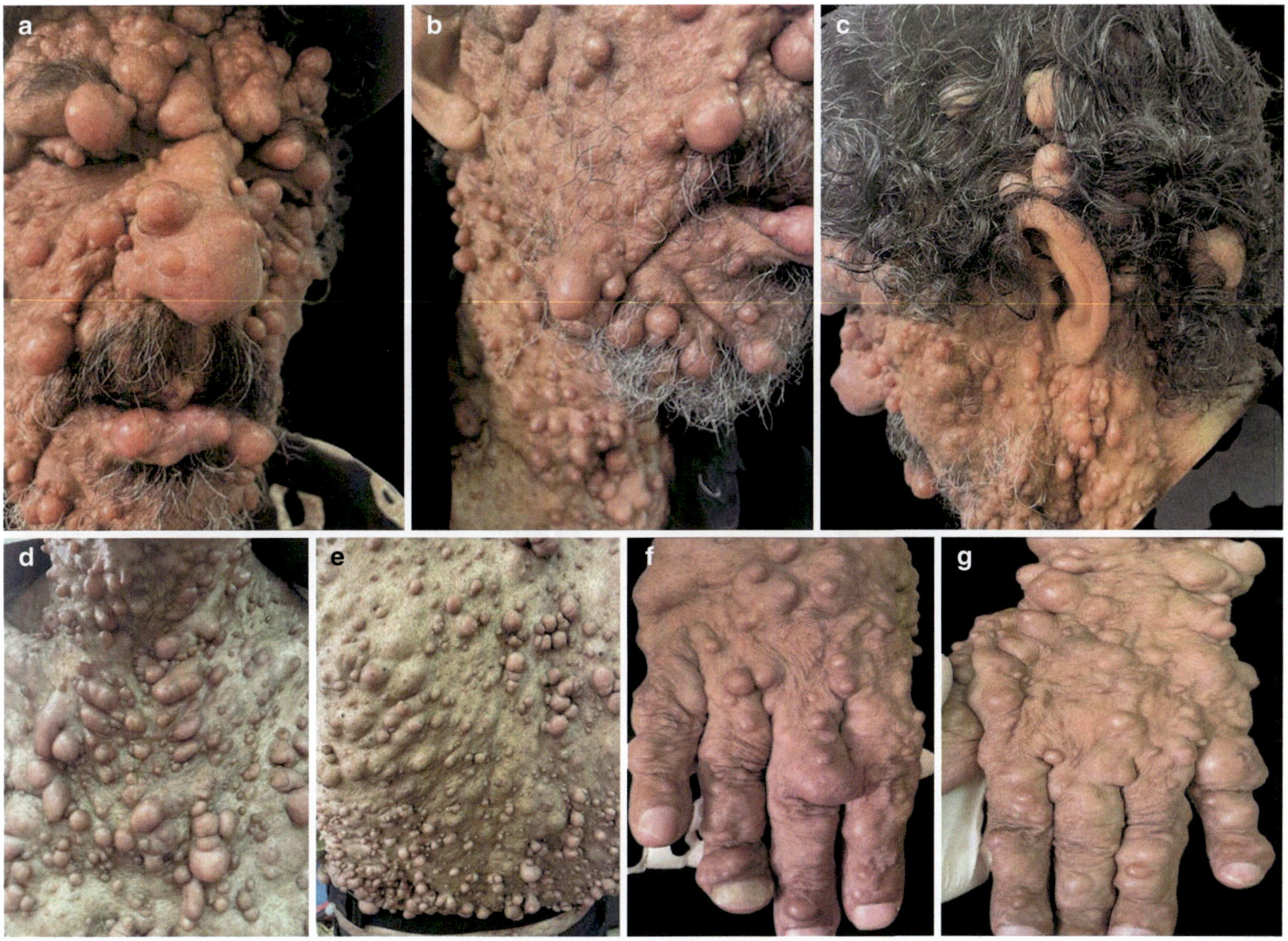

Fig. 5.12 Neurofibromatosis. Multiple neurofibromas on the face (**a**), neck (**b**), and scalp (**c**) impairing proper vision function with cosmetic disfigurement and psychological upset. Multiple neurofibromas on the neck, trunk (**d**, **e**), and hands (**f**, **g**)

Fig. 5.13 Neurofibromatosis. A child with plexiform neurofibroma appearing at birth overlying large café-au-lait macules on upper back. It may be misdiagnosed as a congenital melanocytic nevus

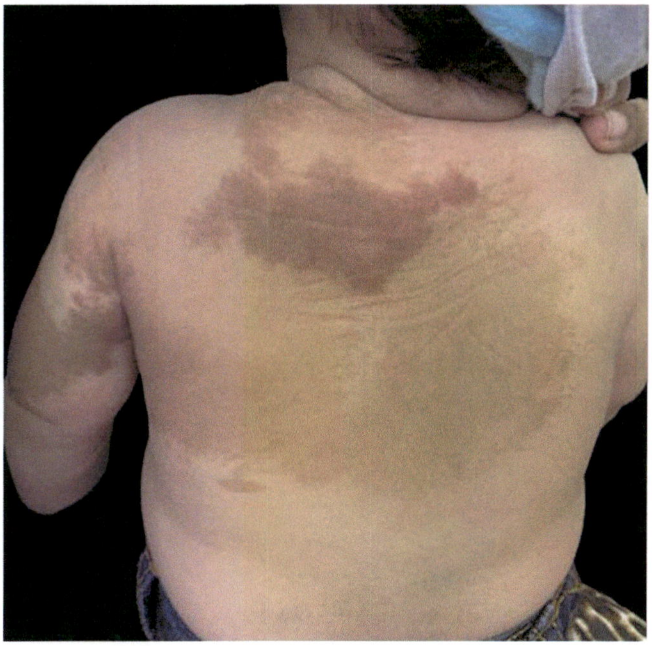

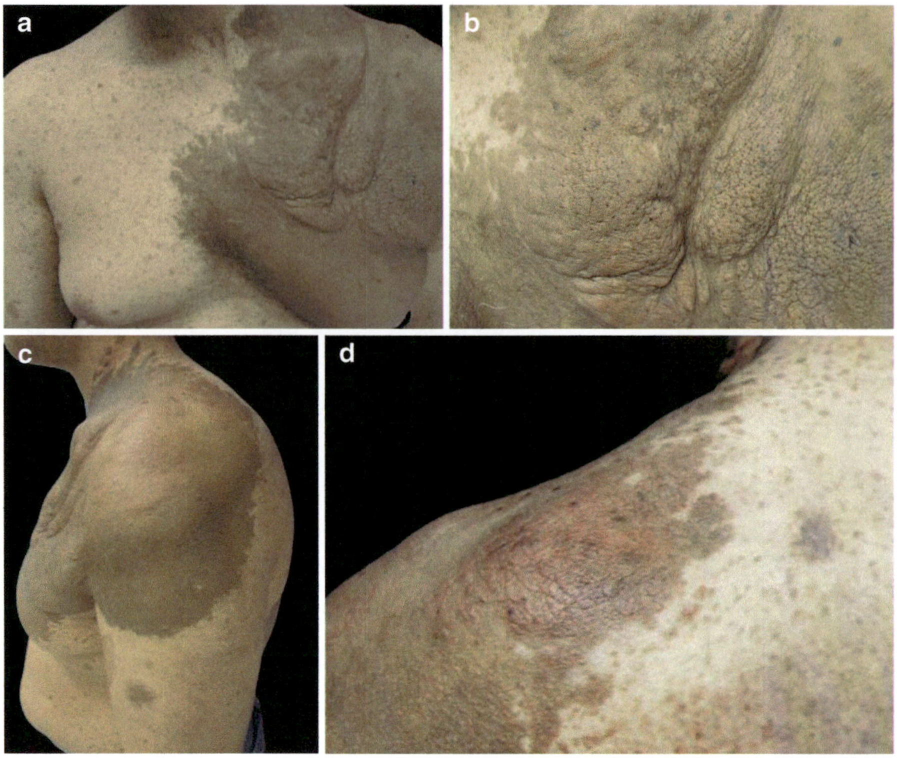

Fig. 5.14 Neurofibromatosis. Adult patient with plexiform neurofibroma dating since birth and multiple café-au-lait patches (**a–d**)

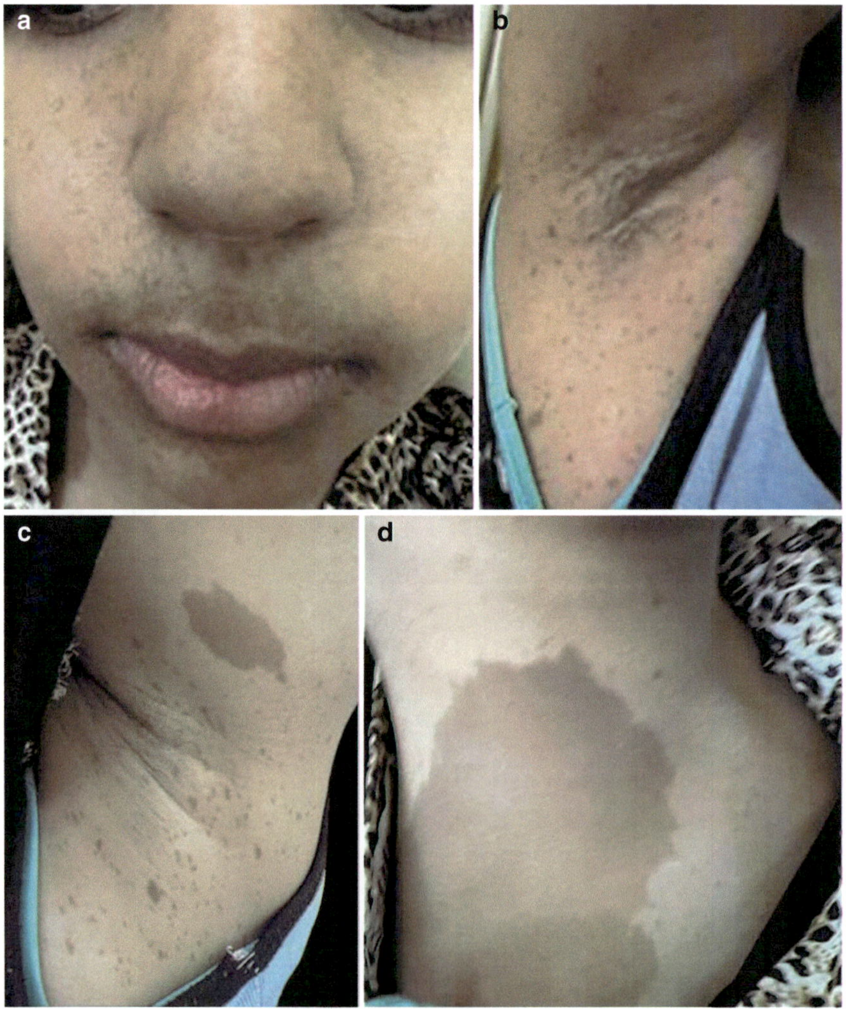

Fig. 5.15 Neurofibromatosis. Multiple facial (**a**) and axillary freckles (**b**) with café-au-lait patches on the forearm (**c**) and the neck (**d**)

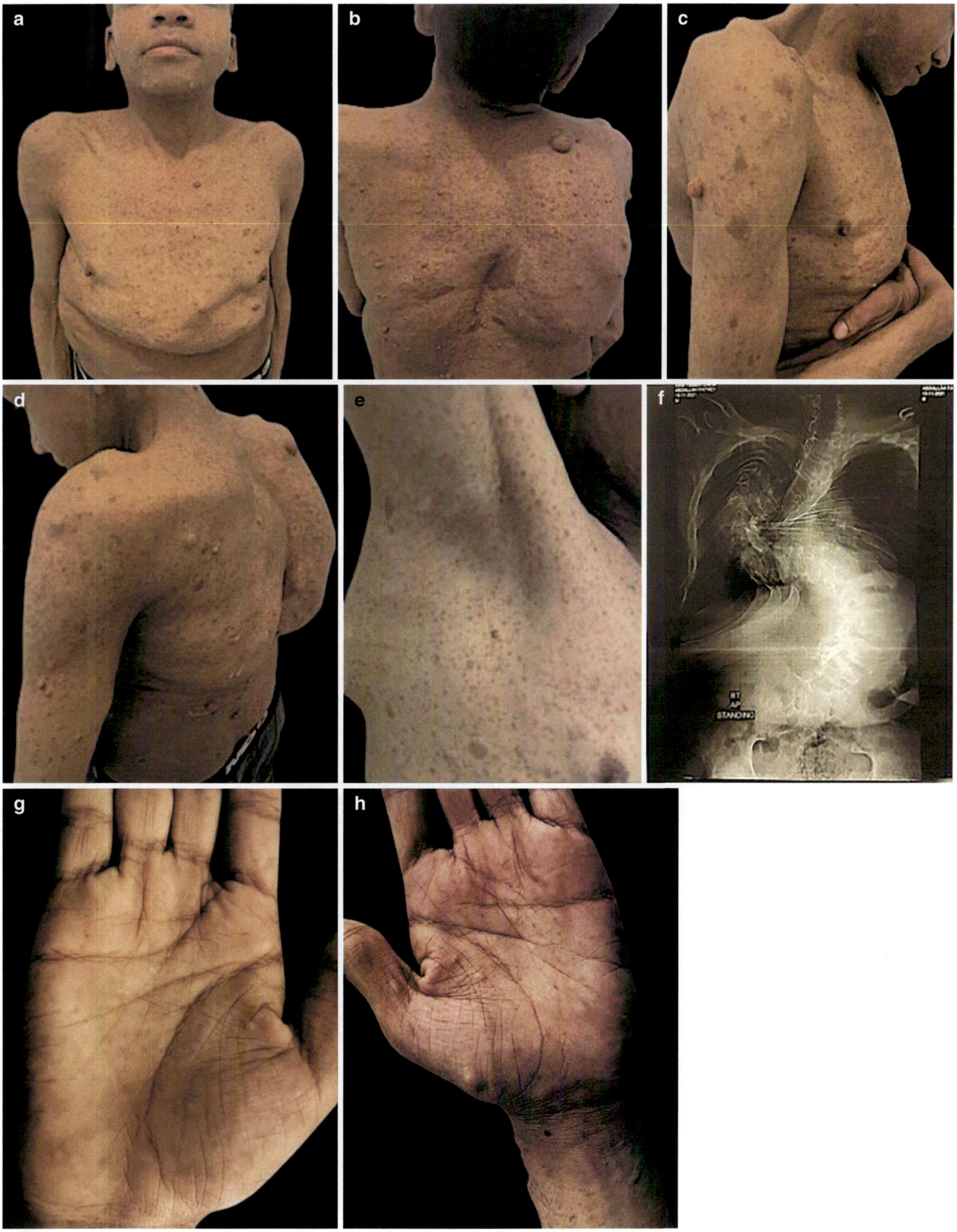

Fig. 5.16 Neurofibromatosis. Multiple freckles with neurofibromas on the trunk and the upper arms (**a–d**) with axillary freckles (**e**) and thoracic cage asymmetry (kyphoscoliosis) (**a**, **b**), proven by X-ray (**f**). Palmar melanocytic macules (Patrick-Yesudian sign) with palmar neurofibromas (**g**, **h**)

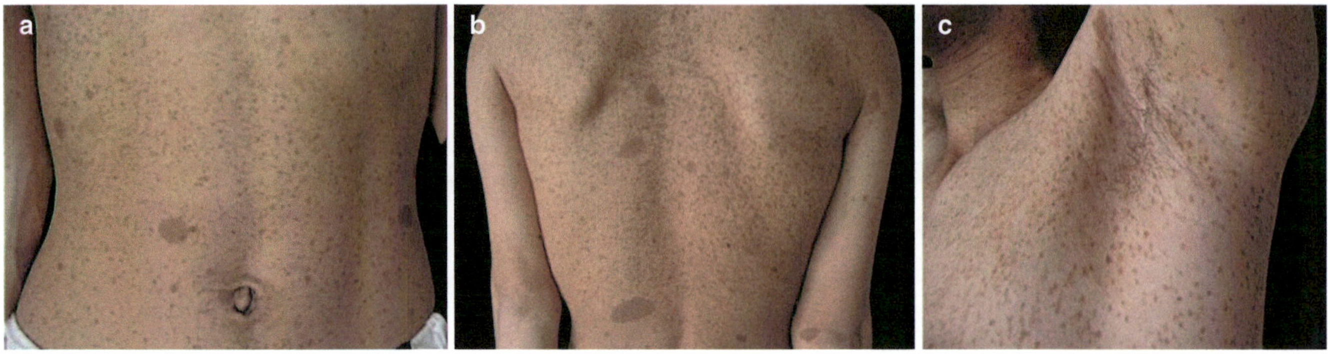

Fig. 5.17 Neurofibromatosis. Multiple café-au-lait macules on the trunk (**a**) and the back (**b**) with axillary freckles (**c**)

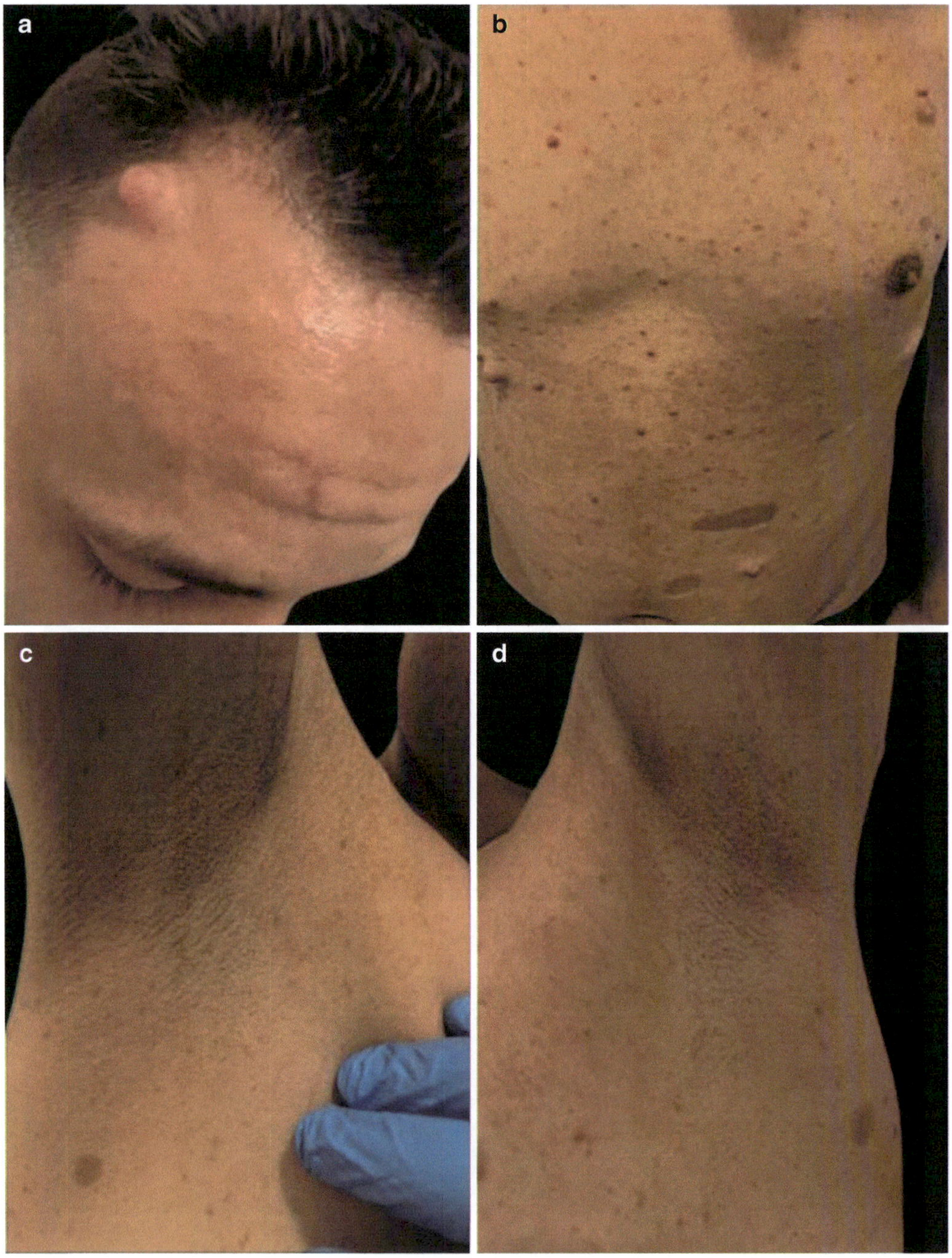

Fig. 5.18 Neurofibromatosis. Multiple neurofibromas on the forehead and abdomen, (**a**, **b**) café- au- lait macules and a nevus anemicus on the chest with axillary freckles "Crowe's sign" (**b**–**d**)

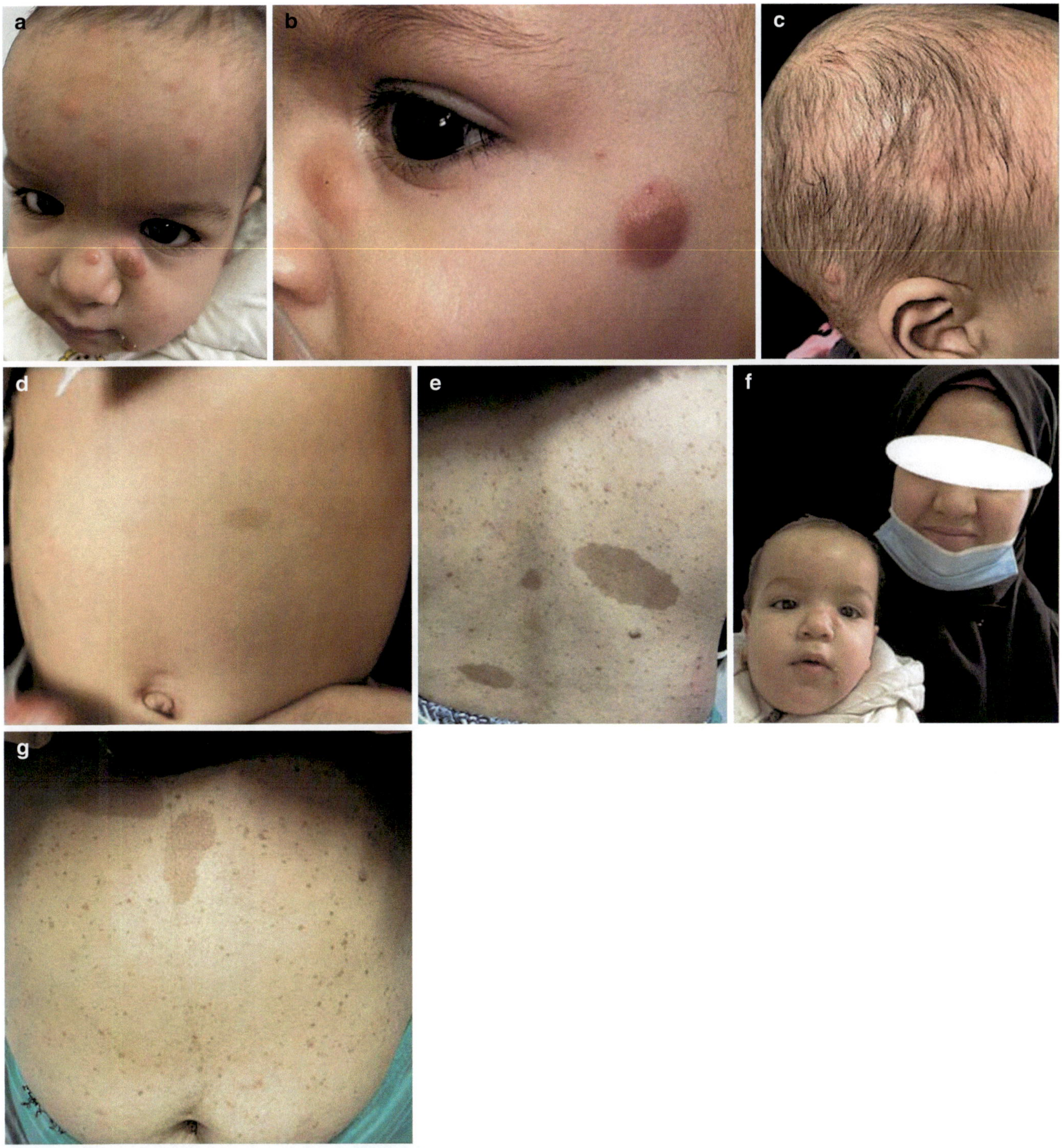

Fig. 5.19 Neurofibromatosis with juvenile xanthogranuloma. A 5-month-old female patient with red nodules on face and scalp diagnosed histopathologically as juvenile xanthogranuloma (**a–c**) with café-au-lait macules on the abdomen (**d**) and the back (**e**). Regular follow-up by CBC showed marked leucocytosis and myelomonocytic leukemia. The mother has neurofibromatosis (**f–g**). The infant is diagnosed as neurofibromatosis type I associated with juvenile xanthogranuloma and juvenile myelomonocytic leukemia

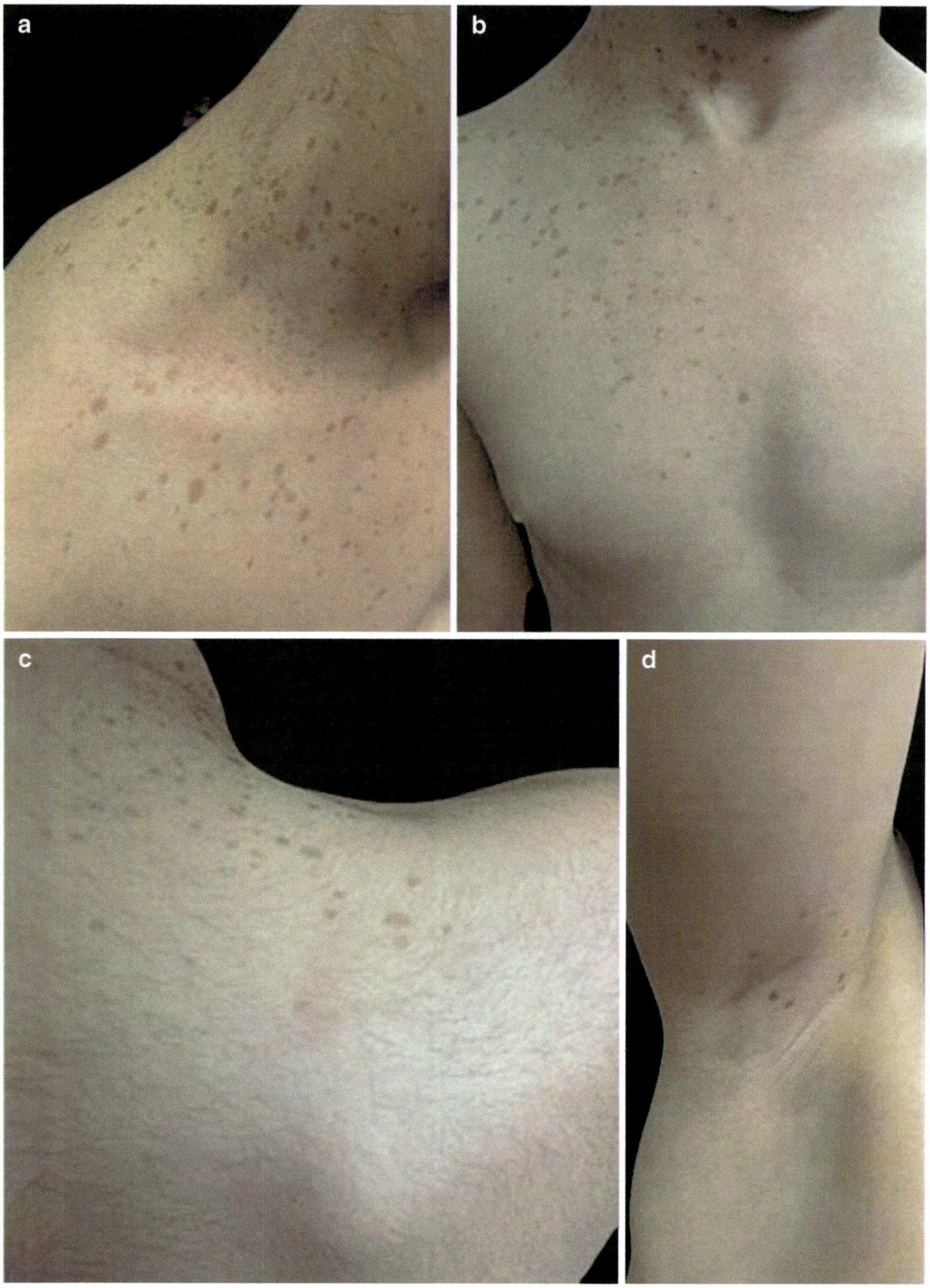

Fig. 5.20 Neurofibromatosis (segmental type). Unilateral café-au-lait macules on the neck and upper trunk (**a**–**c**) and unilateral axillary freckles (**d**)

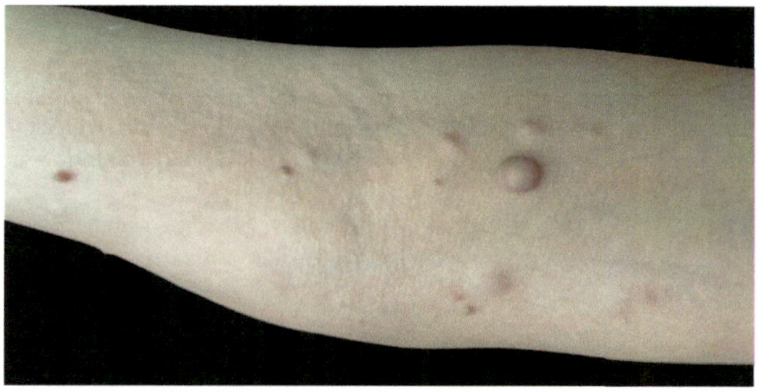

Fig. 5.21 Neurofibromatosis (segmental type). Multiple neurofibroma, segmental type

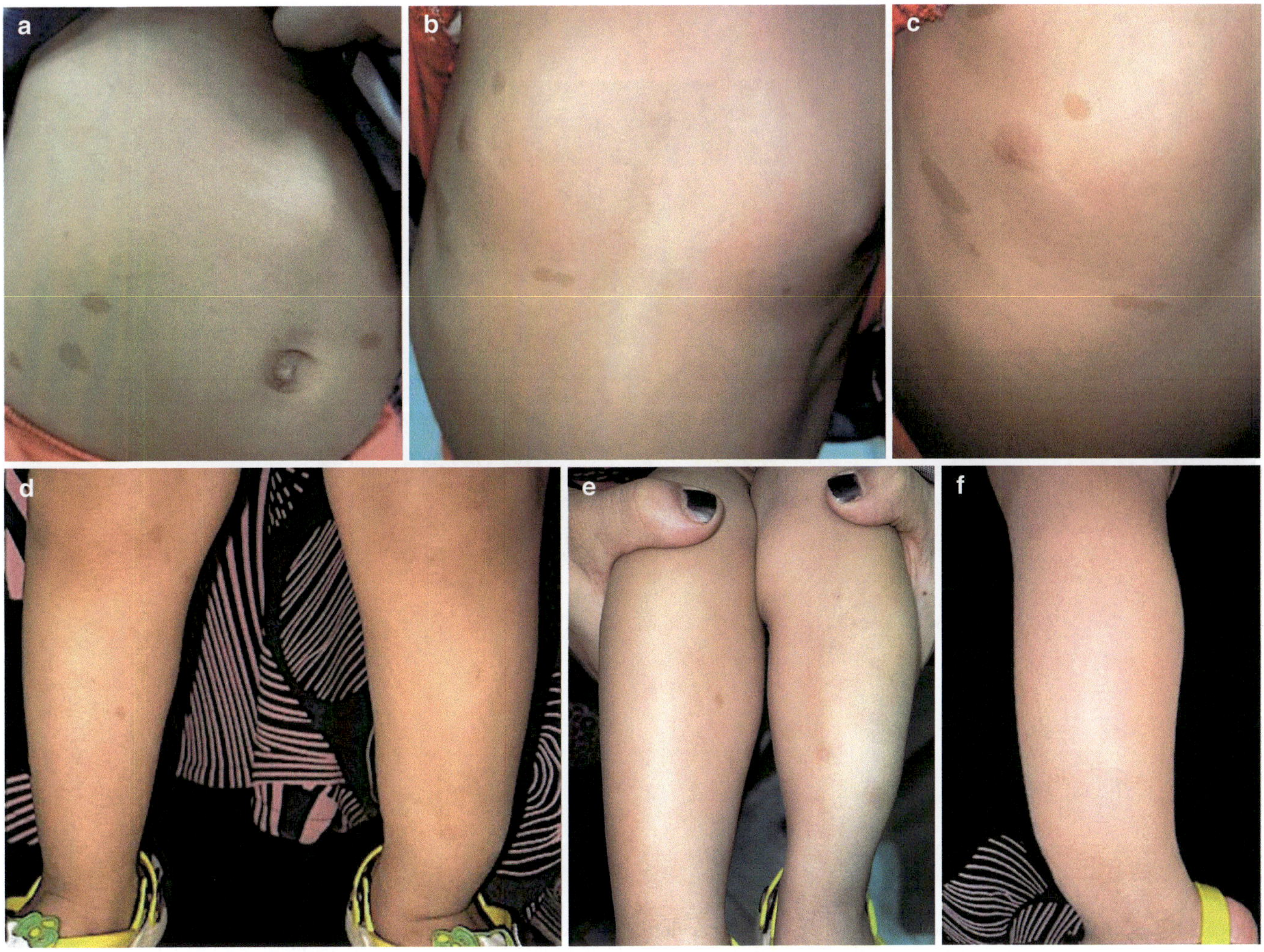

Fig. 5.22 Neurofibromatosis. Café-au-lait macules (**a–c**) and congenital pseudarthrosis of the tibia (**d–f**)

- Congenital pseudarthrosis of the tibia is a rare pathology, which is usually associated with NF1. The tibia shows area of segmental dysplasia resulting in anterolateral bowing of the bone and shortening of the limb (Fig. 5.28).
- Prognosis:
  - Although most individuals have relatively long and healthy lives, the overall life expectancy may be reduced by on average 8 years. The major causes for this increased morbidity and subsequent mortality are hypertension, sequelae of spinal cord lesions, and malignancy.
  - Prompt attention to complications of NF1 and early detection of medical problems may significantly reduce the overall morbidity and mortality rates.
  - NF1 represents a major risk factor for development of malignancy, particularly malignant peripheral nerve sheath tumors, optic gliomas, other gliomas, and leukemias.

Birt–Hogg–Dubé Syndrome (BHDS) (AD) [2, 11, 12] (Figs. 5.23 and 5.24)

- Mutation in in the tumor suppressor folliculin (*FLCN*) gene.
- Characterized by the development of multiple benign skin tumors, lung cysts, spontaneous pneumothorax and an increased risk of kidney lesions (cysts, benign tumors, and kidney cancer). Symptoms of BHDS generally do not appear until adulthood.

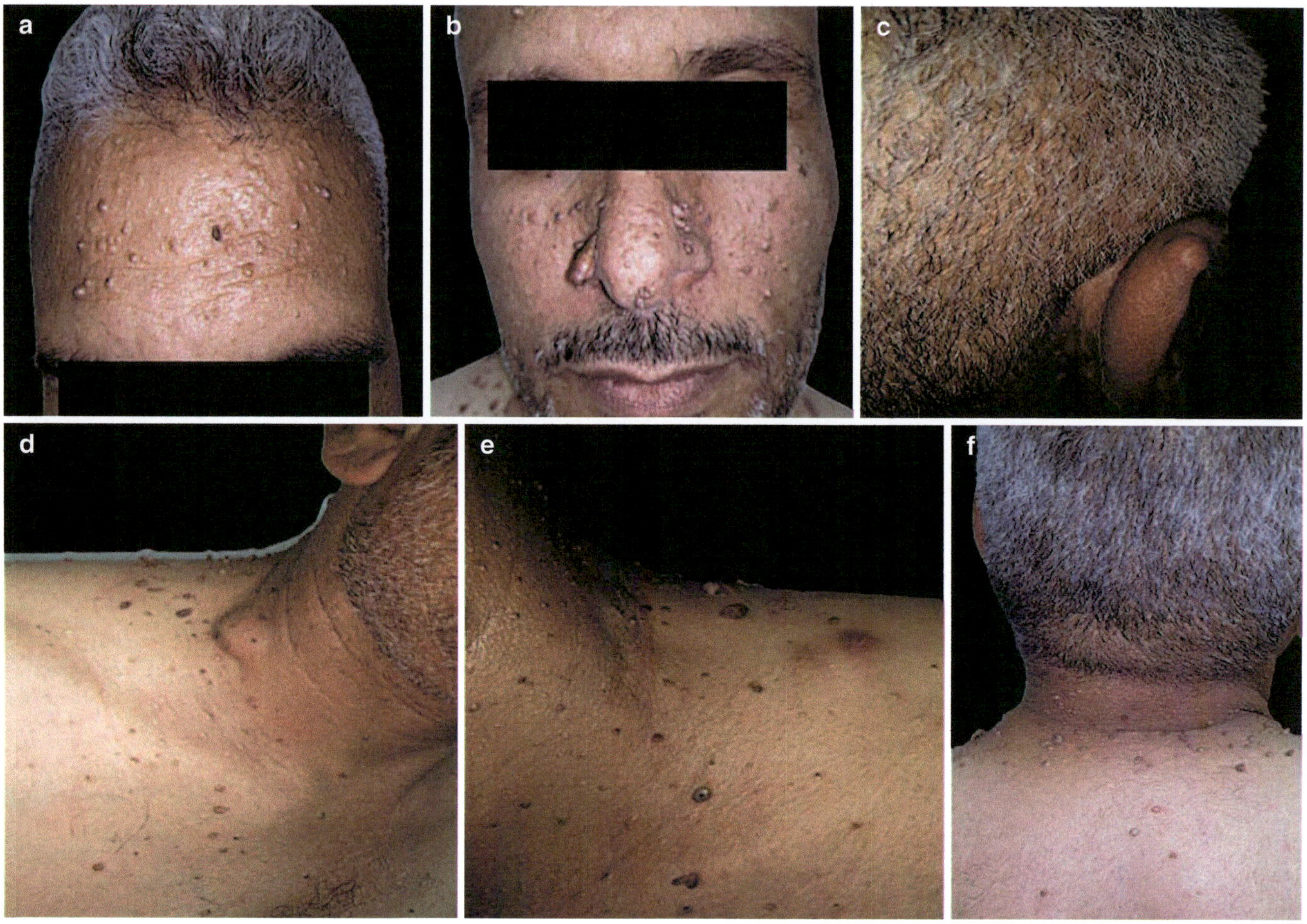

Fig. 5.23 Birt-Hogg-Dubé syndrome. Multiple flesh-colored papules on the face (fibrofolliculoma and trichodiscoma diagnosed by histopathological examination) (**a**, **b**), multiple cysts on the helix and on the right side of neck associated with multiple skin tags around the neck (**c**–**f**)

- Cutaneous manifestations:
  - Fibrofolliculoma: the most common cutaneous manifestations and are present in more than 80% of patients older than age 40 years. They appear as multiple pale or flesh-colored papules predominantly on the nasal and paranasal areas, neck, and trunk.
  - Trichodiscoma: now considered to be scarred remnants of fibrofolliculomas.
  - Angiofibroma.
  - Oral fibroma.
  - Acrochordon, oral papules, cutaneous collagenomas, and epidermal cysts.
- Appropriate laboratory and radiographic tests are recommended regularly to check for internal complications such as pulmonary cysts, pneumothorax, and renal carcinoma.

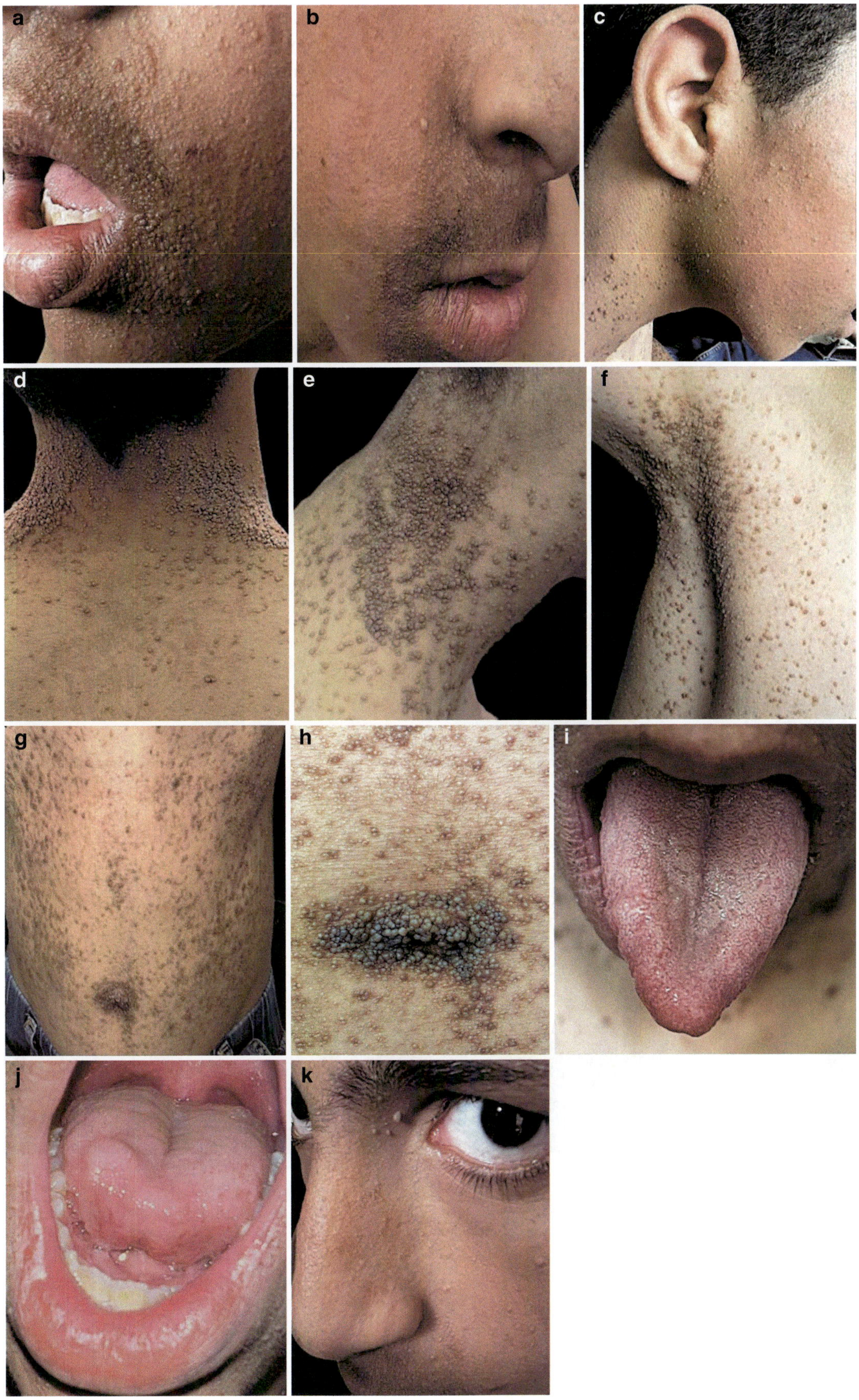

Fig. 5.24 Birt-Hogg-Dubé syndrome. Multiple fibrofolliculomas on the face, the ears, and the neck, axillae (**a**–**g**). Multiple trichodiscoma on the trunk confirmed by histopathology (**g**, **h**).Oral fibroma of the tongue (**i**, **j**) with skin tags around the eyes (**k**)

Cowden Syndrome (AD) [2, 13] (Fig. 5.25)

- Mutations in the phosphatase and tensin homolog (*PTEN*) tumor suppressor gene.
- Characterized by multiple hamartomas and a predisposition to malignant tumors.
- Characteristic skin lesions include:
  - Trichilemmomas (skin colored or yellow-brown, flat topped, 1–5- mm warty papules on the central face surrounding the eyes, nose, and mouth).
  - Acral keratosis, located primarily on the dorsum of the hands and feet, and are wart-like, skin-colored flat-topped papules, 1–4 mm in diameter.
  - Palmoplantar keratoses are translucent hard papules with or without a central pit.
  - Mucocutaneous neuromas.
  - Oral papillomas.
  - Penile macules.
- Skin lesions are often the first clues to the underlying diagnosis.
- Cowden syndrome is characterized by a high risk of both benign and cancerous tumors of the breast, thyroid, uterus, colorectal, kidney, and melanoma.

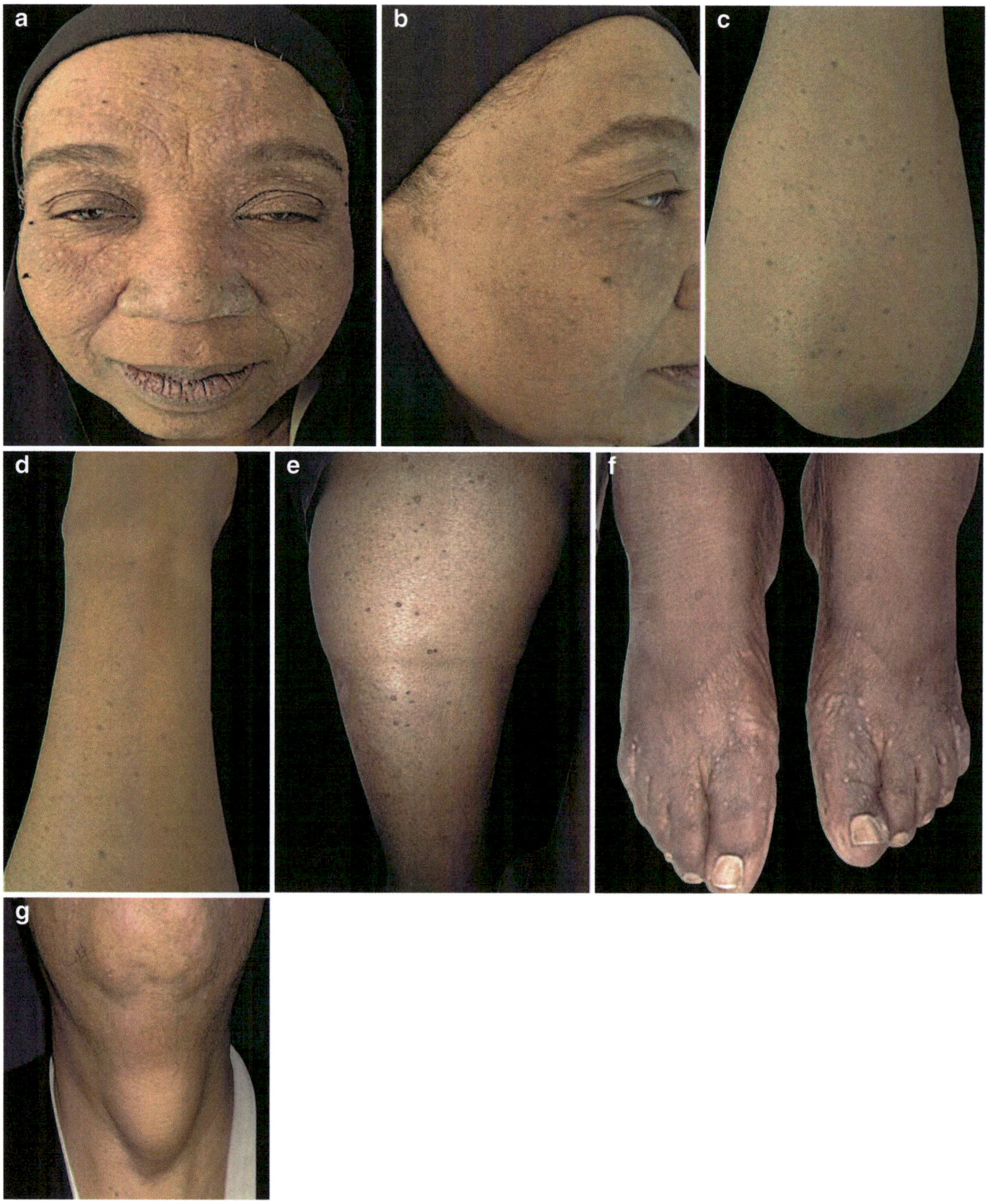

Fig. 5.25 Cowden syndrome. Skin colored and yellow-brown warty papules (trichilemmoma) on the face, eyelids, and nose (**a**, **b**), forearm (**c**, **d**), legs (**e**), and dorsal surface of feet (**f**). Thyroid enlargement in the neck (**g**)

Gorlin Syndrome (AD) [2, 14–16] (Fig. 5.26)

Nevoid Basal Cell Carcinoma Syndrome

- Also called Gorlin-Goltz syndrome or basal cell nevus syndrome (BCNS).
- Mutation of the tumor suppressor patched 1 (*PTCH1*) gene.
- Characterized by numerous basal cell carcinomas (BCCs), along with skeletal, ophthalmologic, and neurologic abnormalities. Multiple neoplasms arise starting in childhood.
- Diagnosis requires the presence of two major or one major and two minor clinical criteria.
- Major criteria include: multiple (>2) BCCs or 1 BCC by ≤20 years of age, odontogenic keratocysts of the jaw proven by histology, palmar or plantar pitting, bilamellar calcification of the falx cerebri, bifid/fused/splayed ribs, first-degree relative with BCNS.
- Minor criteria include: medulloblastoma, increased circumference of the head, congenital malformations (frontal bossing, coarse facies, cleft lip/palate, moderate or severe hypertelorism), other skeletal abnormalities (Sprengel deformity, marked pectus deformity, marked syndactyly of the digits), radiologic abnormalities (bridging of the sella turcica, hemivertebrae, fusion or elongation of the vertebral bodies, modeling defects of the hands and feet, or flame-shaped lucencies of the hands or feet), ovarian, and cardiac fibromas.
- Genetic testing for *PTCH1* is suggested for the following situations: (1) diagnosis confirmation in patients lacking sufficient clinical diagnostic criteria; (2) predictive testing for patients at risk with an affected family member but not meeting clinical criteria; (3) prenatal testing if there is a known familial mutation.
- A multidisciplinary approach is required to manage patients with Gorlin syndrome.
- Numerous baseline examinations are recommended in pediatric patients:
  - A baseline MRI scan of the brain (repeated yearly until 8 years of age then discontinue).
  - Baseline jaw X-rays as soon as tolerated and repeated annually until first jaw cyst then every 6 months until no jaw cysts for 2 years or until the patient is 21 years of age.
  - Baseline spine X-rays at 1 year of age and repeat if symptomatic or per scoliosis protocol every 6 months if abnormal.
  - A baseline cardiac ultrasound to evaluate for cardiac fibromas.
  - Girls should have a pelvic ultrasound at menarche or age 18 to evaluate for ovarian fibromas.
  - Annual speech, vision, and hearing screening along with routine developmental screening.

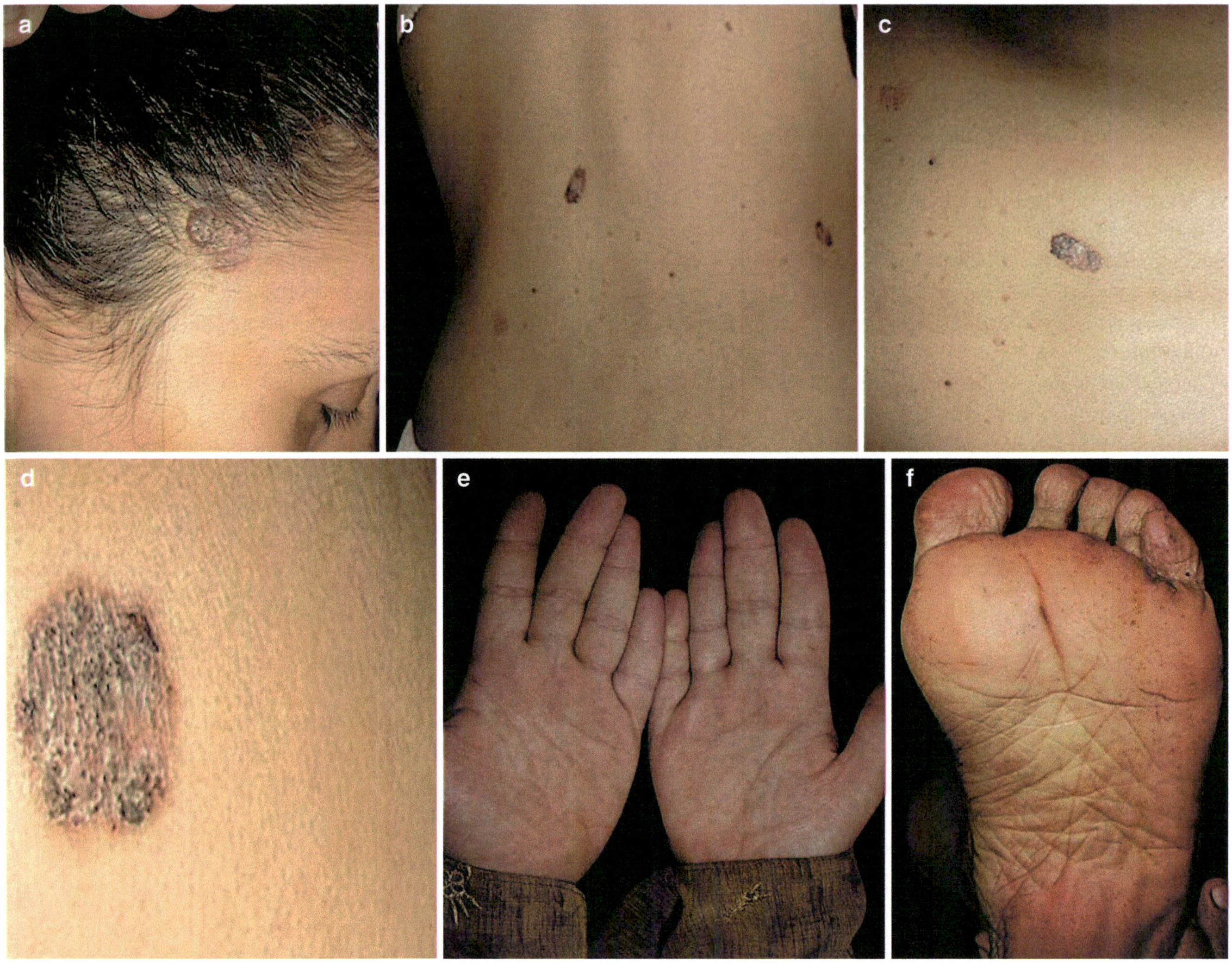

Fig. 5.26 Gorlin Syndrome. Solitary brownish circular plaque on right temporal area with beaded border (**a**), multiple basal cell carcinomas on the trunk, skin tags, and melanocytic naevi (**b**, **c**). Pigmented plaque with beaded border (**d**), palmoplantar pits (**e**, **f**)

Bazex–Dupré–Christol Syndrome (XLD) [17] (Fig. 5.27)

- Sometimes called "follicular atrophoderma-basal cell carcinoma" and "Bazex syndrome"; the latter is best avoided as acrokeratosis neoplastica is also known as "Bazex syndrome," an unrelated rare paraneoplastic syndrome.
- Mutation in the *ACTRT1* gene causing depletion of the tumor suppressor ARP-T1, a non-coding mRNA. ARP-T1 is required for the assembly of cilia, microtubule organelles.
- A rare genodermatosis that manifests with the classical triad of basal cell carcinoma, follicular atrophoderma, and hypotrichosis; yet it may be accompanied by milia, ichthyosis, neurological symptoms, and visceral malignancies.
- **Clinical characteristics:**
  - **Follicular atrophoderma**
    Present at birth
    Ice pick scars
    On backs of hands, elbows, feet, and face
  - **Hair abnormalities**
    Present at birth
    Hypotrichosis of body and scalp hair
    May be mild or absent in females
    Hair shaft abnormalities including pili torti may be also found
  - **Basal cell carcinomas**
    Onset in early adult life
    Develop on the face
    Multiple

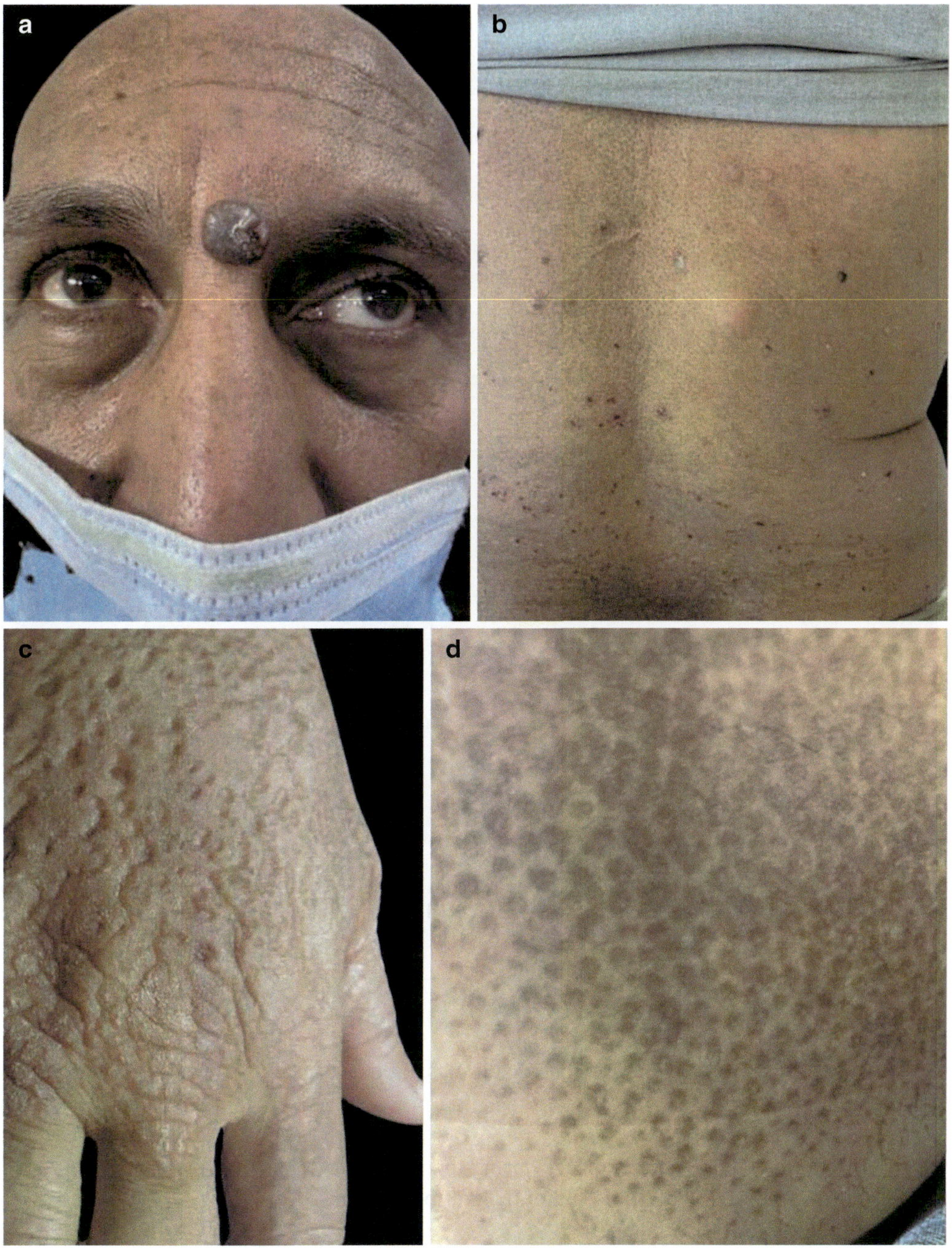

Fig. 5.27 Bazex-Dupré-Christol syndrome. Pigmented nodular basal cell carcinoma on the glabella (**a**), multiple BCC on the back (**b**), and follicular atrophoderma on dorsum of hand and back with ice pick scars (**c**, **d**)

Rombo Syndrome (AD) [18] (Fig. 5.28)

- A very rare genetic disorder, characterized by vermiculate atrophoderma, milia, hypotrichosis, trichoepitheliomas, peripheral vasodilation with cyanosis, and basal cell carcinomas.
- The defective gene is unknown.
- **Clinical pictures:**
  - Hypotrichosis
  - The eyebrows and eyelashes may either show an irregular, patchy distribution with distorted and maldirected growth, or may be missing completely
  - Blepharitis
  - Telangiectasia
  - Acral erythema
  - Multiple BCCs
  - Acral hyperhidrosis.

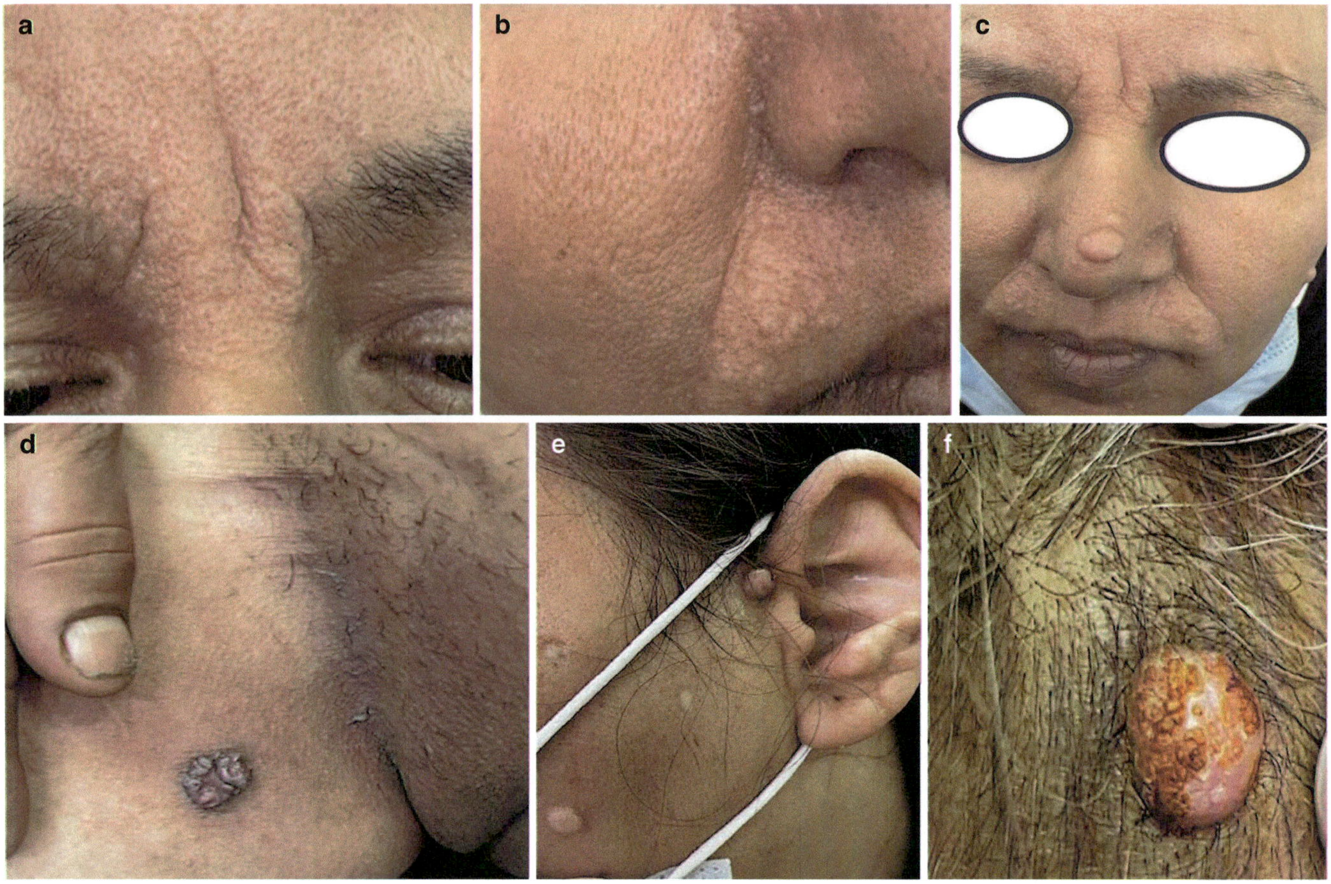

Fig. 5.28 Rombo syndrome. Atrophoderma vermiculatum with ice pick scars on forehead and cheeks (**a**, **b**), solitary trichoepithelioma on tip of nose (**c**), pigmented BCC on medial aspect of right thigh (**d**). Trichoepithelioma in front of left ear, on the left cheek (**e**) and scalp (**f**)

Reed Syndrome (AD) [19] (Fig. 5.29)

- Mutation of fumarate hydratase gene that is classified as a tumor suppressor gene.
- **Clinical features:**
  - **Cutaneous leiomyomas:** appear during the second to fourth decade as multiple painful, grouped, skin-colored to red-brown papules.
  - **Uterine leiomyomas:** >90% of affected women; menorrhagia and pelvic pressure or pain.
  - **Renal cell cancer:** 10–16% of patients; most commonly type 2 papillary renal cell carcinomas that are often early-onset and aggressive (metastases in >50% of patients).

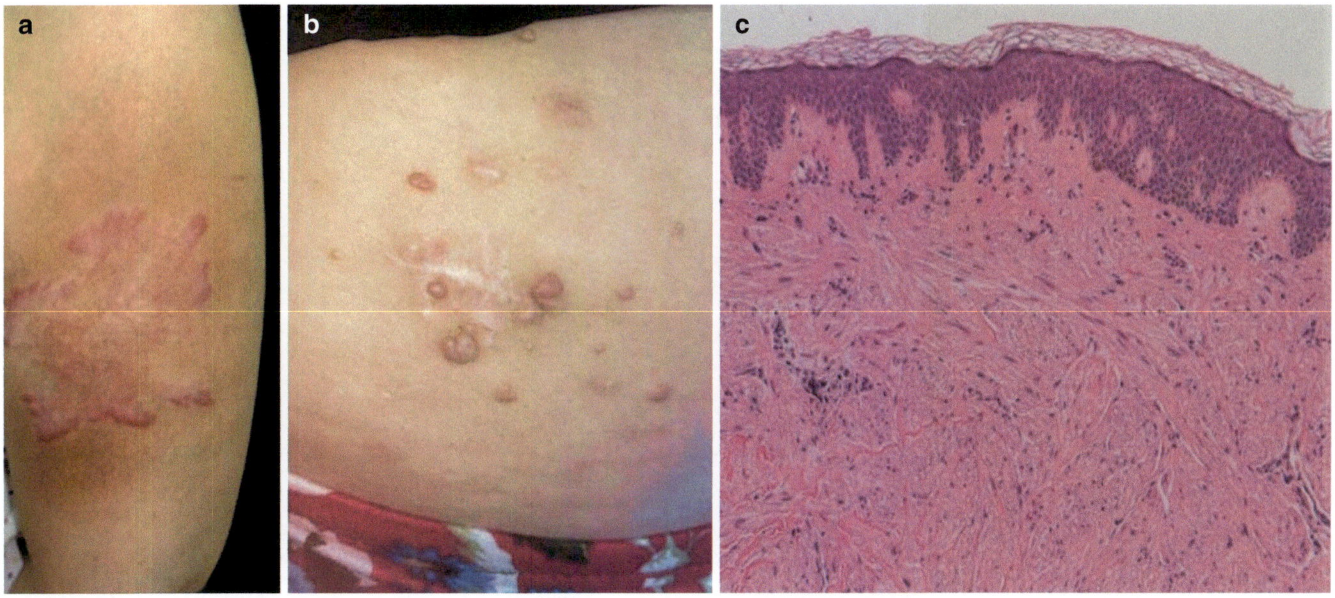

Fig. 5.29 Reed syndrome. Multiple painful red papules on left arm (**a**) and multiple painful, grouped, red-brown papules on the back (**b**) diagnosed as leiomyoma histopathologically (**c**). The patient has associated leiomyoma in the uterus surgically excised by myomectomy

Brooke-Spiegler Syndrome (AD) [20] (Figs. 5.30 and 5.31)

- A rare genetic condition resulting in a range of tumors derived from skin appendages (hair follicle tumors and sweat gland tumors).
- The syndrome includes the limited variants, familial cylindromatosis, and multiple familial trichoepitheliomas.
- Mutations in cylindromatosis tumor-suppressor gene (*CYLD*).
- Characterized by multiple adnexal neoplasia particularly cylindromas, trichoepitheliomas, spiradenomas located on head and neck. Women are commonly affected, usually in third or fourth decade of life. They are occasionally present in association with basal cell adenomas of the parotid glands, milia, organoid nevi, and basal cell carcinomas.
- **Clinical features:**
  - Cylindromas occur as numerous papules, nodules, or tumors distributed over the scalp and sometimes on face and trunk. Malignant transformation to cylindrocarcinomas is rare.
  - Trichoepitheliomas are skin-colored papules distributed on face with a predilection for nasolabial folds, forehead, chin, and preauricular area.
- Brooke–Spiegler syndrome is a devastating condition with no widely accepted standard of treatment. Because Brooke–Spiegler syndrome is characterized by diffuse involvement and numerous adnexal tumors of the head and neck, surgical excision is often difficult.

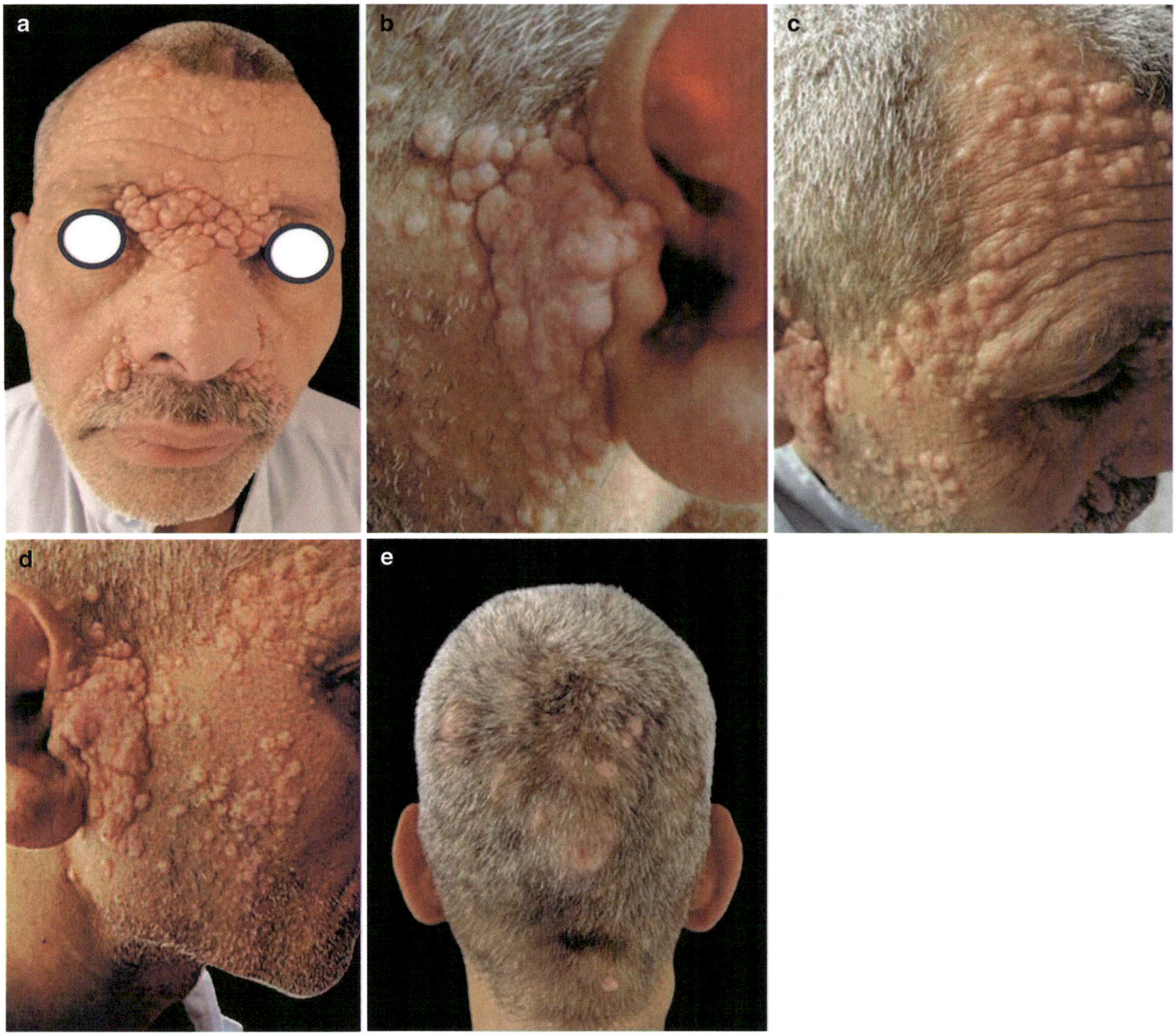

Fig. 5.30 Brooke-Spiegler syndrome. Multiple skin-colored papules and nodules on the face and scalp proved to be trichoepithelioma histopathologically (**a**–**e**)

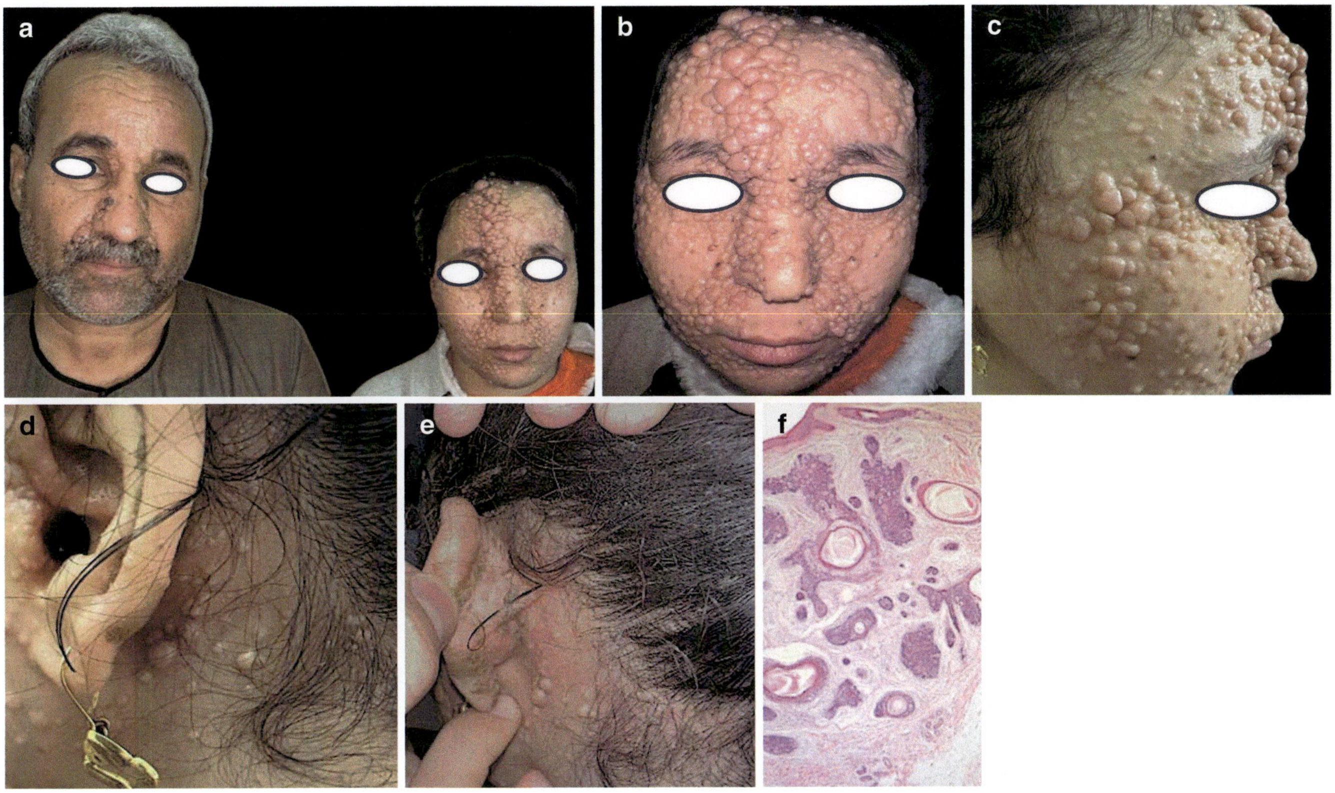

Fig. 5.31 Brooke-Spiegler syndrome (familial multiple trichoepithelioma syndrome). Multiple skin-colored papules and nodules on the face of the father and his daughter (**a**). The daughter shows multiple skin-colored papules and nodules on the face, behind the ear and on the scalp (**b**–**e**) diagnosed histopathologically as trichoepithelioma (**f**)

References

1. Holman JD, Dyer JA. Genodermatoses with malignant potential. Curr Opin Pediatr. 2007;19(4):446–54.
2. Carley H, Kulkarni A. Genodermatoses-opportunities for early detection and cancer prevention. Curr Genet Med Rep. 2022;10(1):1–13.
3. Gerstenblith MR, Goldstein AM, Tucker MA. Hereditary genodermatoses with cancer predisposition. Hematol Oncol Clin North Am. 2010;24(5):885–906.
4. Cardis MA, DeKlotz CMC. Cutaneous manifestations of tuberous sclerosis complex and the paediatrician's role. Arch Dis Child. 2017;102:858–63.
5. Northrup H, Aronow ME, Bebin EM, et al. Updated international tuberous sclerosis complex diagnostic criteria and surveillance and management recommendations. Pediatr Neurol. 2021;123:50–66.
6. Bell SD, Macdonald DM. The prevalence of café au lait patches in tuberous sclerosis. Clin Exp Dermatol. 1985;10(6):562–5.
7. Legius E, Messiaen L, Wolkenstein P, et al. Revised diagnostic criteria for neurofibromatosis type 1 and Legius syndrome: an international consensus recommendation. Genet Med. 2021;23(8):1506–13.
8. Ozarslan B, Russo T, Argenziano G, et al. Cutaneous findings in neurofibromatosis type 1. Cancer. 2021;13(3):463–79.
9. Marque M, Roubertie A, Jaussent A, et al. Nevus anemicus in neurofibromatosis type 1: a potential new diagnostic criterion. J Am Acad Dermatol. 2013;69(5):768–75.
10. Korf BR. Malignancy in neurofibromatosis type 1. Oncologist. 2000;5(6):477–85.
11. Kayhan G, Yılmaz Demirci N, Turktas H, et al. Birt-Hogg-Dube syndrome with a novel mutation in the FLCN gene. Genet Test Mol Biomarkers. 2017;21:632–4.
12. Khoo SK, Giraud S, Kahnoski K, et al. Clinical and genetic studies of Birt-Hogg-Dubé syndrome. J Med Genet. 2002;39:906–12.
13. Lim A, Ngeow J. The skin in Cowden syndrome. Front Med. 2021;8:658842.
14. Hasan A, Akintola D. An update of Gorlin-Goltz syndrome. Prim Dent J. 2018;7(3):38–41.
15. Spiker AM, Troxell T, Ramsey ML. Gorlin syndrome. In: StatPearls. Treasure Island: StatPearls Publishing; 2023. Available from: https://www.ncbi.nlm.nih.gov/books/NBK430921.
16. Bay C, Ousager LB, Jelsig AM. Patients with basal cell naevus syndrome should be offered an early multidisciplinary follow-up and treatment. Ugeskr Laeger. 2015;177(29):12140701.
17. AlSabbagh MM, Baqi MA. Bazex-Dupré-Christol syndrome: review of clinical and molecular aspects. Int J Dermatol. 2018;57(9):1102–6.
18. Michaëlsson G, Olsson E, Westermark P. The Rombo syndrome: a familial disorder with vermiculate atrophoderma, milia, hypotrichosis, trichoepitheliomas, basal cell carcinomas and peripheral vasodilation with cyanosis. Acta Derm Venereol. 1981;61(6):497–503.
19. Almeida FT, Santos RP, Carvalho SD, et al. Reed's syndrome. Indian J Dermatol. 2018;63(3):261–3.
20. Manchanda K, Bansal M, Bhayana AA, et al. Brooke-spiegler syndrome: a rare entity. Int J Trichol. 2012;4(1):29–31.

6 Genodermatoses with Defective Excision Repair

- Xeroderma pigmentosum (XP)
- Pigmented xerodermoid
- DeSanctis–Cacchione syndrome
- Cockayne Syndrome
- Dyskeratosis Congenita
- Rothmund-Thomson Syndrome

Xeroderma Pigmentosum (XP) (AR) [1–4] (Figs. 6.1, 6.2, 6.3, 6.4 and 6.5)

- Autosomal recessive disorder due to mutations in genes involved in the DNA repair, leading to deficient repair of DNA damaged by ultraviolet radiation (UVR).
- Associated with mutations in nucleotide excision repair genes: *XPA, ERCC1, ERCC3 (XP-B), XPC, ERCC2 (XP-D), DDB2 (XP-E), ERCC4 (XP-F)*, and *ERCC5 (XP-G)* and also with mutations in the DNA bypass polymerase *POLH.*
- **Cutaneous manifestations:**
  - Photosensitivity
  - Lentigines (freckle-like pigmentation) in sun-exposed areas, developed in all the patients by the age of 2 years.
  - Dry, rough, and atrophic skin
  - Telangiectasia
  - Stucco keratoses
  - Increased skin cancer susceptibility as actinic keratosis, multiple basal cell carcinomas, invasive squamous cell carcinomas, and less commonly melanomas.
- **Ocular manifestations:**
  - Early dry eye, photophobia, conjunctival injection, severe keratitis, leading to corneal opacification and vascularization, and neoplasms (epithelioma, squamous cell carcinoma, and melanoma).
- **Oral manifestations:**
  - Increased frequency of oral cavity tumors and squamous cell carcinoma of the tip of the tongue.
- **Neurological abnormalities:**
  - Progressive neuronal degeneration resulting in sensorineural deafness, ataxia, areflexia, microcephaly, and intellectual deficiency as well as impaired eyesight.
- **Internal malignancies:**
  - 10:20-fold increase in the incidence of internal malignancies including brain tumors, lung, GIT, kidney, and hematopoietic system.
- **Diagnosis:**
  - Measurement of unscheduled DNA synthesis in cultured skin fibroblasts.
  - The DNA repair tests can be carried out on chorionic villus-derived cells or on amniocytes in affected families.
- **Prognosis**
  - For patients without neurological abnormalities, the prognosis is good.
  - The neurological abnormalities are progressive, leading to progressive disabilities.

N. Moftah et al., *Atlas of Common and Rare Genodermatoses*, https://doi.org/10.1007/978-3-031-60788-2_6

Fig. 6.1 Xeroderma pigmentosum. Early presentation of XP with dry skin and diffuse freckle like pigmentation on the face

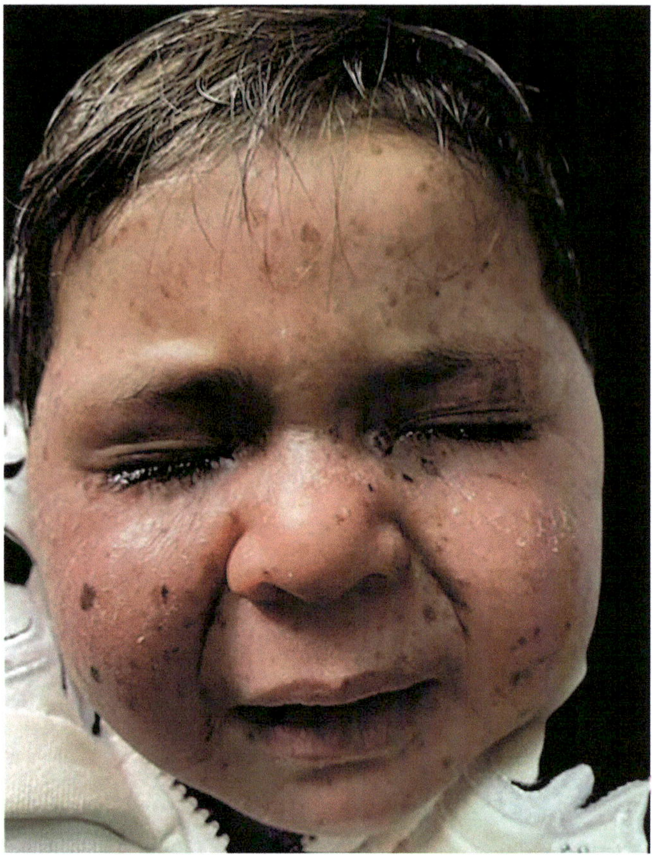

Fig. 6.2 Xeroderma pigmentosum. Dry skin with diffuse freckle like pigmentation on the face (**a**, **b**)

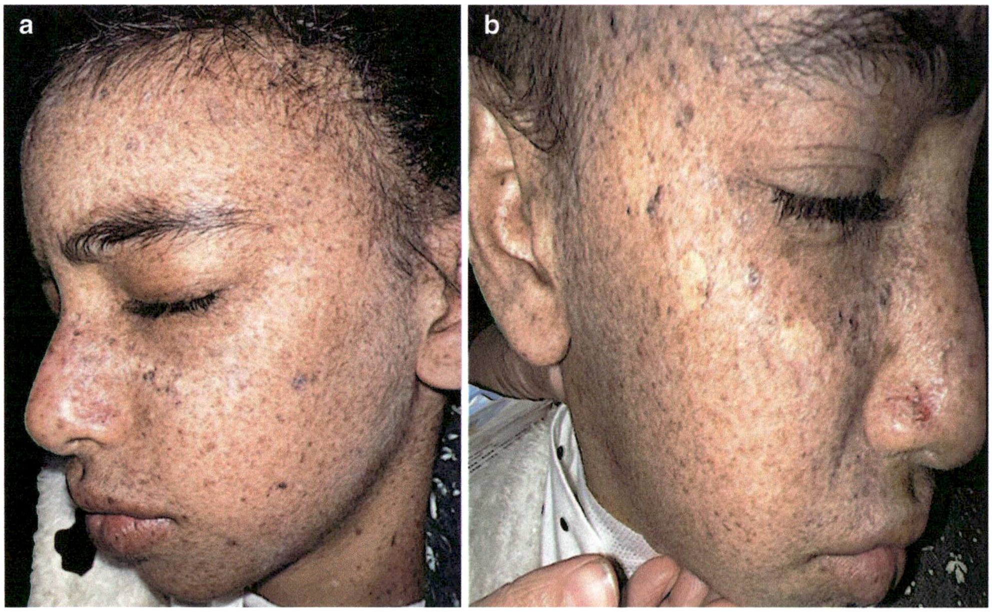

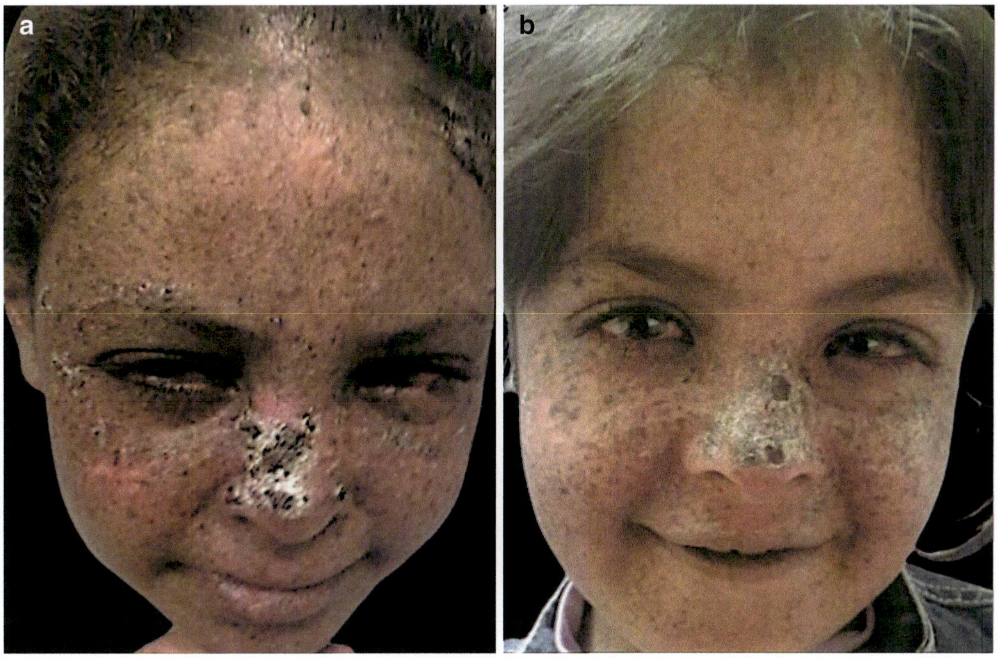

Fig. 6.3 Xeroderma pigmentosum. Squamous cell carcinoma on the lower lip (**a**), upper lip (**b**)

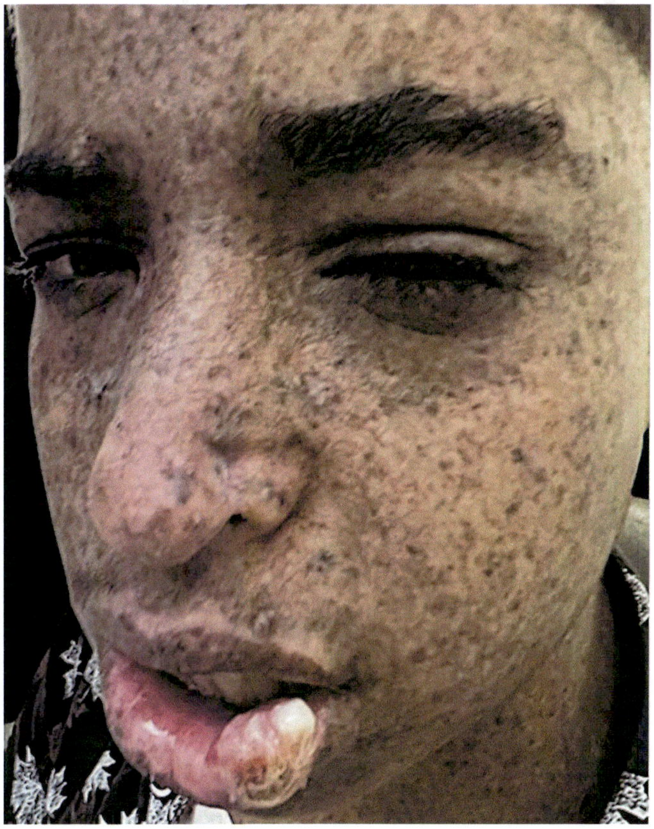

Fig. 6.4 Xeroderma pigmentosum. Multiple tumors as solar keratoses, squamous cell carcinoma in the face and lower lip, respectively

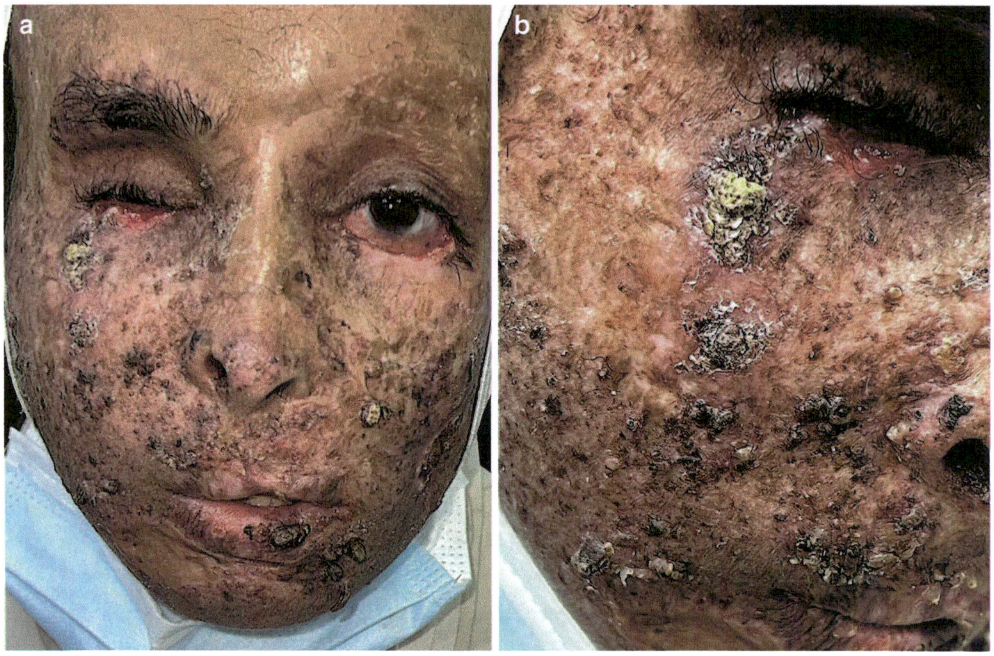

Fig. 6.5 Xeroderma pigmentosum. Ulcerated basal cell carcinoma on the nose (**a**), pigmented basal cell carcinoma on the neck (**b**)

Pigmented Xerodermoid [5, 6] (Fig. 6.6)

- A rare variant of Xeroderma pigmentosum (XP-V) with few reports in the literature.
- (XP-V) has normal nucleotide excision repair of UV-damaged DNA, but they have a defect in the error-prone polymerase, DNA polymerase eta (encoded by *POLH*).
- Cutaneous and ocular manifestations similar to XP, but neurologic involvement is rare.
- Late manifestation of photosensitivity, dyschromic and poikilodermatic skin changes and multiple malignant skin tumors in light exposed areas.
- Clinical features may be mild in some and severe in others.

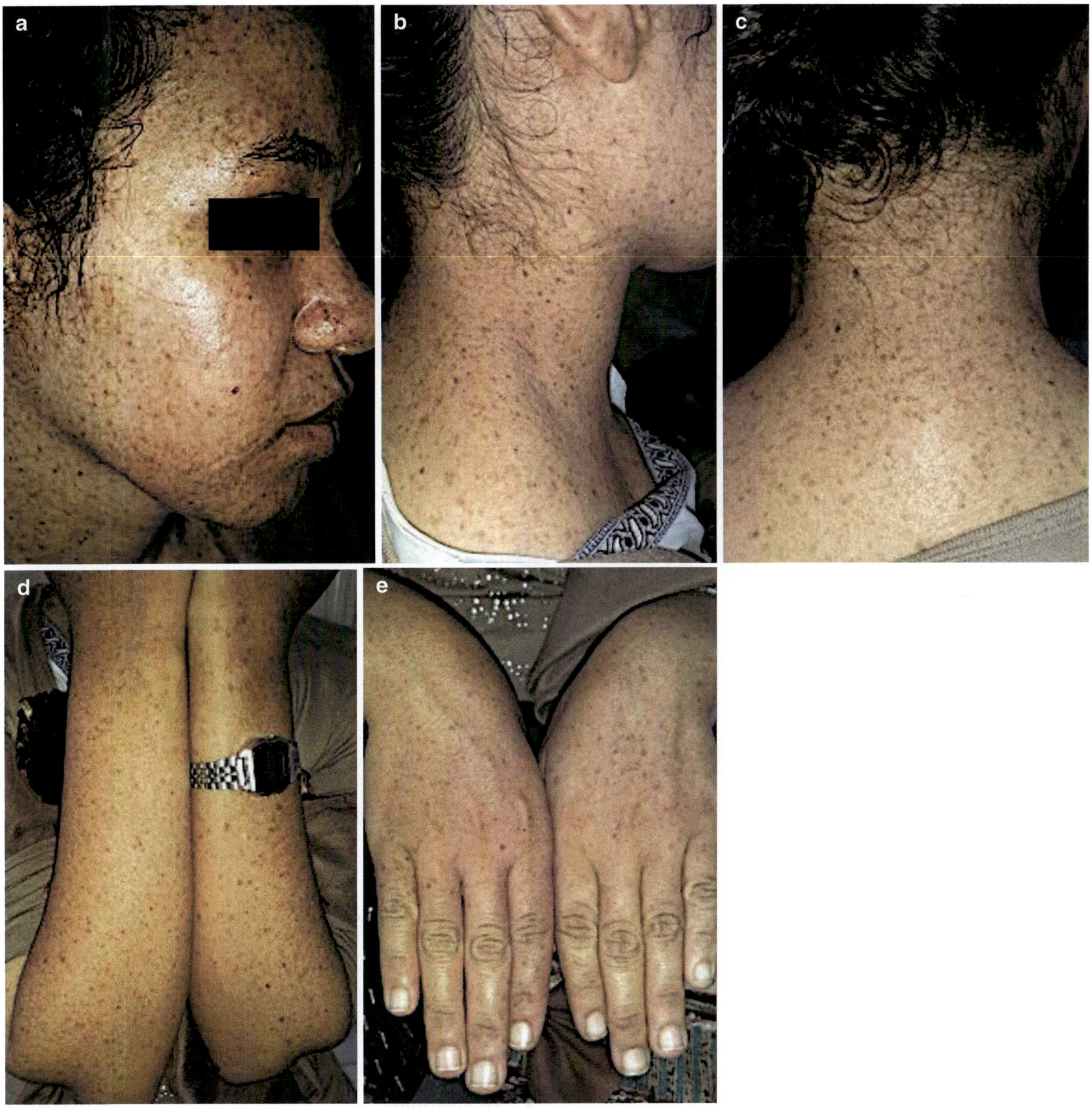

Fig. 6.6 Pigmented xerodermoid. Freckle like pigmentation on the face (**a**), neck (**b**, **c**), forearms (**d**), dorsum of the hands (**e**) in an adult patient

DeSanctis–Cacchione Syndrome (DSC) (AR) [7, 8] (Fig. 6.7)

- One of the rarest manifestations of XP with the most severe DNA repair impairment.
- Due to mutation in the *CSB* gene. It can be associated with *ERCC6* mutation.
- **Cutaneous manifestations:**
  - Dry pigmented skin.
  - Extreme skin sensitivity to ultraviolet radiation (UVR).
  - Abnormal skin pigmentation.
  - High incidence of skin cancers on sun-exposed areas as giant squamous cell carcinoma (SCC) that covered the eye and multiple facial SCCs.
  - Progressive neurologic degeneration.
  - Short stature.
  - Deafness and ataxia.

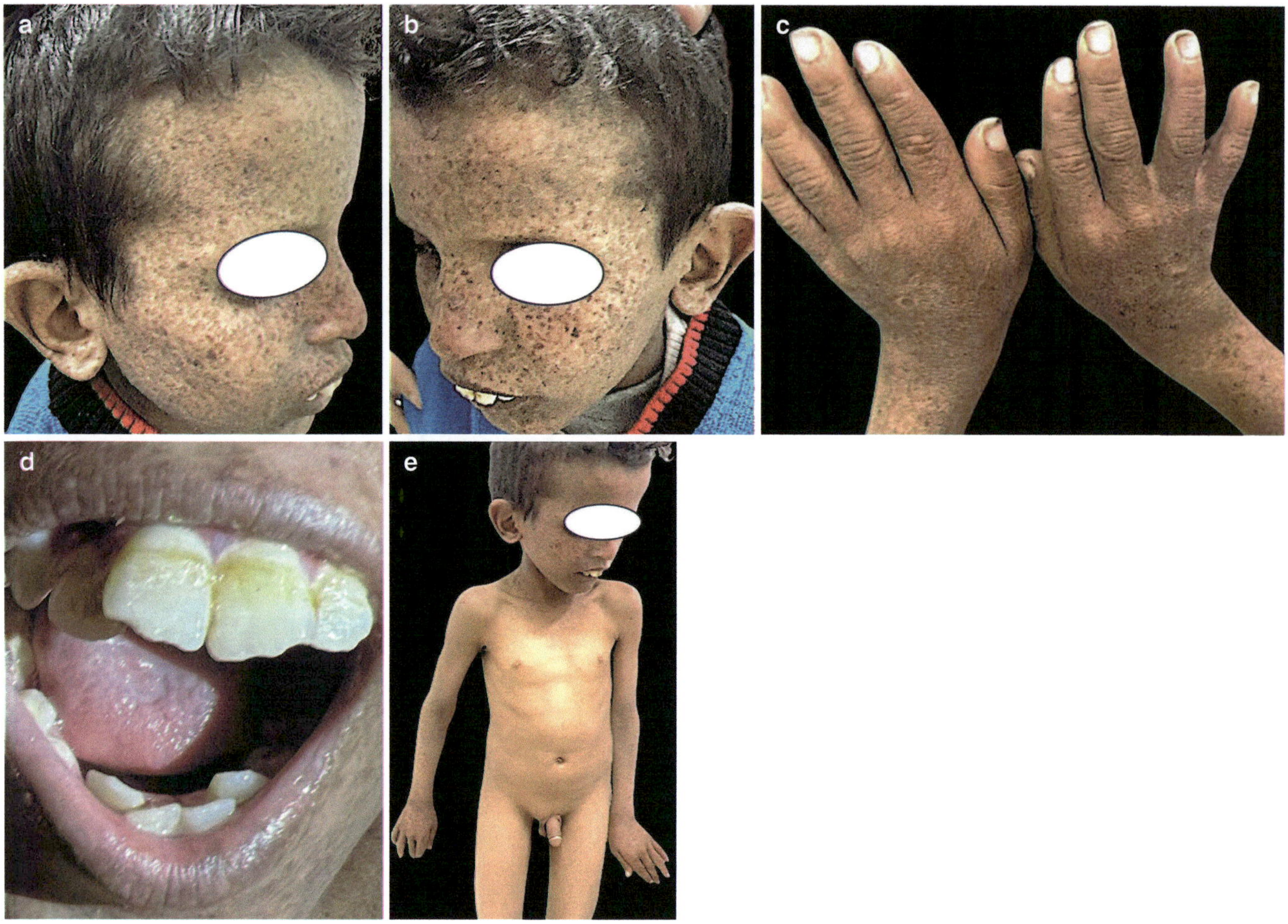

Fig. 6.7 DeSanctis–Cacchione syndrome. Microcephaly, freckle like pigmentation on the face and arms (**a**–**c**), dental crowding (**d**), short stature and hypogonadism (**e**)

Cockayne Syndrome (CS) (AR) [9] (Fig. 6.8)

- It is classified into mainly two different complementation groups:
  - CS-A, due to a mutation on *ERCC8* on chromosome 5q12-q31
  - CS-B, due to a mutation on *ERCC6* on chromosome 10q11
- **Clinical characteristics:**
  - Cachectic dwarfism.
  - Shriveled and wrinkled skin.
  - Loss of subcutaneous fat.
  - Beaked nose.
  - Stooped posture.
- **Hearing:**
  - Sensorineural hearing loss.
- **Eye manifestations**:
  - Cataracts.
  - Pigmentary retinopathy.
- **Cutaneous manifestation:** an extreme sensitivity to sunlight; even a small amount of sun exposure can cause sunburn.
- **Dental caries**
- **Associations:**
  - Cognitive dysfunction
  - Advanced atherosclerosis and vasculopathy
  - Premature onset of hypertension, which often leads to strokes.
  - Renal and cardiac dysfunction.

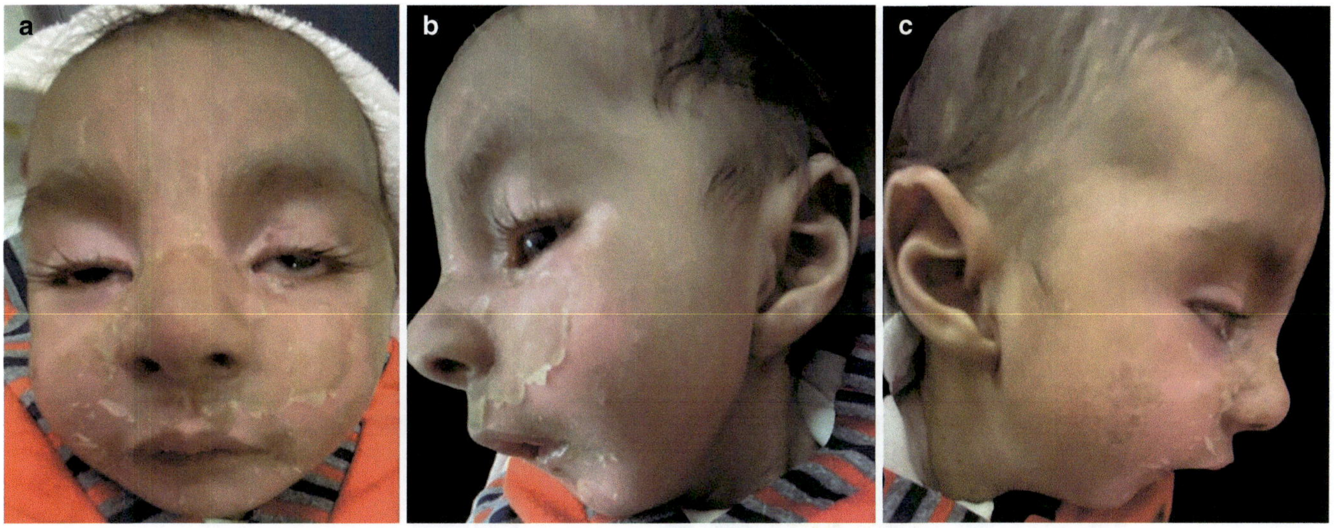

Fig. 6.8 Cockayne syndrome. Photosensitivity with desquamation of facial skin (**a**) Bird-like facies, Mickey Mouse ears, prominent nose, sunken eyes) (**b**, **c**)

Dyskeratosis Congenita (DC) (Zinssser-Engman-Cole syndrome) (X-linked Recessive, AD or AR) [10, 11] (Figs. 6.9 and 6.10)

- Majority of DC patients have a defect in *DKC1* gene encoding the dyskerin protein which is involved in telomere maintenance. It has two other severe variants: Hoyeraal-Hreidarsson syndrome and Revesz syndrome.
- **Incidence**: 1/1,000,000 neonates, with a 13:1 male predominance.
- **Clinical manifestations:**
  - Signs and symptoms usually start to manifest in childhood between the ages of 5 and 10 years.
  - **Presents with a classic triad** of reticulate hyperpigmentation, nail dystrophy, and leukoplakia.
- **Cutaneous manifestations:**
  - Reticulate hyperpigmentation, atrophy, and poikiloderma with telangiectasia.
  - Nail dystrophy.
  - Oral leukoplakia.
  - Premature hair graying or loss.
  - Palmoplantar hyperkeratosis.
  - Skin cancer including basal cell carcinoma, squamous cell carcinoma, and high-grade cervical intraepithelial neoplasia, white striae, and hyperhidrosis.
- **Extra-cutaneous manifestations:**
  - Bone marrow failure.
  - Bones: avascular necrosis of the femoral head, fractures, and osteoporosis.
  - Amblyopia
  - Cardiovascular system: mitral valve prolapse and absence of inferior vena cava.
  - Ear, nose, and throat: bilateral choanal atresia, chronic otitis media, and bilateral non-progressive sensorineural hearing loss.
  - Endocrine: hypogonadism (5.9 %), primary amenorrhea, hypothyroidism, normal thyroid profile and cortisol level, and type 1 diabetes.
  - Gastrointestinal tract: anal stricture, diarrhea, dysphagia, hepatosplenomegaly, and ascites.
  - Genitourinary tract: genital leukoplakia, phimosis, renal agenesis, and undescended testes.
  - Malignancies: actinic keratosis and carcinoma of the gastrointestinal tract.
  - Ocular manifestations: blepharitis, conjunctival leukoplakia, conjunctivitis, and ectropion.
  - Oral cavity: alveolar bone loss, dental abnormalities, and ulceration that precedes to leukoplakia.
- **Prognosis**: The mean age of death in dyskeratosis congenita is the third to fifth decade of life except in cases of Hoyeraal-Hreidarsson syndrome and Revesz syndrome, where life expectancy does not exceed the twenties.

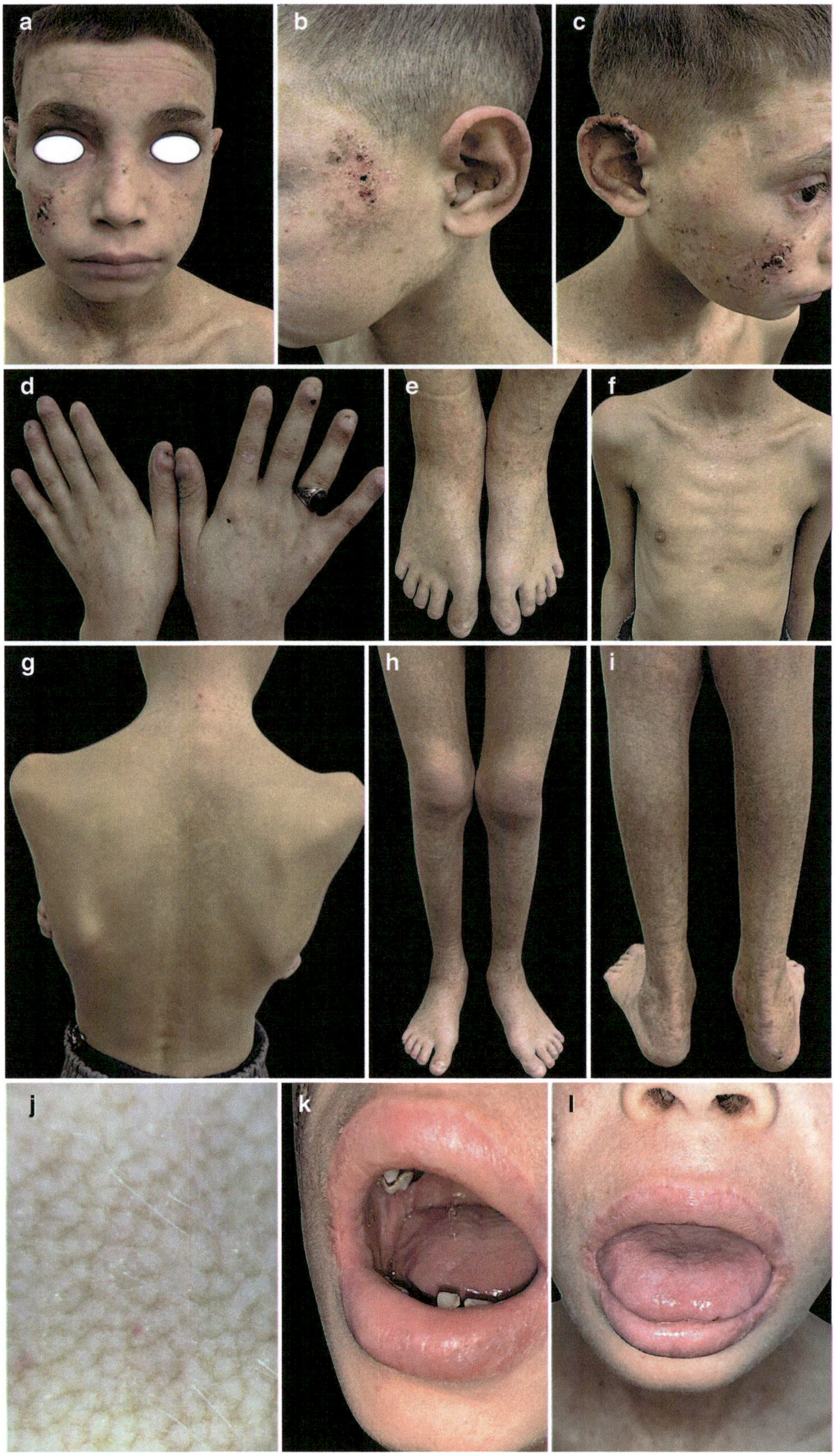

Fig. 6.9 Dyskeratosis congenita. Reticulate hyperpigmentation with multiple actinic keratosis lesions on the face (field cancerization) (**a**–**c**), nail dystrophy (**d**, **e**), reticulate hyperpigmentation allover the chest, back, limbs (**f**–**i**), and by dermoscopy (**j**). Oral leukoplakia on the tongue (**k**, **l**). (*Courtesy, Youmna El-Sayed*)

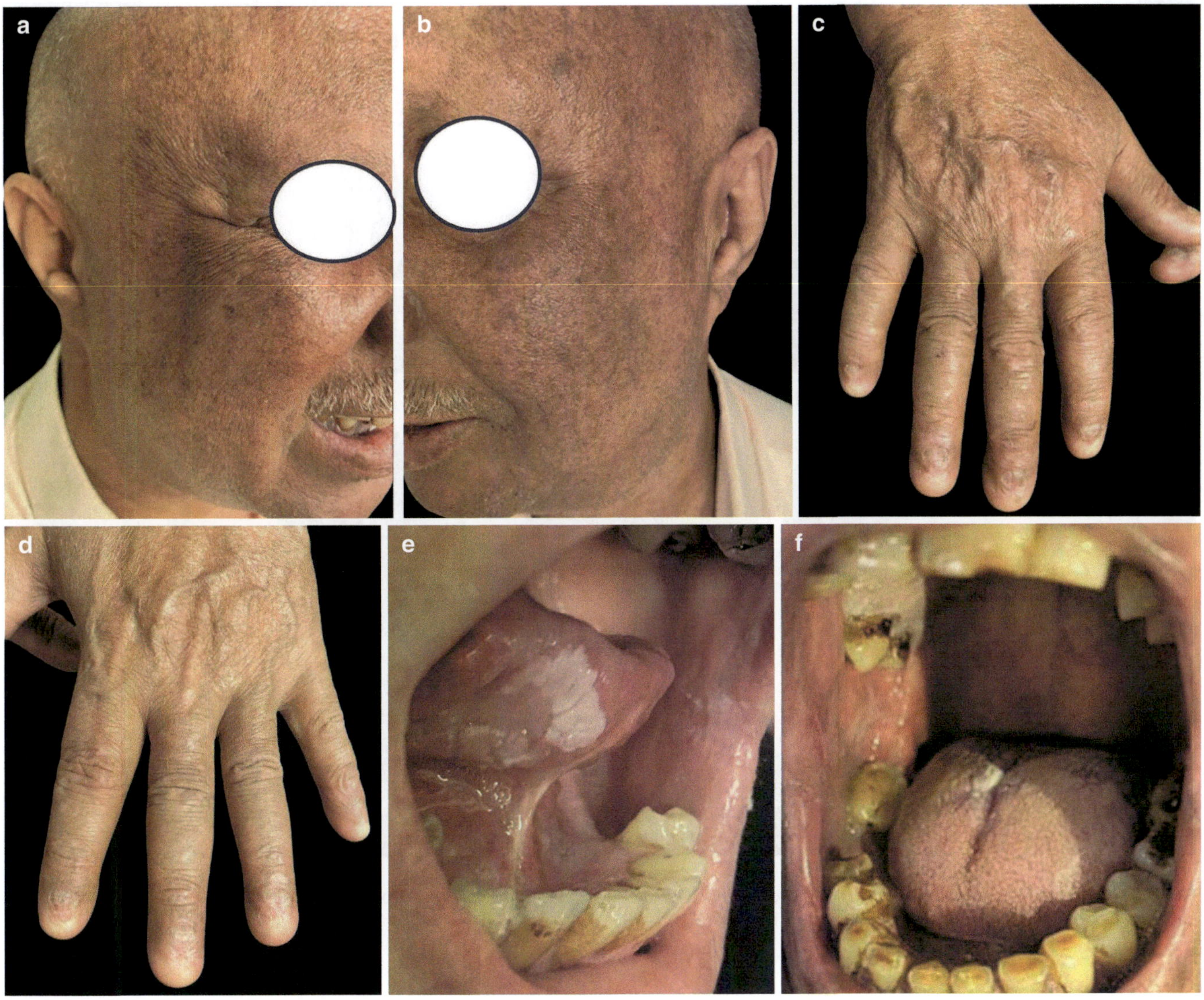

Fig. 6.10 Dyskeratosis Congenita. Reticulate hyperpigmentation on the face (**a**, **b**), nail dystrophy with pterygium formation (**c**, **d**), oral leukoplakia on palate and tongue (**e**, **f**)

Rothmund-Thomson Syndrome (AR) [12] (Fig. 6.11)

- Rare autosomal recessive disorder with equal male-to-female ratio.
- **Classification:**
  - Type II RTS, characterized by poikiloderma and skeletal defects is caused by homozygous or compound heterozygous mutations in the *RECQL4* (also named *RECQ4*) helicase gene.
  - Type I RTS, characterized by poikiloderma and juvenile cataracts is negative for the *RECQL4* mutation.
- **Clinical characteristics:**
  - The first signs usually affect the skin, hair, nails, and teeth.
  - Growth delay and the resulting short stature is the second major clinical sign.
- **Cutaneous manifestation:**
  - Poikiloderma.
  - Café-au-lait spots.
  - Worsening of the erythema following sun exposure.
  - Palmoplantar hyperkeratosis.
  - Calcinosis cutis and porokeratosis are uncommon.

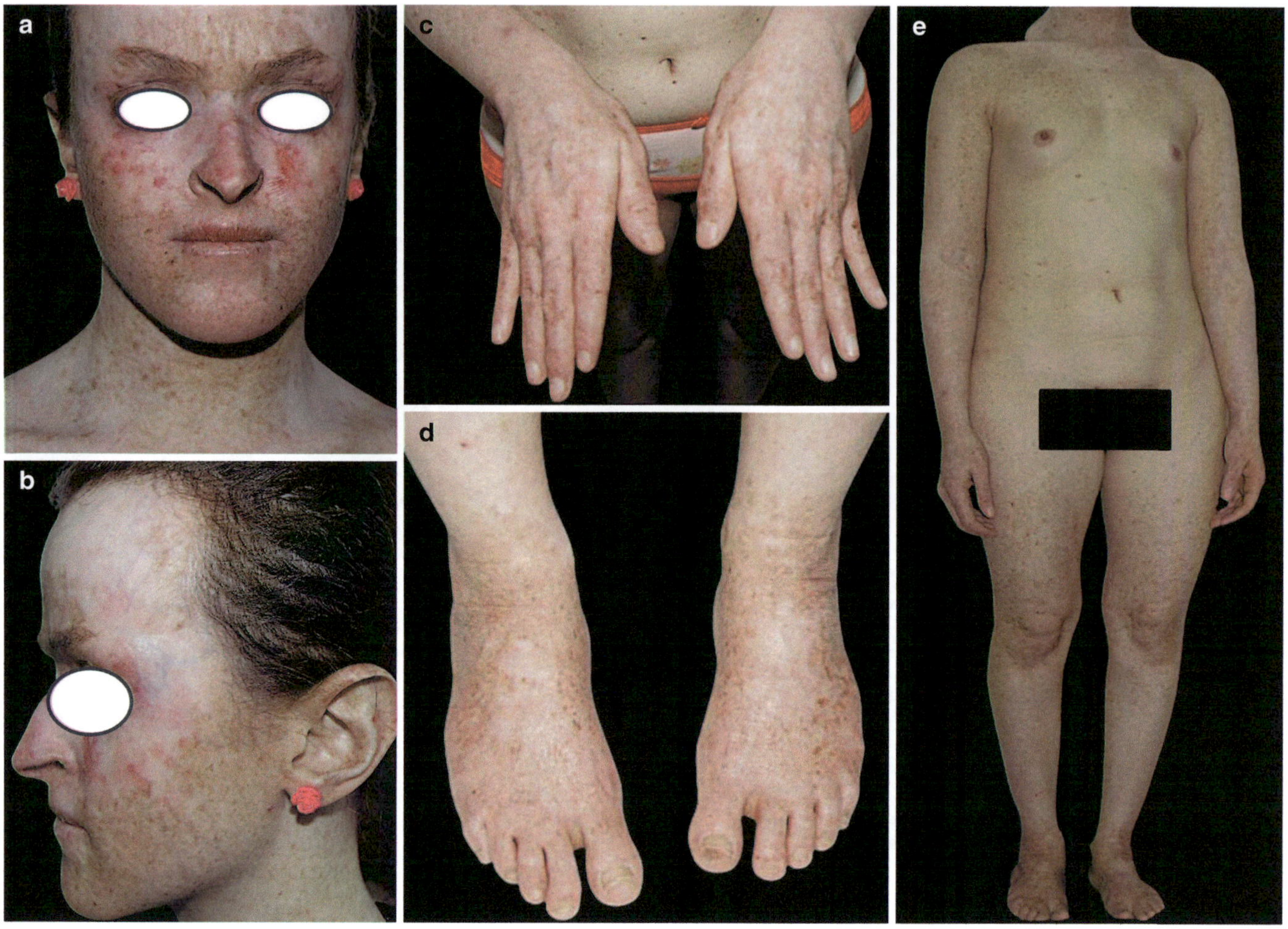

Fig. 6.11 Rothmund-Thomson syndrome. Photosensitivity with poikiloderma in the face (**a**), frontal bossing, saddle nose (**b**) pigmentation in hands, feet (**c**, **d**), and short stature (**e**). The patient has cataract

- **Hair:**
  - Sparse, brittle, thin or absent scalp hair and sparse hair on eyelashes and/or eyebrows.
- **Nails:**
  - Dystrophic or poorly formed nails are common.
  - Pachyonychia is also a frequent sign.
- **Teeth:**
  - Microdontia, rudimentary or hypoplastic teeth.
- **Growth:**
  - Low birth weight, slow weight gain, and short stature.
- **Neurocognitive development:**
  - Neurologic cognitive milestones and intelligence are usually normal.
- **Hearing:**
  - Sensorineural deafness.
- **Bone:**
  - Frontal bossing, saddle nose, and abnormalities of the long bones.
- **Eye manifestations:**
  - Bilateral cataracts, exophthalmos, corneal atrophy/scleralization, congenital bilateral glaucoma, retinal atrophy/coloboma, strabismus, photophobia, and blue sclerae.
- **Gastrointestinal system:**
  - Esophageal or pyloric stenosis, anal atresia, annular pancreas, and rectovaginal fistula
- **Respiratory system:**
  - Lower respiratory tract infections, bronchiectasis
- **Hematological signs:**
  - Progressive leukopenia and chronic microcytic hypochromic anemia
- **Malignancy:**
  - Osteosarcoma occurs in childhood.
  - Cutaneous epithelial neoplasms (squamous cell carcinoma, basal cell carcinoma, and Bowen's disease) occur later.

References

1. Abeti R, Zeitlberger A, Peelo C, et al. Xeroderma pigmentosum: overview of pharmacology and novel therapeutic strategies for neurological symptoms. Br J Pharmacol. 2019;176(22):4293–301.
2. Harper JL, Champion RD, Burton JL, Burn DA, et al. Genetics and genodermatoses Rook/Wilkinson/Ebling textbook of dermatology. 16th ed. Oxford: Blackwell Science Ltd; 1998. p. 407–12.
3. Srivastava G, Srivastava G. Xeroderma pigmentosum. Oxf Med Case Rep. 2021;11:107.
4. Piccione M, Belloni FA. Xeroderma pigmentosum: general aspects and management. J Pers Med. 2021;11(11):1146–52.
5. Deb S, Dhar S. Pigmented xerodermoid. Indian J Paediat Dermatol. 2015;16(3):139–41.
6. Armenta AM, Paul R, Sikandar G, et al. Variant subtype of xeroderma pigmentosum diagnosed in a 77-year-old woman. JAAD Case Rep. 2018;4:1074–6.
7. Rahbar Z, Naraghi M. De Sanctis–Cacchione syndrome: a case report and literature review. Int J Women's Dermatol. 2015;1(3):136–9.
8. Colella S, Nardo T, Botta E, et al. Identical mutations in the CSB gene associated with either Cockayne syndrome or the de Sanctis-Cacchione variant of xeroderma pigmentosum. Hum Mol Genet. 2000;9(8):1171–5.
9. Karikkineth AC. Cockayne syndrome: clinical features, model systems and pathways. Ageing Res Rev. 2017;33:3–17.
10. Al Sabbagh MM. Dyskeratosis congenita: a literature review. JDDG. 2020;18(9):943–67.
11. Walne AJ, Dokal I. Advances in the understanding of dyskeratosis congenita. Br J Haematol. 2009;145(2):164–72.
12. Larizza L, Roversi G. Rothmund-thomson syndrome. Orphanet J Rare Dis. 2010;5:1–16.

7 Vascular Disorders

Vascular disorders may be congenital or acquired. No evidence of inheritance in vascular disorders. Although they are not genodermatoses, it is included in this atlas of geneodermatoses as they are common in the neonate and although most of these disorders are benign and self-limited, some may be part of complex syndromes or systemic disorders or may be associated with complications. Vascular disorders include vascular neoplasms and vascular malformations. They comprise capillary, venous, lymphatic changes or a mixture of them. In this chapter, we discuss classification of these vascular disorders, the common clinical criteria for each one with their photos of the patients. This chapter includes the following diseases:

1. Port-wine stain
2. Sturge–Weber syndrome
3. Klippel–Trenaunay syndrome
4. Proteus syndrome
5. Fabry disease
6. Venous lake
7. Maffucci syndrome
8. Blue Rubber Bleb syndrome
9. Hereditary hemorrhagic telangiectasia
10. Hemangioma
11. Lumbar syndrome
12. Pelvis syndrome
13. Phace syndrome
14. Lymphangioma circumscripta

Capillary Malformations

Port-Wine Stain (Nevus Flammeus) [1–3] (Figs. 7.1, 7.2, and 7.3)

- Port-wine stain (PWS) is a low-flow capillary malformation.
- It is a type of birthmark.
- Incidence: one of the most common vascular anomalies, affecting 0.3–0.5% of newborns with no gender predilection.
- Typically present at birth and dose not involute spontaneously.
- Clinical characteristics:
  - Well demarcated, irregular, bright red or erythematous patch with smooth surface.
  - Site: PWS may affect any site but the most common location is the face in the distribution of the sensory dermatomes of trigeminal nerve.
- Complications:
  - Overgrowth of facial bones underlying PWS.
  - Lip and gingival hypertrophy with recurrent bleeding.
  - Lumbo-sacral PWS may indicate occult spinal dysraphism.
  - Association with other syndromes.
- Investigations: Computed tomography, magnetic resonance imaging, and magnetic resonance angiography can be used to detect any superficial or deep tissue anomalies associated with PWS in the setting of a combined vascular malformation or a syndrome.
- Pathology: widely dilated, thin-walled capillaries scattered throughout the upper dermis or reticular deep dermis. There is no proliferation of endothelial cells or vessels. With age, progressive vascular dilatation occur with or without perivascular fibrosis, which is clinically evident as the hypertrophy and nodularity developing during the natural evolution of PWS.
- Treatment: pulsed dye laser/cosmetic camouflage.

Sturge–Weber Syndrome [4, 5] (Fig. 7.4)

- Sturge–Weber syndrome (SWS) is caused by somatic mutation in the *GNAQ* gene.
- Incidence: rare and the exact incidence is unknown. SWS has no gender predilection.

N. Moftah et al., *Atlas of Common and Rare Genodermatoses*, https://doi.org/10.1007/978-3-031-60788-2_7

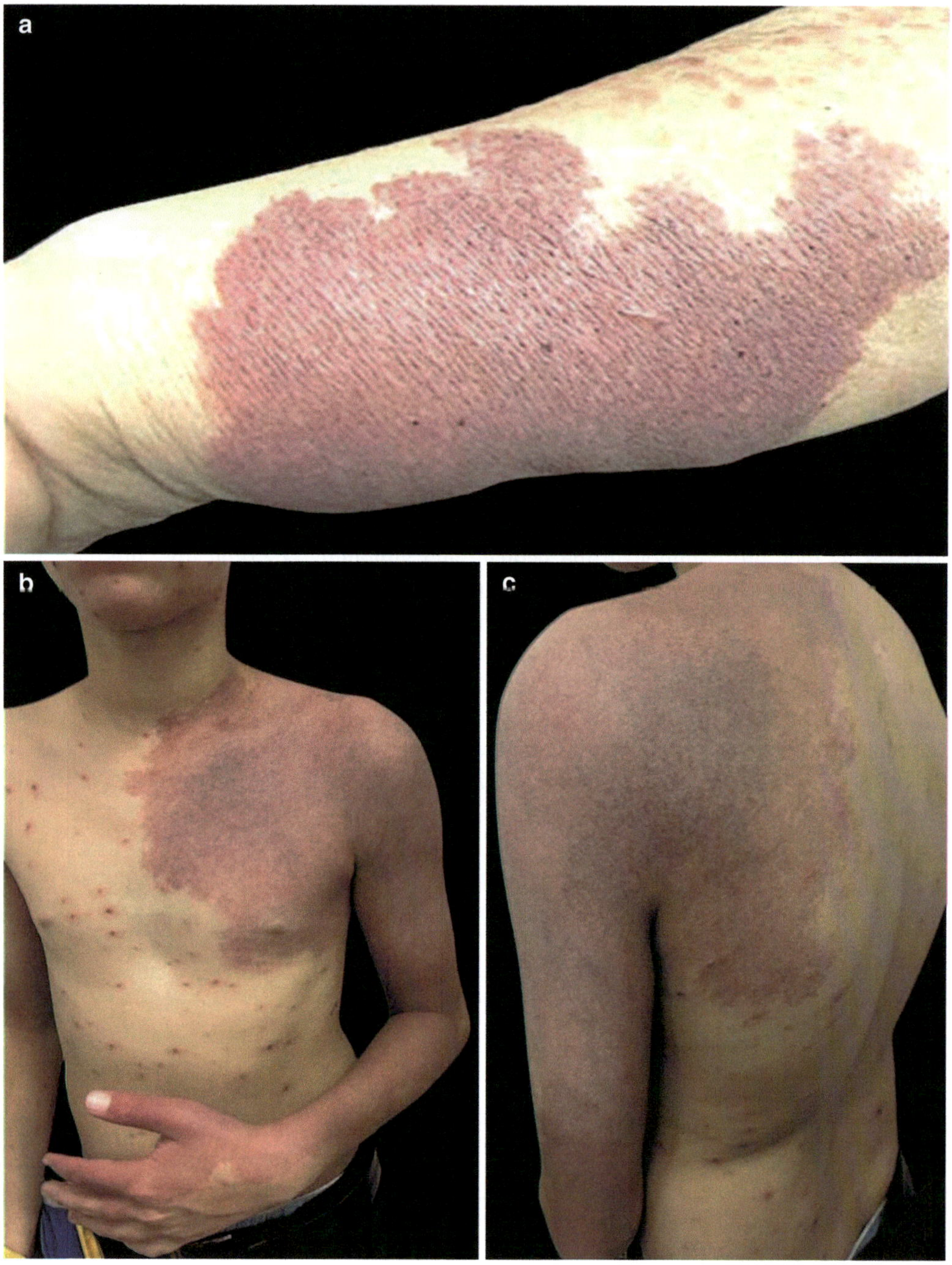

Fig. 7.1 Port-wine stain. Well-demarcated deep red patch and macules in the left forearm (**a**), in segmental pattern in the chest, shoulder, and left arm (**b**, **c**)

- It is considered as one of the Phakomatosis (combination of skin, eye and neurological lesions).
- Cutaneous manifestations:
  - Facial segmental port-wine stain in the ophthalmic division of trigeminal (V1 alone or V1/V2/V3) nerve.
- Ocular: ipsilateral angiomas of the conjunctiva, iris and choroid, congenital glaucoma that may cause buphthalmos.
- CNS: Ipsilateral leptomeningeal angiomas, seizures in the first year of life, mental retardation, contralateral hemiparesis, epilepsy, headache, ischemic attacks, stroke and attention deficit disorder.
- Growth hormone deficiency and hypothyroidism
- Investigations: radiological image: skull CT scan and MRI (Intracranial "tram-track" calcification within first 2 years of life)/intraocular pressure follow-up/an electroencephalogram (EEG) can be used to evaluate and localize seizure activity.
- Treatment: it requires coordinated efforts of a team of specialists. Pediatricians, neurologists, neurosurgeons, dermatologists, and ophthalmologists/pulsed dye laser or cosmetic camouflage for PWS/anti-convulsant for seizures/medical treatment for glaucoma/physical therapy/surgical treatment for resistant seizures.

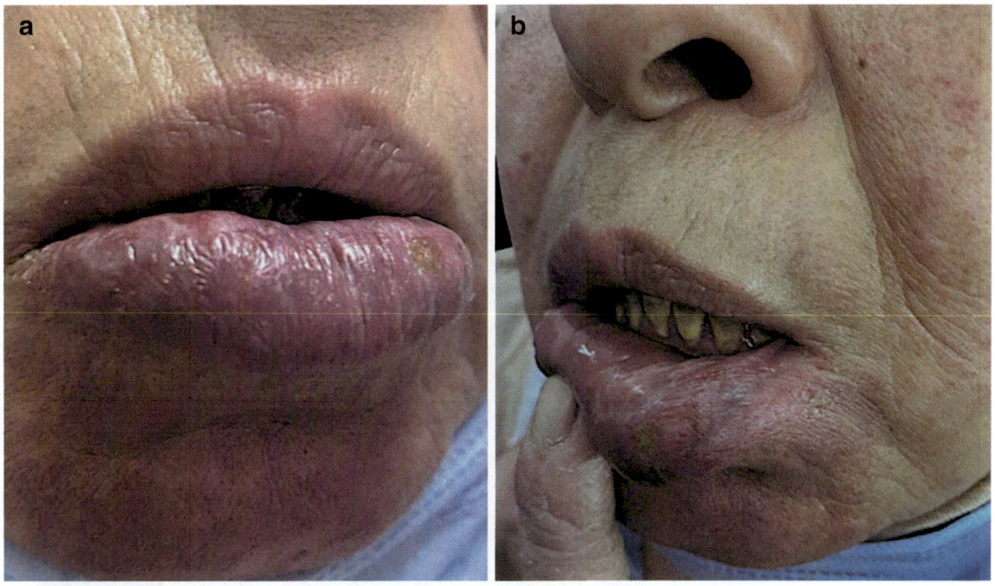

Fig. 7.2 Port-wine stain. Well-demarcated red patch and macules in the chin, lips (**a**, **b**) with actinic cheilitis of the lower lip (**b**)

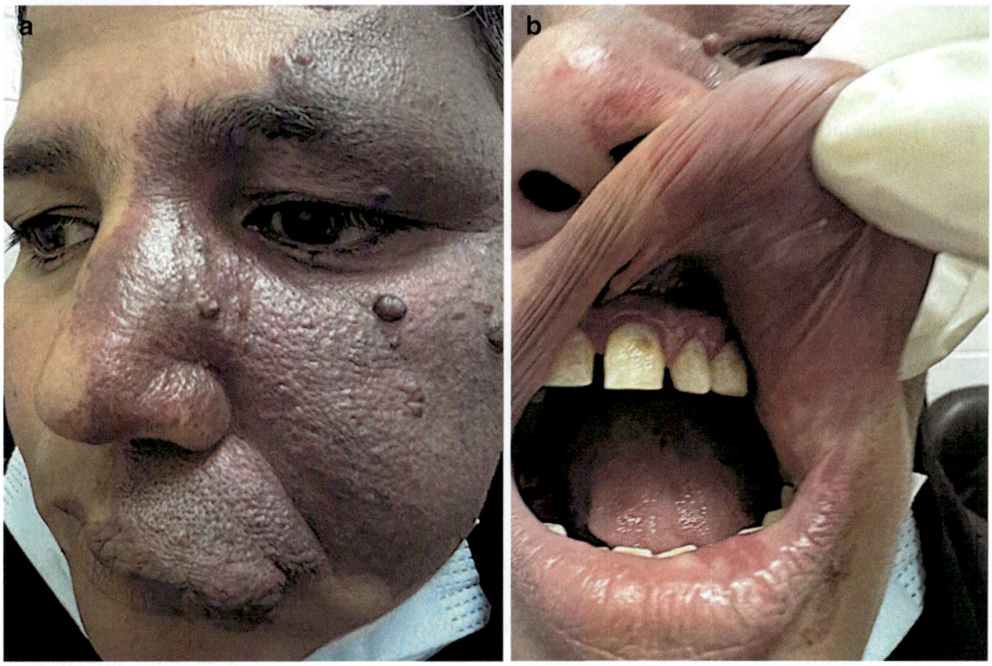

Fig. 7.3 Port-wine stain. Well-demarcated red patch in the trigeminal nerve distribution, with increased skin pigmentation, thickening and nodularity (**a**), gingival hyperplasia (**b**)

Klippel–Trenaunay Syndrome [6, 7] (Figs. 7.5, 7.6, and 7.7)

- Klippel–Trenaunay syndrome (KTS) is a complex congenital disorder defined as the triad of capillary malformation, venous malformation, and limb overgrowth, with or without lymphatic malformation and without AV fistula.
- Severe cases of KTS are caused by mosaic activating variants in the *PIK3CA* gene, experts have proposed that KTS should not be labeled as a distinct diagnostic entity but as part of the *PIK3CA*-related overgrowth spectrum (PROS).
- Cutaneous manifestations:
  - Capillary malformations (CM): port-wine stain is usually the first sign of KTS. With age, the surface of the CM becomes studded with tiny lymphatic vesicles that often ooze clear fluid and turn black due to intralesional bleeding.
  - Venous malformations (VM): varicosities in the superficial and deep venous systems, persistent embryonic veins, and aplasia/hypoplasia with valvular incompetence. Venous malformations can occur in the GI tract, especially in the colon. Dilated tortuous veins can be seen in the affected limb with swelling and discoloration.

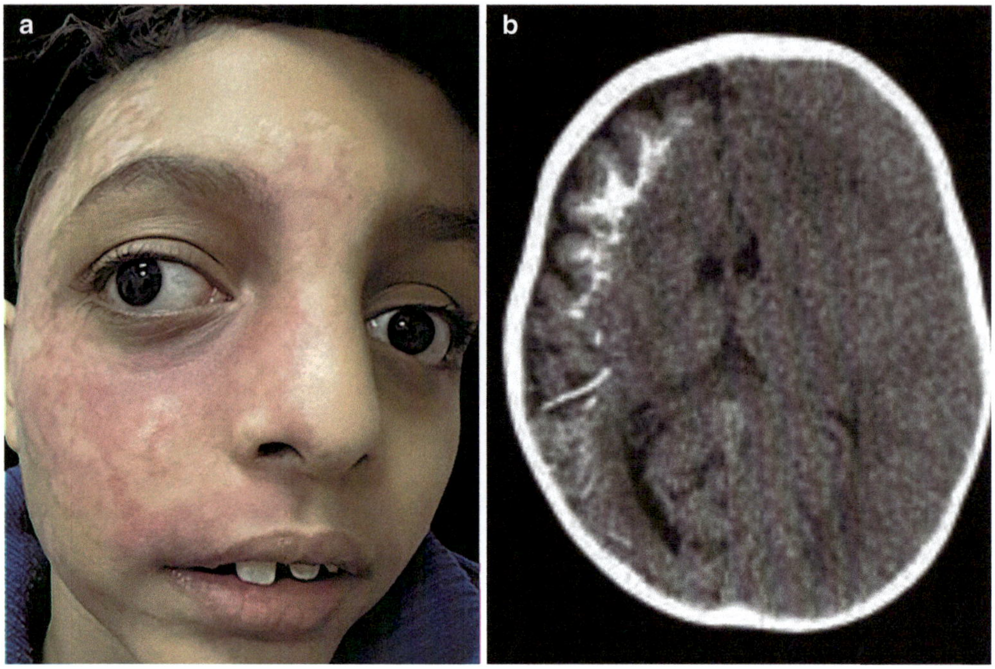

Fig. 7.4 Sturge–Weber syndrome. Port-wine stain in ophthalmic and maxillary division of trigeminal nerve with buphthalmos (**a**), ipsilateral calcification in CT scan (**b**). (*Courtesy, Shaymaa Hosny Elgabry*)

  - Lymphatic malformations: in 15–50% of cases and consist of lymphedema and cystic lymphatic collections.
- Musculoskeletal manifestations: soft tissue and bone hypertrophy in an extremity leading to the limb-length discrepancy.
- Other manifestations: syndactyly, polydactyly, and clinodactyly, seizures, developmental delay, and genitourinary abnormalities presenting as hematuria.
- Complications:
  - Cellulitis due to stasis and lymphatic leak.
  - Bleeding from GI tract vascular malformations which can be chronic and occult.
  - Recurrent pulmonary embolism secondary to deep venous thrombosis.
  - Limb hypertrophy may require de-bulking surgeries for mobility and ambulation.
- Diagnosis: the diagnosis is based on physical signs and symptoms. Computed axial tomography (CAT), magnetic resonance imaging (MRI) scans, and color Doppler studies may be useful in determining the extent of the condition and how best to manage it.
- Treatment: medical by anticoagulant and elastic stocking
  - Rapamycin works in KTS by inhibition of PI3K/AKT/mTOR pathway. Rapamycin-protein complex inhibits the action of mTOR1, leading to the arrest of cell growth, thereby preventing tissue overgrowth
  - Capillary malformation: laser/sclerotherapy
  - Venous malformation: sclerotherapy
  - Overgrowth: Surgical closure of the growth plate at the knee (epiphysiodesis) is often needed to equalize leg length.

Proteus Syndrome [8–10] (Figs. 7.8 and 7.9)

- Extremely rare genetic disorder caused by mosaic alteration or mutation in the *AKT1* gene.
- The first manifestations occur between the age of 6 and 18 months.
- Clinical features: progressive segmental or patchy overgrowth most commonly affecting the bone, skin, adipose tissue, and central nervous systems.
- Skin and connective tissue manifestations:
  - Cerebriform connective tissue nevi especially on the sole, hand, alae nasi, and ear, are present in most of the cases (nearly pathognomonic).
  - Linear verrucous epidermal nevi.
  - Café-au-lait macules are often present.
  - Overgrowth of fat (lipomas) or invasive lipomas that produce large intra-abdominal or intrathoracic lesions.
  - Fatty infiltration of the myocardium, particularly the intraventricular septum.
  - Vascular malformations are common, port-wine stains is the commonest followed by venous malformations with varicosities and arterial malformations, which are less common.
- Bone and soft tissue manifestations:
  - Overgrowth of limbs, digits, and skull, which is usually disproportionate and asymmetric.

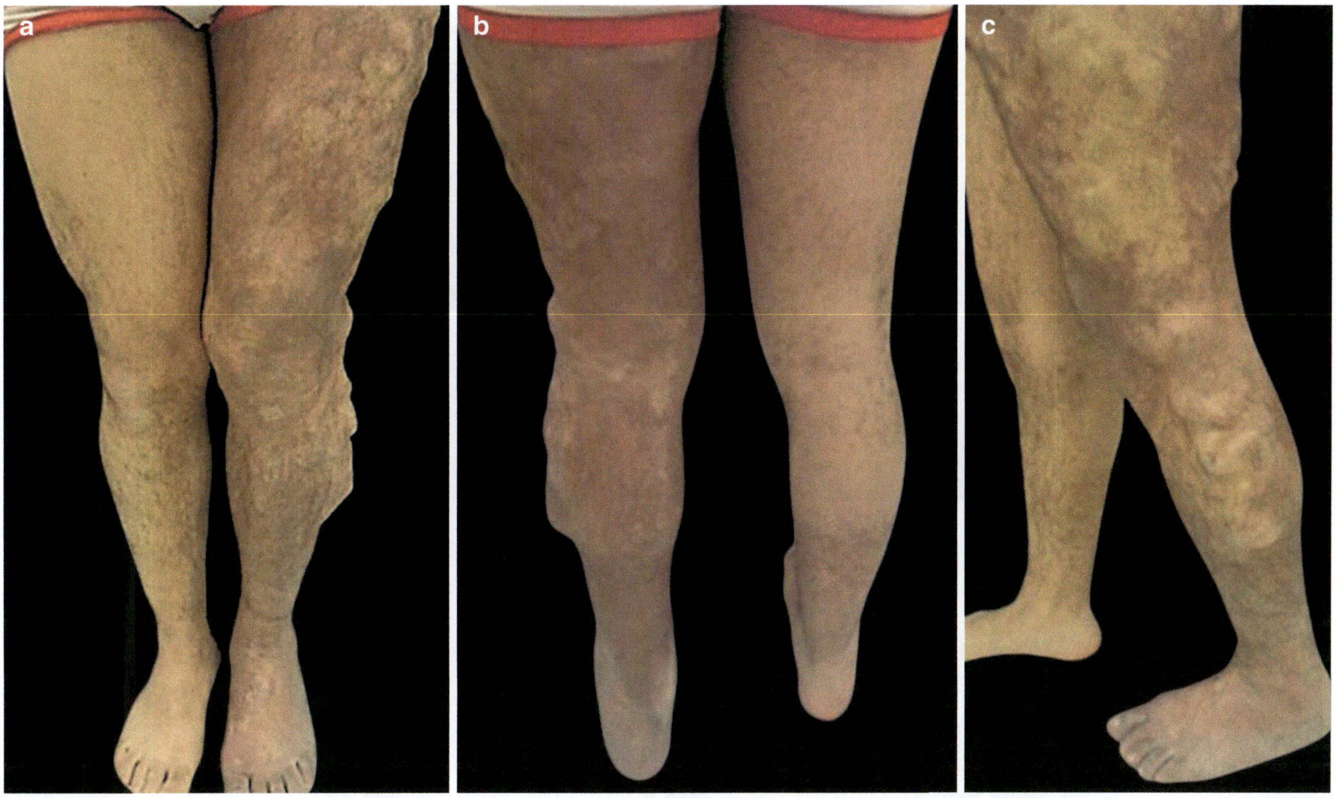

Fig. 7.5 Klippel–Trenaunay syndrome. Large port-wine stain in the left lower leg and thigh with unilateral hypertrophy over the affected limb with engorged and tortuous vessels (**a**–**c**)

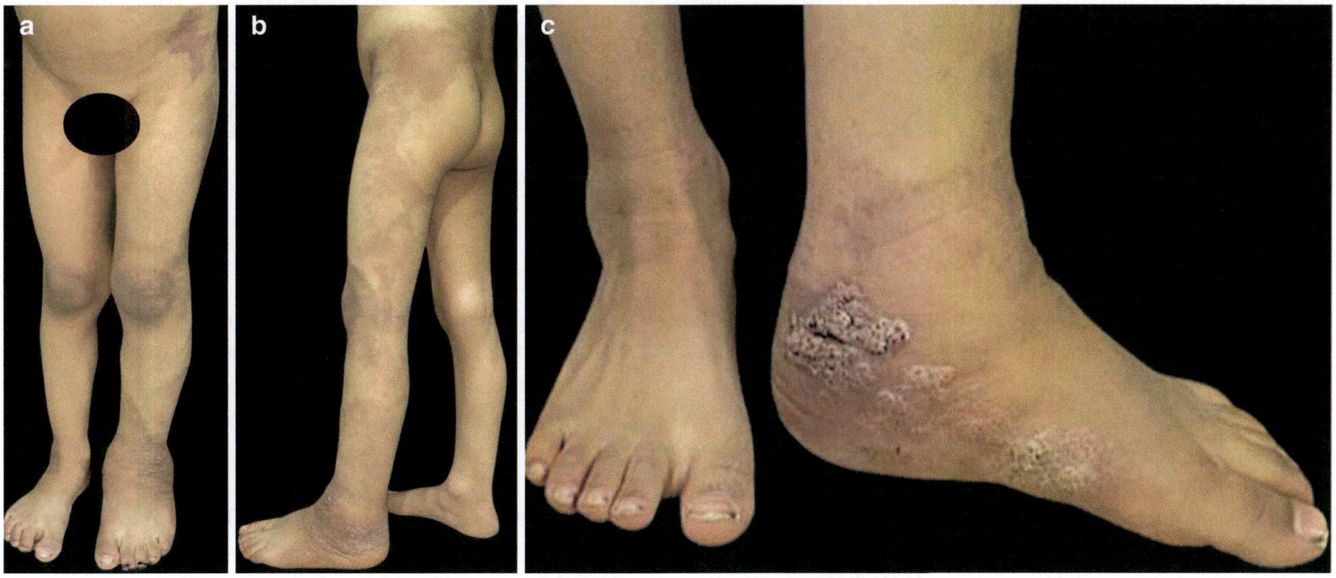

Fig. 7.6 Klippel–Trenaunay syndrome. Large port-wine stain in the lower abdomen, left lower leg, and thigh with unilateral hypertrophy over the affected area (**a**, **b**), verrucous warty keratotic lesion on the left foot (lymphatic malformation) (**c**). After 3 months: infection, oozing, and crustation (**d**)

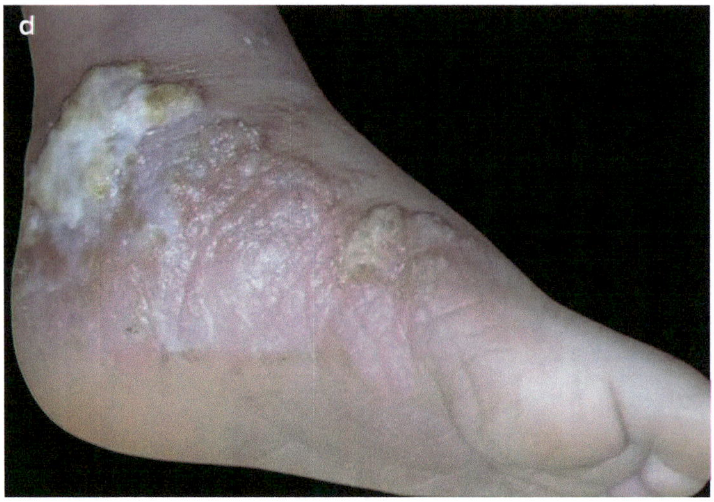

Fig. 7.6 (continued)

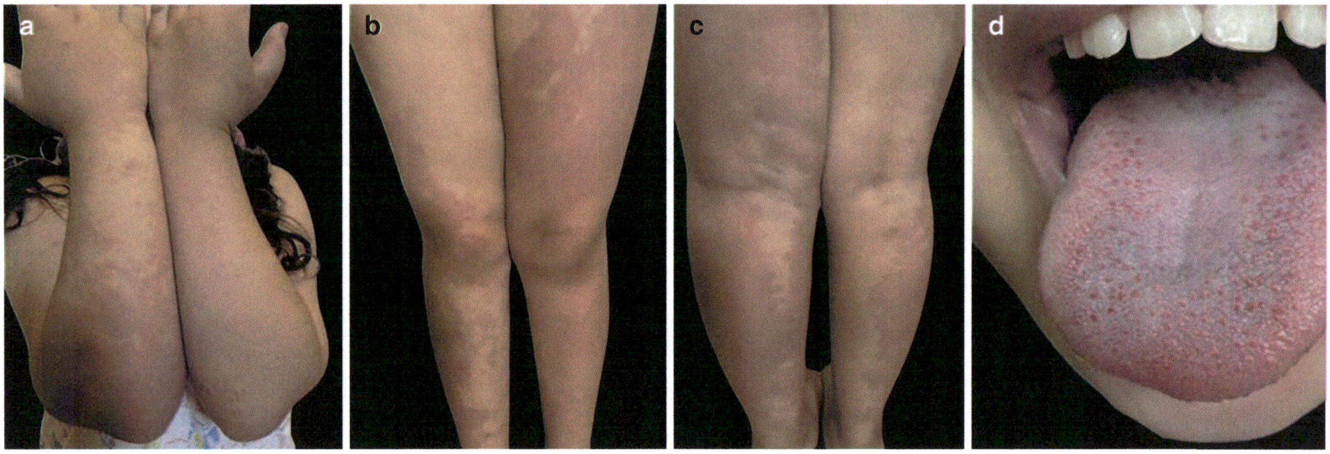

Fig. 7.7 Klippel–Trenaunay syndrome. Large port-wine stain involving the right upper limb, both lower limbs and tongue with prominent papillae (**a**–**d**)

  - Disproportionate overgrowth and focal atrophy of the upper arm muscles and neck, leading to the "hunched-over" look.
  - Scoliosis
- Dysmorphic facial features: dolichocephaly, long face, downslanting palpebral fissures, and/or minor ptosis, depressed nasal bridge, wide or anteverted nares, and open mouth at rest.
- Associated tumors: benign tumors include lipomas, ovarian cystadenomas, and monomorphic parotid adenomas.
  - Malignant neoplasm includes testicular papillary adenocarcinoma, mesothelioma of the tunica vaginalis, and peritoneal mesothelioma.
- Treatment: A multidisciplinary team of doctors is required including orthopedist, craniofacial surgeon, plastic surgeon, dermatologist, dentist, neurosurgeon, and psychologist.
  - Management of skin manifestations: Periodic evaluation of lesions/laser treatment for port-wine stain/surgical excision of lesions if they interfere with functional activities or for cosmetic purposes.

Fabry Disease [11–13] (Figs. 7.10 and 7.11)

- X-linked recessive sphingolipidosis.
- Due to mutations in the *GLA* gene with subsequent deficiency of the lysosomal enzyme α-galactosidase.
- Incidence: 1 in 1000 to 9000 people worldwide.
- Types:
  - Classic type: clinical symptoms appear early during childhood. Symptoms get progressively worse over time.

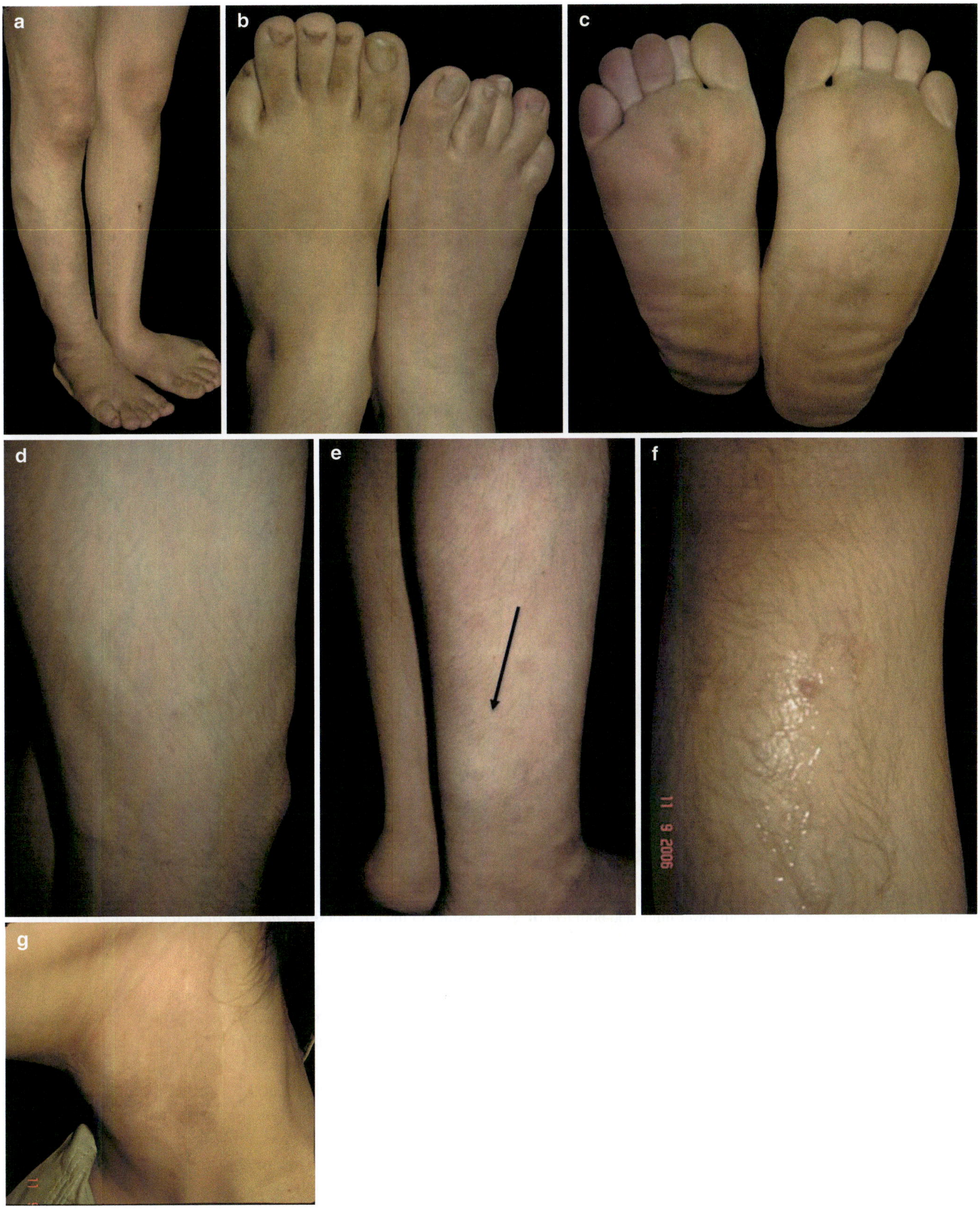

Fig. 7.8 Proteus syndrome. Asymmetry between the length of both lower limbs, feet, and toes (**a**–**c**), port-wine stain, prominent dilated veins and lipoma (arrow) in the right lower limb (**d**, **e**), lymphorrhea (**f**), and café-au-lait patches in the neck (**g**). (*Courtesy, Shaymaa Hosny Elgabry*)

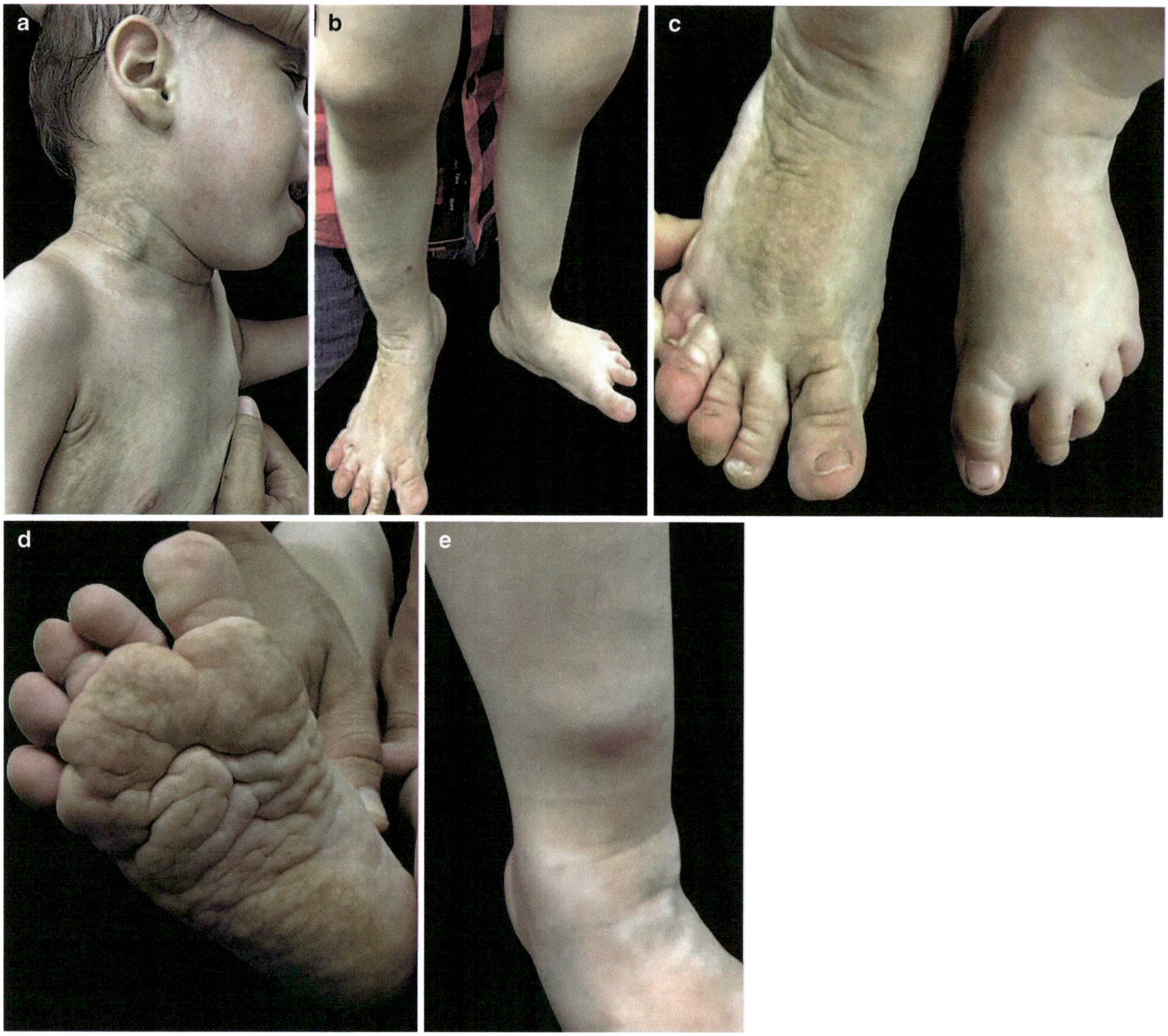

Fig. 7.9 Proteus syndrome. Linear unilateral epidermal nevus (**a**), asymmetry between the length of both lower limbs and both feet (**b**, **c**), cerebriform connective tissue nevi on the right sole (deep brain-like grooves and whorls) (**d**), subcutaneous lipoma in the left leg and varicosities of the left foot (**e**). (*Courtesy, Hala Abd El Salam Fayed*)

  - Late-onset/atypical type: patient does not have symptoms until they are in their 30s or older. The first indication of the disease may be kidney or heart failure.
- Clinical manifestations of classic type:
  - Acroparesthesias: may occur as early as 2–8 years of age in male patients, particularly associated with fevers. Affected individuals may experience episodes of severe burning pain in the hands and the feet. Fabry's crises (episodes of severe pain) may last for hours to days and are frequently triggered by exercise, fatigue, stress, and/or fever.
  - Anhidrosis or hypohidrosis: associated with heat intolerance in warm temperatures, with exercise, or fevers.
  - Angiokeratomas: small red to black papules affecting mainly the area between the hips and the knees (bathing trunk distribution).
  - Gastrointestinal problems: early manifestation of type 1 Fabry, abdominal cramping, frequent bowel movements, and diarrhea may also occur.
  - Corneal dystrophy
  - Additional symptoms: chronic fatigue, dizziness, headache, generalized weakness, nausea, and/or vomiting, delayed puberty, lack of or sparse hair

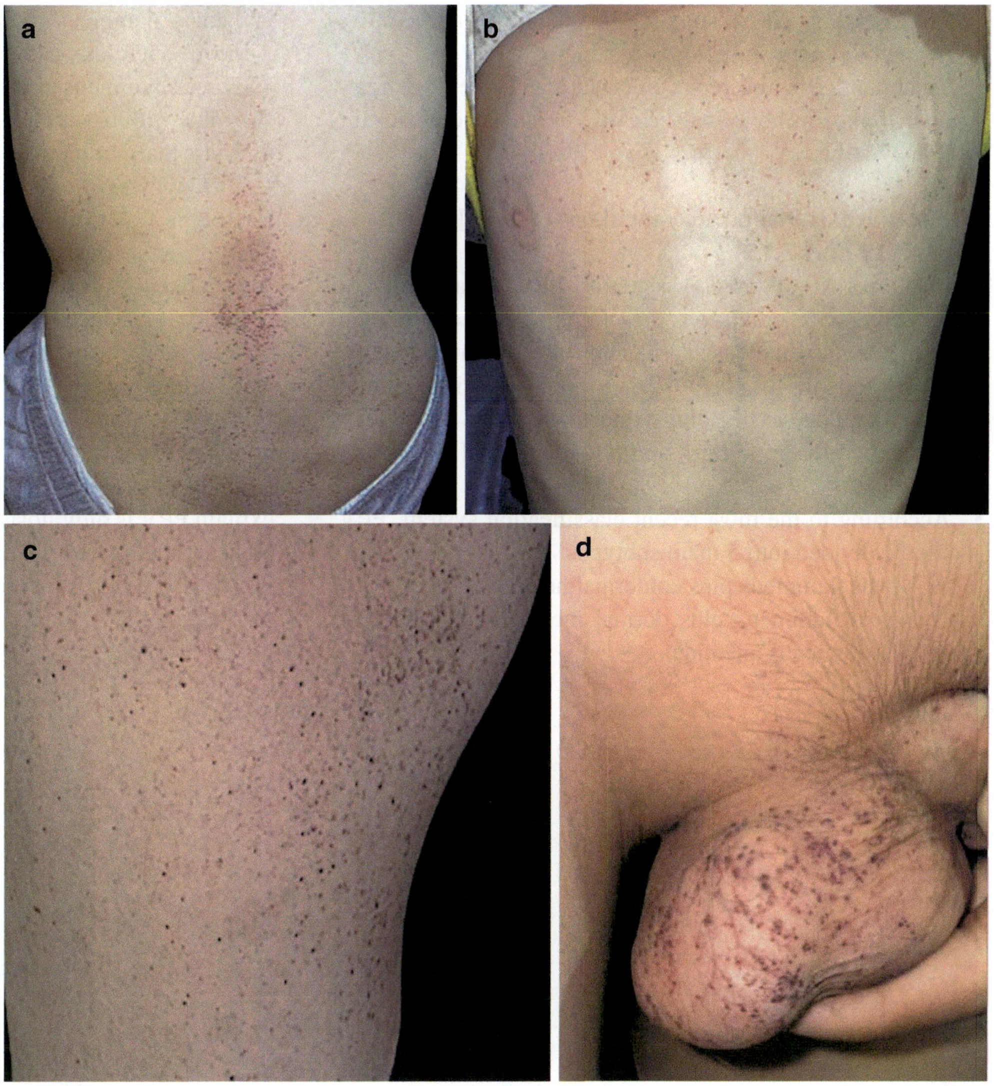

Fig. 7.10 Fabry disease. Numerous angiokeratomas in back (**a**), chest (**b**), and bathing suit area (**c**, **d**)

growth, rarely malformation of the joints and lymphedema.

- Clinical manifestations of classic and late onset males:
  - Renal dysfunction: progressive decrease in renal function is due to the progressive accumulation of globotriaosylceramide (GL-3) in the kidneys, particularly in the endothelial cells, smooth muscle cells, and podocytes
  - Cardiac disease: include heart enlargement, typically left ventricular hypertrophy leading to hypertrophic cardiomyopathy, arrhythmias, and heart failure.
  - Cerebrovascular complications. As a result of atrial fibrillation, about 7% of males and 4% of females with Fabry disease, experience ischemic or hemorrhagic strokes, occurring typically in the fourth decade of life or later.
  - Respiratory abnormalities: accumulation of glycosphingolipids and consequent fibrosis can cause interstitial lung disease, restrictive lung disease, obstructive airway disease, or a mixture of obstructive and restrictive disease.
  - Additional symptoms: hearing loss, tinnitus, dizziness and vertigo and depression.
- Patients with later-onset subtype typically do not have angiokeratoma, sweat normally, do not experience the Fabry pain or crises, and do not have heat intolerance or corneal involvement. But they develop heart or kidney disease later in adult life.
- Prognosis: mortality is usually due to cardiovascular disease, and kidney failure.
- Diagnosis: enzyme assay**:** this test measures alpha-GAL enzyme activity in your blood. Measurements of 1% or lower indicate disease

– Genetic: genetic testing (DNA sequencing) to identify the *GLA* gene mutation
- Treatment: enzyme replacement therapy/ medical treatment for pain, abnormal heart rhythms and dialysis for kidney failure.

Phakomatosis Pigmentovascularis [14–16] (Figs. 7.12 and 7.13)

- Phakomatosis pigmentovascularis (PPV) is a family of rare congenital conditions presenting with a combination of pigmentary and vascular lesions of different types.
- Most probably it is due to postzygotic somatic mutation rather than due to hereditary transmission
- Typically present at birth and affect all racial and ethnic groups.
- According to the most recent classification system, PPV can be divided into 5 main subtypes:
  – Nevus flammeus plus epidermal nevus
  – Nevus flammeus plus dermal melanocytosis with or without nevus anemicus
  – Nevus flammeus plus nevus spilus with or without nevus anemicus
  – Nevus flammeus plus dermal melanocytosis plus nevus spilus with or without nevus anemicus
  – Cutis marmorata telangiectatica congenita plus dermal melanocytosis
- Each type was further subdivided according to the presence of cutaneous-only manifestations (subtype a) or if associated to systemic manifestations (subtype b), the majority of which are ocular, vascular, skeletal, and neurological.
- The pathogenesis of PPV is not fully known yet, but it is believed to be an abnormality in the development of melanocytic nevus cells and vasomotor neural cells derived from the neural crest. The best accepted genetic model to explain PPV is didymosis (twin spots) where two areas of adjacent cutaneous lesions, formed by mutant tissues which also differ from the normal surrounding tissue.

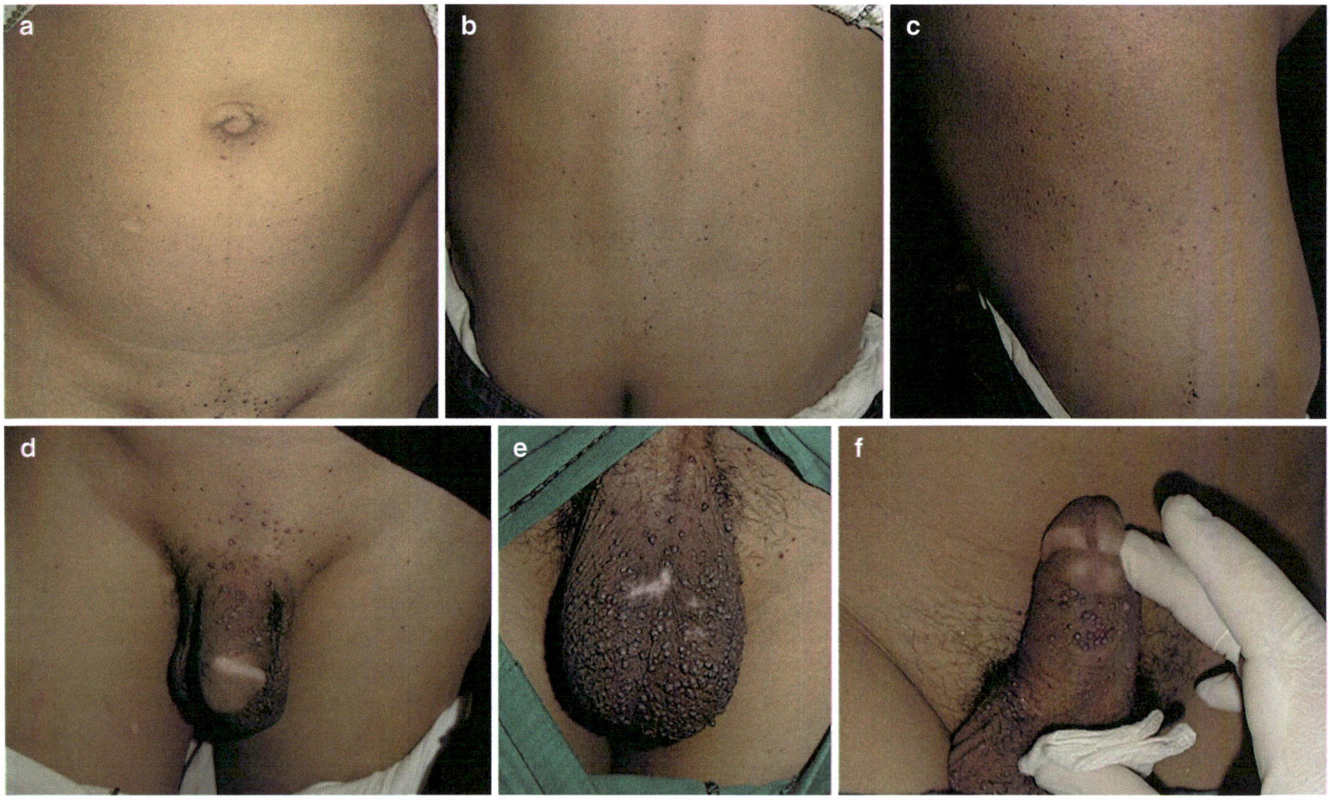

Fig. 7.11 Fabry disease. Numerous angiokeratomas in the bathing suit area (**a**–**f**)

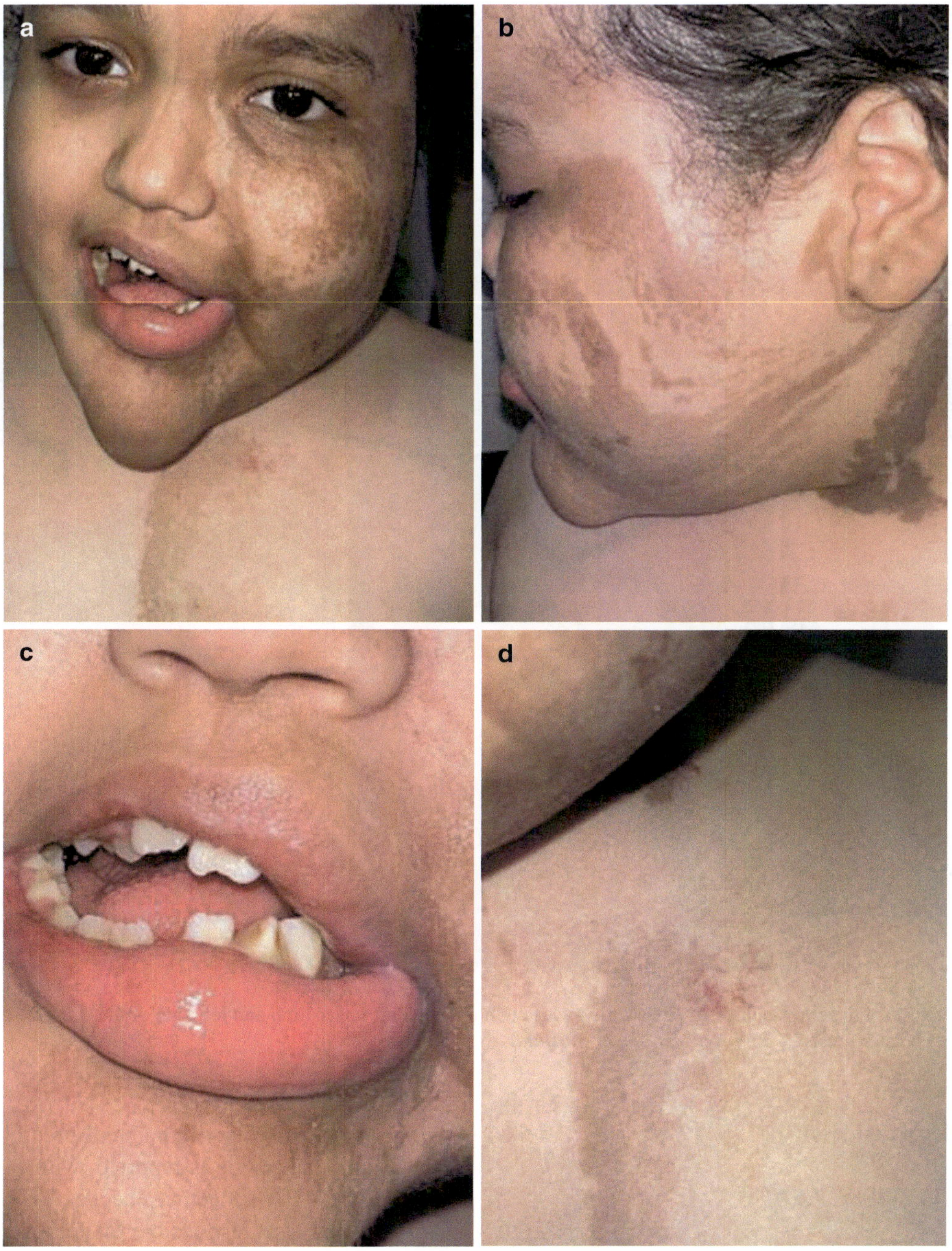

Fig. 7.12 Phakomatosis pigmentovascularis (type 1b). Capillary malformation on the left chest with systematized epidermal nevus syndrome. Hemimegalencephaly leading to asymetry of the face (**a–d**). The patient has epilepsy and intellectual disability

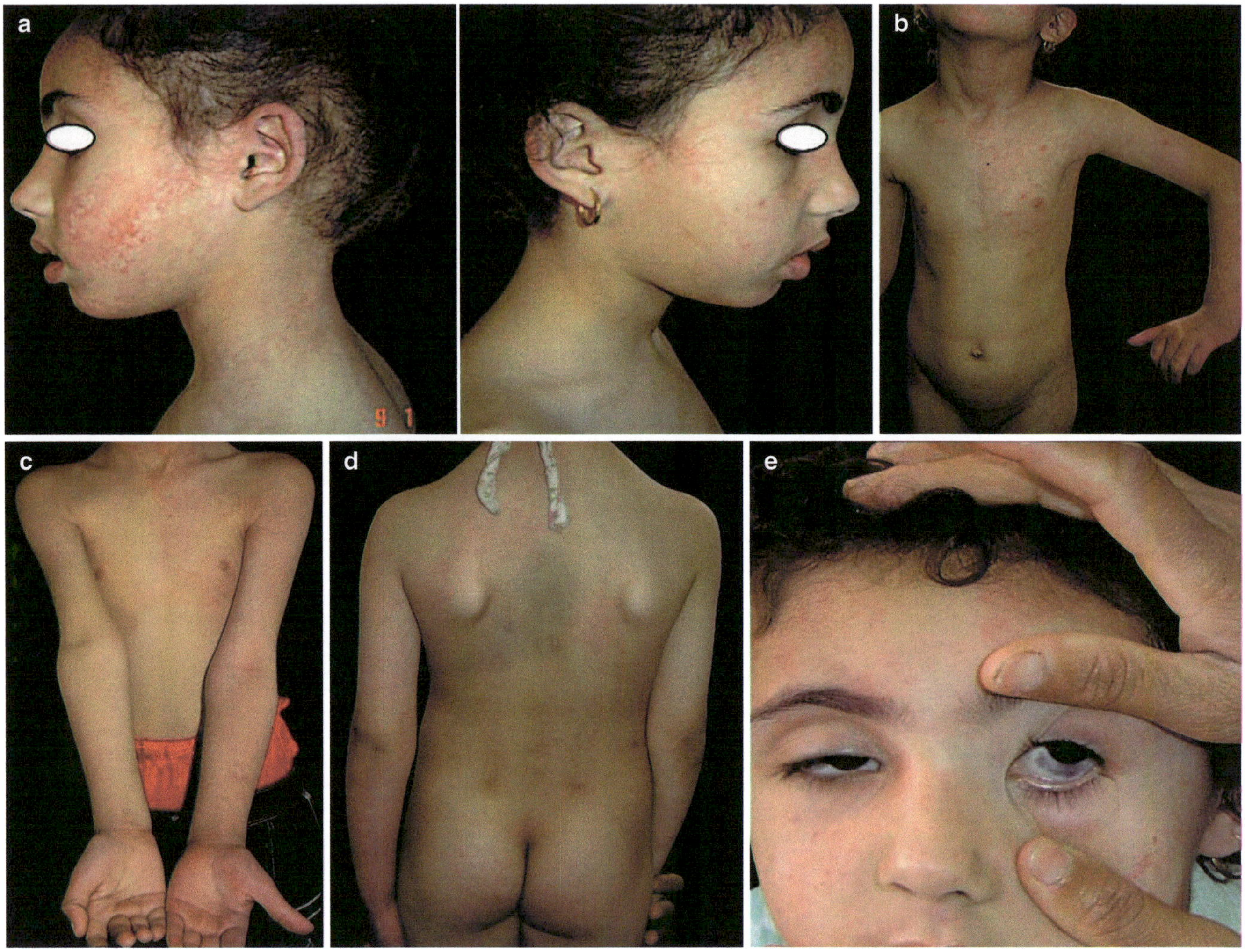

Fig. 7.13 Phakomatosis pigmentovascularis (type 2a): port-wine stain on face, left upper limb and left side of the chest, Mongolion spot on the back and left ocular melanocytosis (**a**–**e**). (*Courtesy, Abeer Mostafa*)

Venous Malformations

Venous Lake [17] (Fig. 7.14)

- Venous lake is a venous dilatation usually appearing as soft, compressible, dark blue to violaceous papules, in the lower lip in middle-aged or older men and women of any race.
- The color disappears on compression of the macule or papule due to the clearance of blood from the dilated venule.
- Treatment: light electrocautery, laser ablation, liquid nitrogen cryosurgery, and rarely surgical removal.

Blue Rubber Bleb Nevus Syndrome (Sporadic/AD) [18, 19] (Fig. 7.15)

Bean Syndrome

- It is a rare syndrome of venous malformations that arise in skin, GIT, and other organs.
- Inheritance: usually a sporadic disorder; however, autosomal dominant mode is reported, with somatic mutations in TEK (*TIE2*) gene that encodes TEK tyrosine kinase protein receptor, responsible for angiogenesis.
- Prevalence: approximately 200 cases have been reported in literature, with no sexual predisposition.
- Onset: cutaneous manifestations present at birth or early childhood; however, visceral involvement appears in early adulthood.
- Clinical characteristics:
  - A dominant subcutaneous nodular lesion (few millimeters up to 4 or 5 cm) appears on skin, mucous membranes or various body locations [heart, spleen, liver, CNS, eye, and GIT (mostly, small bowel)], with increase in size and number with time.
  - It is blue to violaceous, painful, soft compressible with tenderness on palpation and rubbery in consistency.
  - Focal areas of hyperhidrosis overlying these lesions.
- Investigations:

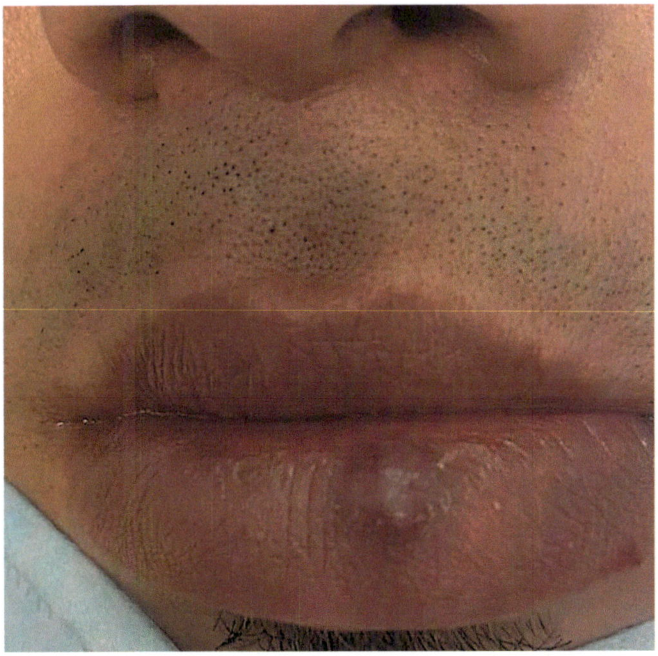

Fig. 7.14 Venous lake. Nevus showing blue to violaceous, soft compressible nodule

- Imaging techniques [endoscopic ultrasound, magnetic resonance imaging (MRI), computed tomography (CT), and barium studies].
- Fecal occult blood tests, complete blood count (CBC), and iron panels.
- Dermoscopy: superficial and light red arborizing veins, maculae with undefined borders on palms and soles, and blue-purple nodules with lacunae divided by white linear structures.
- Skin biopsy: non-specific, with features of venous malformations (large, tortuous, dilated vessels with a single endothelial lining, and smooth muscle in the vessel walls).

- DD: other congenital vascular malformations (diffuse neonatal hemangiomatosis, Klippel–Trenaunay–Weber syndrome, Maffucci syndrome, and mucosal venous malformation syndrome).
- Complications:
  - Recurrent GIT hemorrhage, with iron deficiency anemia or intestinal intussusception.
  - Thrombosis presents in venous malformations (slow-flow lesions) as tender, erythematous, warm swelling.
- Prognosis: normal lifespan as long as GIT bleeding is controlled.

Maffucci Syndrome [20, 21] (Figs. 7.16 and 7.17)

- Maffucci syndrome is a rare disorder showing infantile hemangioma (infantile hemangioma) and enchondroma (benign cartilage enlargement).
- Inheritance: non-hereditary congenital condition, with no genetic pattern of inheritance. However, somatic mutations in isocitrate dehydrogenase (*IDH*)-1 and -2 genes may occur.
- Prevalence: affects 1 in every 100,000 people, with no sexual or ethnic predisposition.
- Onset: at the age of 4–5 years old.
- Clinical characteristics:
  - Infantile hemangiomas (IHs):

    Bluish soft subcutaneous nodules appear in hands (32%) and feet (23%), blanching with pressure.

    Phleboliths (calcifications), forming micro thrombi, are important diagnostic findings.
  - Bony lesions:

    Enchondromas appear usually in the metaphysis of short bones such as metacarpals and phalanges of hands, and infrequently in short bones of feet and long bones of upper and lower limbs.
- Investigations:
  - X-ray:

    Multicentric radiolucent osteolytic areas with significant cortical thinning and endosteal scalloping.

    Phleboliths are easily identified as small calcifications.
  - Skin biopsy: hemangiomas.
  - Doppler: soft tissue hemangiomas show hyper echoic areas and modest marginal blood flow.
- D.D.: Ollier disease, diseases with unilateral enchondroma but without hemangiomas, blue rubber bleb nevus syndrome, Gorham's syndrome (bone and soft tissue angiomatous lesions) and Kaposi's sarcoma.
- Complications: pathological fractures, skeletal deformities, vascular overgrowth, limb-length discrepancies, and malignant transformations (52–57%) including chondrosarcomas.

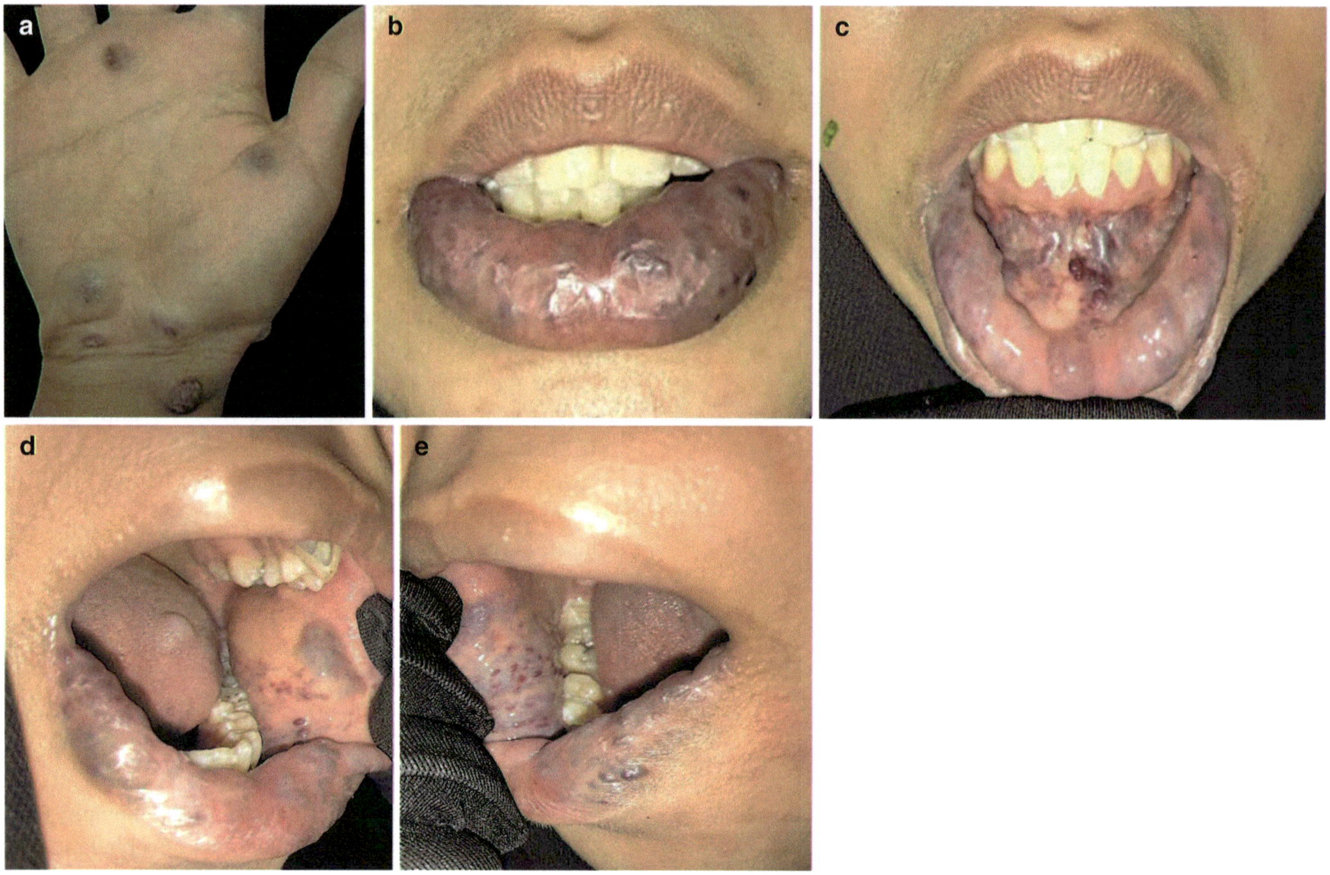

Fig. 7.15 Blue rubber bleb nevus. Multiple blue to violaceous, soft compressible nodules on hands (**a**) lips (**b**) and oral mucous membrane (**c**–**e**)

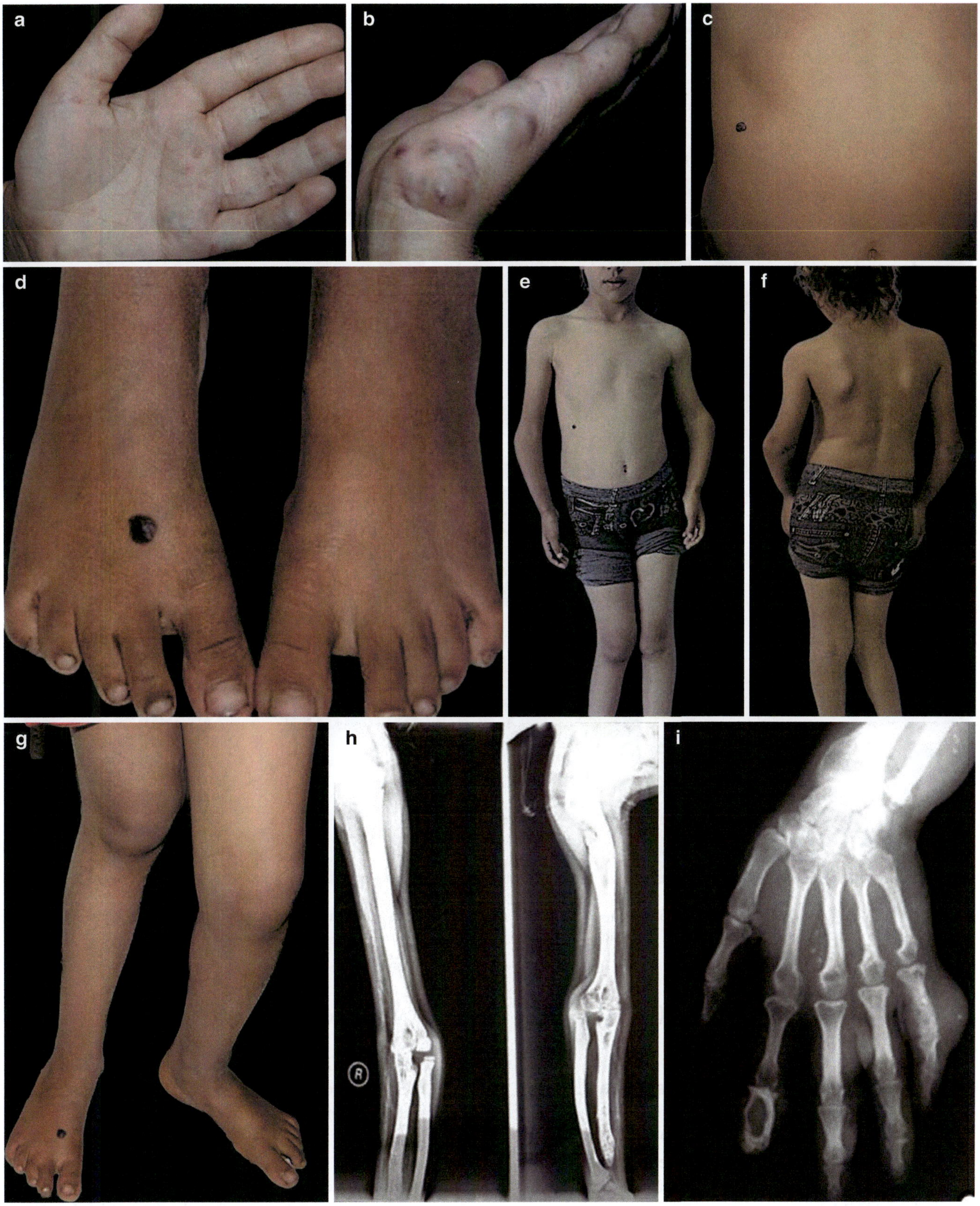

Fig. 7.16 Mafucci syndrome. Multiple, compressible dark blue nodules on the hands (**a**, **b**), abdomen (**c**), and feet (**d**). Assymetry between lengths of right and left sides of both upper and lower limbs (**e–g**). X ray showing metaphyseal distortions due to multiple enchondromas and soft tissue masses due to venous maformations (**h**, **i**)

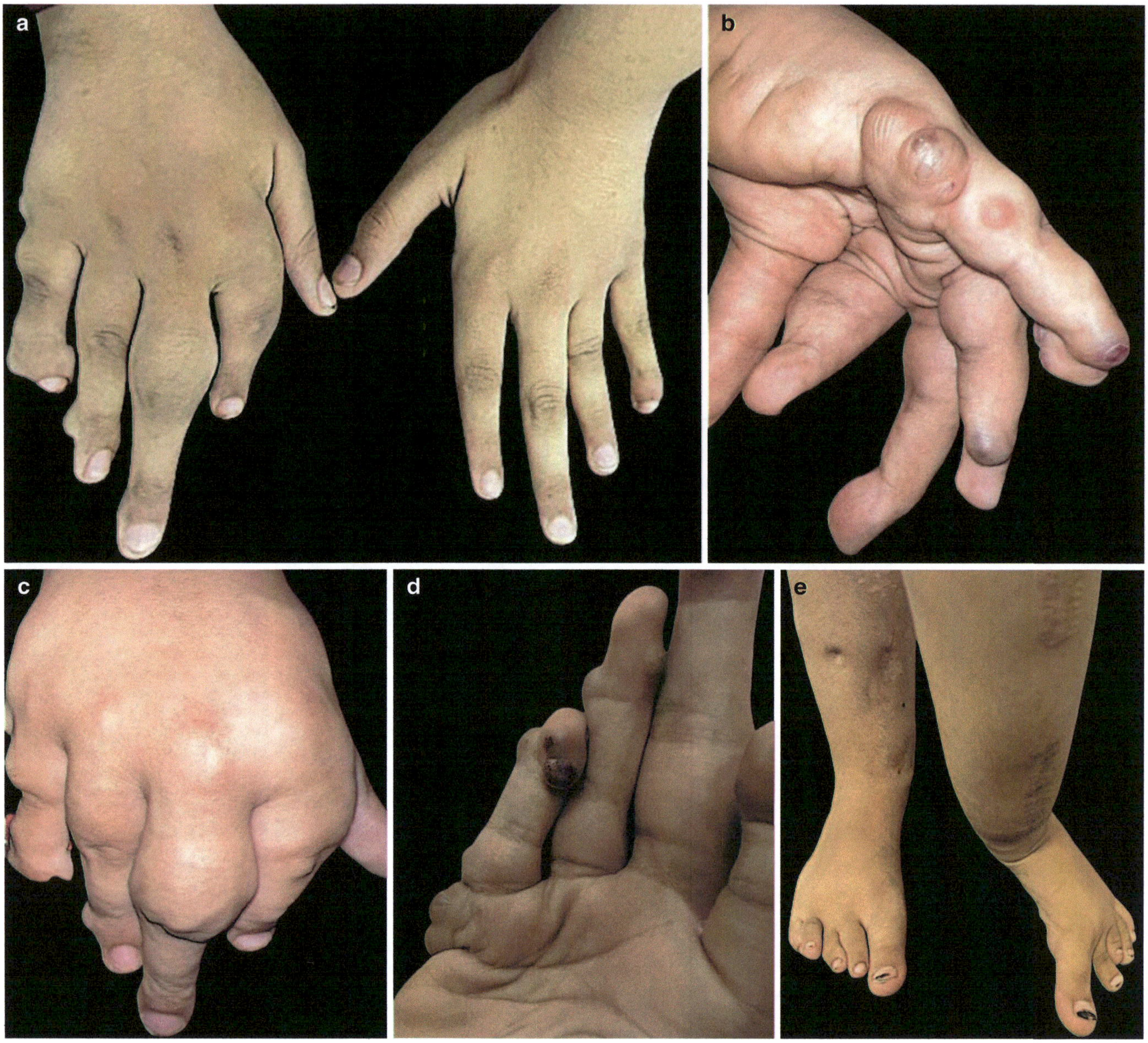

Fig. 7.17 Mafucci syndrome showing multiple enchondromas and soft compressible dark blue nodules on the hands with asymmetry of the extrimities (**a**–**e**). Scars of previous excision of enchondromas (**e**)

Osler-Weber-Rendu Syndrome (AD) [22–24] (Fig. 7.18)

Hereditary Hemorrhagic Telangiectasia

- Osler-Weber-Rendu disease (OWRD), hereditary hemorrhagic telangiectasia (HHT), is a rare disorder that shows mucocutaneous telangiectases and arteriovenous malformations (AVMs).
- Inheritance: autosomal dominant, with mutations of endoglin (*ENG*) gene, activin receptor like kinase (*ALK*)-1 gene or *SMAD4 gene*.
- Clinical characteristics: four clinical criteria as follows [5]:
  - Epistaxis (90%):
    Spontaneous and recurrent epistaxis from telangiectases of nasal mucosa at the of age 21 years, resulting in fatigue and anemia. It increases with age.
  - Mucocutaneous lesions (75%):
    Often appear 1 year after the first episode of epistaxis at multiple characteristic sites (e.g., face, lips, oral cavity, tongue, nares, ears, hands, chest, and toes), and the number increases with age.

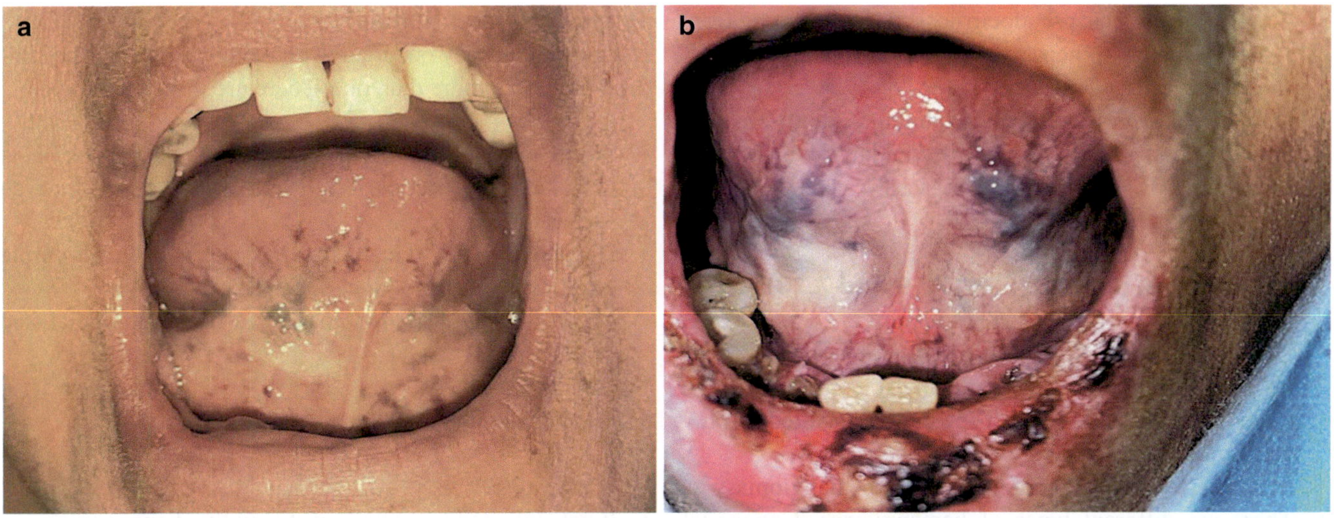

Fig. 7.18 Two cases of Osler–Weber–Rendu syndrome. Multiple dark red linear, punctate telangiectasias and hemorrhagic blisters on the lips, undersurface of the tongue and floor of mouth (**a**, **b**). Associated recurrent epistaxis is the main complaint in them

Dark red lines, punctate and pulsating vascular papules or non-pulsating, star-shaped telangiectases resembling spider angiomas (1–3 mm in diameter).

Lesions blanch partially with pressure.

- Visceral lesions (30%):

  Lung:

  Pulmonary AVMs, with right-to-left pulmonary shunting, cause transient ischemic attack, brain abscess, and ischemic stroke because of embolization of bland or septic material into cerebral vasculature.

  Symptoms of pulmonary AVMs include dyspnea, fatigue, cyanosis, hypoxemia, clubbing, secondary polycythemia, and pulmonary hypertension; however, most patients have no significant symptoms.

  Central nervous system (CNS):

  Arteriovenous anastomoses and aneurysms may lead to, stroke, brain abscess or intracerebral hematoma, with focal neurologic signs (migraine headache, paresthesia, seizures, and paralysis).

  Gastrointestinal tract (GIT):

  GIT bleeding (from stomach and small bowel) at the fifth or sixth decade.

  Thrombosis of AVMs causes abdominal pain.

  Liver:

  It is often asymptomatic; however, hepatomegaly, right upper-quadrant pain, jaundice, high-output cardiac failure, bleeding from esophageal varices, portal hypertension, encephalopathy, and liver failure are the most clinical patterns.

  Cardiovascular system (CVS):

  Deep vascular abnormalities in digits appear using a handheld illuminator.

  Patients with anemia may be pale, and hyperdynamic circulation may be exacerbated by anemia.

  Eyes:

  Visual disturbances caused by intraocular hemorrhage and retinal telangiectasias.

  Bloody tears due to conjunctival telangiectases.

- Family history: A first-degree relative, who has HHT.

The HHT diagnosis is classified as definite if three or four criteria are present, possible or suspected if two criteria are present, and unlikely if fewer than two criteria are present.

- Investigations: for identifying specific complications;
  - CBC: decreased hemoglobin, polycythemia, increased white blood cell in infections (e.g., brain abscess).
  - Abnormal liver enzymes and coagulation profile [prothrombin time (PT) and activated partial thromboplastin time (aPTT)] in liver involvement.
  - Urine and stool analysis: for detection of blood.
  - Arterial blood gas and oximetry: for pulmonary AVMs.
  - Imaging modalities for identification of telangiectases or AVMs: (ultrasonography, CT, chest radiography, contrast echocardiography, MRI, barium enema, and upper and lower GIT endoscopy and angiography).
  - Punch biopsy: telangiectases manifest as focal dilatation of the postcapillary venules in dermal upper-horizontal plexus, perivascular lymphocytic infiltrate, multiple layers of thickened smooth muscle cells around connecting venules. Markedly dilated arterioles and venules connect directly in a tortuous network, without intervening capillary bed.

- Liver specimens: pseudocirrhosis due to shunting from hepatic artery to hepatic or portal vein.
- Genetic tests.
- D.D.: Cockayne syndrome, Rothmund–Thomson syndrome, Louis–Bar syndrome, essential telangiectasia, actinic keratosis, scleroderma, rosacea.

Hemangiomas [25–28] (Figs. 7.19 and 7.20)

- Hemangiomas, also known as hemangiomas of infancy or infantile hemangiomas, are the most common benign tumor of infancy (5–10%). They are often called “strawberry marks” due to their clinical appearance.
- Endothelial cell proliferation results in hemangiomas.
- There are different types of hemangiomas. Congenital hemangiomas are visible at birth whereas infantile hemangiomas appear later in infancy. Infantile angiomas are characterized by early, rapid growth followed by spontaneous involution.
- The etiology includes several hypotheses.
  - The most likely hypothesis: hypoxic stress upregulates expression of GLUT 1 and VEGF leading to the mobilization of endothelial progenitor cells. The progenitor cells are positive for CD133 and CD31.
  - Another hypothesis suggests that placental trophoblasts serve as the origin of stem cells for hemangiomas.
  - A third hypothesis suggests that inflammatory hemangioma development involves vasculogenesis from progenitor cells (de novo formation) as well as the formation of new vessels from existing ones (angiogenesis). Angiogenic factors have been suggested to act on endothelial cells and pericytes to initiate the formation of a capillary network.
- Hemangiomas are more common in girls than in boys.
- They are more common in premature infants and twins.
- Most hemangiomas go through several phases of growth.
  - Most appear during the first weeks of life and grow fast for the first 2–3 months.
  - For the next 3–4 months, the hemangioma may grow more slowly.
  - Then, there is usually a period of no change to the hemangioma.
  - At around 1 year of age, the hemangioma begins to slowly shrink and fade in color. This happens over the next 1–10 years. Many go away completely during this time. By the time a child is 5 years old, half of all hemangiomas will be flat and lighter in color. By age 10, many are gone or only faintly visible.

Types of Hemangiomas

Hemangiomas may occur anywhere on the body. Some children may have more than one. There are three main types:

- **Superficial** (on the surface of the skin): These look flat at first, and then become bright red with a raised, uneven surface.
- **Deep** (under the skin): These appear as a bluish-purple swelling with a smooth surface.
- **Mixed:** These hemangiomas have both superficial and deep components.

The hemangioma may need intervention if:

- If ulcerates
- It gets infected (especially if it is in the diaper area).
- It causes problems with any of the following:
  - Vision
  - Breathing
  - Hearing
  - Eating
  - Diaper changes
- It is very large or it is a cosmetic concern, such as on the face.

Treatment

Most hemangiomas go away over time without any treatment. If the hemangioma is causing a problem, there are different treatment options. This may depend on the size, location, and behavior of hemangioma. Treatments may include the following:

- **Topical:**
  - Topical beta blockers: These may help lighten the hemangioma and slow its growth. This works best on smaller, superficial hemangiomas.
  - Topical antibiotic: These are applied when there are open sores with concern for infection.
- **Oral:**
  - Propranolol (2 mg/kg/day) is now the first-line treatment option for concerning hemangiomas.
  - Prednisone is used in select cases that may be resistant to other treatment or if propranolol cannot be used.
- **Surgery:** This may be considered once the hemangioma has stopped growing or other treatments have failed. Surgery may be used to remove markings left over from hemangiomas.
- **Pulsed dye laser**

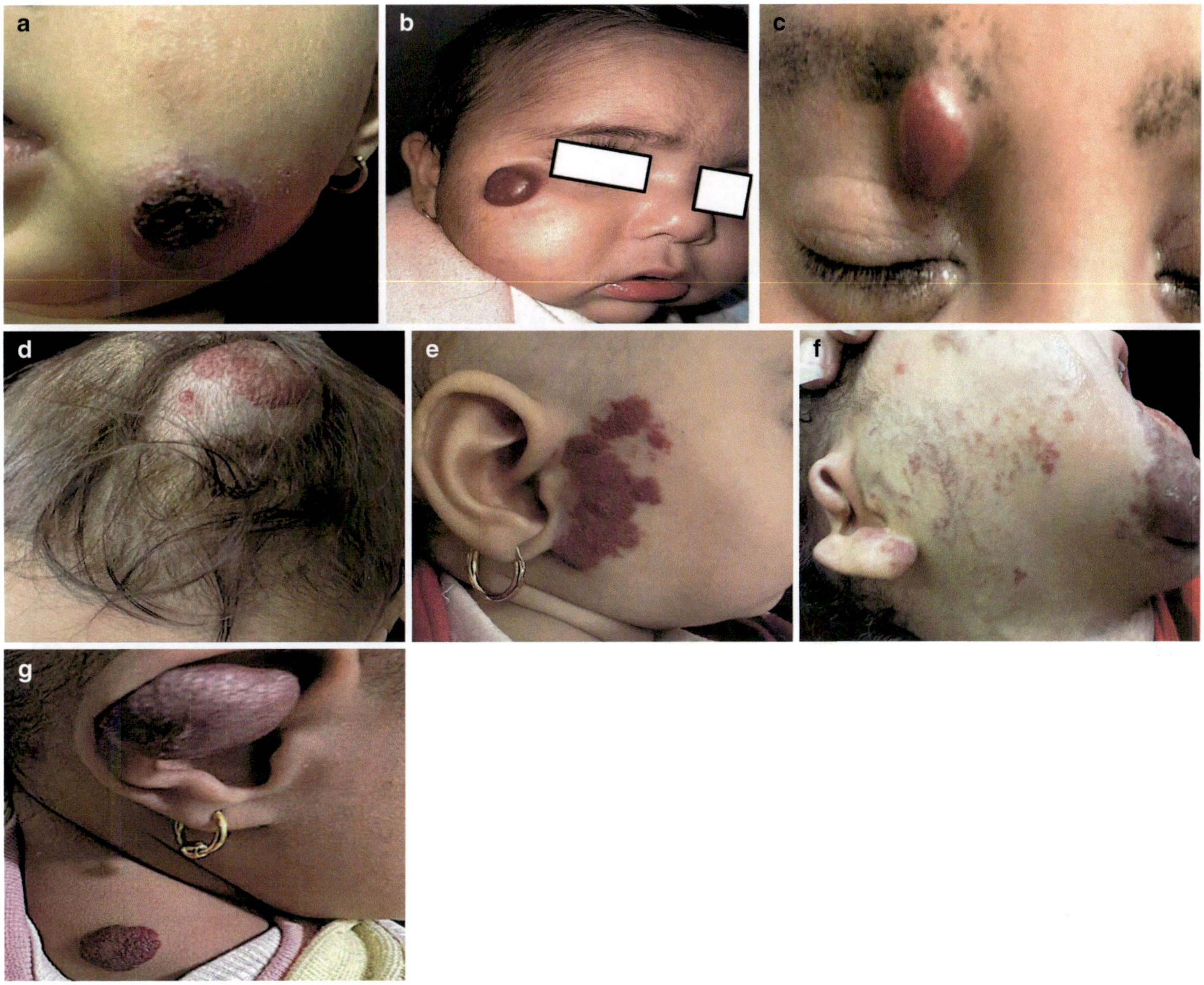

Fig. 7.19 Cases of infantile hemangiomas. Hemangioma on lower left cheek with ulceration (**a**), on right cheek (**b**), on right eye brow (**c**) on scalp with deep component (**d**) red hemangiomatous plaque in front of ear (**e**). Hemangioma in the right side of the face with deep component leading to ear deformity (**f**) and on the external auditory canal and upper back (**g**)

PHACES Syndrome [29–31] (Fig. 7.21)

- Inheritance: no evidence of genetic abnormalities, however, defective embryogenesis can occur between weeks 3 and 12 of gestation, before or during vasculogenesis, because certain malformations and infantile hemangioma can affect the same side of the body.
- The acronym of PHACES syndrome, the most frequent neurocutaneous vascular disorders in childhood, can represent the most representative features of the syndrome (**P**osterior fossa malformations, **H**emangioma, **A**rterial anomalies, **C**oarctation of the aorta/**C**ardiac defects, **E**ye abnormalities, and **S**ternal malformations).
- Prevalence: 2–3% of all infantile hemangioma cases, and in 20–31% of large or segmental facial infantile hemangioma.
- Clinical characteristics:
  - Skin (IHs):

    At birth, IHs can be absent or present as slightly erythematous or telangiectatic area. At the end of first month of life, they are already visible as telangiectasias, solitary lesions, confluent plaques, small papules, and tumors with deeper involvement.

    Three phases of progression include; proliferation in the first 5 months of life, stabilization, and spontaneous involution after years.

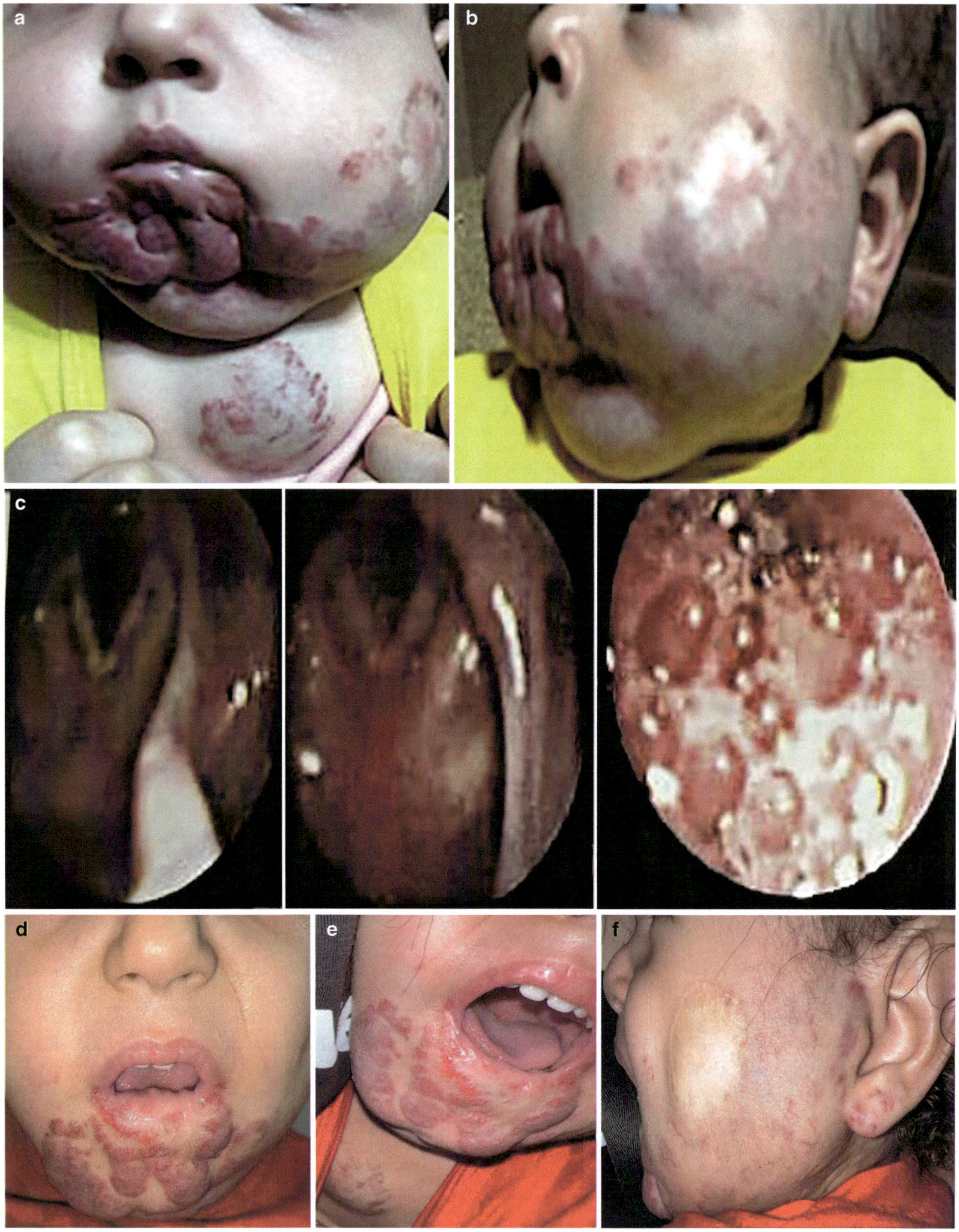

Fig. 7.20 (**a**) Facial infantile hemangioma on beard area and reaching to anterior chest with deep component (**a**, **b**). Subglottic laryngeal hemangioma revealed by flexible transnasal pharyngo-laryngo eosophagoscopy examination (**c**), Regression of hemangioma after 9 months treatment by propranolol (**d–f**)

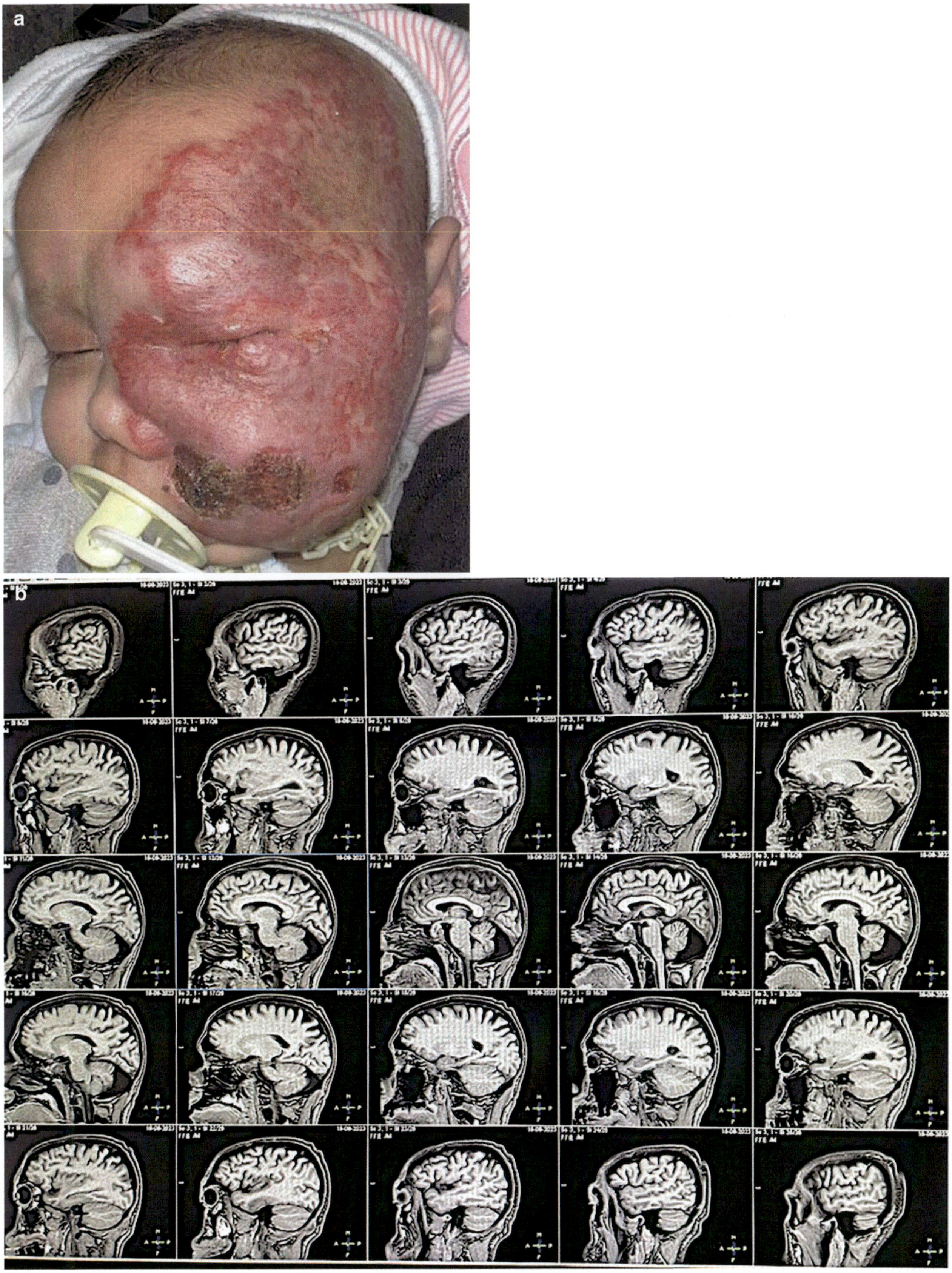

Fig. 7.21 PHACES syndrome. Left segmental facial infantile hemangioma with central crustation (**a**). MRI brain sagittal cuts showing a posterior fossa midline arachnoid cyst (**b**). (*Courtesy, Belal Muwafak*)

The most common affected sites include face, scalp, and postauricular and cervical regions in the descending order.

Suggestion of systemic involvement occur in large IHs (>5 cm in diameter) or segmental ones on face (frontotemporal and frontonasal segments bear a higher risk of ocular and CNS involvement, whereas those on mandibular segment are linked to a greater risk of midline and cardiovascular defects).

- Vascular and structural involvement of the brain:
  Brain changes and cutaneous IH tend to be on the same side of the body.
  Cerebrovascular accident (CVA): vascular stenosis and occlusion of cerebral vessels that are related to Circle of Willis, with subsequent reduction in blood flow and thromboembolism, interfering with brain perfusion causing chronic and silent ischemia with significant headache.
  Structural brain changes: signs and symptoms of neuropsychomotor developmental delay, seizures, and headaches. Posterior fossa malformations include dysphagia, feeding difficulties, and speech delays.
- Cardiac involvement: Aortic arch anomalies: coarctation of aorta, narrowing with subsequent aneurysmatic dilatation of adjacent segments in transverse, and descending portion
- Aberrant origin of subclavian artery.
- Other involvement: endocrine abnormalities, enamel hypoplasia if infantile hemangioma is in oral cavity.
- Investigations: CT, MRI, MRA of brain, neck and aortic arch and brachiocephalic vessels.
- Echocardiogram
- Treatment: Propranolol is the preferred medication for IH when systemic treatment is indicated.
- The initial dose is 0.5–1 mg/kg/day in the first week, increasing progressively to 2–3 mg/kg/day b.i.d. or t.i.d. It can be administered during the day, followed immediately by food. Propranolol should be discontinued if upper airway infections develop with bronchospasm and reduced food intake
  Prognosis: Neurological and cognitive impairments are potential causes of morbidity in these patients.

Lumbar (Sacral) Syndrome (XL) [32, 33] (Fig. 7.22)

- LUMBAR syndrome is a rare developmental malformation characterized by infantile hemangioma of lower half of body and malformations in pelvic region (urogenital anomalies and ulceration, myelopathy, bony deformities, anorectal malformations and arterial and renal anomalies).
- Inheritance: X-linked mode, with mosaic mutation of *AKT3*, *PIK3R2*, and *PIK3CA* genes, which are involved in visceral, skeletal and vascular malformations.
- Clinical characteristics:
  - Hemangioma (IH):
    IH may be extensive (>2.5 cm) or segmental in sacral region, followed by lumbar area, perineum/genitals, and lower extremities.
    Ulceration was more likely when IH was extensive (3 or 4 regions involved).
    IH are usually associated with regional hyperplasia or atrophy.
    Other cutaneous defects such as skin tags and sacral dimples.
  - Myelopathy (80%): with lumbar infantile hemangioma
  - Urogenital anomalies, anorectal malformations and renal anomalies: with sacral infantile hemangioma
  - Spinal anomalies: with IH >2.5 cm overlying lumbosacral spine.
  - Anomalies of iliac and superficial femoral arteries: with extensive infantile hemangioma in lower limb.
- Investigations:
  - Imaging studies (MRI for myelopathy, MRI angiography and MRI venography, and CT angiography).
- Treatment:
  - Oral propranolol should be used with extreme caution because of risk of occult arterial anomalies. So, investigation for internal vascular anomalies is required before therapy for fear of potential hypotension and reduced perfusion.

Pelvis Syndrome [34] (Fig. 7.23)

- The acronym PELVIS syndrome emphasizes the major features of this syndrome: *p*erineal hemangioma, *e*xternal genitalia malformations, *l*ipomyelomeningocele, *v*esicorenal abnormalities, *i*mperforate anus, and *s*kin tag.
- Large perineal hemangiomas should be recognized as indicators of underlying pathologic conditions. Although not all the components of the acronym are necessary to fit the malformation sequence.
- Systematic pelviperineal imaging (ultrasound, CT scan, and spine MRI) should be performed to detect occult urogenital abnormalities or visceral hemangiomatosis even without obvious external malformations.

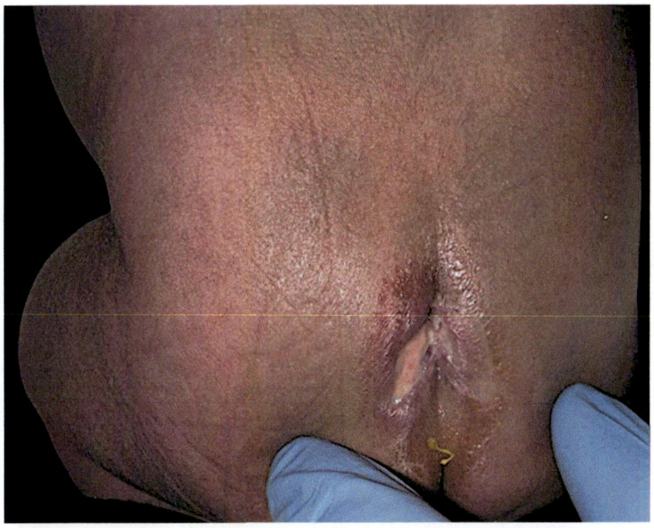

Fig. 7.22 Lumbar syndrome. Perineal hemangioma with ulceration. The infant has mongolion spot. (*Courtesy, Ammar Aldujally*)

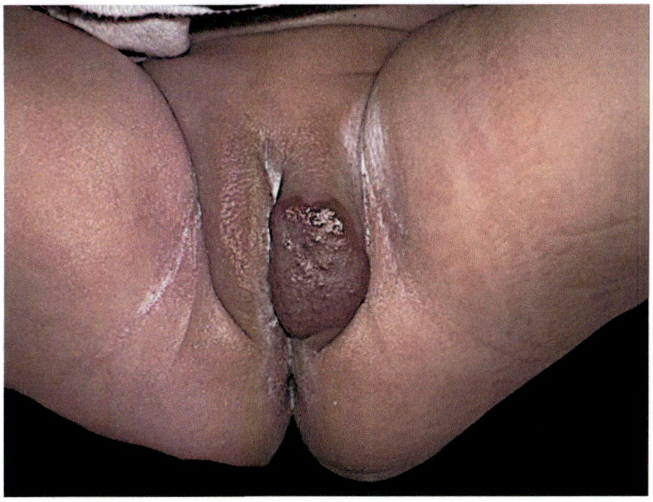

Fig. 7.23 Infantile perineal hemangiomas in a female infant with no systematic pelviperineal imaging abnormalities. Infantile perineal hemangiomas should be investigated to exclude "Pelvis syndrome." The acronym PELVIS syndrome emphasizes the major features of this syndrome: *p*erineal hemangioma, *e*xternal genitalia malformations, *l*ipomyelomeningocele, *v*esicorenal abnormalities, *i*mperforate anus, and *s*kin tag

Lymphangioma Circumscriptum (LC) [35, 36] (Figs. 7.24 and 7.25)

- Lymphangioma circumscriptum is a benign lymphatic malformation characterized by dilation of lymphatic vessels with feeding cisterns in subcutaneous tissue.
- It is congenital or acquired as a result of damage to lymphatic vessels secondary to various etiologies with no evidence of inheritance.
- Onset: at birth or early childhood, but lesions can occur at any age.
- Clinical characteristics:
  - Isolated or grouped translucid, thin-walled vesicles filled with a clear liquid.
  - These vesicles often resemble frog spawn and tend to increase in number and size with occasional rupture leading to bleeding or super infection with *Staphylococcus aureus*, recurrent cellulitis and lymphedema of the limb that may cause subcutaneous thickening or cyst formation.
  - Chest, mouth, axilla and tongue are the commonly affected sites.
- Investigations:
  - Dermoscopy: red and pale homogenous area resembling vascular lagoons and whitish and yellowish areas with thin linear vessels.
  - Skin biopsy: acanthosis, hyperkeratosis, and multiple dilated lymph vessels in deep dermis. The lumen of all involved vessels is filled with lymphatic fluid and often blood cells. The dermis often has numerous lymphocytes with evidence of fibroplasia.
- Complications:
  - It depends upon the location of LC such as obstruction of airways and esophagus in case of oral lesions, secondary infections, cellulitis and hemorrhage. Psychosexual abnormalities may develop in genital lesions.

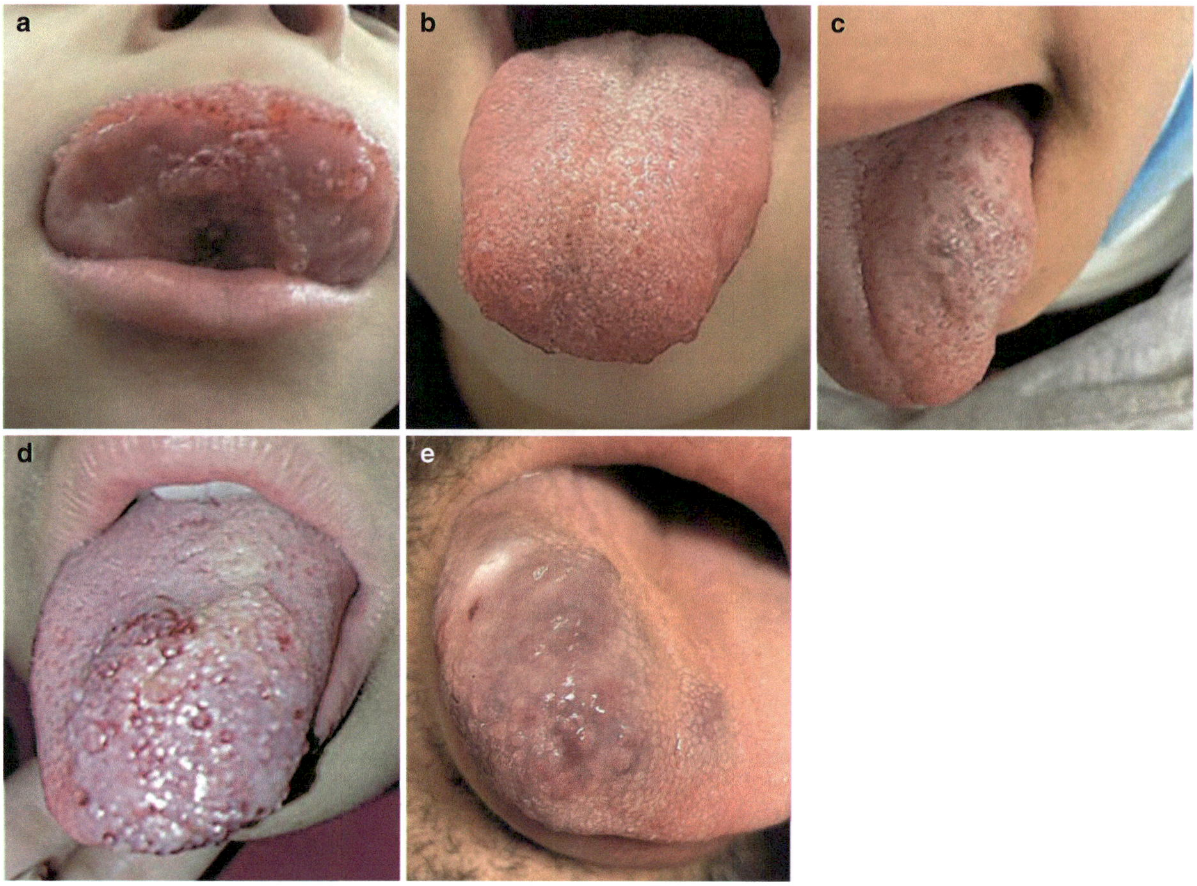

Fig. 7.24 Five cases of lymphangioma circumscriptum of lips and tongue. Asymptomatic deep grouped seated vesicles and papulovesicles (Frog spawn) (**a**–**e**)

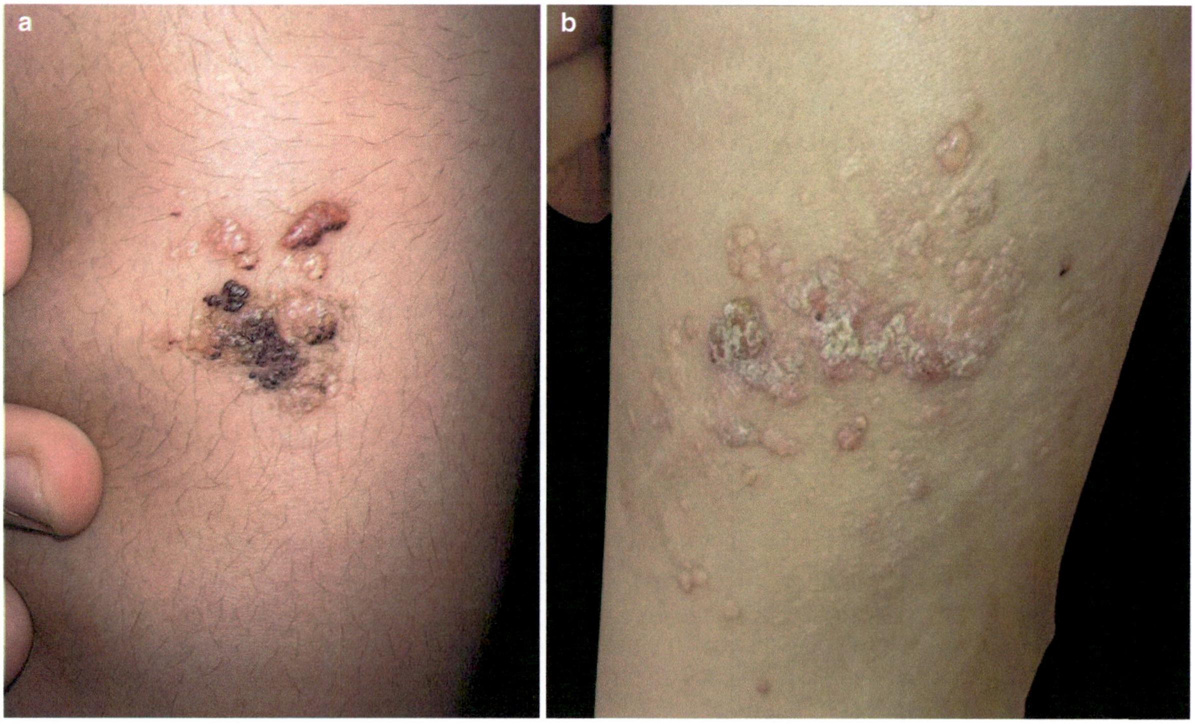

Fig. 7.25 Lymphangioma circumscriptum. Asymptomatic deep seated clustered skin colored and hemorrhagic vesicles and papulovesicles (Frog spawn) on extremities on normal skin (**a**) and previous old linear scar with recurrence (**b**)

- D.D.:
  Lymphangiectasis (lymphatic obstruction) with previous surgery or radiation therapy in the affected area, smaller CLC can resemble warts, molluscum contagiosum, hemangioma, angiokeratoma, or lymphangioendothelioma.

References

1. Lee JW, Chung HY. Capillary malformations (portwine stains) of the head and neck: natural history, investigations, laser, and surgical management. Otolaryngol Clin N Am. 2018;51:197–211.
2. Yu J, Streicher JL, Medne L, et al. EPHB4 mutation implicated in capillary malformation-arteriovenous malformation syndrome: a case report. Pediatr Dermatol. 2017;34:e227–30.
3. Chen JK, Ghasri P, Aguilar G, et al. An overview of clinical and experimental treatment modalities for port wine stains. J Am Acad Dermatol. 2012;67:289–304.
4. Thorpe J, Frelin LP, McCann M, et al. Identification of a mosaic activating mutation in GNA11 in atypical Sturge-Weber syndrome. J Invest Dermatol. 2021;14:685–8.
5. Smegal LF, Sebold AJ, Hammill AM, et al. Multicenter research data of epilepsy management in patients with Sturge-Weber syndrome. Pediatr Neurol. 2021;119:3–10.
6. Luks VL, Kamitaki N, Vivero MP, et al. Lymphatic and other vascular malformative/overgrowth disorders are caused by somatic mutations in PIK3CA. J Pediatr. 2015;166:1048–54.
7. Kihiczak GG, Meine JG, Schwartz RA, et al. Klippel-Trenaunay syndrome: a multisystem disorder possibly resulting from a pathogenic gene for vascular and tissue overgrowth. Int J Dermatol. 2006;45:883–90.
8. Turner JT, Cohen MM Jr, Biesecker LG. Reassessment of the proteus syndrome literature: application of diagnostic criteria to published cases. Am J Med Genet A. 2004;130A:111–22.
9. Sapp JC, Buser A, Burton-Akright J, et al. A dyadic genotype-phenotype approach to diagnostic criteria for Proteus syndrome. Am J Med Genet C Semin Med Genet. 2019;181:565–70.
10. Almeida HL Jr, Fiss RC, Happle R. Macrodactyly with skin hypertrophy: a minimal form of the Proteus syndrome. An Bras Dermatol. 2011;86:557–9.
11. Eng CM, Germain DP, Banikazemi M, et al. Fabry disease: guidelines for the evaluation and management of multi-organ system involvement. Genet Med. 2006;8:539–48.
12. Desnick RJ, Brady R, Barranger J, et al. Fabry disease, an under-recognized multisystemic disorder: expert recommendations for diagnosis, management, and enzyme replacement therapy. Ann Intern Med. 2003;138:338–46.
13. Baig S, Vijapurapu R, Alharbi F, et al. Diagnosis and treatment of the cardiovascular consequences of Fabry disease. QJM. 2019;112:3–9.
14. Catter L, Burgin S. Phakomatosis pigmentovascularis. https://www.visualdx.com/visualdx/diagnosis/phakomatosis+pigmentovascularis. Accessed 2 October 2023.
15. Hasegawa Y, Yasuhara M. Phakomatosis pigmentovascularis type VIa. Arch Dermatol. 1985;121:651–5.
16. Segatto MM, Schmitt EU, Hagemann LN, et al. Phakomatosis pigmentovascularis type IIa–case report. An Bras Dermatol. 2013;88(6):85–8.
17. Goldman MP. Laser treatment of cutaneous vascular lesions. In: Goldman MP, editor. Cutaneous and cosmetic laser surgery. St. Louis: Mosby; 2006. p. 31–91.
18. Soblet J, Kangas J, Nätynki M, et al. Blue rubber bleb nevus (BRBN) syndrome is caused by somatic TEK (TIE2) Mutations. J Invest Dermatol. 2017;137:207–16.
19. Jin XL, Wang ZH, Xiao XB, et al. Blue rubber bleb nevus syndrome: a case report and literature review. World J Gastroenterol. 2014;20:17254–9.
20. Kaplan RP, Wang JT, Amron DM, et al. Maffucci's syndrome: two case reports with a literature review. J Am Acad Dermatol. 1993;29:894–9.
21. Hussain SF, Kadir MF, Ahmed RU, et al. Maffucci syndrome: a rare case report. Bangladesh Med Coll J. 2019;24:35–8.
22. Shovlin CL, Guttmacher AE, Buscarini E, et al. Diagnostic criteria for hereditary hemorrhagic telangiectasia (Rendu-Osler-Weber syndrome). Am J Med Genet. 2000;91:66–7.
23. Hammill AM, Wusik K, Kasthuri RS. Hereditary hemorrhagic telangiectasia (HHT): a practical guide to management. Hematol Am Soc Hematol Educ Program. 2021;2021:469–77.
24. McDonald J, Bayrak-Toydemir P, et al. Hereditary hemorrhagic telangiectasia: an overview of diagnosis, management, and pathogenesis. Genet Med. 2011;13:607–16.
25. Yu Y, Flint AF, Mulliken JB, Wu JK, Bischoff J. Endothelial progenitor cells in infantile hemangioma. Blood. 2004;103:1373–5.
26. Holland KE, Drolet BA. Infantile hemangioma. Pediatr Clin N Am. 2010;57:1069–83.
27. Takahashi K, Mulliken JB, Kozakewich HP, Rogers RA, Folkman J, Ezekowitz RA. Cellular markers that distinguish the phases of hemangioma during infancy and childhood. J Clin Invest. 1994;93:2357–64.
28. Léauté-Labrèze C, Harper JI, Hoeger PH. Infantile haemangioma. Lancet. 2017;390(10089):85–94.
29. Metry D, Heyer G, Hess C, et al. Consensus statement on diagnostic criteria for PHACE syndrome. Pediatrics. 2009;124:1447–56.
30. Metry DW, Haggstrom AN, Drolet BA, et al. A prospective study of PHACE syndrome in infantile hemangiomas: demographic features, clinical findings, and complications. Am J Med Genet A. 2006;140:975–86.
31. Hartemink DA, Chiu YE, Drolet BA, et al. PHACES syndrome: a review. Int J Pediatr Otorhinolaryngol. 2009;73:181–7.
32. Iacobas I, Burrows PE, Frieden IJ, et al. LUMBAR: association between cutaneous infantile hemangiomas of the lower body and regional congenital anomalies. J Pediatr. 2010;157:795–801.
33. Drolet BA, Chamlin SL, Garzon MC, et al. Prospective study of spinal anomalies in children with infantile hemangiomas of the lumbosacral skin. J Pediatr. 2010;157:789–94.
34. Girard C, Bigorre M, Guillot B, et al. PELVIS syndrome. Arch Dermatol. 2006;142(7):884–8.
35. Gopal AP, Robertez AS. Cutaneous lymphangioma circumscriptum: frog spawn on the skin. Int J Dermatol. 2009;48:1290–5.
36. Aggarwal K, Gupta S, Kumar JV, et al. Congenital lymphangioma circumscriptum of the vulva. Indian Pediatr. 2009;46:428–9.

8 Acantholytic Genodermatoses

- **Darier disease (Keratosis follicularis)**
- **Hailey-Hailey disease (Benign familial chronic pemphigus)**

Darier Disease (Keratosis Follicularis) (AD) [1, 2] (Figs. 8.1, 8.2, 8.3, 8.4, 8.5, 8.6, 8.7, 8.8, and 8.9)

- Darier disease is connected with a mutation in the *ATP2A2* gene, encoding sarco/endoplasmic reticulum ATPase type 2 (*SERCA2*).
- The product of this gene is responsible for the transport of calcium in the endoplasmic reticulum of epidermal cells, and its malfunction causes aberrant epidermal keratinization and abnormal cell adhesion.
- The first clinical symptoms of Darier disease usually appear in adolescence or early adulthood and may be associated with pruritus.
- Hyperkeratotic papules in seborrheic regions: strongly corneous red-brown papules covered with a grey keratin plug, located mainly in the seborrheic areas, the forehead, nasolabial folds, neck, scalp, chest, back, and flexural regions as axillae, groins, and submammary skin.
- Superinfection with malodor.
- Hand involvement: Punctate keratosis, palmar pits or hemorrhagic macules. Acrokeratosis verruciformis-like lesions on the dorsum can be found in 50% of patients.
- Nail changes are helpful for diagnosis: red and white longitudinal bands, nail ridges, subungual hyperkeratosis, and V-shaped defects in the free margin of the nail. Rarely, complete nail dystrophy occurs.
- On the mucous membranes, the lesions appear as whitish, clustered papules with central depression, described as the image of "cobblestones."
- Two forms:
  - First type: segmental or linear lesions are located unilaterally along lines of Blashko.
  - Second type (90%): diffuse type occurring in both sides.
- Other subtypes: vesiculobullous type, cornifying type, an acral hemorrhagic form, and comedonal Darier disease.
- Patients with Darier disease often suffer from neuropsychiatric disorders, mental retardation, depression, bipolar disorder, suicidal thoughts, psychoses, and epilepsy. Ophthalmic disorders as recurrent herpetic keratitis, minor ulcerations of the corneal epithelium or conjunctival keratosis may occur.
- Differential diagnosis: seborrheic dermatitis, acanthosis nigricans, transient acantholytic dermatosis (Grover disease), familial benign pemphigus (Hailey-Hailey disease), and pemphigus vegetans.
- The linear variant of Darier disease requires differentiation from the linear verrucous epidermal nevus (ILVEN).

N. Moftah et al., *Atlas of Common and Rare Genodermatoses*, https://doi.org/10.1007/978-3-031-60788-2_8

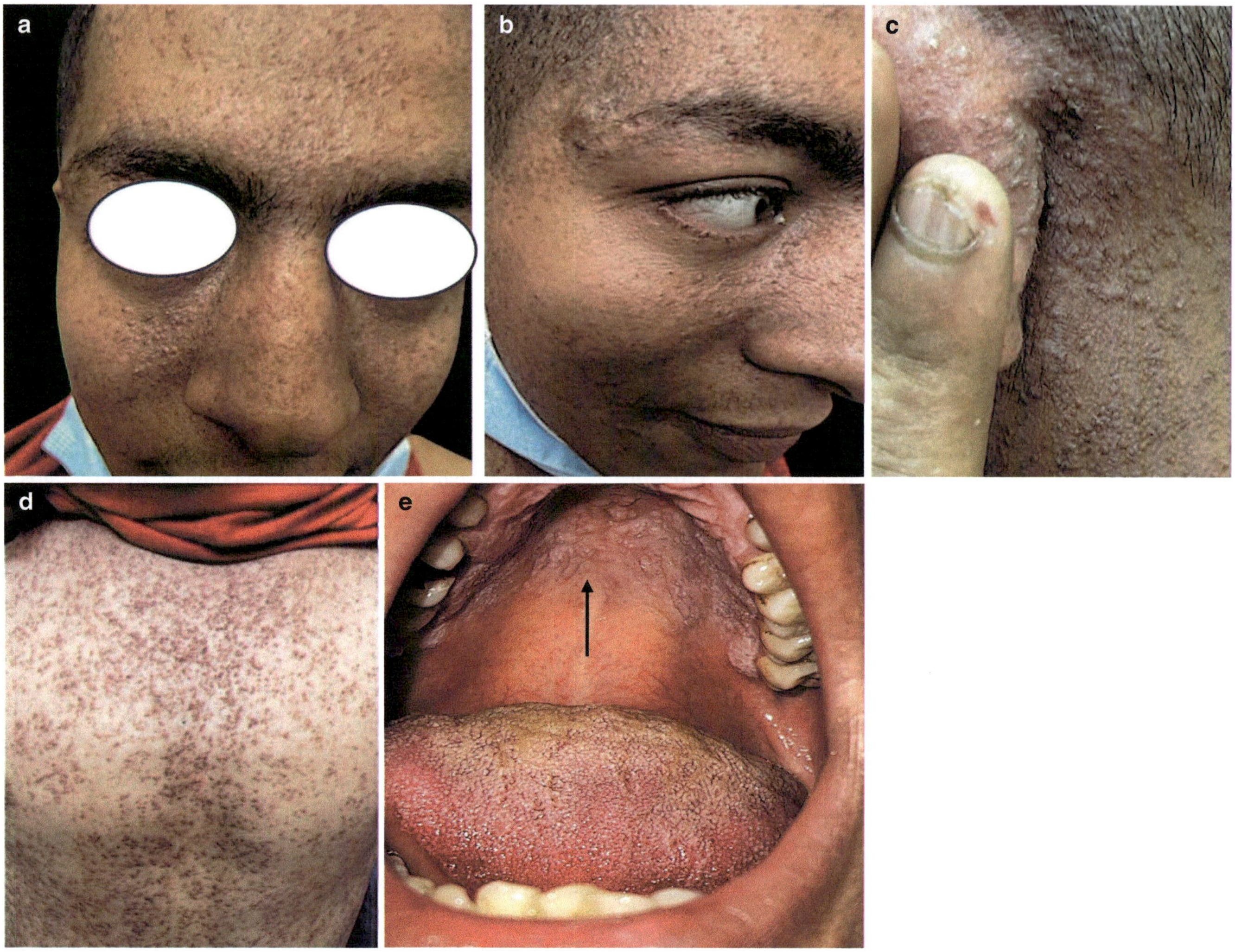

Fig. 8.1 Darier disease. Numerous hyperkeratosis skin-colored to red yellow-brown papules on the face behind the ear and trunk and may become confluent (**a**–**d**). White cobblestone papules with central depression were observed on hard palate (**e**)

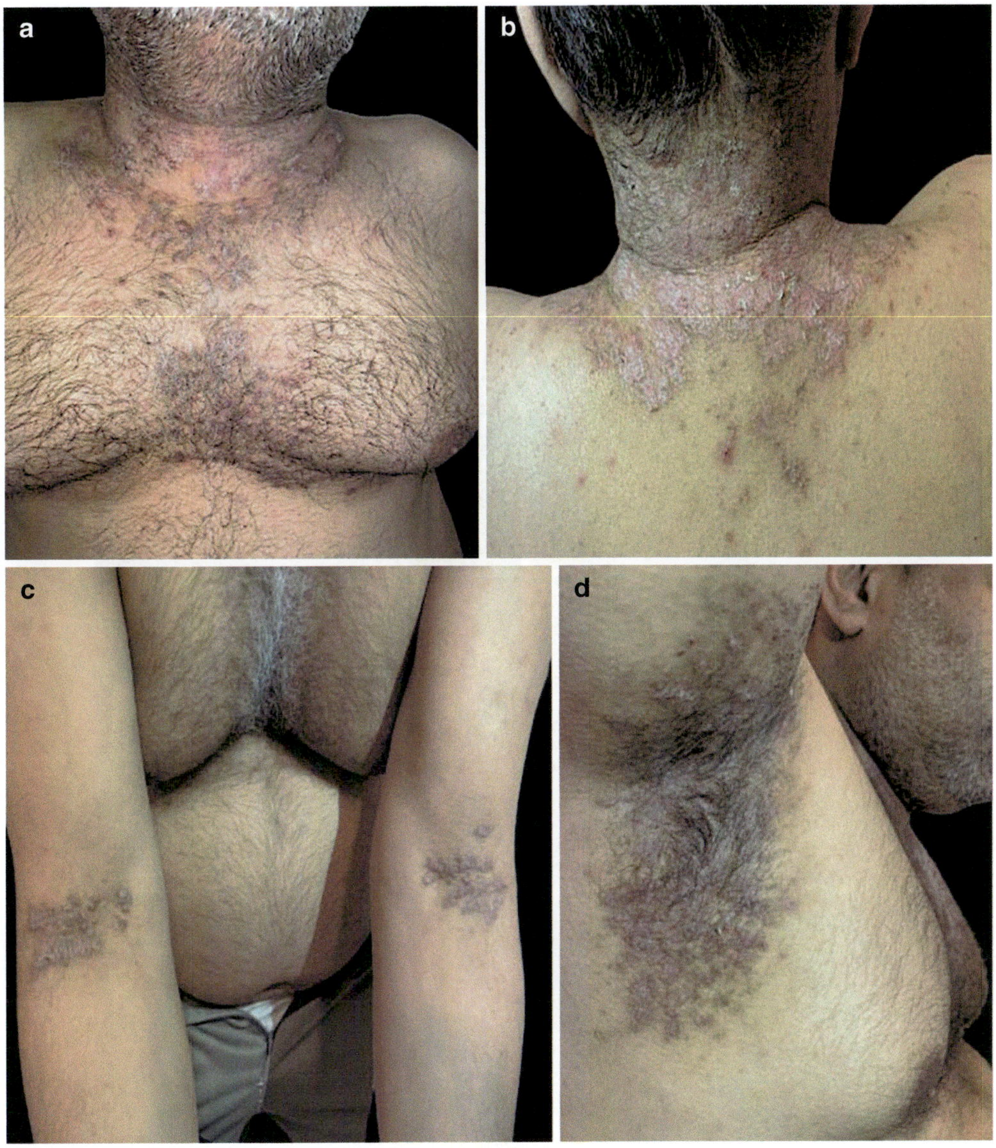

Fig. 8.2 Darier disease. Multiple red yellow-brown papules with crustation on the midsternum and posterior of neck involvement with a predilection for seborrheic areas (**a**–**d**)

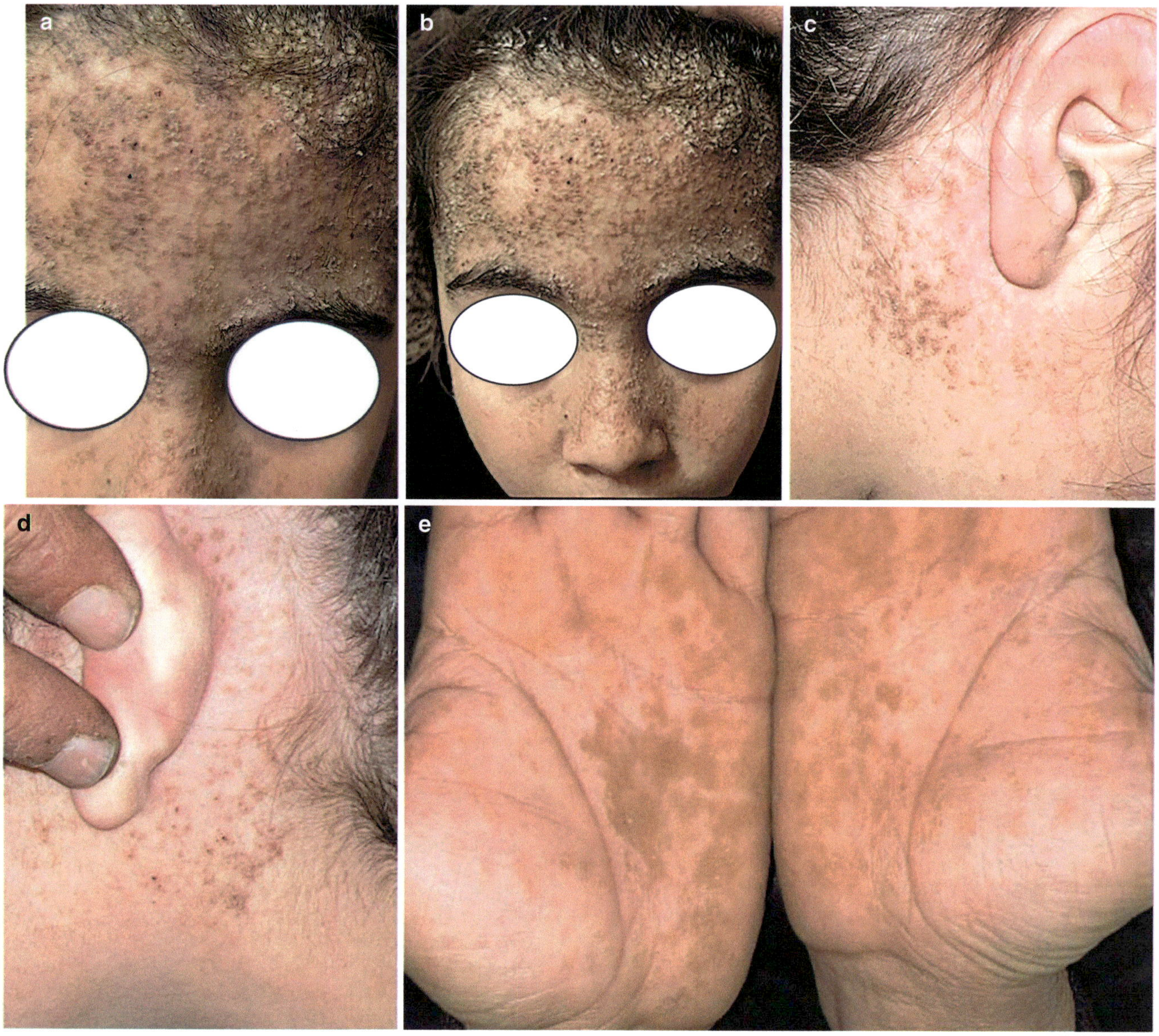

Fig. 8.3 Darier disease. Multiple skin-colored to red yellow-brown crusted papules on face, scalp (**a**, **b**) and behind the ears (**c**, **d**). Hyperkeratosis on palms (**e**). (Courtesy, Samar Ashry)

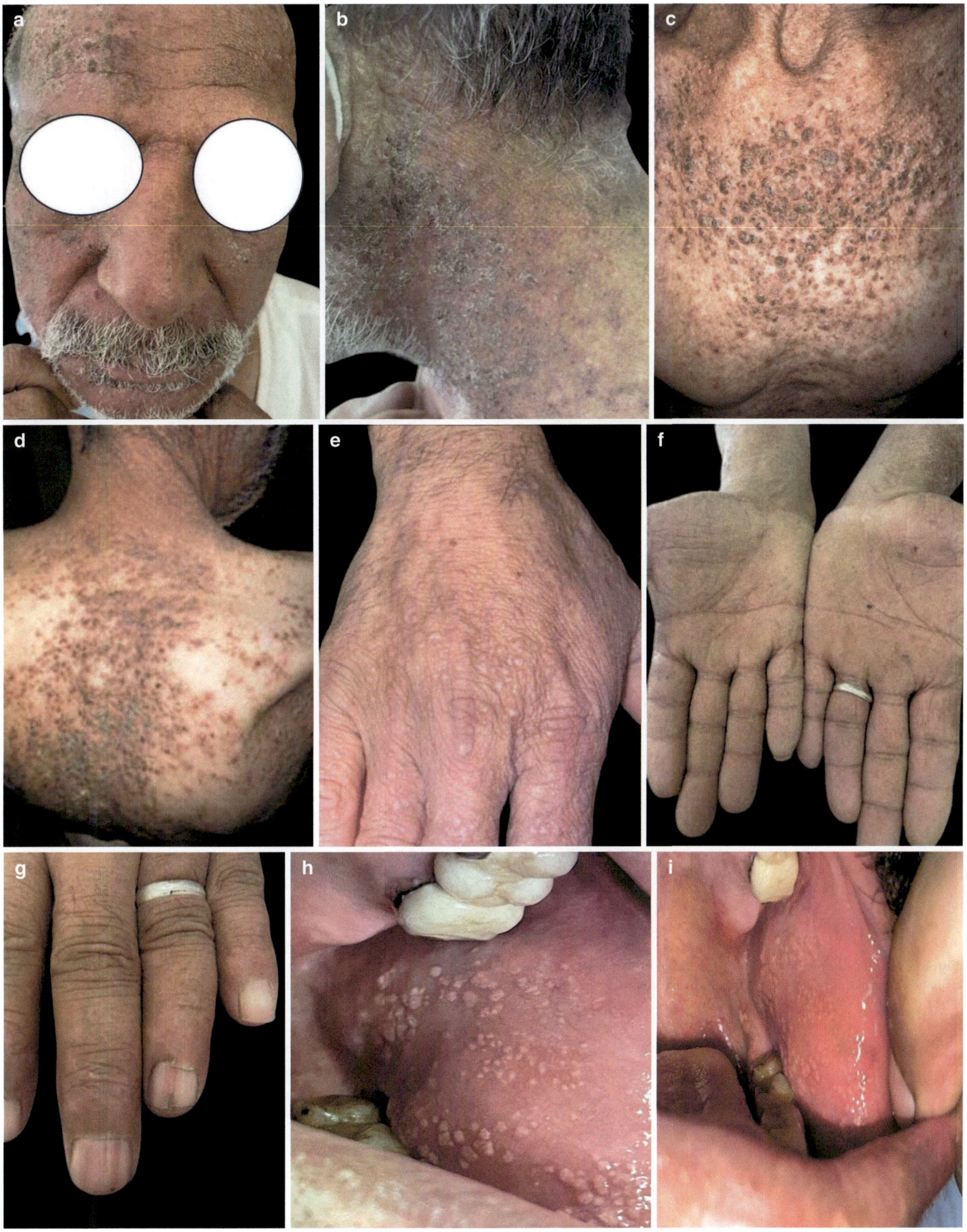

Fig. 8.4 Darier disease. Hyperkeratotic discrete scaly crusted brown funnel-shaped papules on seborrheic area such as, scalp, forehead, nasolabial and behind the ears (**a–d**). Keratotic papules on dorsum of hands and hyperkeratosis of palms (**e**, **f**). Combination of red and white alternating longitudinal bands, distal V-shaped notch on the nail (**g**). Oral white flat umbilicated papules (**h**, **i**)

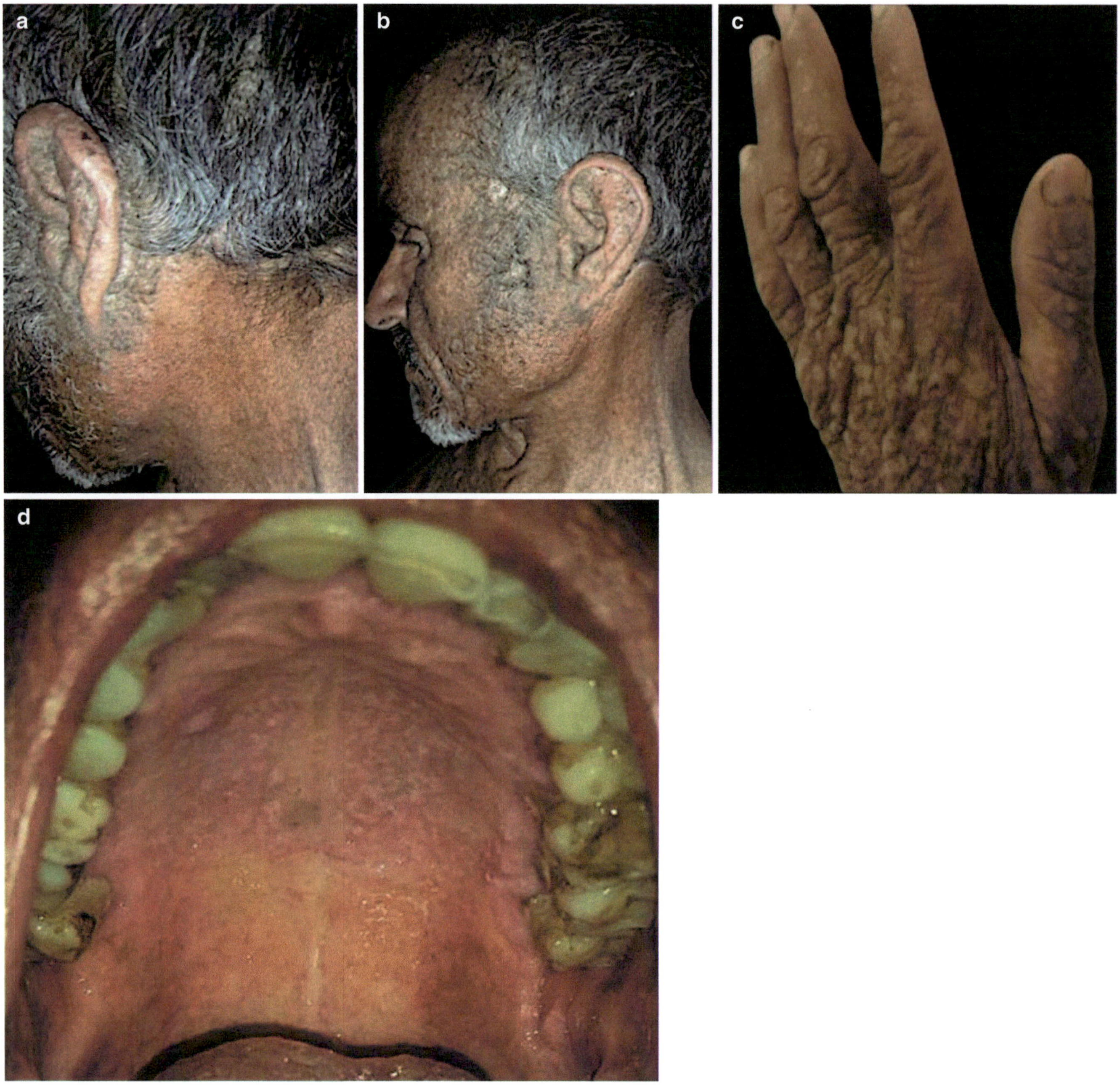

Fig. 8.5 Darier disease. Hyperkeratotic scaly, brown crusted papules on scalp, face, behind the ears (**a**, **b**), multiple flat topped papules on dorsum of hands (Acrokeratosis verruciform-like lesions) (**c**) and white flat multiple umbilicated papules on hard palate (**d**)

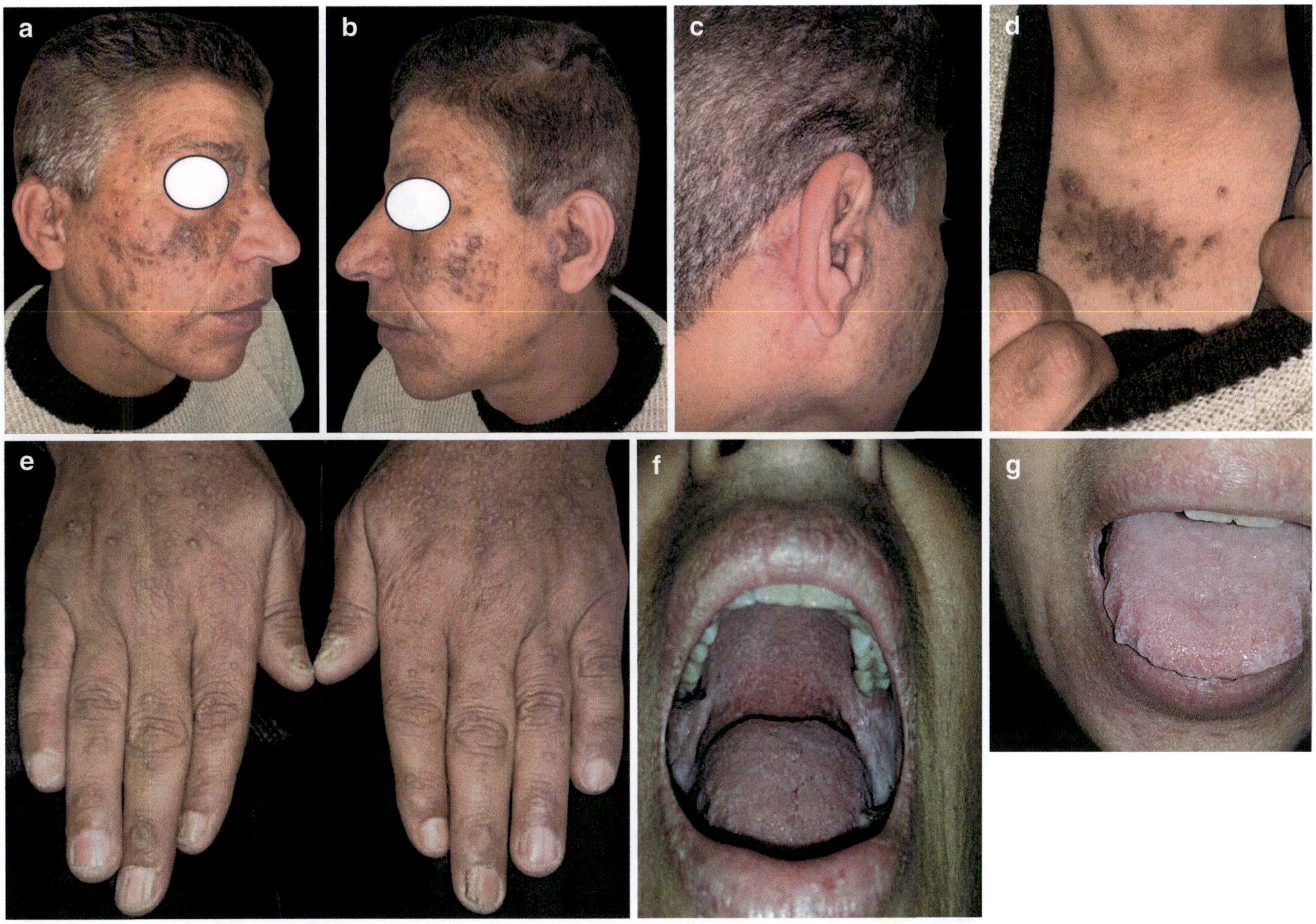

Fig. 8.6 Darier disease (Comedonal type). Erythematous brown greasy papules (comedo like) coalese into plaques on the face, behind the ear and chest (**a**–**d**). Acrokeratosis verruciform-like multiple flat topped papules on dorsum of hands with combination of red and white alternating longitudinal bands, distal V-shaped notch and brittle nails (**e**). Widespread white umbilicated papules over the entire palate (**f**) with indentation of tongue (scalloped tongue) (**g**)

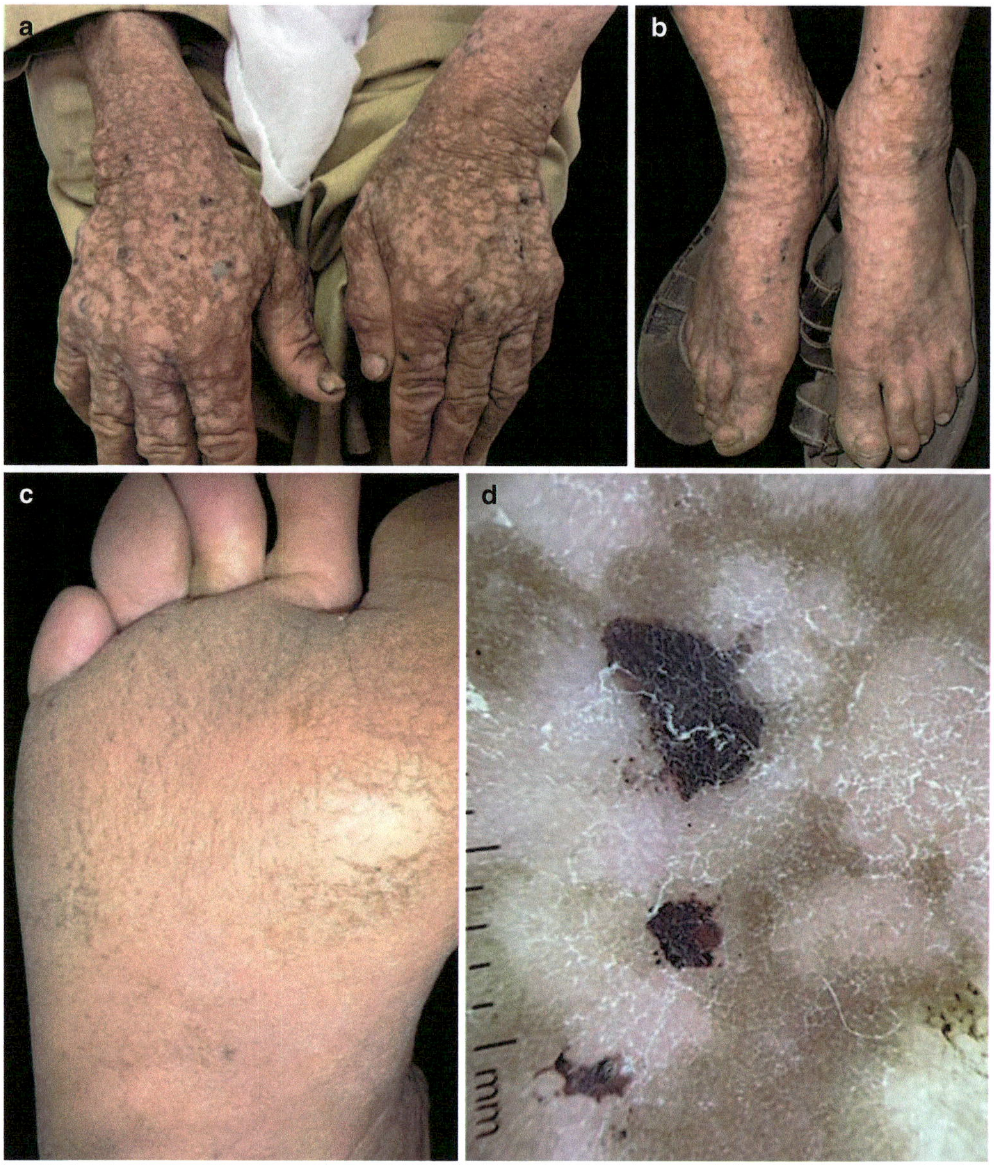

Fig. 8.7 Darier disease (acral type). Multiple flat topped papules on dorsum of hands and legs (acrokeratosis verruciform-like verrucous) with multiple hemorrhagic macules and patches on dorsum of hands (**a**, **b**). Plantar keratoderma (**c**). Dermoscopy shows multiple hemorrhagic macules and patches on dorsum of hands (**d**)

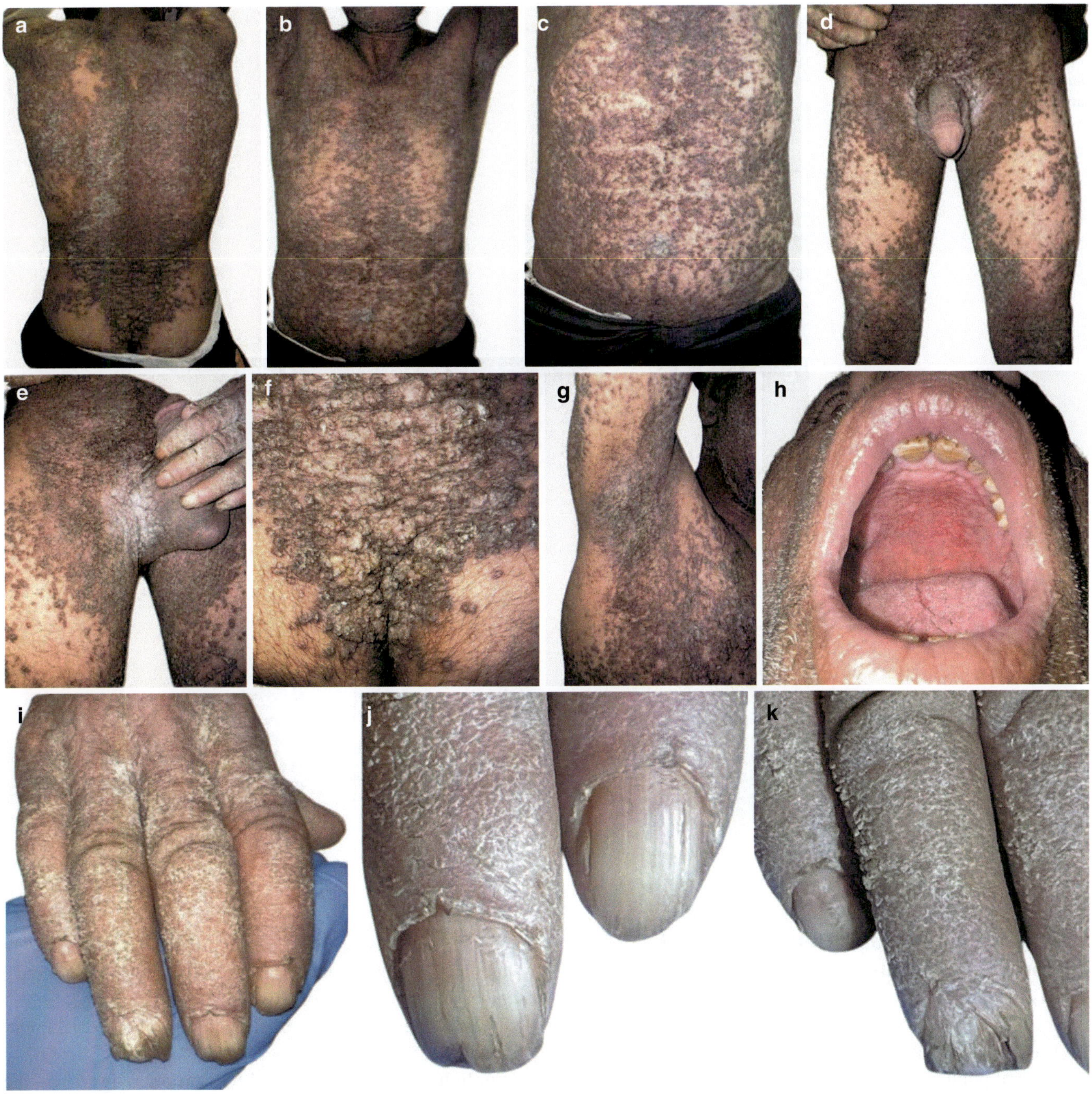

Fig. 8.8 Darier disease. Hyperkeratotic brown plaques on the trunk, groins and lower extremities can vary from red to brown and may become confluent into large plaques (**a**–**g**). Fissures in inguinal region (**d**, **e**). multiple white flat umbilicated papules in hard palate giving a cobblestone appearance (**h**). Distal V-shaped notch, brittle nail, longitudinal ridging, fissuring, subungual hyperkeratosis with scaling dorsum of hand and fingers (**i**–**k**)

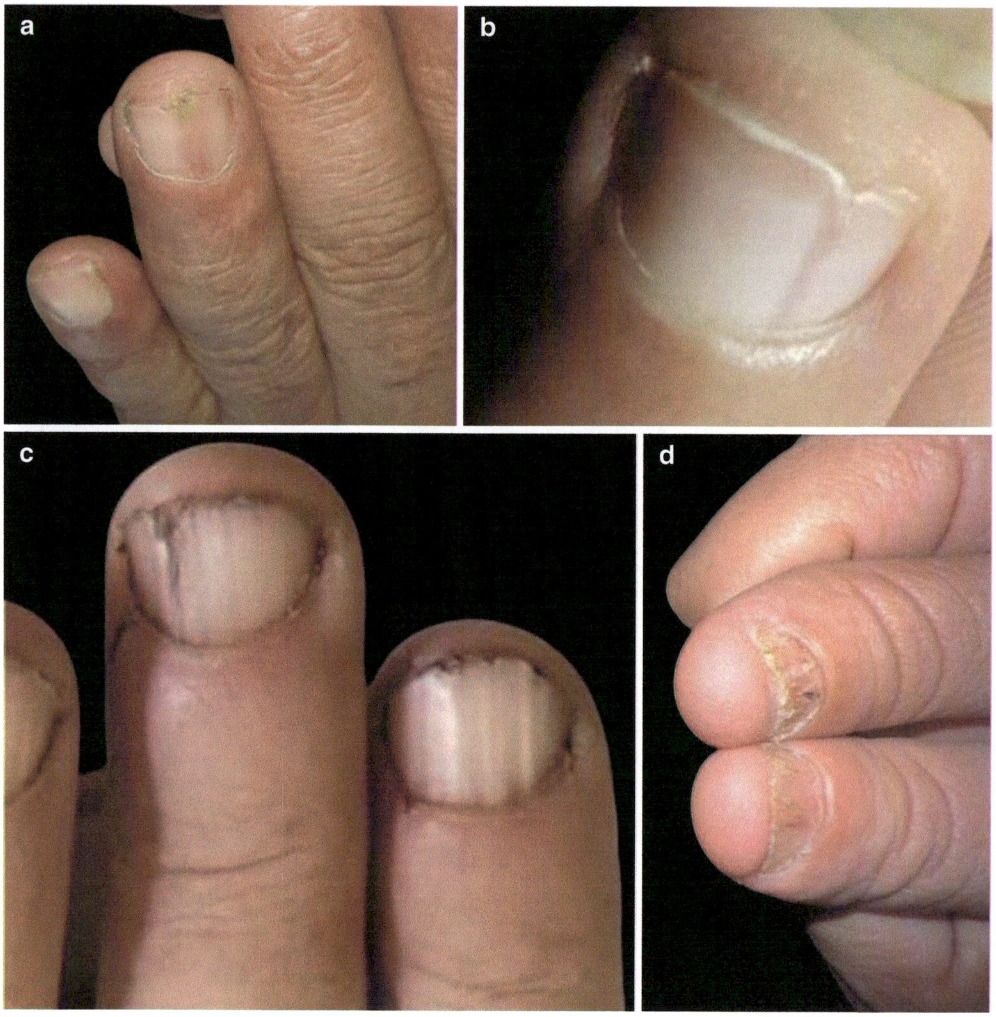

Fig. 8.9 Nail changes of Darier disease. Nails showing red and white longitudinal striations, v-shaped nicking and nails dystrophy (**a**–**d**)

Hailey-Hailey Disease (Benign Familial Chronic Pemphigus) (AD) [3–5] (Figs. 8.10, 8.11, and 8.12)

- Rare skin condition that affects around 1/50,000 of the general population.
- Autosomal dominant, but some cases are due to a mutated gene, *ATP2C1*, and therefore, can occur with patients who do not have a family history of the condition.
- *ATP2C1* gene mutation leads to changes in calcium transport into the Golgi apparatus that result in desmosomal dysfunction and keratinocyte acantholysis.
- Affect both males and females equally.
- The disease usually becomes most noticeable during puberty but may appear later.
- Appear as painful blistering, and varying degrees of erythema most commonly in skin folds, including but not limited to the neck, axilla, and groin.
- Flaccid vesicles or bullae are the primary lesions, but they are hardly noticeable as they easily rupture and leave macerated erosions, sometimes with crusting.
- The disease shows exacerbation and remissions and usually heals without scarring.
- Sunlight, heat, sweating, and friction often aggravate the disorder.
- Involvement of the buccal, vaginal or conjunctiva mucosae is rare.
- Two forms:
  - The segmental form is usually unilateral and linear (along the lines of Blaschko).
  - The generalized form is rare.
- Common complication is secondary infection by fungi and bacteria.
- The main differential diagnoses are pemphigus vulgaris, Darier disease, inverse psoriasis, seborrheic dermatitis, intertrigo, and erythrasma.

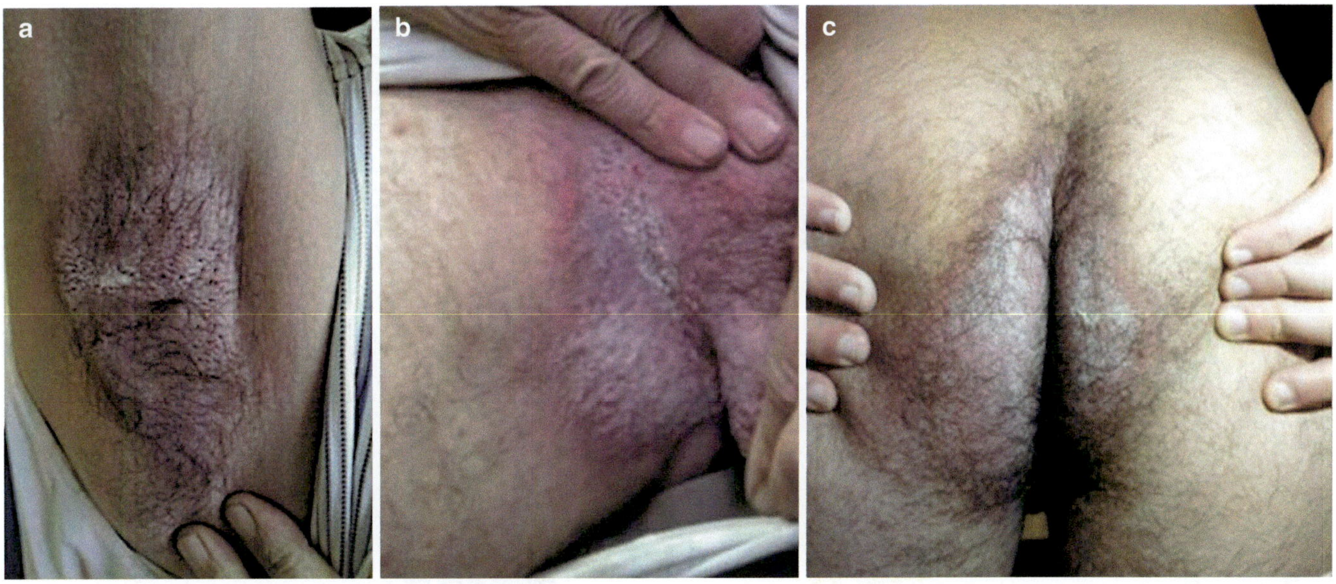

Fig. 8.10 Hailey-Hailey disease. Erythematous, eroded plaques and vegetative lesions in the intertriginous areas (axilla, groin, and intergluteal regions) with macerations (**a**–**c**)

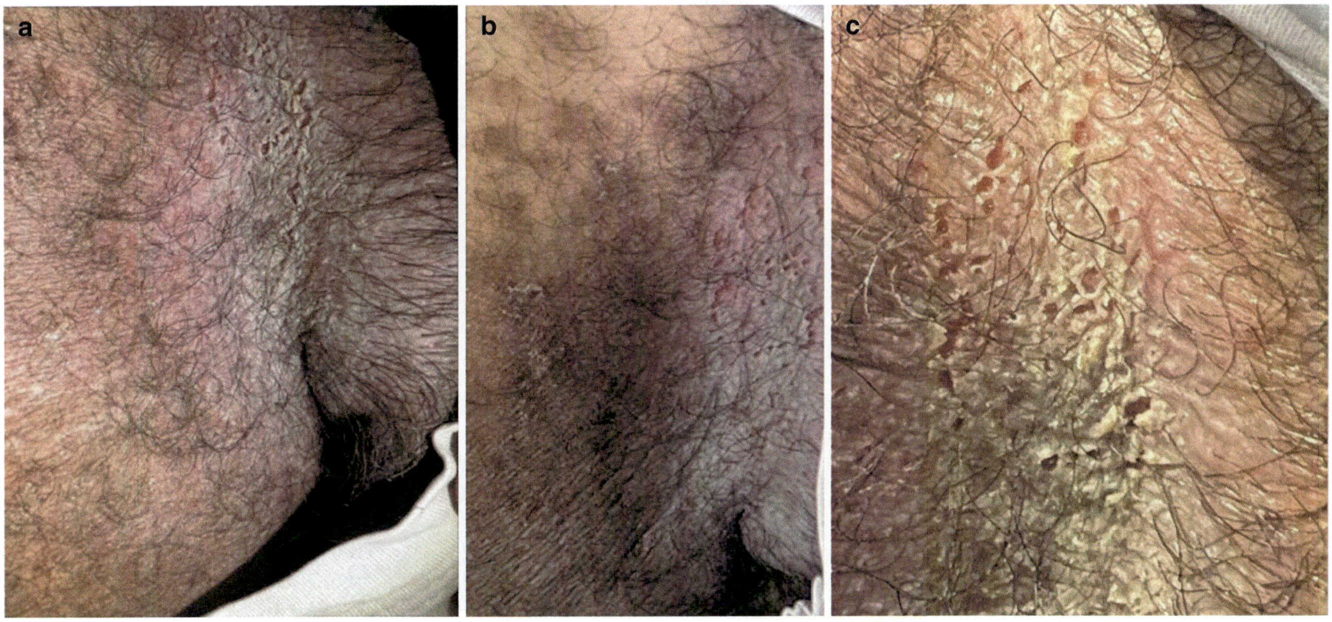

Fig. 8.11 Hailey-Hailey disease. Erythematous, eroded plaques and vegetations with erosive, crusted lesions in inguinal area (**a**–**c**)

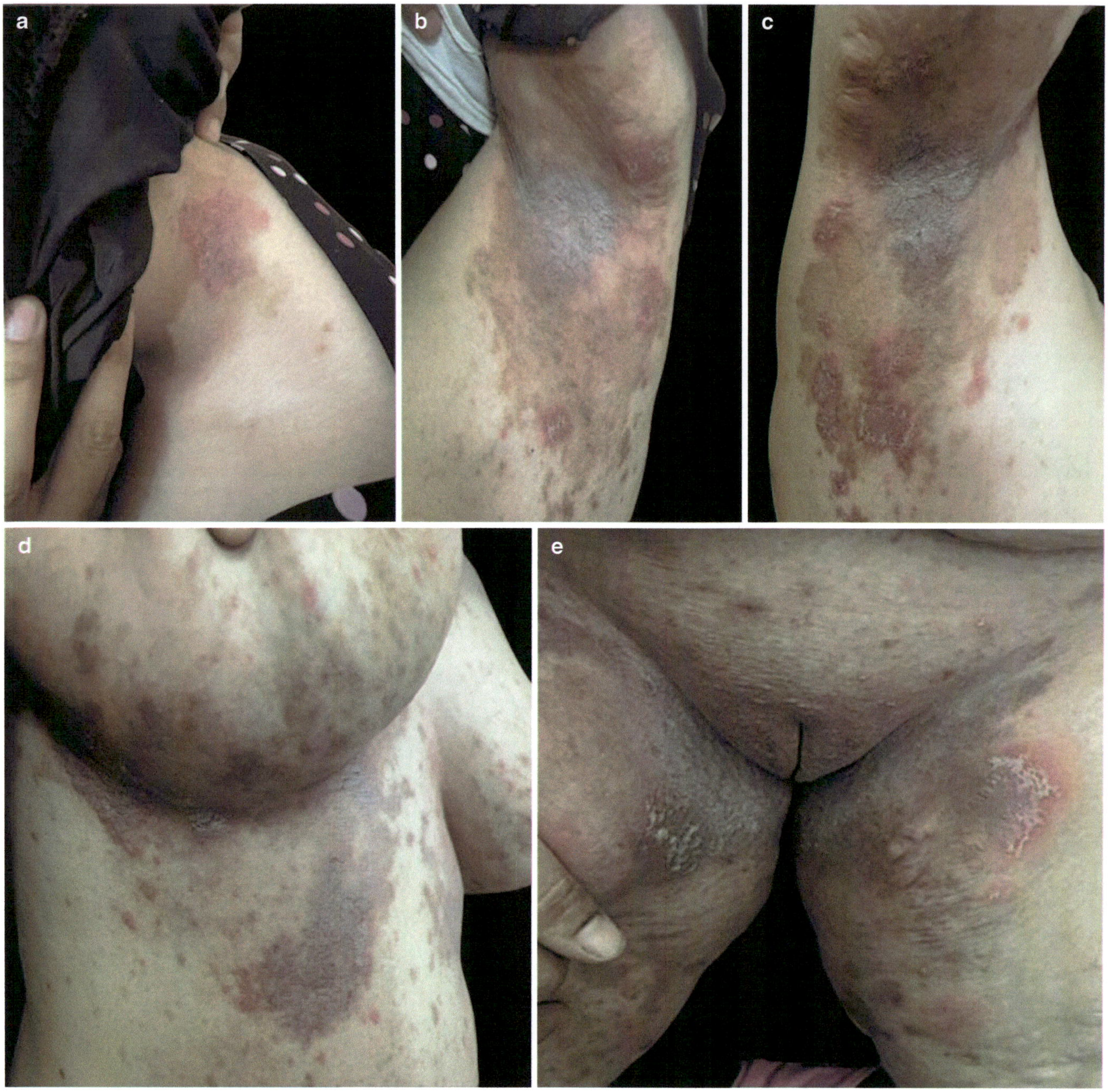

Fig. 8.12 Hailey-Hailey disease. Erythematous, eroded plaques with erosive, crusted lesions in neck, axillae, under breasts, inguinal area (**a–e**). Circinate plaques on the neck with erosions and crusting in the active borders (**a**). Erythematous, eroded plaque, intact flaccid vesicles and blisters and erosive, crusted lesions on the axillae (**b**, **c**) and under breasts with vegetations and macerations (**d**). Circinate plaques in the inguinal region with erosions and crusting in the borders with vegetations (**e**)

References

1. Sakuntabhai A, Ruiz-Perez V, Carter S, et al. Mutations in ATP2A2, encoding a Ca2+ pump, cause Darier disease. Nat Genet. 1999;21:271–7.
2. Chyl-Surdacka K, Borzęcki A, Latifa J, et al. Keratosis follicularis (Darier disease)—clinical characteristics and treatment—a review and update. Postepy Dermatol Alergol. 2023;40:337–40.
3. Reddy S, Brahmbhatt H. A narrative review on the usage of surgical skin grafting, acitretin, and tacrolimus in the treatment of Hailey-Hailey disease. Cureus. 2021;13:e19704. https://doi.org/10.7759/cureus.19704.
4. Burge SM. Hailey–Hailey disease: the clinical features, response to treatment and prognosis. Br J Dermatol. 1992;126:275.
5. Tansini PB, Boff AL, Weber MB, et al. Familial "benign" pemphigus? Erythroderma and fatal outcome. An Bras Dermatol. 2020;95:75–7.

9 Dermal Disorders

- **Cutis laxa**
- **Ehlers-Danlos syndrome**
- **Pseudoxanthoma Elasticum**
- **Marfan syndrome**
- **Buschke-Ollendorff Syndrome**
- **Lipoid proteinosis**
- **Focal dermal hypoplasia** (**Goltz syndrome**)
- **Juvenile hyaline fibromatosis**

Cutis Laxa (AD, AR, XLR) [1, 2] (Fig. 9.1)

- A group of rare heritable and acquired conditions characterized by sparse and fragmented elastic fibers (Table 9.1).
- Clinical characteristics (apparent at birth or early childhood):
  - Skin: loose, sagging skin with reduced elasticity.
  - Face: aged facial appearance with down-slanting palpebral fissure and long philtrum.
  - Pulmonary emphysema, diverticula, inguinal or umbilical hernias.
  - Cardiac or arterial abnormalities.
  - Skeletal or joint anomaly.
  - Delayed growth and development.
- Pathology: sparse and/or fragmented elastic fibers. Complete absence of elastic fibers may occur in severe cases.
- Prognosis: morbidity and mortality are usually due to pulmonary complications.
- Treatment: reconstructive surgery for sagging skin and multidisciplinary approach for internal organs affection.

N. Moftah et al., *Atlas of Common and Rare Genodermatoses*, https://doi.org/10.1007/978-3-031-60788-2_9

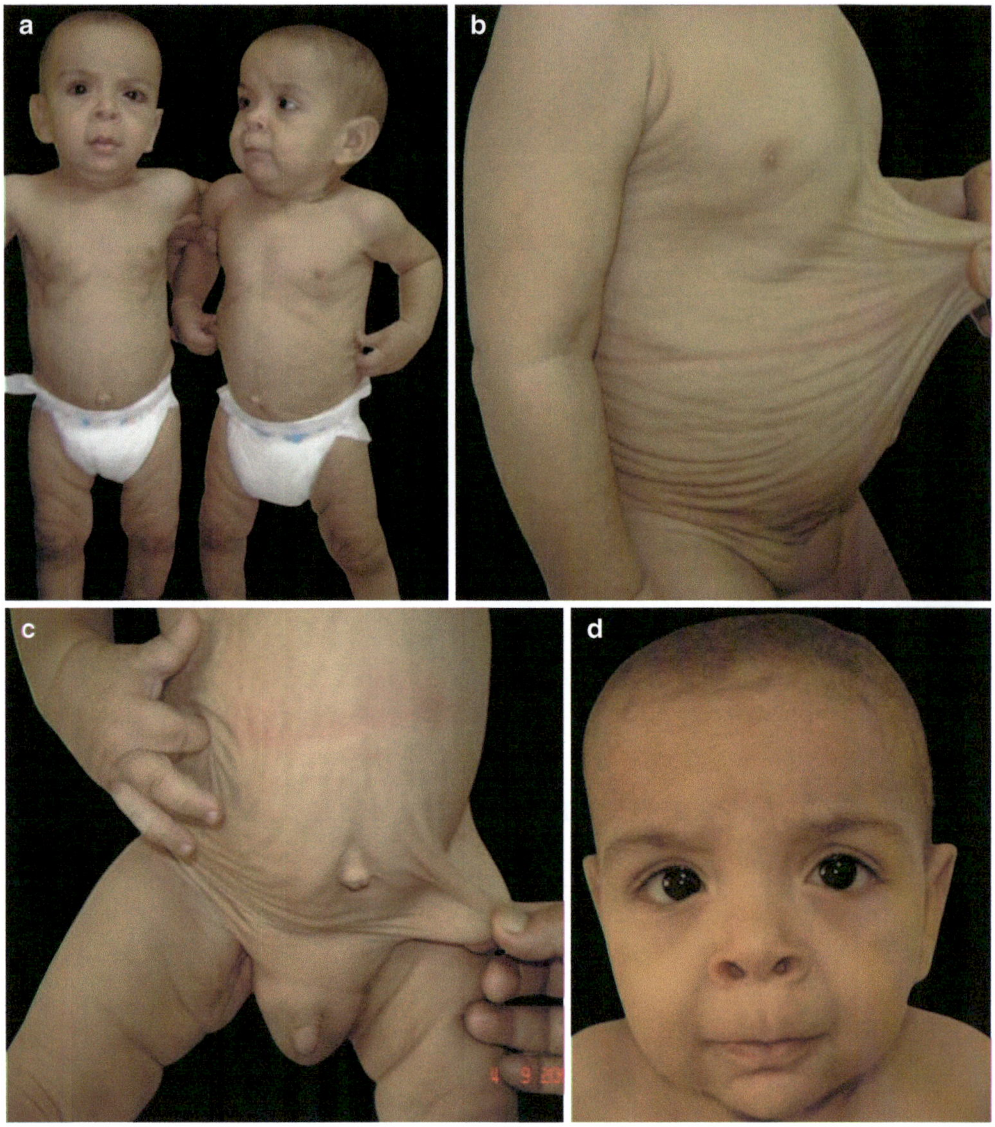

Fig. 9.1 Cutis laxa in twins. Loose, sagging skin with reduced elasticity on the abdomen (**a–c**), down slanting palpebral fissure, dropping jowls and long philtrum (**d**). (*Courtesy, Hala Abd El Salam Fayed*)

Table 9.1 Cutis laxa mode of inheritance, gene defect, affected protein, and extracutaneous features

Inheritance	Gene defect	Protein	Extracutaneous features
AD	*ELN*	Elastin	Cardiac valve anomaly, aortic dilatation Emphysema Hernias
	FBLN5	Fibulin 5	
	ALDH18A1	Pyrroline-5 carboxylate synthetase	Corneal opacity and cataract Cranial arterial tortuosity
AR	*FBLN4*	Fibulin 4	Arterial or aortic tortuosity/aneurysms Emphysema Bladder diverticula Joint laxity/fractures Micrognathia
	FBLN5	Fibulin 5	Arterial or aortic stenosis Emphysema Bladder diverticula
	LTBP4	Latent TGF-β binding protein-4	Pulmonary malformation/arterial stenosis GIT malformations Micrognathia Joint laxity
	ATP6V0A2	Vacuolar H^+-ATPase A2 subunit	Ocular anomaly and strabismus Microcephaly Neurological degeneration O- and N-glycosylation defect
	ATP6V1E1 *ATP6V1A*	Vacuolar H^+-ATPase V1 subunits E1 and A	Pneumothoraces Cardiac anomaly Triangular face Hypotonia/hip dysplasia
	PYCR1	Pyrroline-5 carboxylate reductase1	Translucent skin Corneal opacity/cataract Triangular face/absent corpus callosum Hip dysplasia/joint laxity Cranial arterial tortuosity
	ALDH18A1	Pyrroline-5 carboxylate synthetase	Corneal opacity/cataract Cranial arterial tortuosity
	GORAB	Golgin, RAB6-interacting	Malar hypoplasia/prognathism Joint laxity/osteoporosis/fracture
	RIN2	RAS and RAB interactor2	Sparse hair Gingival hypertrophy Macrocephaly Scoliosis/joint laxity
XLR	ATP7A	ATPase, Cu^{2+}-transporting α-polypeptide	Easy bruising Coarse hair/long face with hooked nose Occipital calcifications Chronic diarrhea/bladder diverticula

Ehlers-Danlos Syndrome (EDS) (AD, AR) [3, 4] (Figs. 9.2 and 9.3)

- Defective function of collagens, collagen processing enzymes, and/or collagen associated proteins.
- Cutaneous manifestations:
  - Hyperextensible skin.
  - Fragile skin of knees, elbows, shins, and forehead.
  - Poor wound healing with cigarette paper appearance and easy bruising.
  - Molluscoid pseudo tumors on knees and elbows.
  - Sub-cutaneous multiple small hard nodules over the bony prominences.
- Associations:
  - Elastosis perforans serpiginosa and piezogenic papules.
- Extracutaneous manifestations (variable according to the subtype):
  - Joint hypermobility.
  - Scoliosis.
  - Spontaneous arterial, intestinal or utrine rupture in vascular type.
- Classification:
  - Classic type (AD): mutation in *COL5A1, COL5A2/α1* and *α2* chains of type V collagen.
    Cutaneous features: hyperextensible and fragile skin with easy bruising and atrophic scar.
    Extracutaneous features: joint hypermobility, ability to touch the nose with tongue (Gorlin sign).
  - Hypermobile (AD): unknown.
    Cutaneous features: hyperextensible skin.

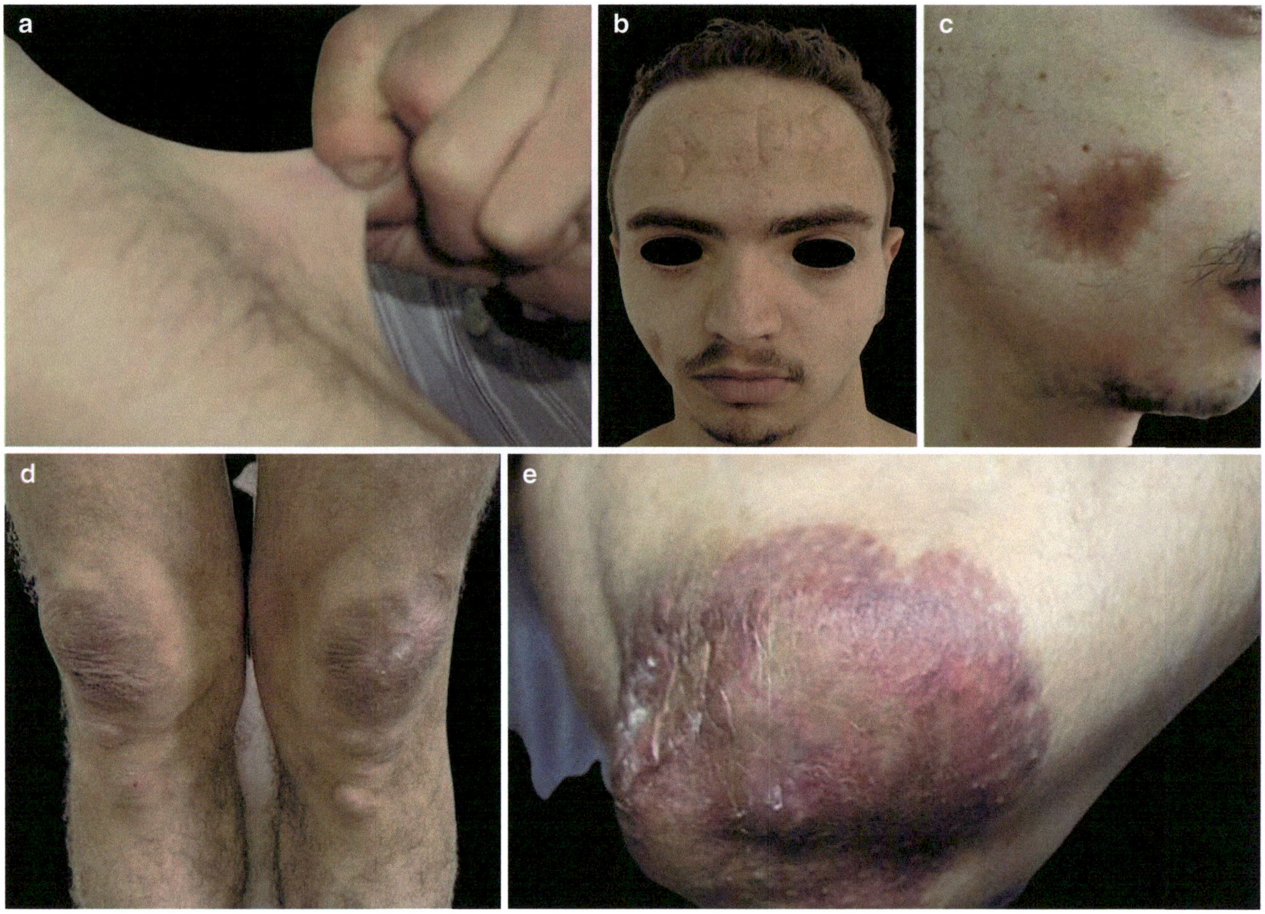

Fig. 9.2 Ehlers-Danlos syndrome (Classic type). Hyperextensible skin in the arm (**a**), atrophic linear scars on the forehead (**b**), atrophic scar with cigarette paper appearance on the right cheek and knees (**c**, **d**), extensive bruising on the elbow (**e**)

Extracutaneous features: joint hypermobility, dislocations, and variable autonomic dysfunction.

- Vascular (AD): mutation in *COL3A1/α1* chain of type III collagen.
  Cutaneous features: thin translucent skin with excessive bruising.
  Extracutaneous features: joint hypermobility, arterial, gastrointestinal, and uterine rupture.
- Kyphoscoliotic (AR): mutation in *PLOD1/lysyl hydroxylase* or *FKBP14/FK506* binding protein 14.
  Cutaneous features: hyperextensible and fragile skin.
  Extracutaneous features: joint hypermobility, kyphoscoliosis, osteopenia, congenital hypotonia, and blue sclera.
- Musculocontractural (AR): mutation in *CHST14/dermatan-4-sulfotransferase*.
  Cutaneous features: hyperextensible and fragile skin with wrinkled palms.
  Extracutaneous features: joint hypermobility, contracture, scoliosis, craniofacial anomaly, and ocular fragility.
- Arthrochalasia (AD): mutation in *COL1A1, COL1A2/α1,* and *α2* chains of type 1 collagen.
  Cutaneous features: hyperextensible and fragile skin.
  Extracutaneous features: severe joint hypermobility with scoliosis and congenital hip dislocation.
- Dermatosparaxis (AR): mutation in *ADAMTS2/procollagen 1N-peptidase.*
  Cutaneous features: severe skin fragility with sagging and easy bruising.
  Extracutaneous features: hernias, puffy eyelids, and delayed closure of fontanelles.
- Periodontal (AD): mutation in *C1R, C1S/complement C1r, C1s.*
  Cutaneous features: mild hyperextensible skin and easy bruising.
  Extracutaneous features: early onset periodontitis, gingival recession, and marfanoid features.
- Cardiac valvular (AR): mutation in *COL1A2/α1* chains of type 1 collagen.
  Cutaneous features: hyperextensible and fragile skin with easy bruising and atrophic scar.
  Extracutaneous features: cardiac valve defect.

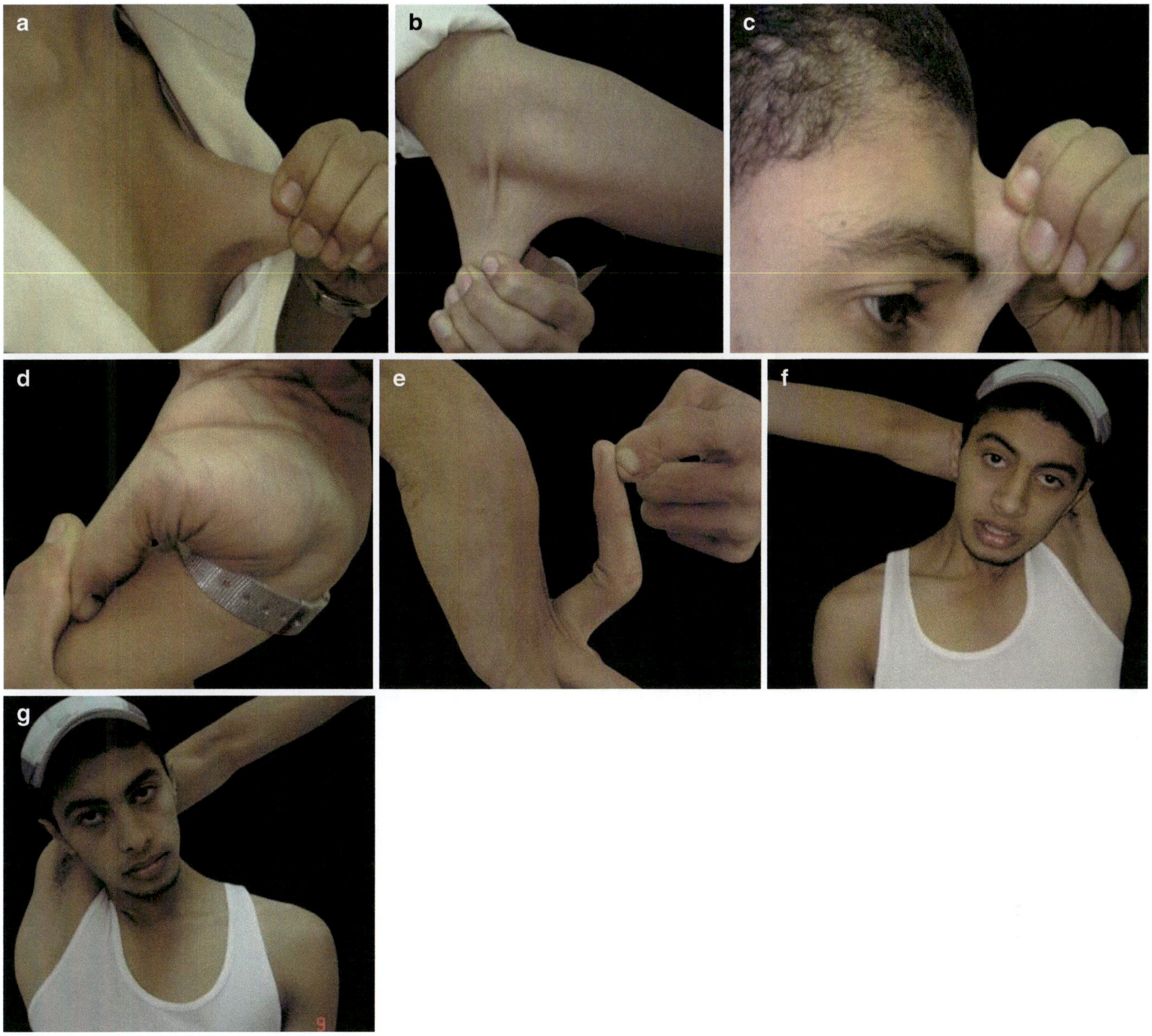

Fig. 9.3 Ehlers-Danlos syndrome (Hypermobile type). Hyperextensible skin in the chest (**a**), arm (**b**), and forehead (**c**), Joint hypermobility at the wrist (**d**), fingers (**e**), and shoulders (**f**, **g**)

- Brittle cornea syndrome (AR): mutation in *COL1A2/ α1* chains of type I collagen.
  Cutaneous features: soft, translucent skin with variable hyperextensibility and acral wrinkling.
  Extracutaneous features: ocular fragility, keratoconous, blue sclera, and impaired hearing.

Pseudoxanthoma Elasticum (PXE) (AR) [5, 6] (Figs. 9.4 and 9.5)

- Loss of function mutations in ATP-binding cassette subfamily C member 6 gene (*ABCC6*).
- Autosomal recessive with slight female predominance.
- Affects the elastic fibers of the skin, eyes, and cardiovascular system.
- Cutaneous manifestations:
  - Flexural small thin yellowish papules that coalesce to form cobble-stone-like plaques with characteristic plucked chicken skin appearance.
  - Starts during first or second decade of life and the lateral neck is usually affected first.
  - Sagging skin in axillae and groin.
  - Yellowish papules on lower lip.
  - Perforating PXE due to increased dermal calcium deposition with extrusion of yellowish material in advanced condition.
- Ocular manifestations:

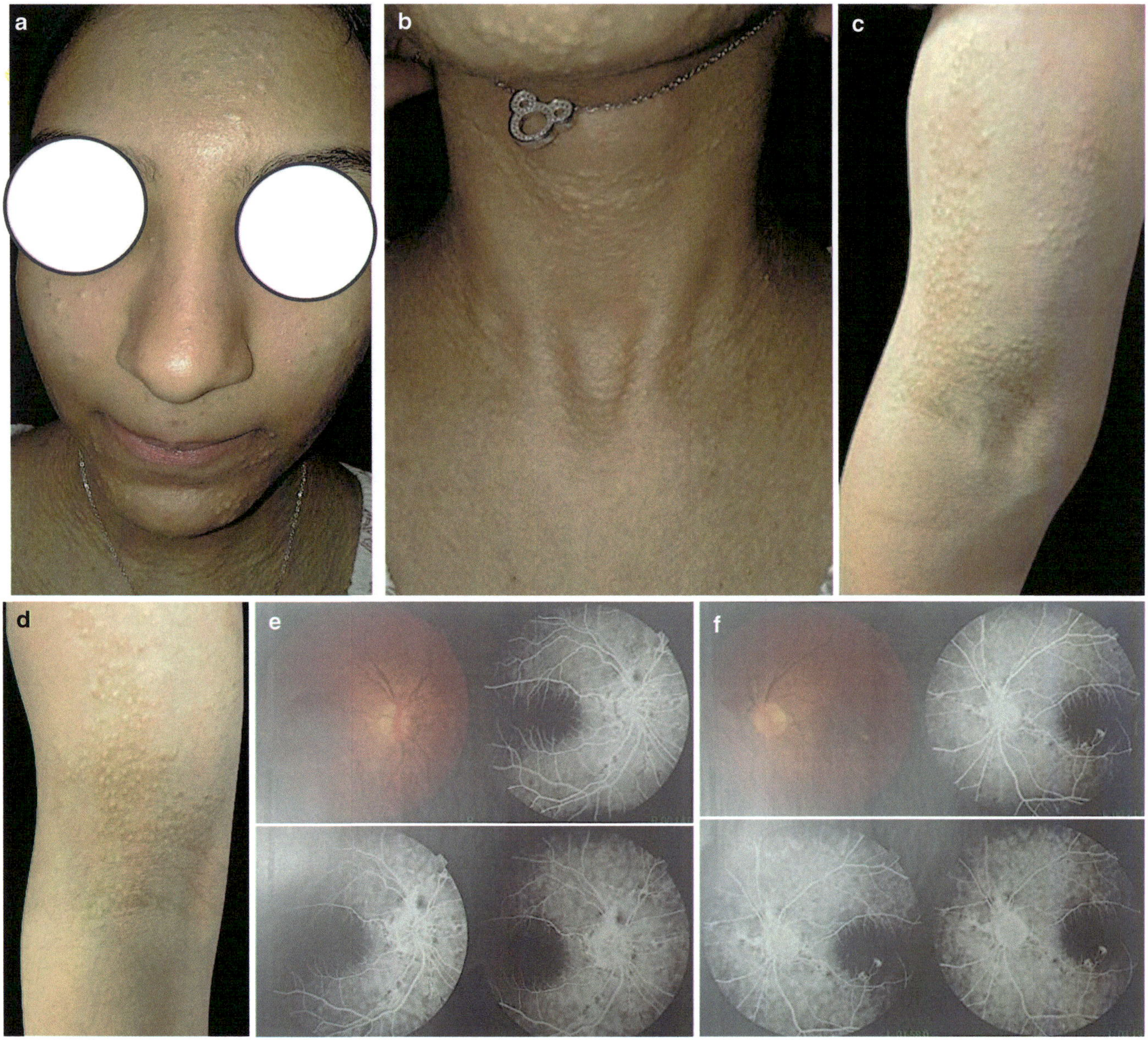

Fig. 9.4 Pseudoxanthoma Elasticum. Yellowish papules in the face, neck (**a**, **b**), antecubital fossae (**c**, **d**), angioid streaks (**e**, **f**)

- Angioid streaks (breaks in the calcified elastic lamina of Bruch membrane).
- Cardiovascular manifestations:
  - Calcification of elastic media and intima of medium sized arteries with atheromatous plaques formation.
  - Gastrointestinal bleeding from the stomach duo to calcified mucosal blood vessels.
  - Angina, mitral valve prolapse and myocardial infarction.
  - Renovascular hypertension.

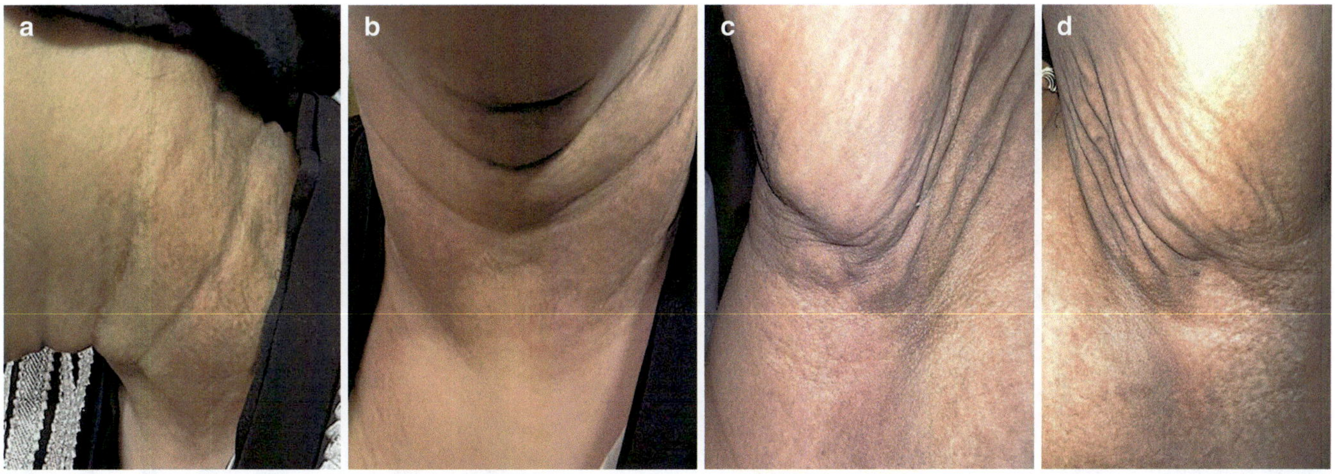

Fig. 9.5 Pseudoxanthoma Elasticum. Cobble-stone-like plaques in the neck (**a**, **b**), thickened, yellowish, sagging skin of both axillae (**c**, **d**)

- Histopathology: distorted, fragmented elastic fibers in the mid and deep reticular dermis.

  Calcium deposits are seen in advanced cases.

  Characteristic changes in elastic fibers can be seen by special stains.

Marfan Syndrome (AD) [7, 8] (Fig. 9.6)

- Autosomal dominant mutation in *FBN1*/fibrillin gene (major component of microfibrils).
- Cutaneous manifestations:
  - Striae, elastosis perforans serpiginosa and decreased subcutaneous fat on extremities.
- Extracutaneous manifestations:

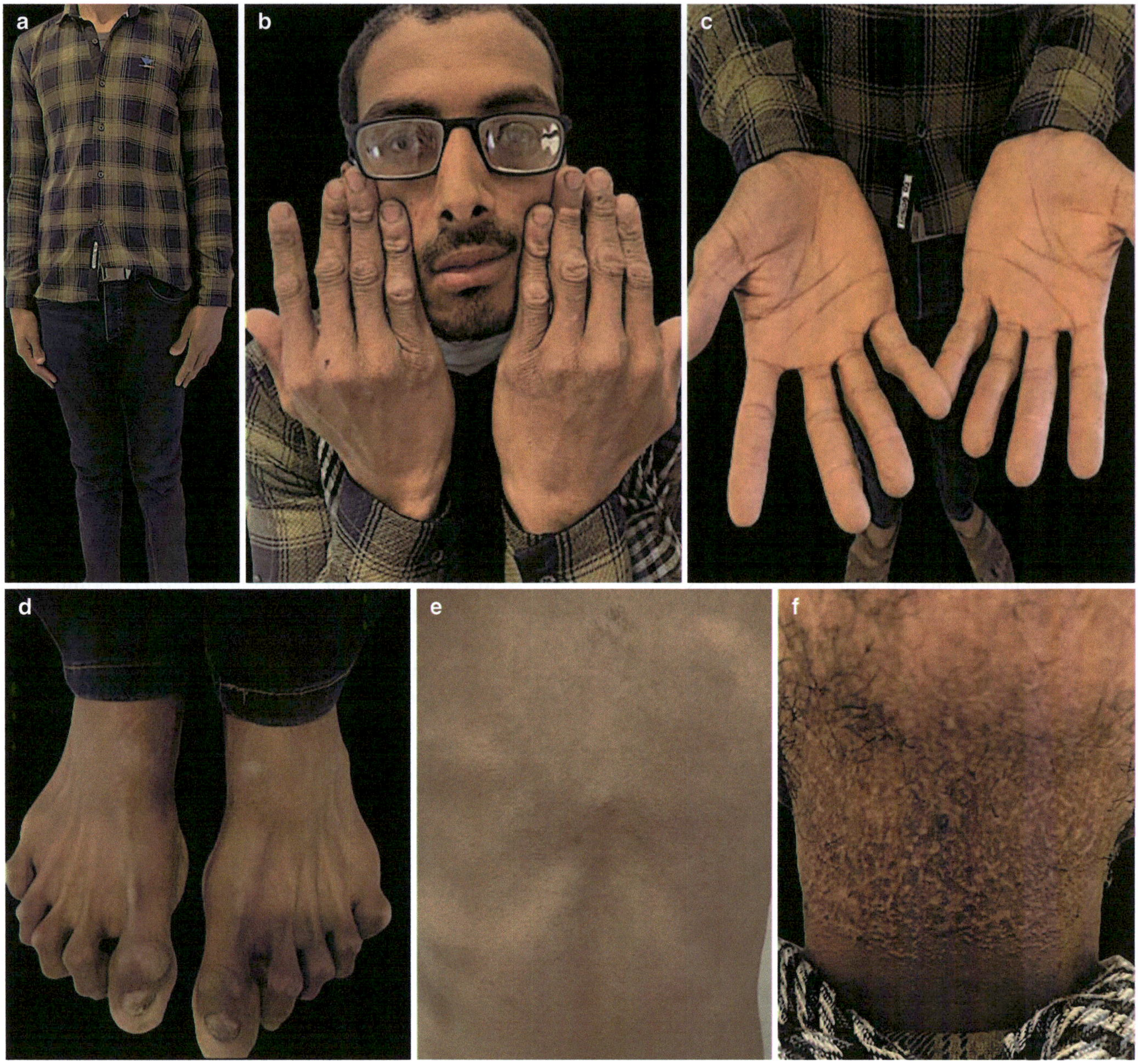

Fig. 9.6 Marfan syndrome. Tall, thin patient with long arms (**a**), long fingers (**b**, **c**), hammer toes (**d**), pectus excavatum (**e**), anetoderma like patches in the neck (**f**)

- Tall patient with disproportionately long limbs.
- Scoliosis.
- Lens sublaxation.
- Aneurysmal dilataion of ascending aorta (most common cause of mortality).
- Wrist sign: positive if the thumb and little finger overlap when wrapped around the opposite wrist.

Buschke-Ollendorff Syndrome (AD) [9, 10] (Fig. 9.7)

- Autosomal dominant mutation of *LEM* domain containing protein 3 (*LEMD3*) gene.
- This mutation reduces the amount of functional LEMD3 protein with subsequent increase in bone morphogenic protein (BMP) and transforming growth factor-beta (TGF-β) pathways resulting in excessive bone and connective tissue growth.
- Incidence: 1:20,000 people worldwide.
- Cutaneous manifestations:

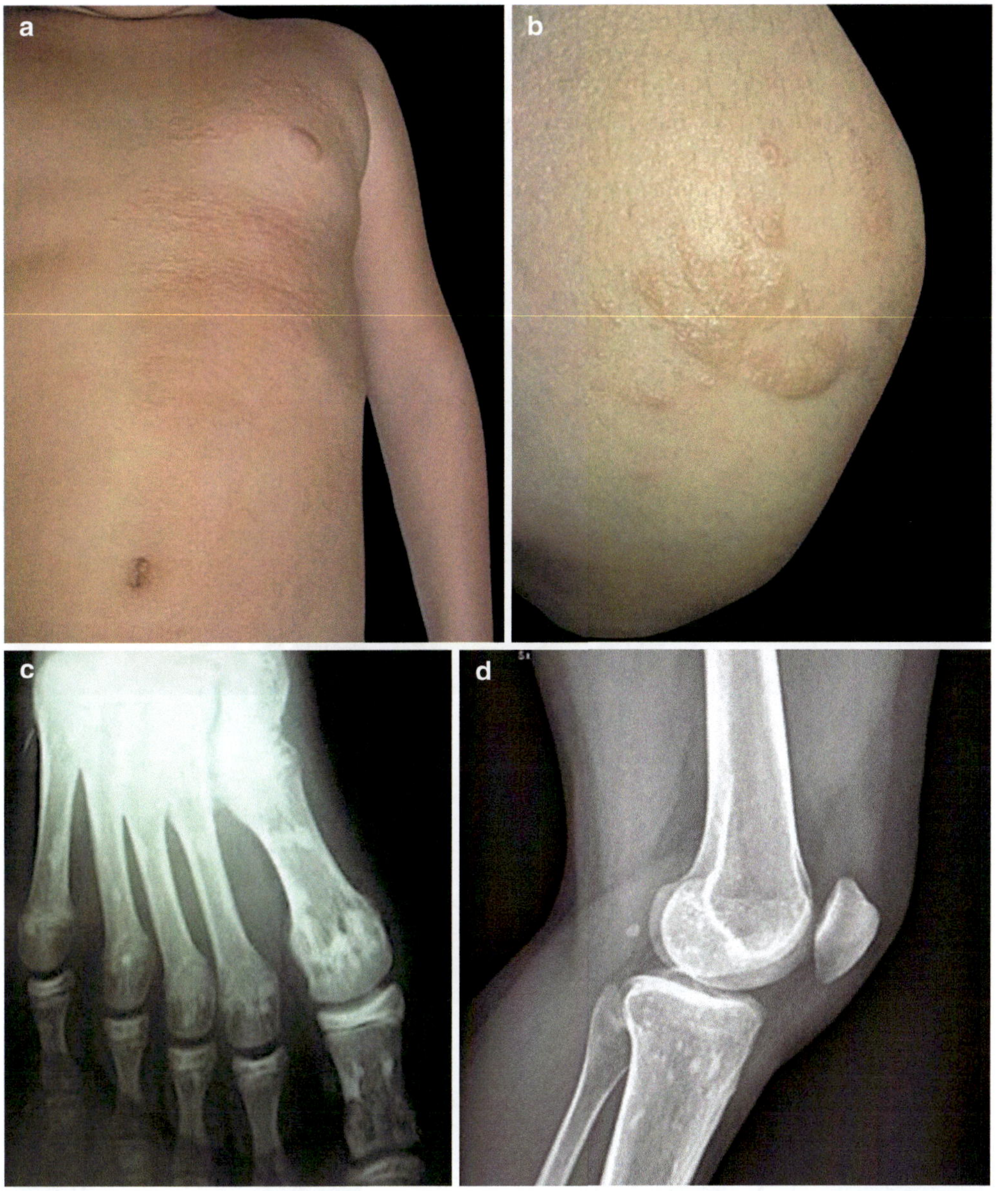

Fig. 9.7 Buschke-Ollendorff Syndrome. Connective tissue nevi (dermatofibrosis lenticularis disseminata) in the chest (**a**), elbow (**b**), sclerotic hand bones (melorheostosis) (**c**), spotted lower limb bone (osteopoikilosis) (**d**)

 - Connective tissue naevi also called dermatofibrosis lenticularis dissemenata (elastomas, collagenomas or fibromas), especially on the torso and extremities.
- Extracutaneous manifestations:
  - Osteopoikilosis (spotted bones due to increased bone density in some areas).
  - Nasolacrimal duct obstruction.
  - Amblyopia.
  - Hearing impairment.
  - Diabetes mellitus.
  - Short stature.
- Prognosis: mortality is usually due to development of osteosarcoma, chondrosarcoma or giant cell tumors in sites of increased bone density.

Lipoid Proteinosis (Hyalinosis Cutis et Mucosae) (AR) [11–13] (Figs. 9.8, 9.9, 9.10, 9.11, 9.12, and 9.13)

- Mutations in extracellular matrix protein 1 (*ECM1*) gene.
- Clinical manifestations:
  - Laryngeal affection (infiltration of laryngeal mucosa):
    Weak cry (the first clinical sign of the disease).
    Hoarseness of voice that may progress to complete aphonia.
  - Cutaneous lesions (appear during the first 2 years of life):
    First stage: vesicles and hemorrhagic crusts on the face and extremities which resolve with ice-pick like scars.

Second stage: papules, plaques, and nodules on the face, neck, axillae, and scrotum with beaded appearance of eye lid margin.

- Verrucous lesions on elbows, knees, and hands.
- Generalized scaling and alopecia of the eyebrows and eyelashes.

– Oral lesions:

Macroglossia.

Restricted tongue motion/cobble-stone appearance of tongue and buccal mucosa.

Dental abnormalities as conical teeth.

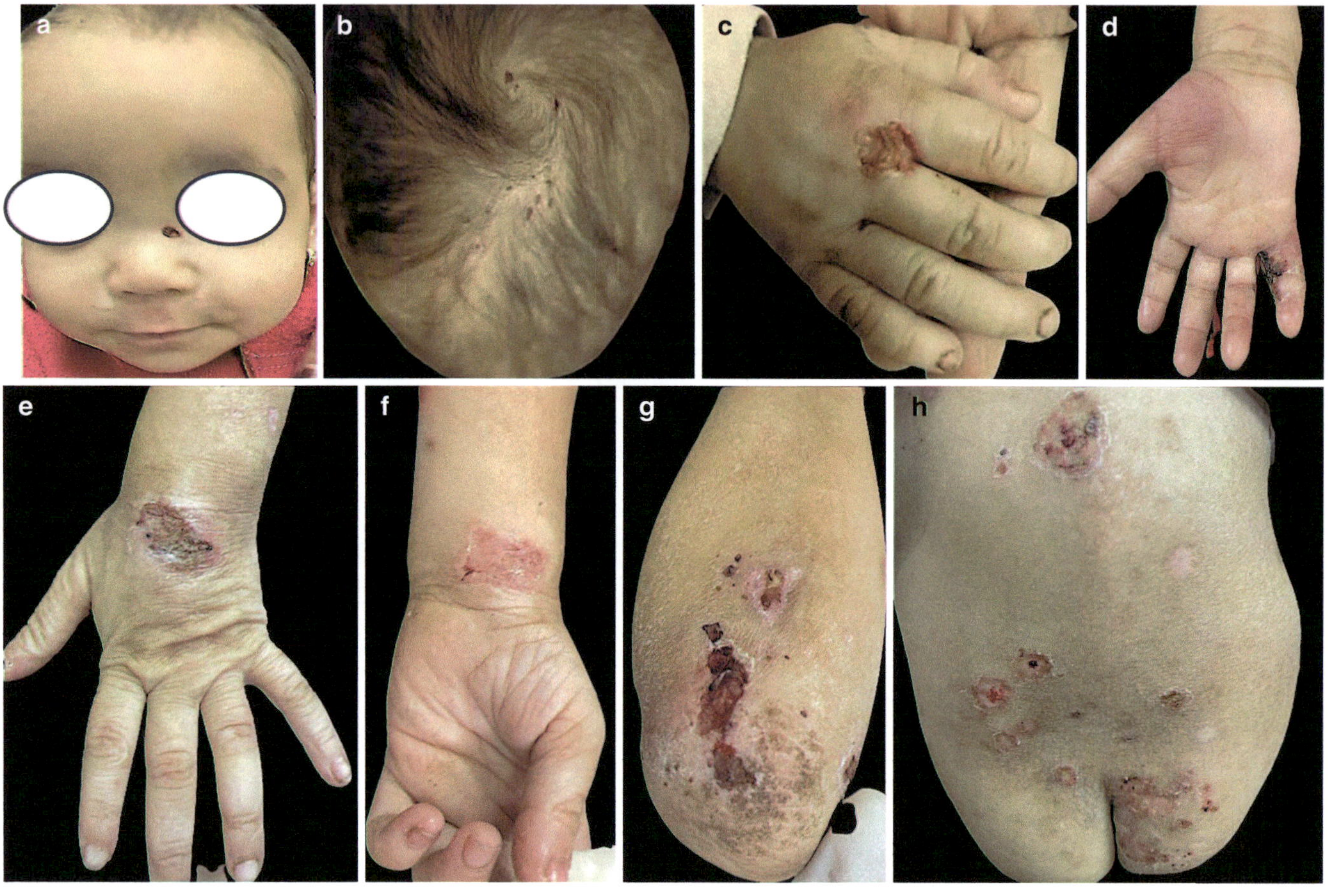

Fig. 9.8 Lipoid Proteinosis. Early crusted vesiculobullous lesions on the face (**a**), scalp (**b**), hands (**c–e**), on the wrist (**f**), elbow (**g**), and the back (**h**)

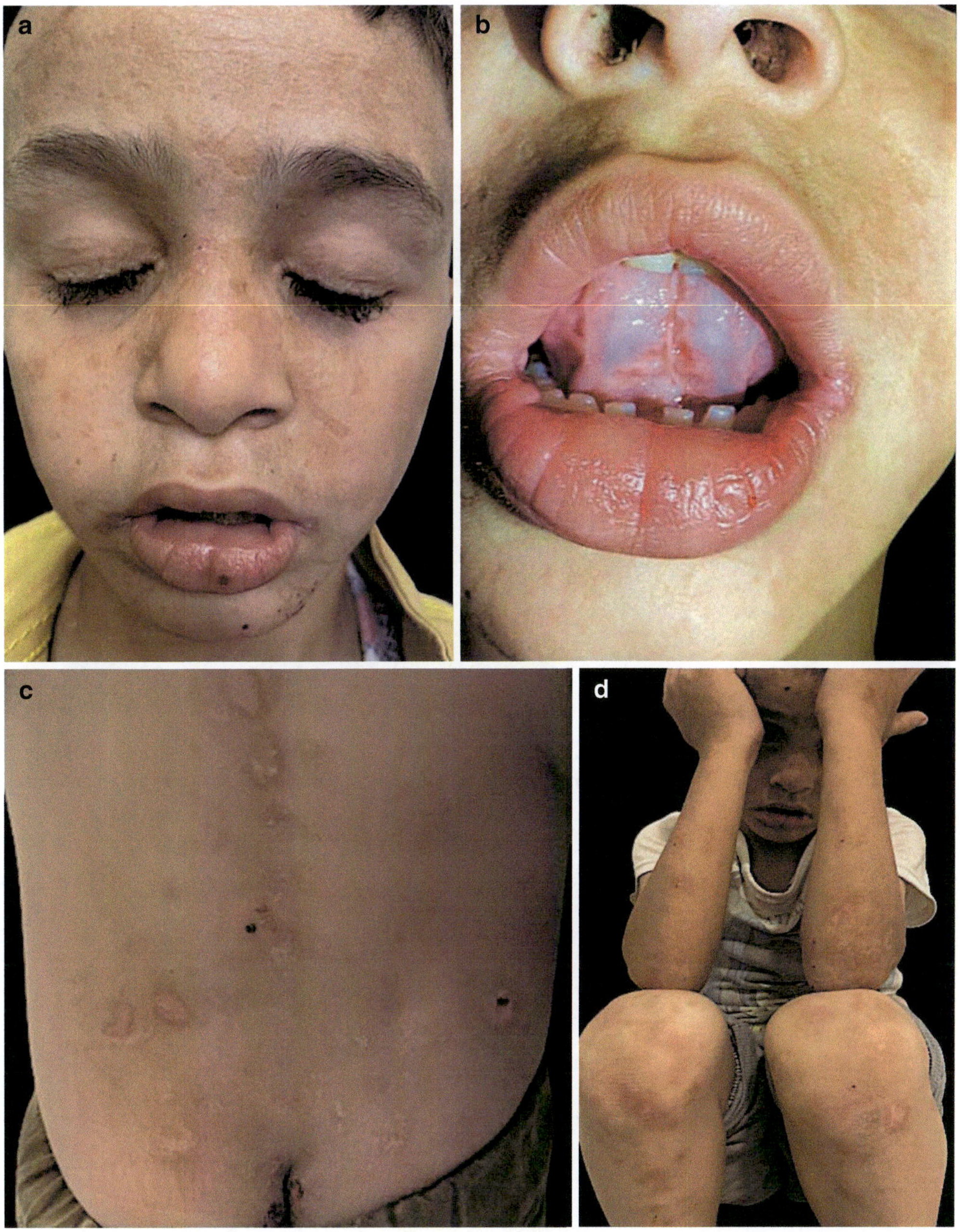

Fig. 9.9 Lipoid Proteinosis. Bilateral small beaded papules on upper eyelid margin with multiple atrophic facial scars (**a**), thickened enlarged lips with conical teeth (**b**), and scars of previous vesiculobullous lesions on the back, elbows, and knees (**c**, **d**)

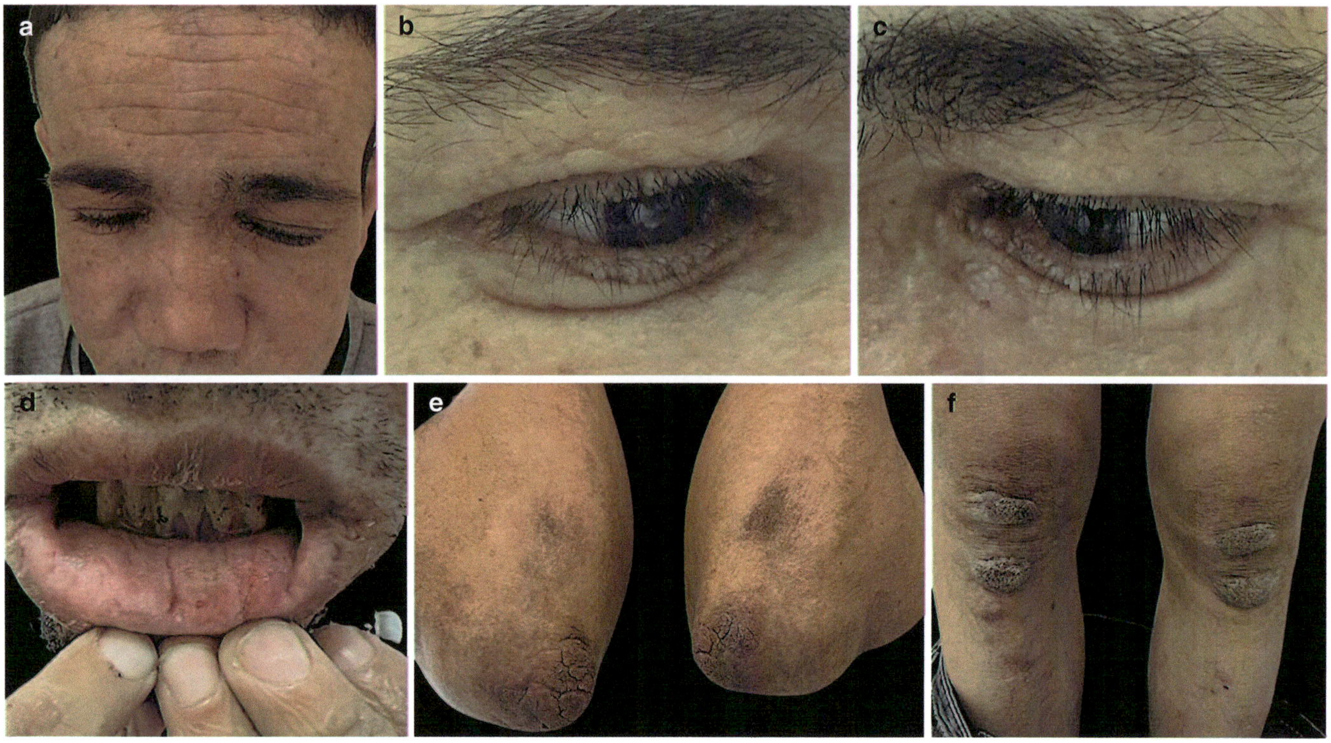

Fig. 9.10 Lipoid Proteinosis. A 15-years-old patient with premature photoaging of the face (**a**), bilateral small beaded papules on eyelid margin (**b**, **c**), cobble-stone appearance of buccal mucosa (**d**), and thickened verrucous lesions on elbows and knees (**e**, **f**)

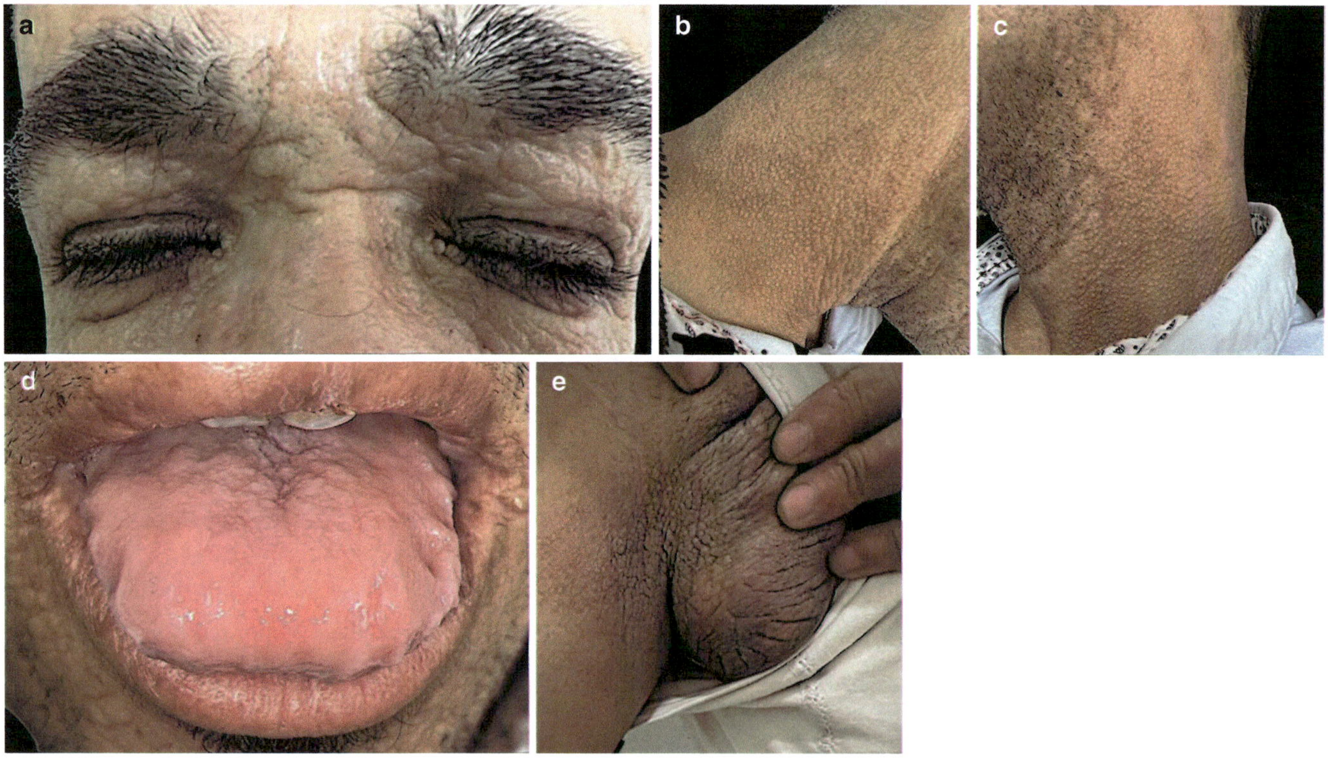

Fig. 9.11 Lipoid Proteinosis. The same patient of Fig. 9.10 when he became 27 years old. Bilateral small beaded papules on eyelid margin (**a**), multiple yellowish papules on the neck (**b**, **c**), thickened, pale, and enlarged crenated tongue (**d**), and thickened scrotal skin (**e**)

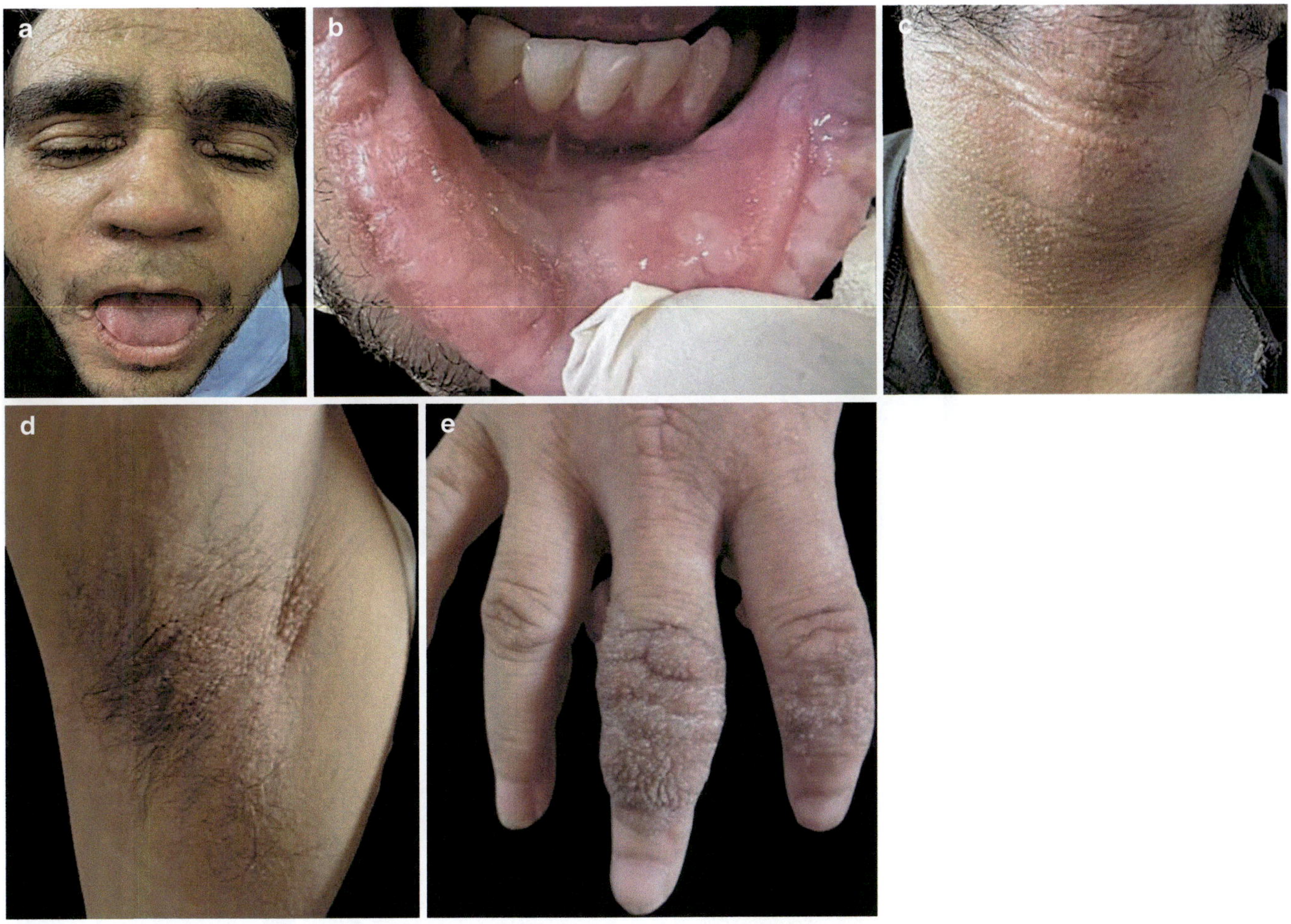

Fig. 9.12 Lipoid Proteinosis. Bilateral yellowish papules and nodules on eyelid margin and lips (**a**), cobble-stone appearance of buccal mucosa (**b**), multiple yellowish papules on the neck and axilla (**c**, **d**), and thickened verrucous lesions on the hand (**e**)

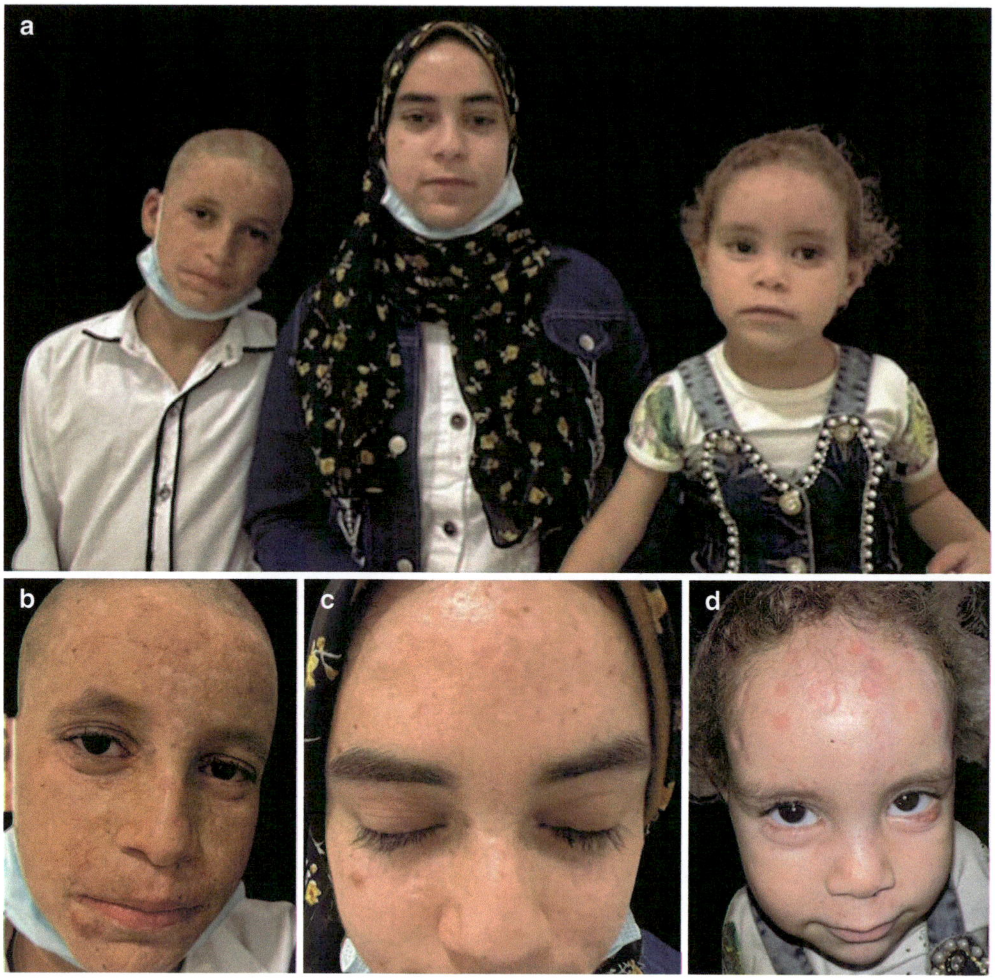

Fig. 9.13 Lipoid Proteinosis in three siblings (**a**–**d**)

Recurrent parotitis.

- Neurological:

  Bilateral, intracranial sickle shaped calcification within the temporal lobes (pathognomonic).

  Seizures and abnormal behavior.

- Histopathology:
  - H&E stain: hyaline like thickening of the capillaries within the papillary dermis in early lesions.

    Hyperkeratosis, papillomatosis, thickened dermis with pink hyaline deposits in bundles perpendicular to the dermo-epidermal junction.
  - PAS positive and diastase resistant.

Focal Dermal Hypoplasia (Goltz syndrome) [14, 15] (Figs. 9.14, 9.15, 9.16, 9.17, 9.18, 9.19, and 9.20)

- X-linked dominant and lethal in utero for males (abnormality in PORCN gene on the X chromosome).
- Incidence: ranges from 1:50,000 to 1:150,000.
- Cutaneous manifestations:
  - Linear areas of cutaneous atrophy following Blaschko lines.
  - Linear or reticulate of hypo or hyperpigmentation with telangectasia simulating poikiloderma.
  - Fat herniation.
  - Soft yellowish papules and nodules.
  - Raspberry like papillomas on the lips, gums, anus, and genitalia.
  - Aplasia cutis congenita.
  - Nail abnormalities.

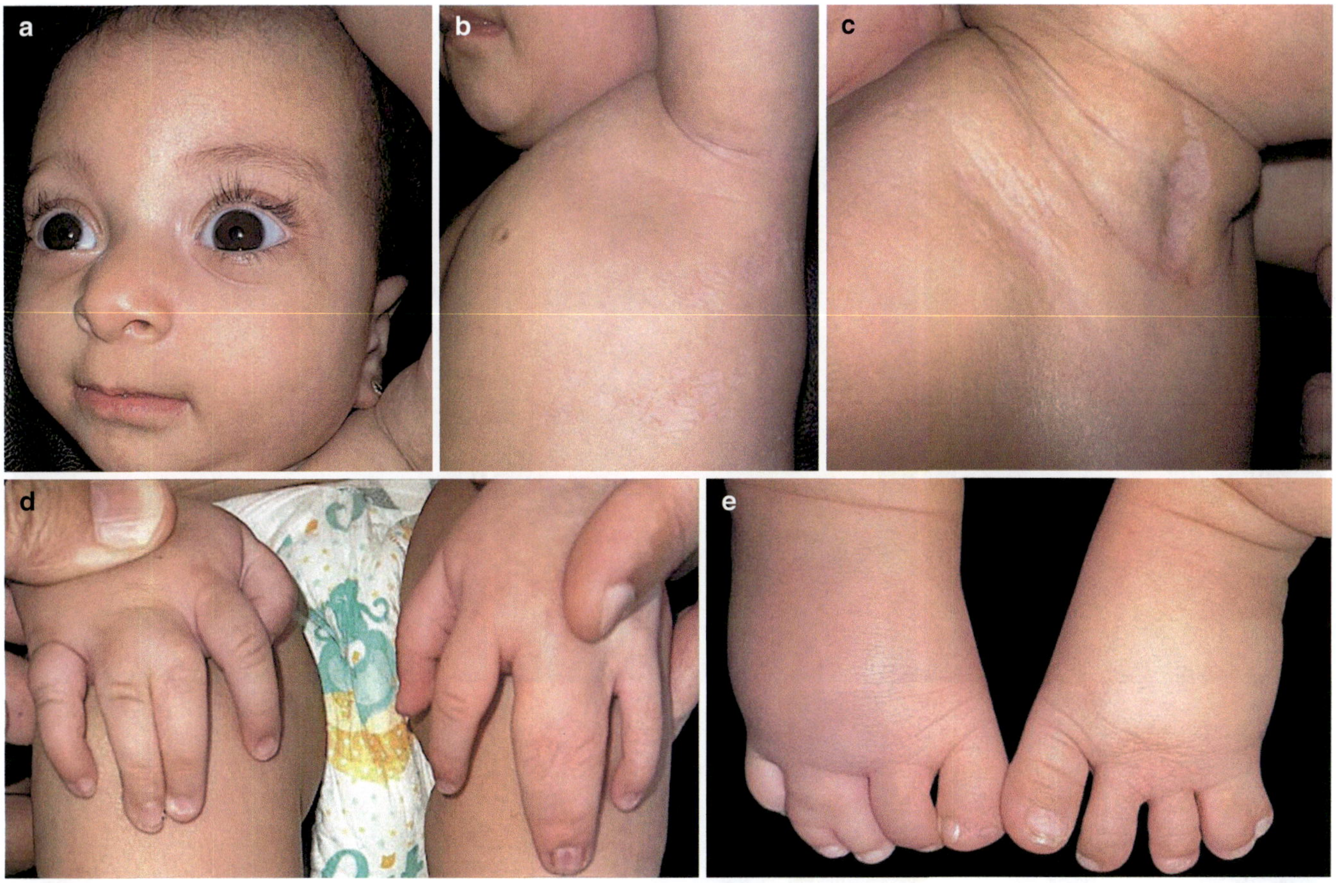

Fig. 9.14 Goltz syndrome. Low set ear (**a**) dermal hypoplasia in the chest and neck (**b**, **c**) and syndactyly of fingers and toes (**d**, **e**)

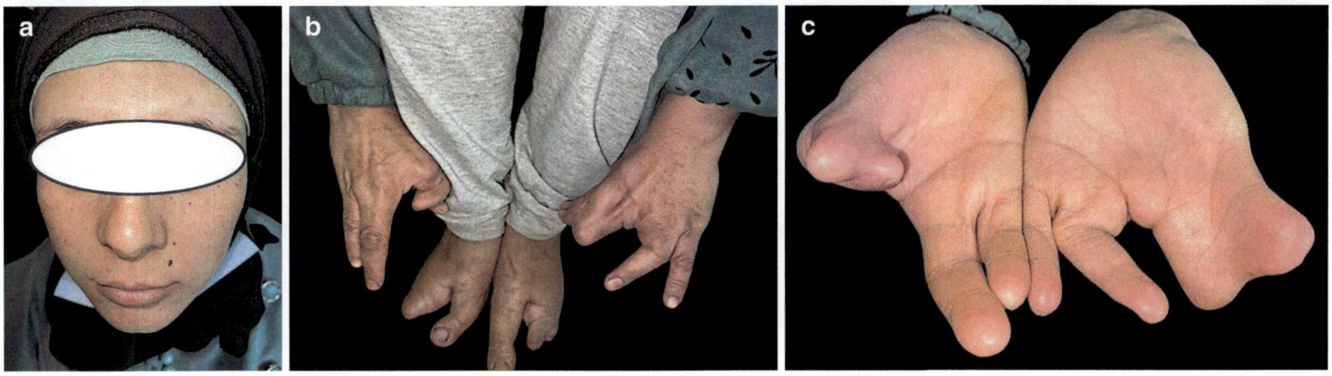

Fig. 9.15 Goltz syndrome. Mother of the infant in Fig. 9.14 showing syndactyly of fingers and toes (**a**–**c**)

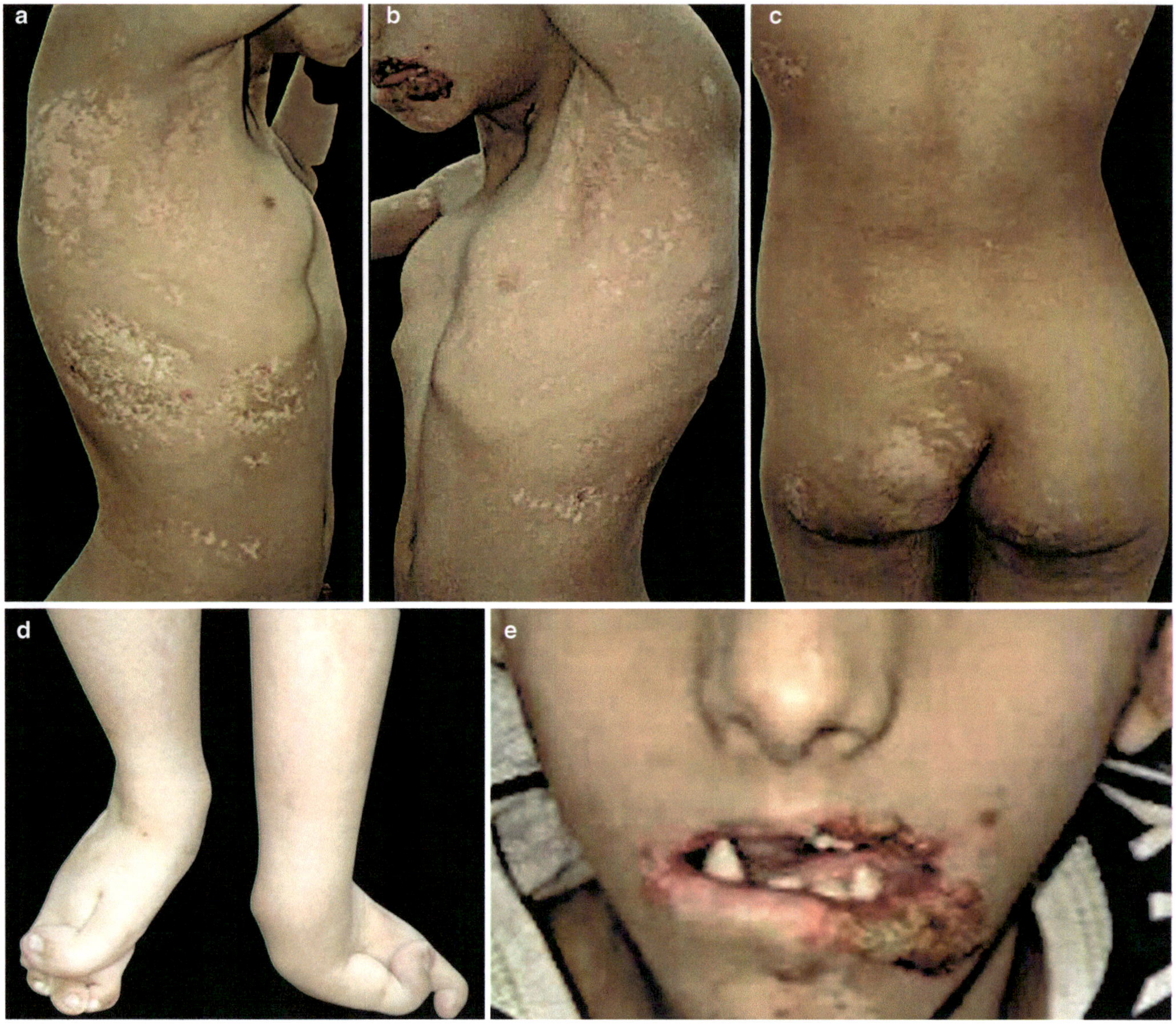

Fig. 9.16 Goltz syndrome. Dermal hypoplasia with poikiloderma like appearance on the chest, abdomen, and buttocks (**a**–**c**), syndactyly of toes (**d**), and Raspberry-like papillomas on the lips (**e**)

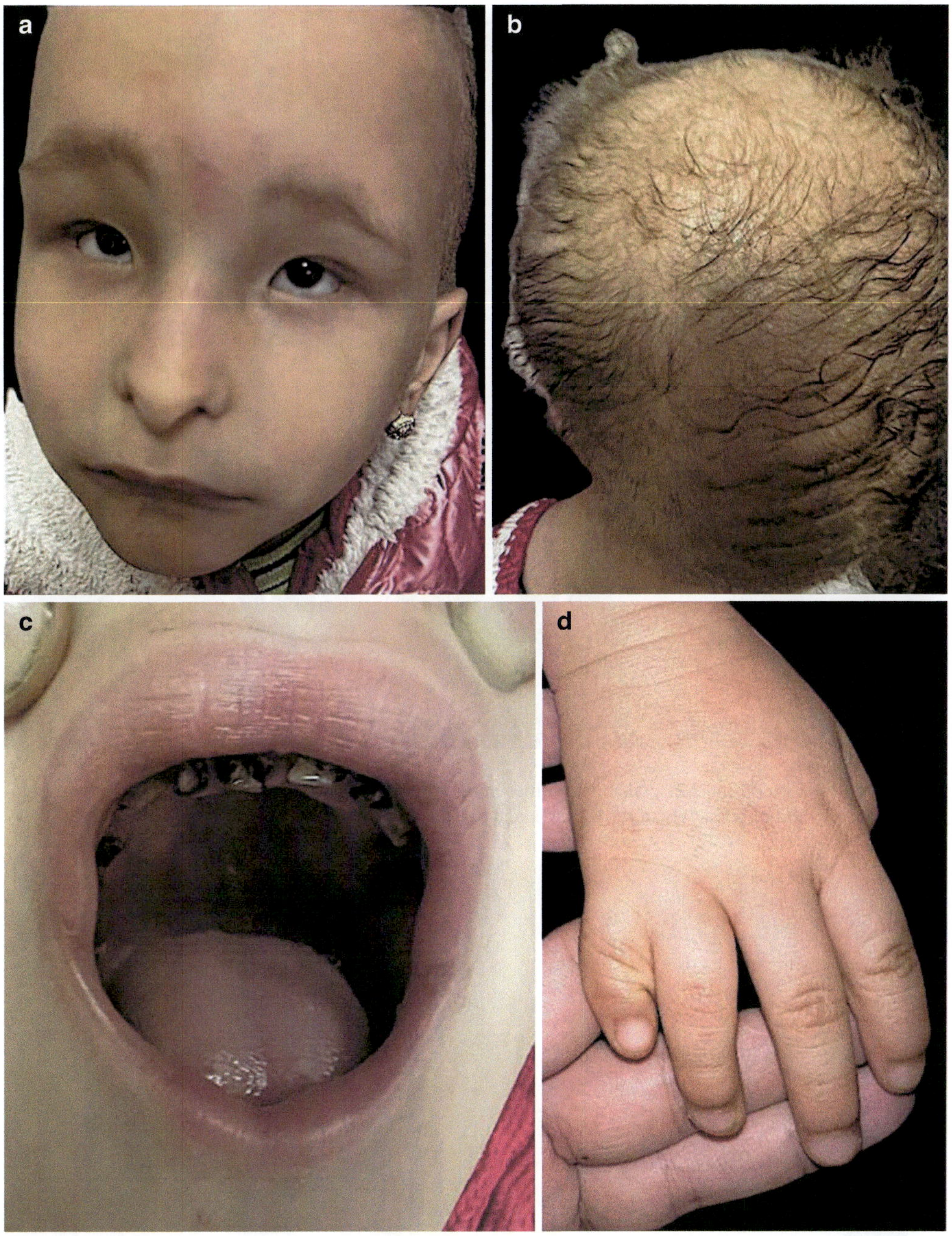

Fig. 9.17 Goltz syndrome. Microphthamia (**a**), alopecia with brittle sparse hair (**b**), small hypoplastic teeth (**c**), and syndactyly of fingers (**d**)

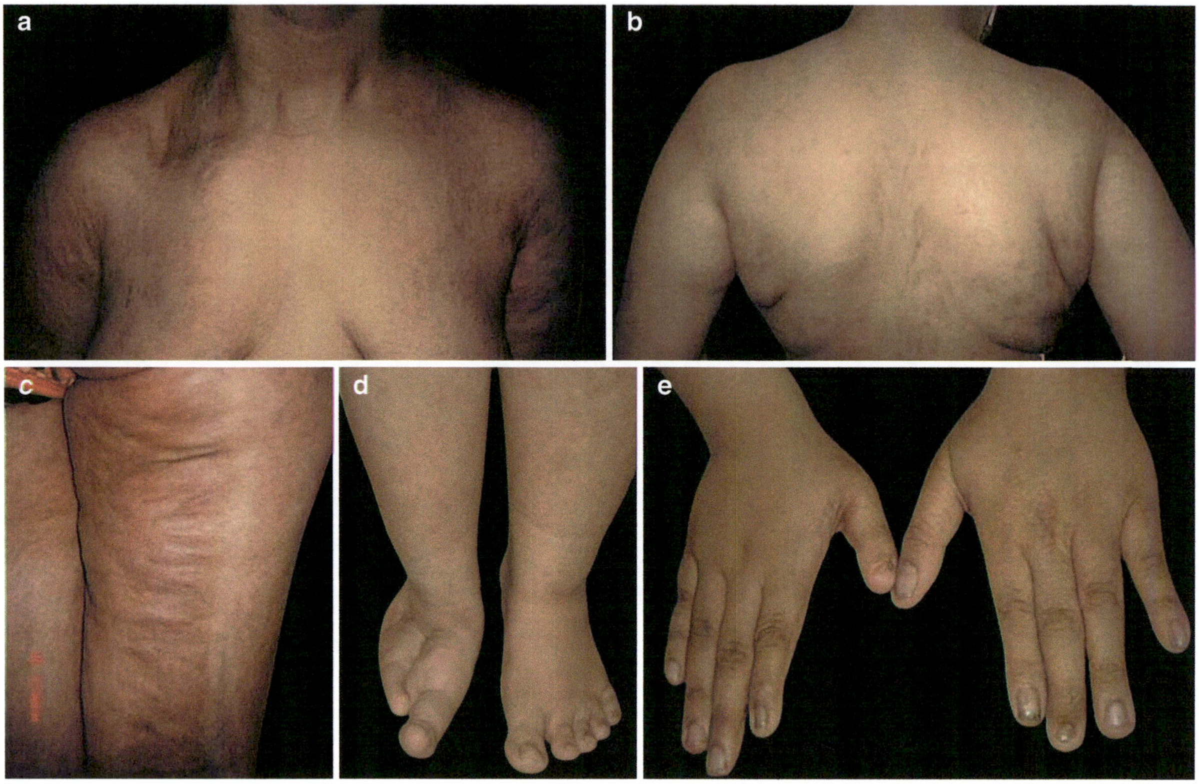

Fig. 9.18 Goltz syndrome. Skeletal abnormalities of the ribs and scapula (**a**, **b**), linear areas of fat herniation following Blaschko lines in the thigh (**c**), syndactyly and oligodactyly of the toes (**d**), and nails dystrophy (**e**)

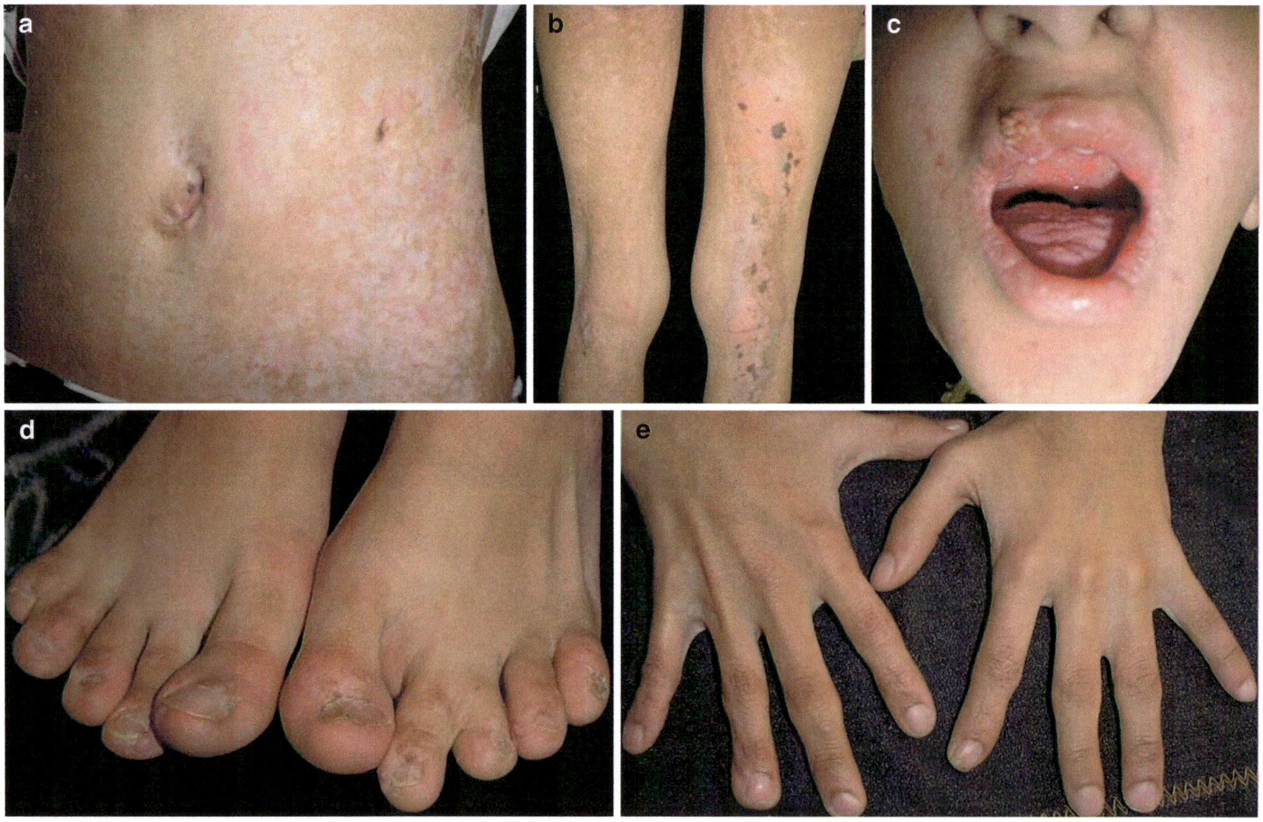

Fig. 9.19 Goltz syndrome. Dermal hypoplasia on the trunk, shoulder, and lower limbs (**a**–**c**), raspberry-like papillomas on the lips (**c**), nails dystrophy, syndactyly of the toes and fingers (**d**, **e**)

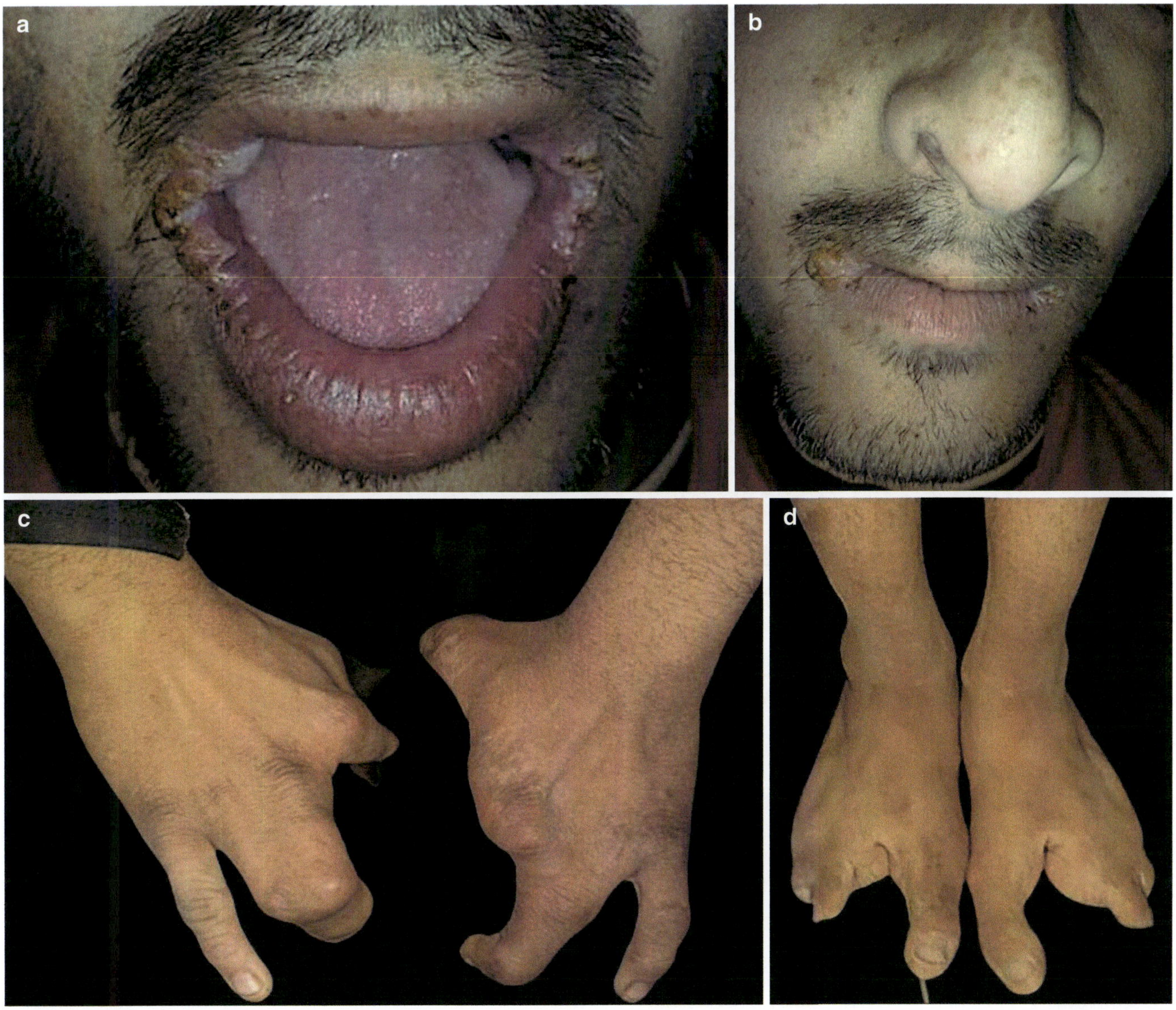

Fig. 9.20 Goltz syndrome (X-linked dominant) in a male. Raspberry-like papillomas on the angles of the lips (**a**, **b**), syndactyly and oligodactyly of the fingers and toes (**c**, **d**)

  - Focal alopecia.
- Skeletal manifestations:
  - Fusion or absence of fingers and toes.
  - Lobster claw hand.
  - Asymmetric development of face, trunk, extremities, and scoliosis sometimes.
  - Parallel, vertical striations in the metaphysis of long bone (Osteopathia striata).
- Ocular manifestations:
  - Coloboma of the eye.
  - Microphthalmia.
  - Ocular agenesis.
- Other manifestations:
  - Agenesis of the teeth.
  - Asymmetry of ears.
  - Abnormality of the kidney and ureter.
- Treatment: vascular lasers for papillomas and telangectasias/surgical excision of papillomas/multidisciplinary approach for internal organs affection.

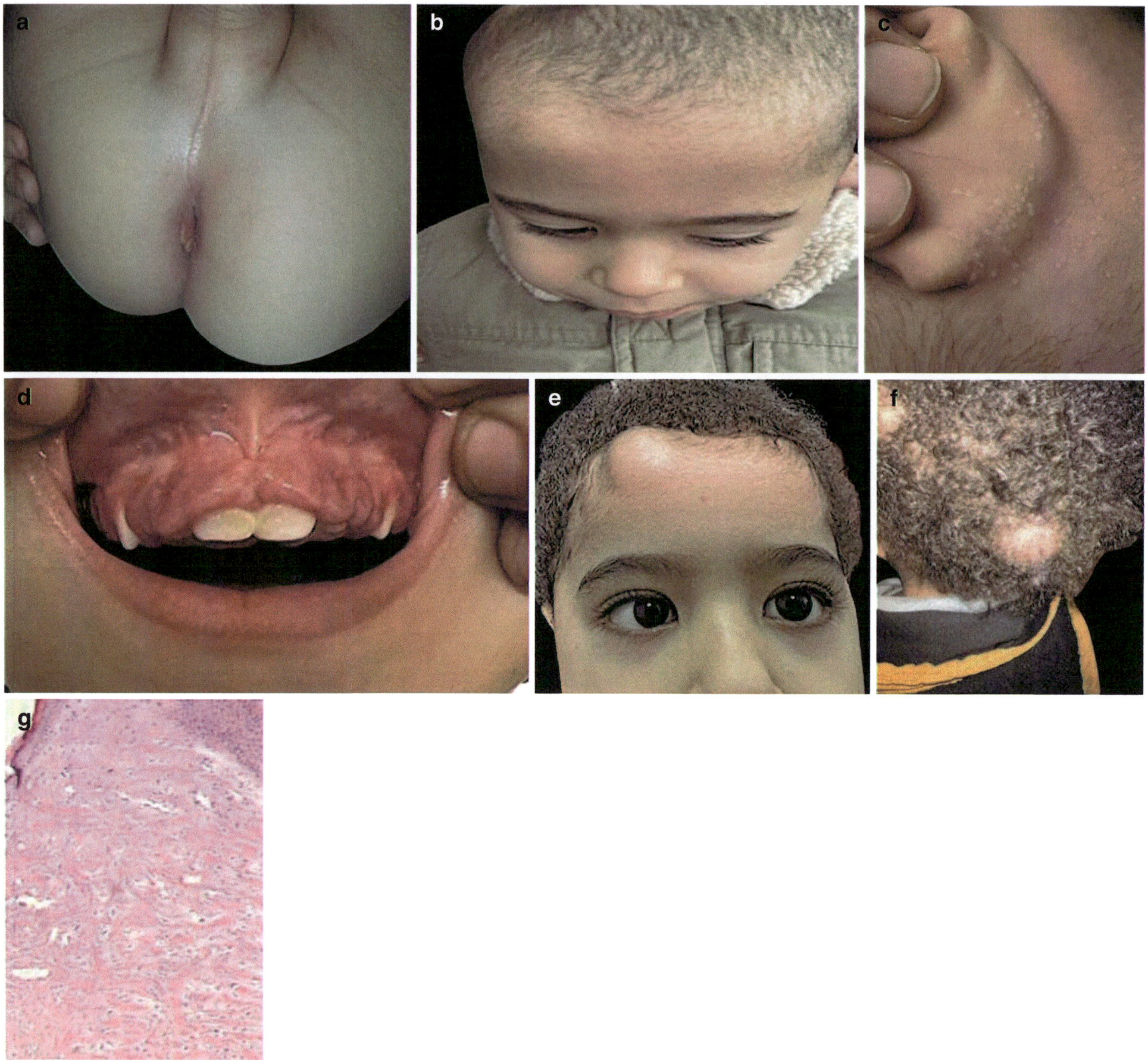

Fig. 9.21 Juvenile hyaline fibromatosis (JHF). A boy first presented with papillomatous perianal lesions at age of 4 months (**a**). At age of 2 years, he developed multiple, painless, variable-sized nodules over forehead and pearly white papules on ear lobules (**b**, **c**) with gingival hyperplasia (**d**). One year later, he developed other painless nodular masses on the face and the scalp (**e**, **f**). Surgical excision of scalp lesions were done, and histopathological examination confirms the diagnosis of JHF (**g**). No systemic or skeletal affection was detected

Juvenile Hyaline Fibromatosis (JHF) (AR) [16, 17] (Fig. 9.21)

- An extremely rare autosomal-recessive hereditary disease.
- Mutation in capillary morphogenesis protein 2 (*CMG2*) also known as anthrax toxin receptor 2″ (ANTXR2).
- JHF is a relatively mild presentation of the hyaline fibromatosis syndrome (HFS) family of diseases, with Infantile hyaline fibromatosis (IHF) being the more lethal form. Currently, literature is considering the presence of a spectrum of presentations rather than two distinct diseases: IHF and JHF.
- The clinical onset is usually noted from birth up to 5 years of age.
- Manifestations can be debilitating, and patients typically present with gingival hypertrophy, nodular skin lesions, papulonodular skin lesions, and osteolytic bone disease.

References

1. Morava E, Lefeber DJ, Urban Z, et al. Defining the phenotype in an autosomal recessive cutis laxa syndrome with a combined congenital defect of glycosylation. Eur J Hum Genet. 2008;16:28–35.
2. Berk DR, Bentley DD, Bayliss SJ, et al. Cutis laxa: a review. J Am Acad Dermatol. 2012;66(5):842.e1–17.
3. Malfait F, Francomano C, Byers P, et al. The 2017 international classification of the Ehlers–Danlos syndromes. Am J Med Genet C Semin Med Genet. 2017;175(1):8–26.
4. Atzinger CL, Meyer RA, Khoury PR, Gao Z, Tinkl, et al. Cross-sectional and longitudinal assessment of aortic root dilation and valvular anomalies in hypermobile and classic Ehlers-Danlos syndrome. J Pediatr. 2011;158:826–30.
5. Marconi B, Bobyr I, Campanati A, et al. Pseudoxanthoma elasticum and skin: clinical manifestations, histopathology, pathomechanism, perspectives of treatment. Intractable Rare Dis Res. 2019;4(3):113–22.
6. Vanakker OM, Martin L, Gheduzzi D, et al. Pseudoxanthoma elasticum-like phenotype with cutis laxa and multiple coagulation factor deficiency represents a separate genetic entity. J Invest Dermatol. 2007;127(3):581–7.
7. Dean JC. Marfan syndrome: clinical diagnosis and management. Eur J Med Genet. 2007;15:724–33.
8. Rangasetty UC, Karnath BM. Clinical signs of Marfan syndrome. Hosp Physician. 2006;42(4):33–8.
9. Ehrig T, Cockerell CJ. Buschke-Ollendorff syndrome: report of a case and interpretation of the clinical phenotype as a type 2 segmental manifestation of an autosomal dominant skin disease. J Am Acad Dermatol. 2003;49(6):1163–6.
10. Pope V, Dupuis L, Kannu P, Mendoza-Londono R, et al. Buschke-Ollendorff syndrome: a novel case series and systematic review. Br J Dermatol. 2016;174(4):723.
11. Chan I, Liu L, Hamada T, et al. The molecular basis of lipoid proteinosis: mutations in extracellular matrix protein 1. Exp Dermatol. 2007;16:881–90.
12. Lee MY, Wang HJ, Han Y, et al. Lipoid proteinosis resulting from a large homozygous deletion affecting part of the ECM1 gene and adjacent long non-coding RNA. Acta Derm Venereol. 2015;95:608–10.
13. Di Giandomenico S, Masi R, Cassandrini D, et al. Lipoid proteinosis: case report and review of the literature. Acta Otorhinolaryngol Ital. 2006;26:162–7.
14. Goltz RW, Henderson RR, Hitch JM, et al. Focal dermal hypoplasia syndrome. A review of the literature and report of two cases. Arch Dermatol. 1970;101(1):1–11.
15. Bree AF, Grange DK, Hicks MJ, et al. Dermatologic findings of focal dermal hypoplasia (Goltz syndrome). Am J Med Genet C Semin Med Genet. 2016;172C:44–51.
16. Braizat O, Badran S, Hammouda A. Juvenile hyaline fibromatosis: literature review and a case treated with surgical excision and corticosteroid. Cureus. 2020;12(10):e10823.
17. Xia L, Hu Y, Zhang C, et al. Juvenile hyaline fibromatosis: a rare oral disease case report and literature review. Transl Pediatr. 2021;10(11):3124–9.

10 Ectodermal Dysplasia

- **Hypohidrotic or anhidrotic ectodermal dysplasia (Christ-Siemens-Touraine syndrome)**
- **Hidrotic ectodermal dysplasia (Clouston syndrome)**
- **Ankyloblepharon-ectodermal dysplasia-clefting syndrome (Hay-Wells syndrome)**
- **Rapp-Hodgkin syndrome**
- **Witkop's syndrome (tooth-and-nail syndrome)**
- **Oculo-mandibulo-facial syndrome (Hallermann-Streiff syndrome)**
- **Monilethrix**
- **Atrichia with papular lesions**
- **Uncombable hair syndrome**
- **Björnstad syndrome**

Hypohidrotic or Anhidrotic Ectodermal Dysplasia [1, 2] (Christ-Siemens-Touraine Syndrome) (XLR) (Figs. 10.1, 10.2, 10.3, 10.4, and 10.5)

- Hypohidrotic or anhidrotic ED is the most common type.
- Inheritance: X-linked recessive (XLR), with mutations in Ectodysplasin gene (*EDA*) that is more observed in males than females.
- Clinical characteristics:
  - Hypohidrosis, intolerance to heat and repeated episodes of unexplained fever before second year of life.
  - Skin:
    Smooth, soft, dry and thin (due to partial or complete absence of sweat and sebaceous glands).
    Increased susceptibility to eczema.
    Palmoplantar hyperkeratosis.
    Fine linear wrinkles, with perioral and periorbital hyperpigmentation.
  - Hair: thin sparse hairs or alopecia [mainly in scalp and sometimes in other areas (e.g., eyebrows, eyelashes, and axillary and pubic areas)].
  - Teeth:
    Dental hypodontia to anodontia of primary or permanent teeth, especially in mandible.
    Conical crown forms of the present teeth (pegged teeth) in anterior region of maxilla and mandible.
  - Nails: normal or somewhat spoon shaped.
  - Facies and craniofacial development:
    Variations in shape of skull with prominent chin and frontal bossing (inverted triangle).
    Prominent supraorbital ridge, depression of nasal bridge (saddle nose) and wide nostrils.
    Protuberant everted lips.
    Maxillary retrusion due to sagittal underdeveloped maxilla, with forward and upward displacement of mandible.
    Large ears.
    High-arched palate and cleft palate.
  - In females: aplastic or hypoplastic mammary glands.
  - Eyes: impaired lacrimal gland function and occasionally, glaucoma.
  - Asthma and frequent respiratory infections.
- Laboratory investigations:
  - Quantitative hypogammaglobulinemia with impaired T-lymphocyte subset populations.
  - Decreased sweating by starch iodine test.
  - Pilocarpine iontophoresis and skin biopsy for detection of hypohidrosis and reduced number of eccrine glands.
  - Prenatal diagnosis using genetic mutation analysis may be performed in case of family history of ED.
- Possible Complications: febrile seizures and brain damage.

N. Moftah et al., *Atlas of Common and Rare Genodermatoses*, https://doi.org/10.1007/978-3-031-60788-2_10

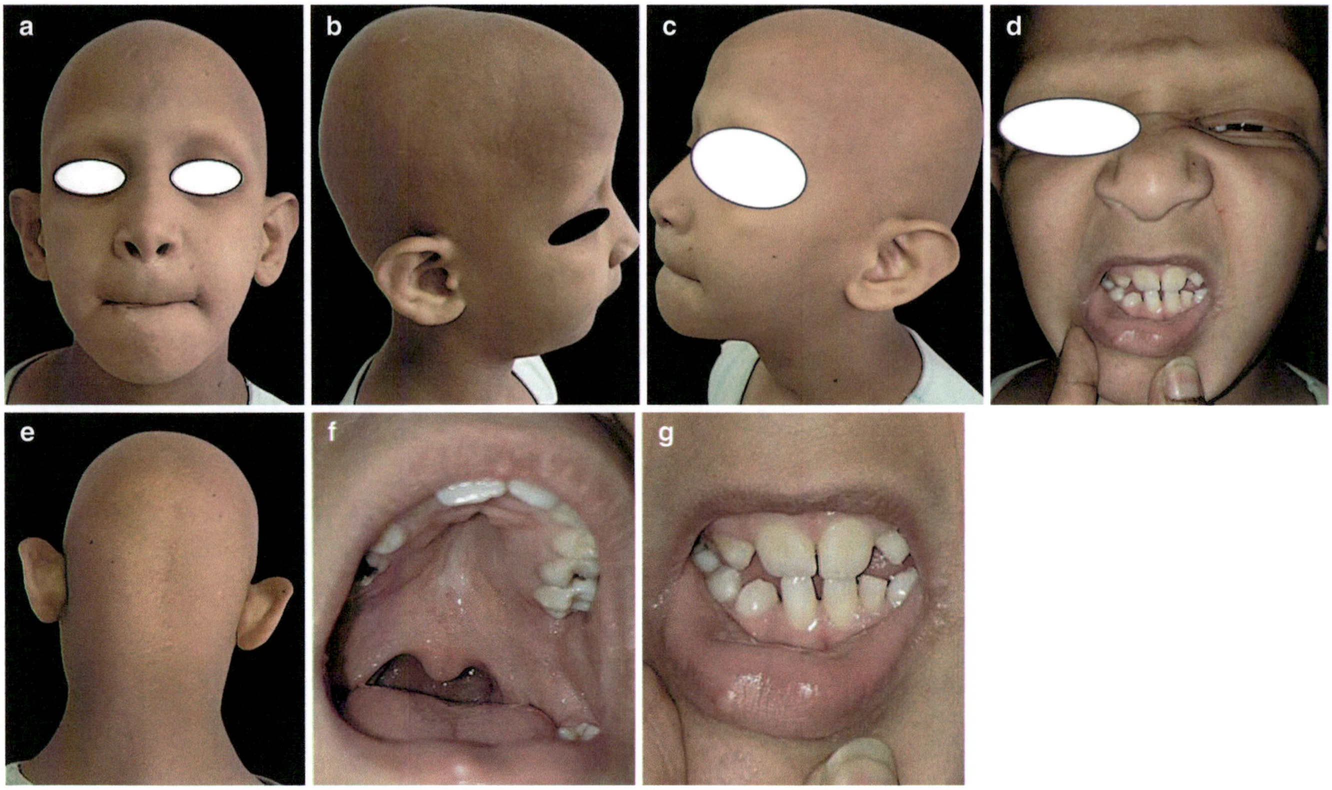

Fig. 10.1 Anhidrotic or hypohydrotic ectodermal dysplasia. Female patient with frontal bossing (**a–c**), saddle nose (**a–d**), large ear (**a–c**, **e**), sunken cheeks (**a–d**), alopecia, loss of eye lashes and eyebrows (**a–e**), periorbital hyperpigmentation (**a–d**), and dental hypoplasia with conical pegged teeth (**f**, **g**)

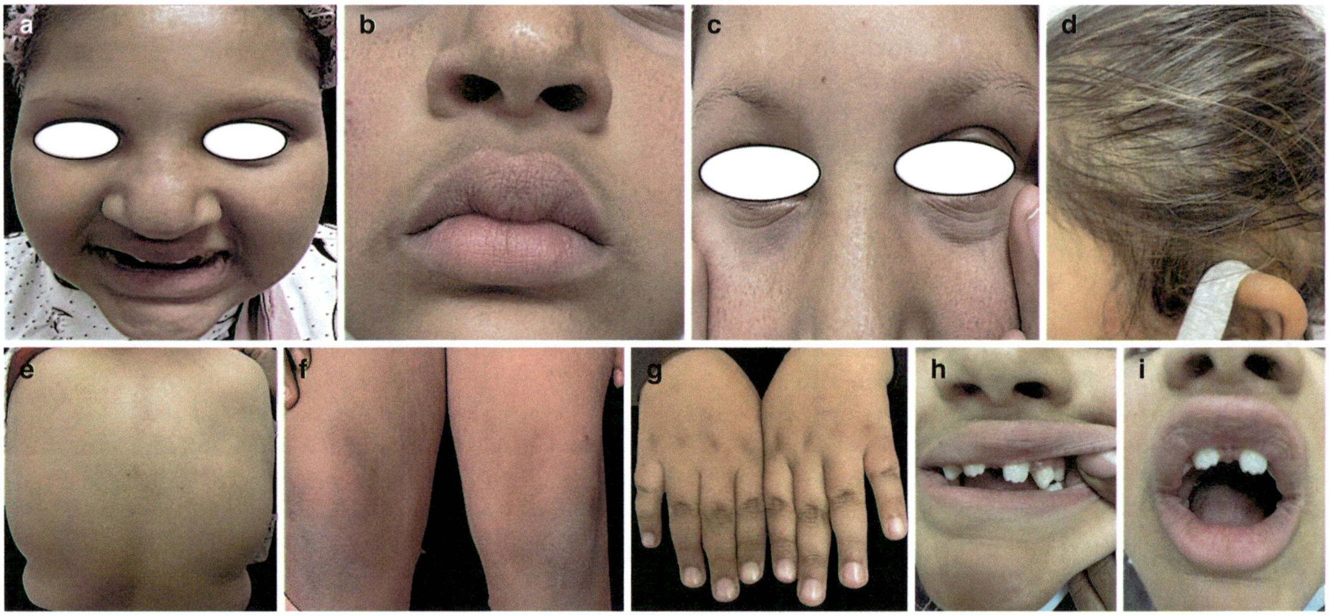

Fig. 10.2 Anhidrotic or hypohydrotic ectodermal dysplasia. Female patient with frontal bossing, elongated thin chin (**a**), wide nostril (**a**, **b**), thick everted lip (**a**, **b**), saddle nose (**a**), perioral and periorbital hyperpigmentation (**b**, **c**), wrinkling (**c**), sparse hairs in scalp, eye brows and eye lashes (**c**, **d**), hypohidrotic and dry skin (atopic like) (**e**, **f**) and normal nail (**g**). Conical (pegged) teeth and hypodontia on lower jaw (**h**, **i**)

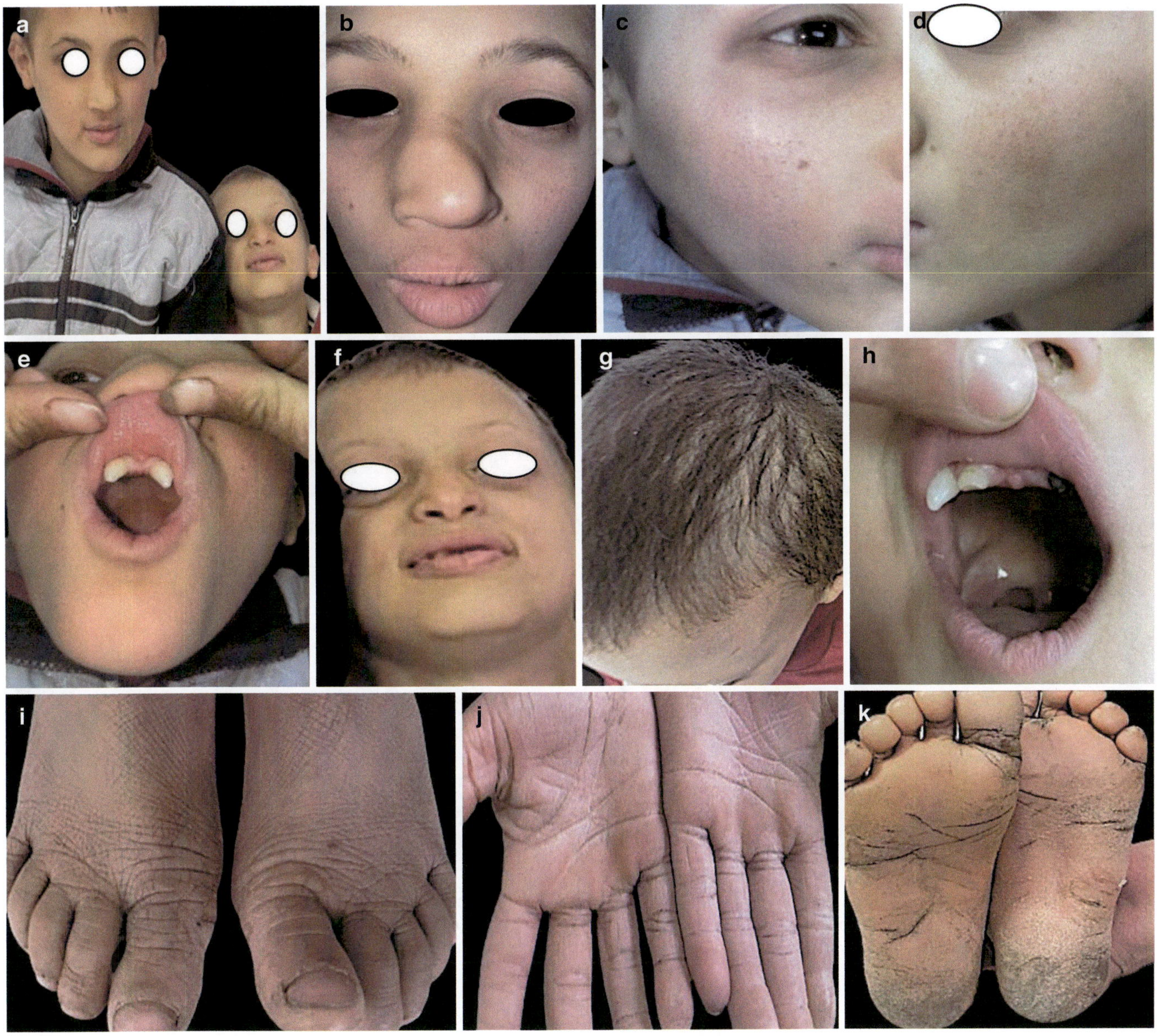

Fig. 10.3 Anhidrotic or hypohydrotic ectodermal dysplasia in two brothers (**a**). The elder boy showing saddle nose with nasal deformity, thick everted lips, thin small chin (**a**, **b**), dry skin (**c**, **d**), periorbital hyperpigmentation (**b**–**d**), hypodontia and conical pegged teeth (**e**). The younger one showing thick everted lip (**f**), sparse hair (**g**), hypodontia (**h**), dry skin (**i**), and palmoplantar hyperkeratosis (**j**, **k**). He is mentally retarded

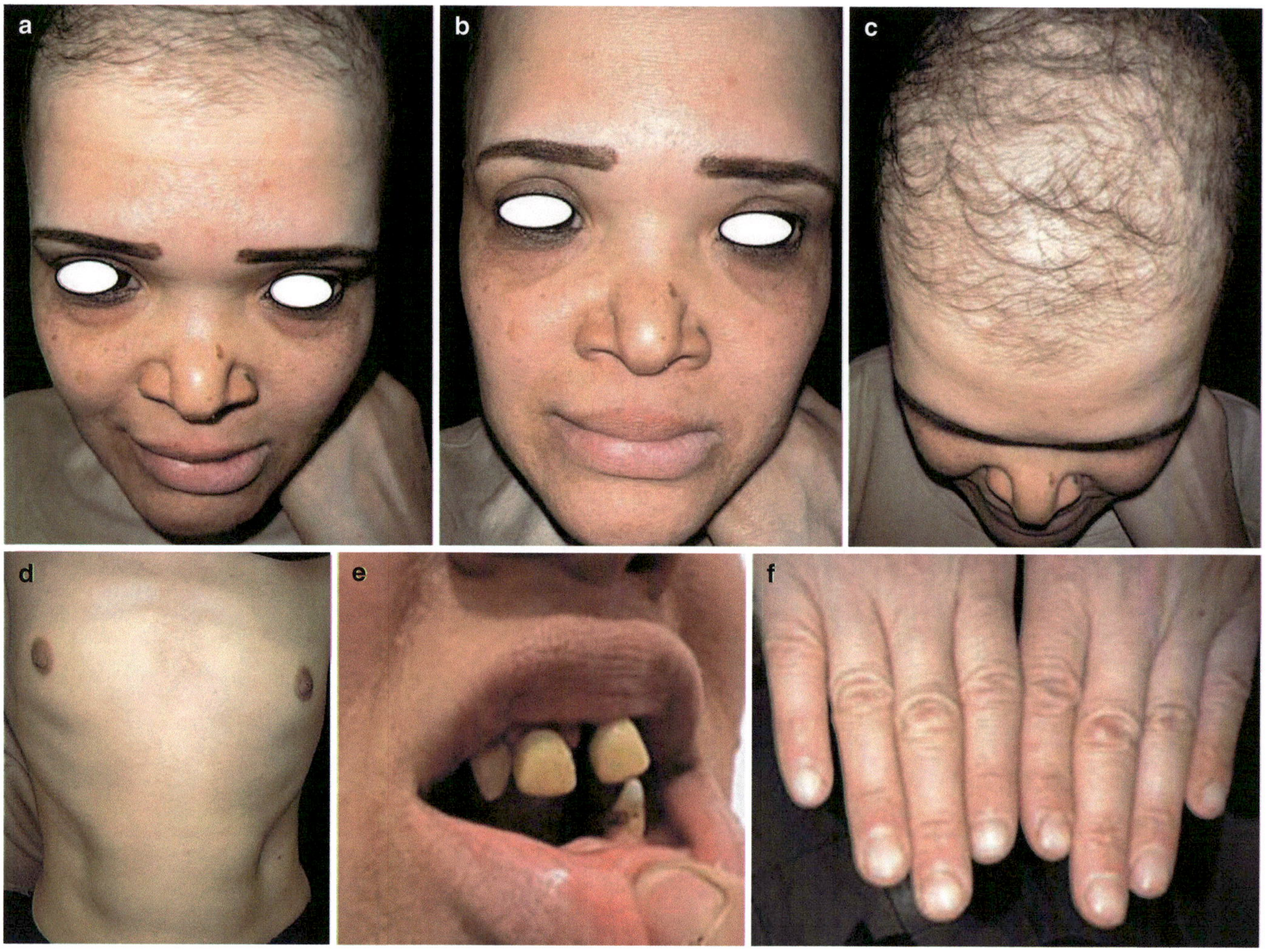

Fig. 10.4 Anhidrotic or hypohidrotic ectodermal dysplasia. Female patient 25 years old showing frontal bossing, saddle nose deformity, periorbital hyperpigmentation, thick everted lips (**a**, **b**), sparse hair in scalp, eyelashes, and eyebrows (**a–c**), small breast (hypoplasia of mammary gland) (**d**), hypodontia, conical pegged teeth, gingival atrophy (**e**), and normal nails (**f**)

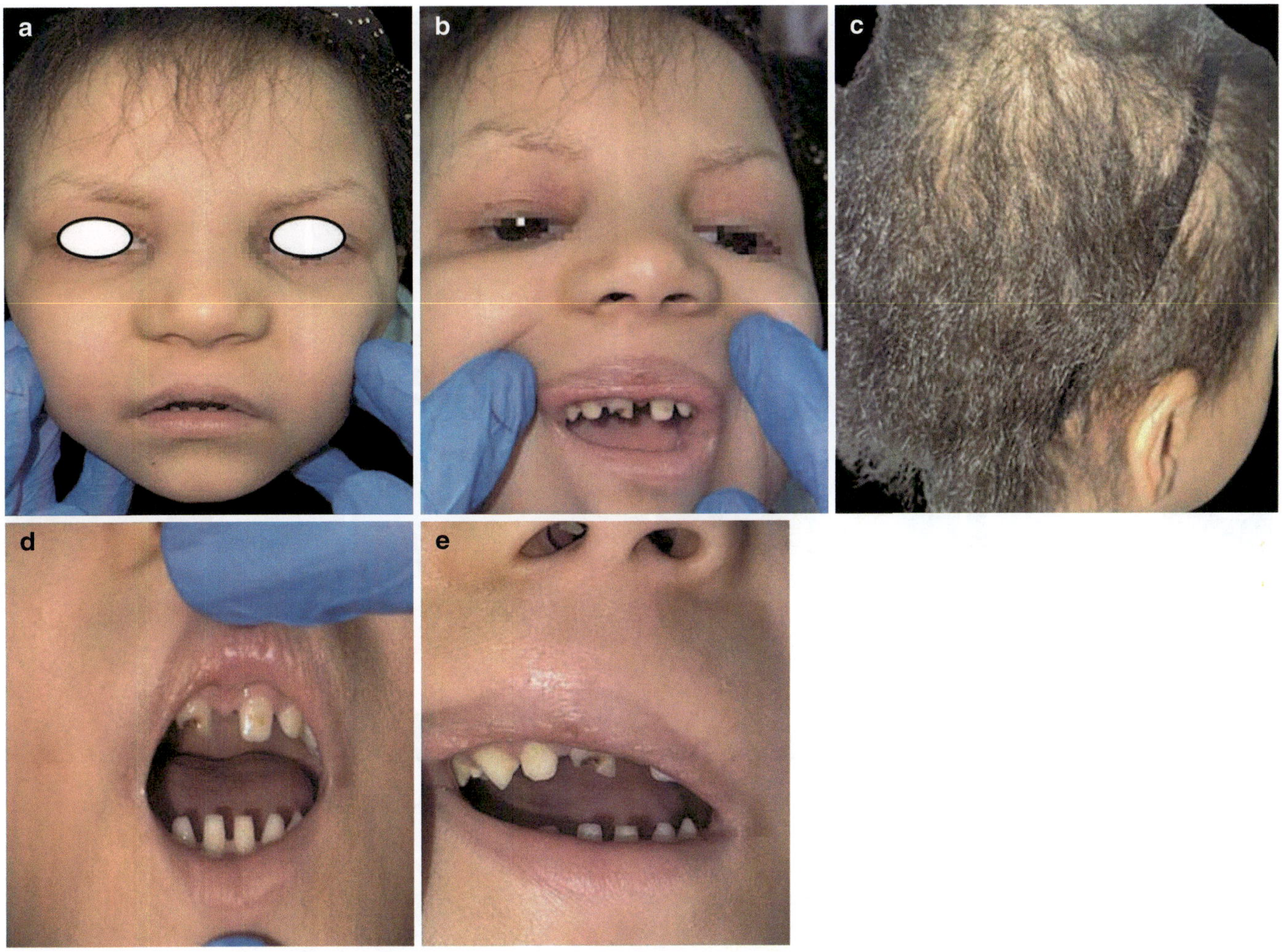

Fig. 10.5 Anhidrotic or hypohydrotic ectodermal dysplasia. Frontal bossing, flat nasal bridge, periorbital hyperpigmentation and wrinkling, sparse hair in scalp, eyelashes, and eyebrows (**a**–**c**), hypodontia and conical pegged teeth (**d**, **e**)

Hidrotic Ectodermal Dysplasia [3, 4] (Clouston Syndrome) (AD) (Figs. 10.6, 10.7, and 10.8)

- Hidrotic ED (Clouston syndrome) is characterized by clinical triad of nail dystrophy, alopecia, and palmoplantar hyperkeratosis, but with normal sweat glands.
- Inheritance: autosomal dominant, with mutations in *GJB6* gene, encoding for protein connexin 30.
- Clinical characteristics:
  - Hidrotic ED is similar to hypohidrotic ED, but hereditary patterns of nails and sweat glands involvement are different.
  - Nail abnormalities are the most consistent feature that manifested at birth or in early infancy:

    Nails are thickened, slow growing, brittle, often hyperconvex and discolored with striation.

    Micronychia and recurrent paronychial infections with onycholysis.
  - Hair involvement manifests at birth or later during infancy or childhood.

    Total or partial, often progressive, alopecia.

    Residual hairs (mostly in scalp, and sometimes in eyebrows, eyelashes, pubic and body areas) are slow growing, sparse, fine, and brittle.
  - Palmoplantar hyperkeratosis begins in childhood and tends to worsen with age.
  - Pebbled skin on dorsal aspect of toes and fingers.

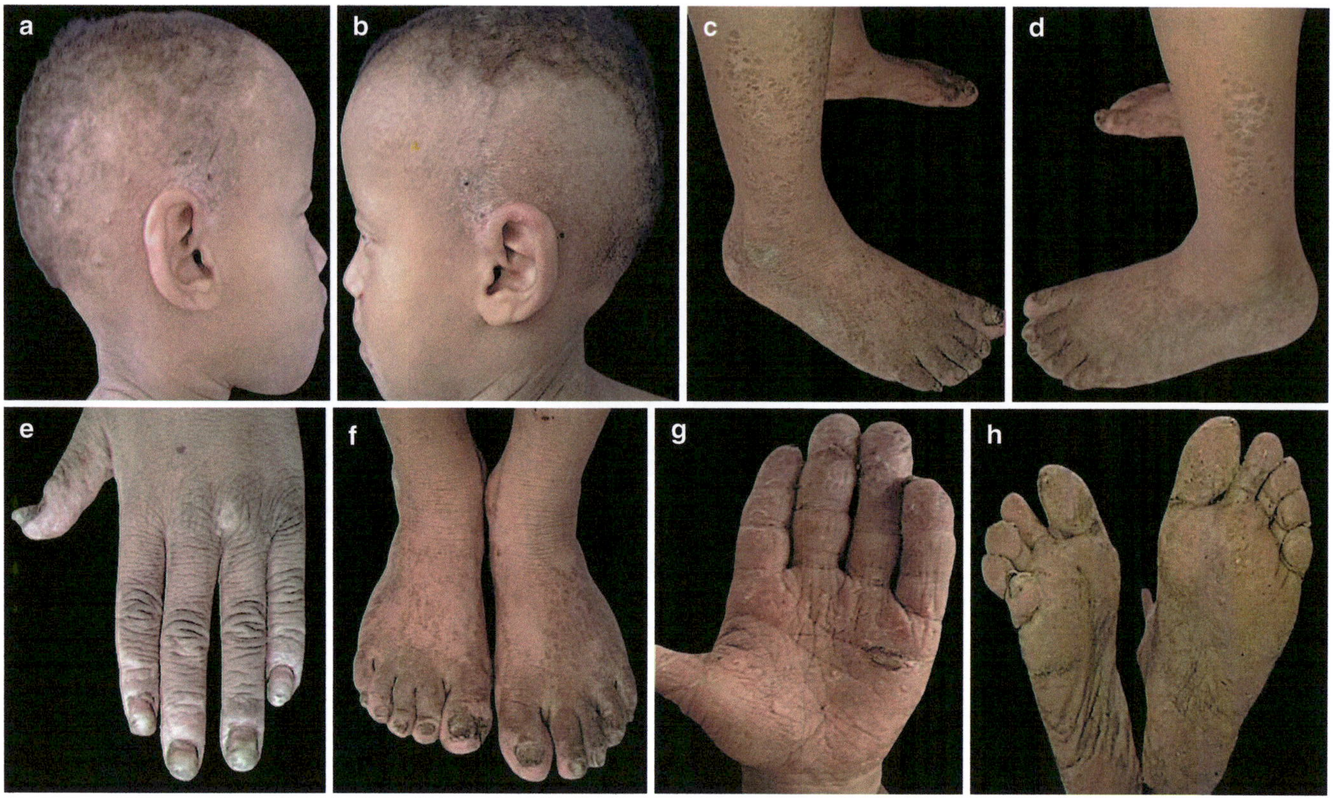

Fig. 10.6 Hidrotic ectodermal dysplasia (clouston syndrome). Sparse hair (**a**, **b**), dry skin (**a–f**), pebbled skin on dorsal aspect of fingers and toes (**c–f**), dystrophic nails (**e**, **f**), and palmoplantar keratoderma (**g**, **h**)

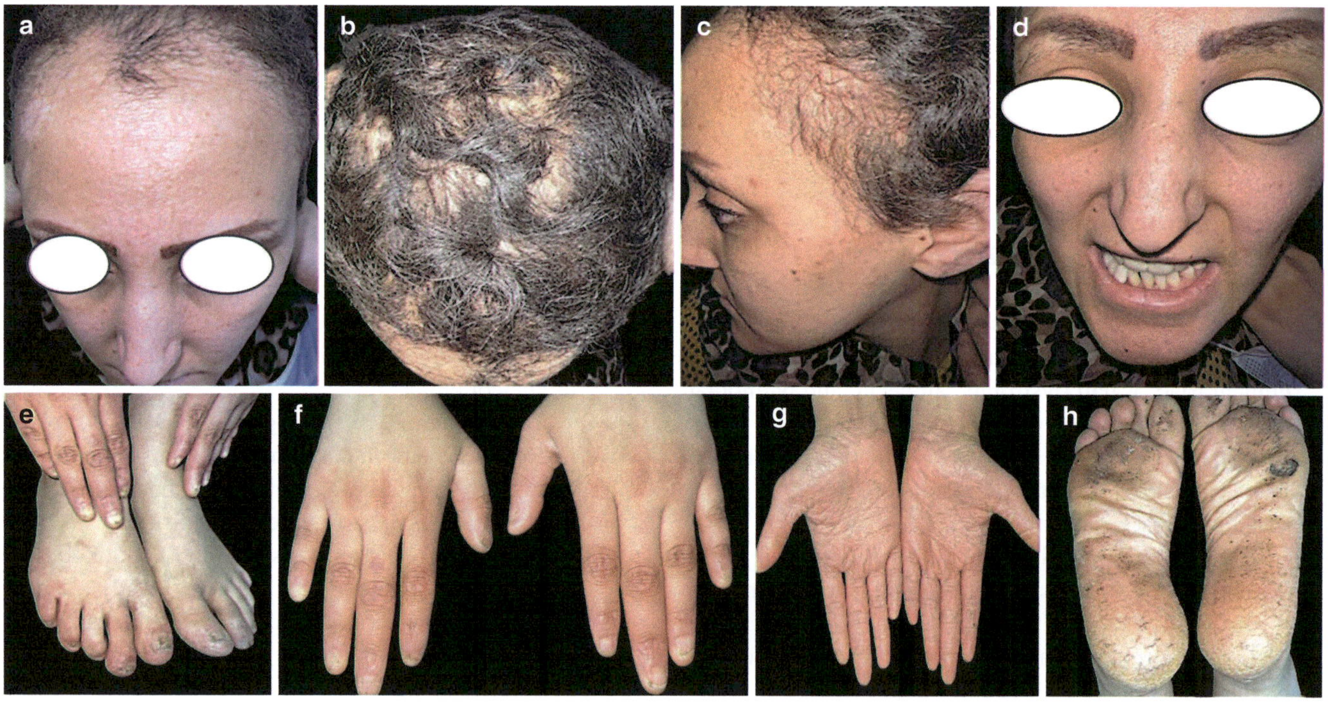

Fig. 10.7 Hidrotic ectodermal dysplasia (Clouston Syndrome). Sparse hair (**a–c**), normal teeth (**d**), pebbled skin on dorsal aspect of fingers and toes (**e–h**), dystrophic nails (**e**, **f**), palmoplantar keratoderma (**g**, **h**)

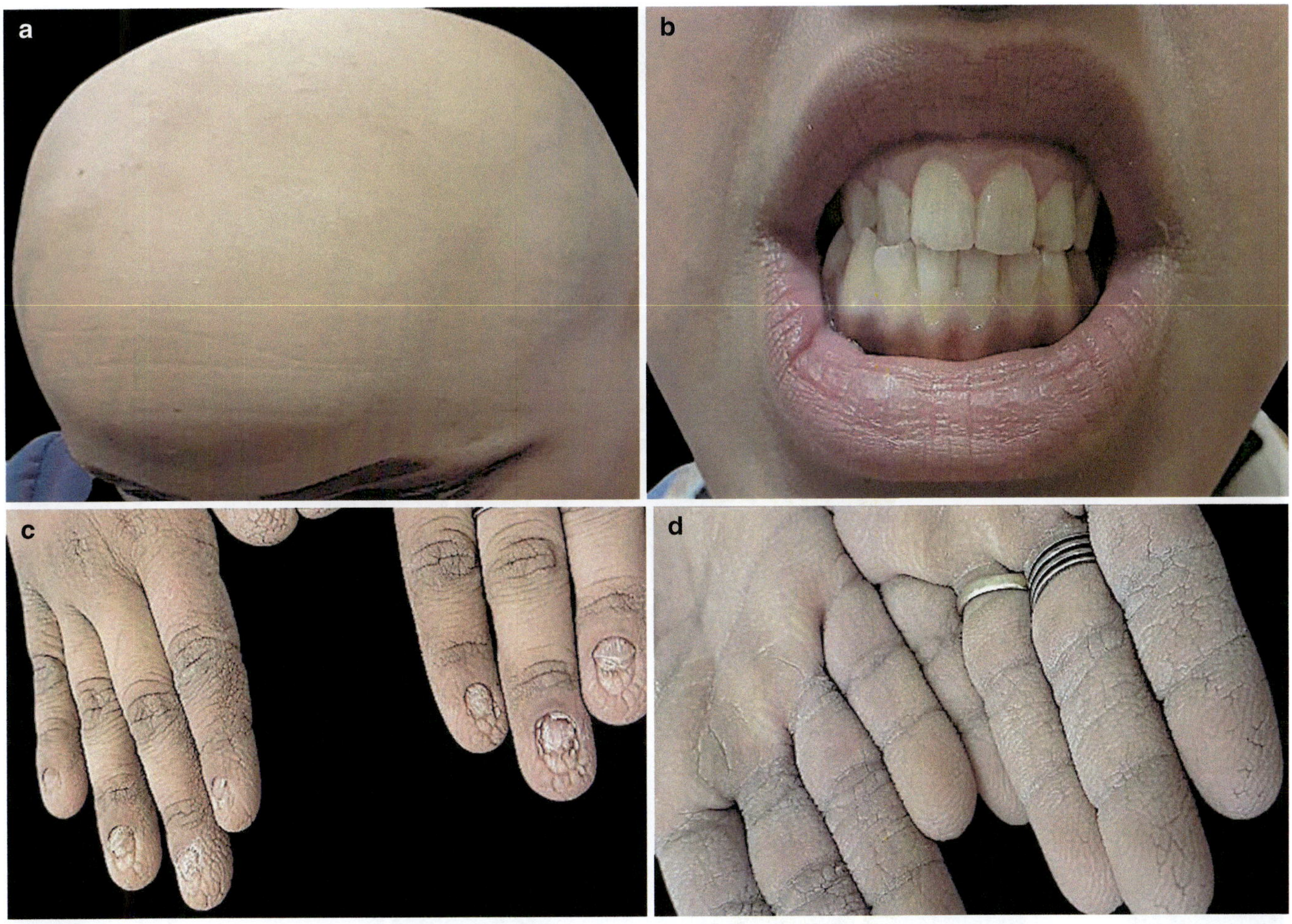

Fig. 10.8 Hidrotic ectodermal dysplasia (clouston syndrome). Alopecia (**a**), normal teeth (**b**), pebbled skin on dorsal aspect of fingers (**c**), dystrophic nails (**c**), and palmar keratoderma (**d**)

Ankyloblepharon-Ectodermal Dysplasia-Clefting Syndrome [5, 6] (Hay-Wells Syndrome) (AD) (Fig. 10.9)

- Ankyloblepharon-ectodermal dysplasia-clefting (AEC) syndrome, Hay-Wells syndrome, is a form of ED, in which there is abnormal development of ectodermal tissues.
- Inheritance: autosomal dominant, with mutations in *TP63* gene that help in making a p63 protein to play an essential role in early development.
- Clinical characteristics:
  - Skin:
    - Mild to severe skin erosions mostly on scalp, neck, hands, and feet in infancy, with recurrence throughout childhood and adulthood, leading to life-threatening infections, scarring, and hair loss.
    - Mottled hypo- and hyper-pigmentation.
    - Erythroderma or bullous lesion resembling epidermolysis bullosa.
  - Eye: ankyloblepharon filiforme adnatum (tissue strands partially or completely fuse upper and lower eyelids).
  - Ectodermal dysplasia:
    - Hypohidrosis.
    - Dental defects and cleft lip/palate.
    - Hair: sparse hairs, with loss of eyebrows and eyelashes.
    - Nail deformity.
  - Limb abnormalities, most commonly fused fingers and toes (syndactyly). Less often, permanently bent fingers and toes (comptodactyly), a deep split in hands or feet, missing fingers or toes and fusion of remaining digits (ectrodactyly).
  - Deafness is common (>90% of patients).
  - Facies:
    - Small jaws that cannot open fully.
    - Narrow space between the upper lip and nose (philtrum).

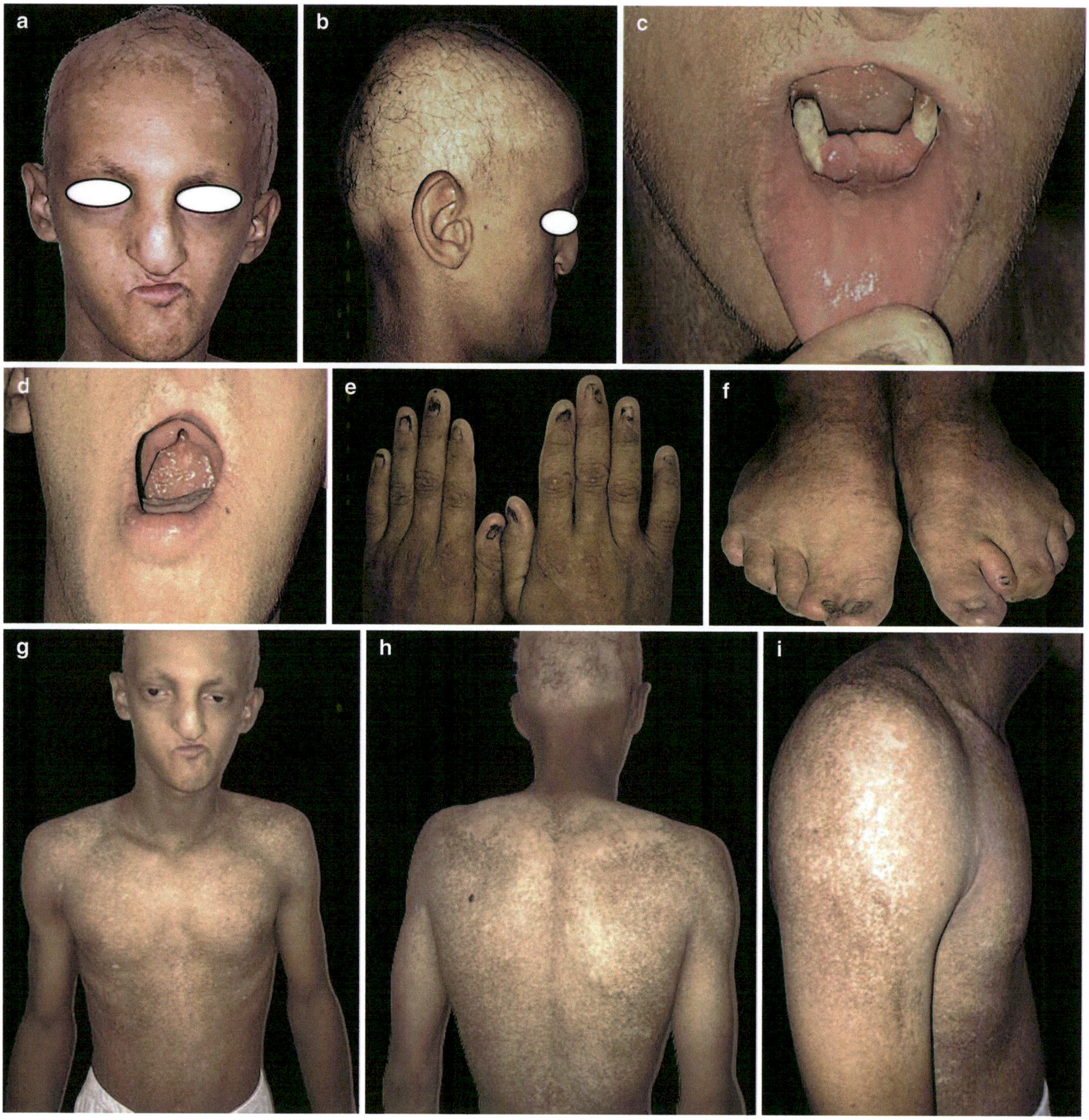

Fig. 10.9 Ankyloblepharon-ectodermal dysplasia-clefting syndrome (Hay-Wells syndrome). Narrow space between upper lip and nose (**a**), sparse hairs of scalp, eyebrows and eyelashes (**a**, **b**), small jaws that cannot open fully (**c**, **d**), dental defects and cleft palate (**c**, **d**), nail dystrophy and syndactyly (**e**, **f**), with mottled hypo and hyperpigmentation (**g**–**k**)

- Others: hypospadias in males, digestive problems, absent tear duct openings in eyes and chronic sinus or ear infections.
- Rapp-Hodgkin syndrome overlaps clinically with AEC syndrome to be considered a part of the same disease spectrum.

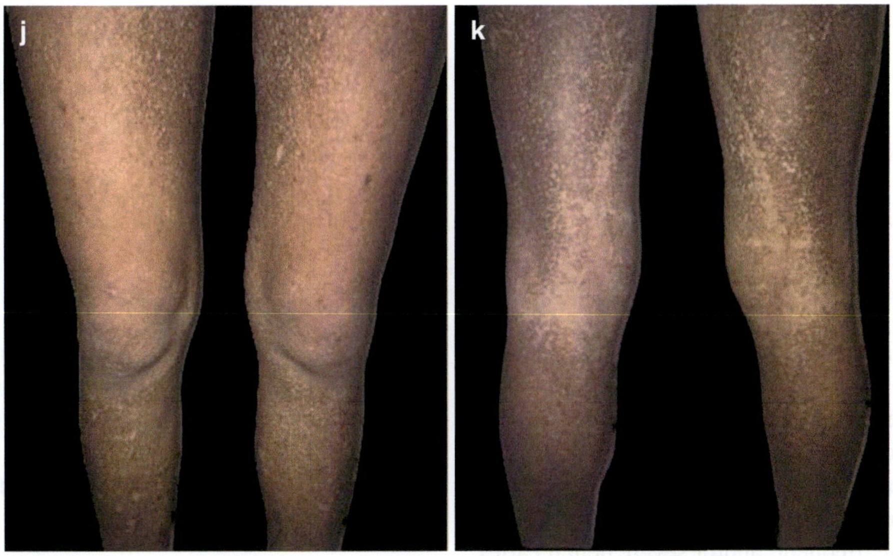

Fig. 10.9 (continued)

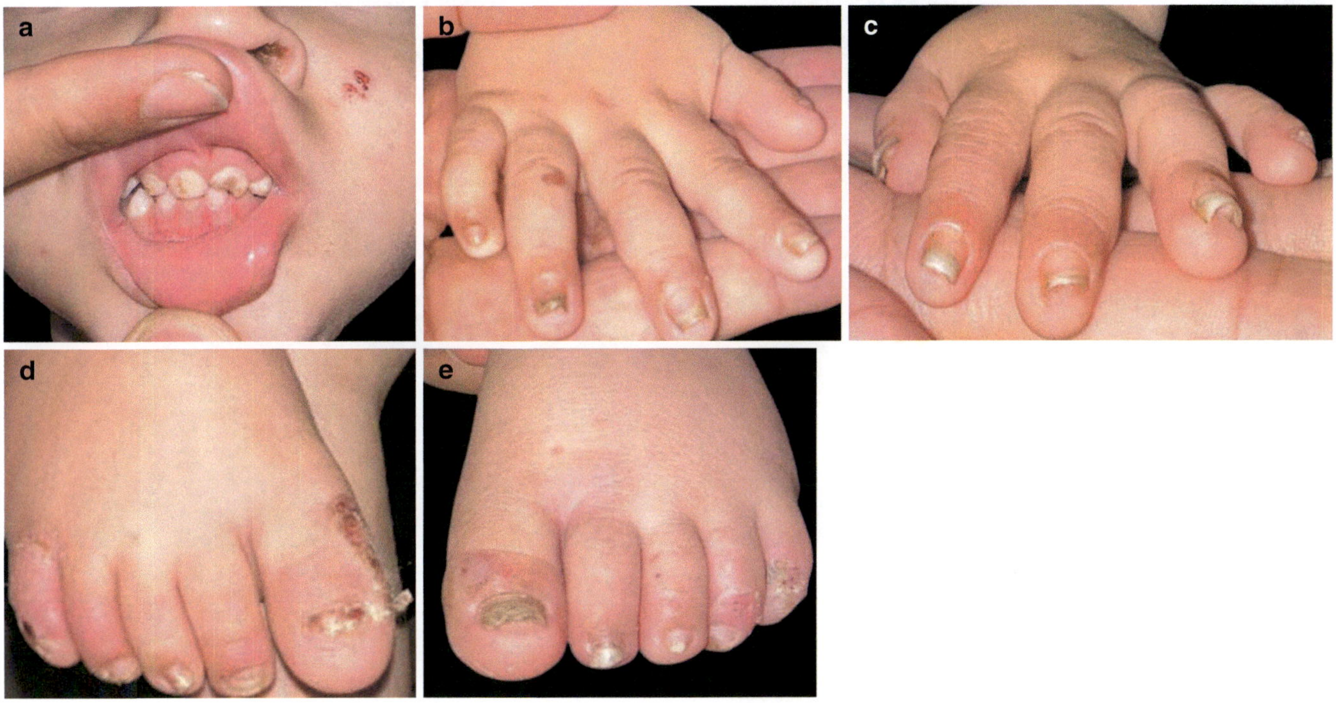

Fig. 10.10 Witkop's syndrome (Tooth-and-Nail syndrome). Hypodontia (**a**) and nail dystrophies (**b**–**e**)

Witkop's Syndrome [7] (Tooth-and-Nail Syndrome) (AD) (Fig. 10.10)

- Witkop syndrome, a rare variant of ED, is characterized by tooth and nail abnormalities.
- Inheritance: autosomal dominant, with mutations in *MSX-1* gene.
- Clinical characteristics:
  - Teeth:

    Hypodontia and, infrequently, anodontia of the permanent teeth (maxillary incisors, second molars, and maxillary canines).

    Agenesis of six or more teeth, excluding third molars, called oligodontia.

    Defects in primary teeth may be so mild to be noted until permanent teeth fail to erupt.
  - Nails:

    Defect or absence of nail plates of fingers and toes at birth, with more severe affection in toenails.
  - Hair: some patients might have fine, diffuse and thin hair, without alopecia.
- DD: hypohidrotic ED; characteristic facies of ED are not seen, with normal sweat glands and less severe features in Witkop's syndrome.

Hallermann-Streiff Syndrome [8, 9] (Oculo-Mandibulo-Facial Syndrome) (Sporadic/AD) (Fig. 10.11)

- Hallermann-Streiff syndrome (HSS) is a rare congenital disorder.
- Inheritance: Most cases of HSS are sporadic, but sometimes, it is autosomal dominant.
- Onset: arises between fifth and seventh week of embryonic life.
- Clinical characteristics:
  - Facies: dyscephaly with bird-face, frontal bossing, beak-like nose, and hypoplasia of the mandible.
  - Proportioned dwarfism.
  - Dental anomalies: absent, malformed, irregularly set teeth, premature eruption and persistence of deciduous teeth, open bite, frequent, and/or severe dental caries.
  - Eyes: bilateral microphthalmia, congenital cataract, blue sclera, anti-mongoloid slanting of palpebral fissures, iris atrophy, anterior and posterior synechiae, vitreous opacities, and pale optic discs.
  - Hypotrichosis in scalp, eyelashes, and eyebrows.
  - Cutaneous atrophy usually affecting scalp and face, especially nose.
  - Ears: normal.
  - Nails: normal.
- D.D.: differentiated from other related mandibulo-facial dysostoses and ED by the absence of anomalies of ears, nails and extremities, musculo-arthritic anomalies, and neuropsychological deficit.
- Complications: lethal pulmonary infections and respiratory and feeding difficulties.

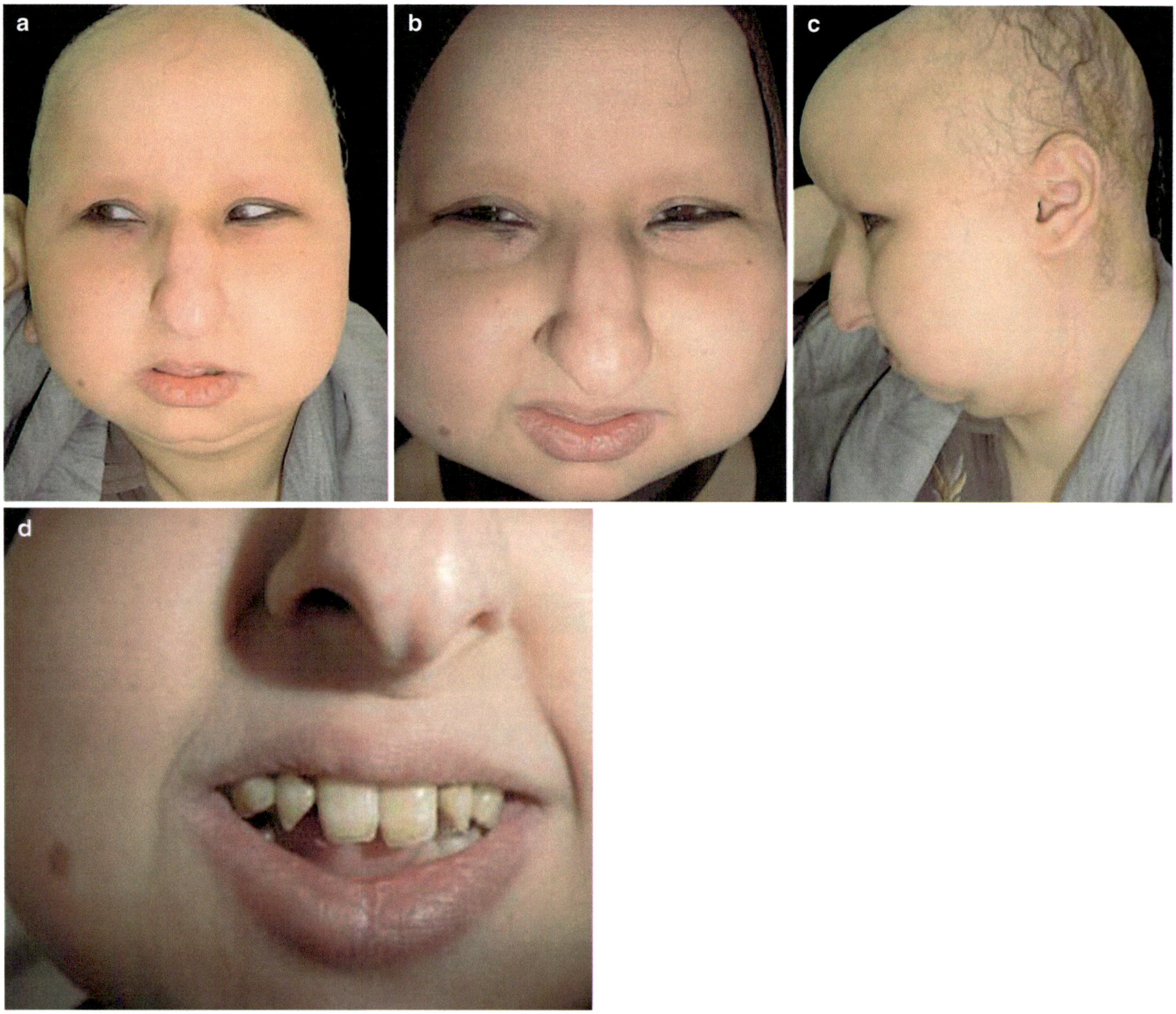

Fig. 10.11 Hallermann-Streiff syndrome (Oculo-mandibulo-facial syndrome). Frontal bossing (**a**), microphthalmia (**a**, **b**), beak-like nose (**b**–**d**), hypoplasia of mandible (**a**, **b**), hypotrichosis (**a**, **c**), and open bite with malformed teeth (**d**)

Monilethrix (AD) [10, 11] (Fig. 10.12)

- Monilethrix is a rare hair shaft disorder characterized by hair fragility with patchy dystrophic alopecia.
- Inheritance: autosomal dominant, with mutations in hair keratin genes (*KRT 81, KRT 83, KRT 86*).
- Onset: during early childhood.
- Clinical characteristics:
  - Hairs:
    Diffuse hypotrichosis of scalp, with short, fragile, and broken hairs that do not grow long enough, especially in friction sites (top of head, nape, and occipital areas).
    In severe forms, eyelashes, eyebrows or secondary sexual hairs may be involved.
    Elliptical beaded nods along hair shaft (trichorrhexis nodosa) due to periodic thinning.
    Large hyperkeratotic follicular papules, most commonly on occiput.
  - Others: keratosis pilaris, syndactyly, nail abnormalities (koilonychia, brittle nails), cataract, dental abnormalities, and epilepsy.
- Trichoscopy and light microscopy of hair: uniform elliptical nodes (normal-hair diameter with medulla) and intermittent constrictions (internodes with no medulla).
- DD: Other hair shaft anomalies such as pseudomonilethrix, congenital alopecia, trichorrhexis invaginata, and ED.
- Prognosis: few cases remit spontaneously in adulthood, whereas most cases are persistent.

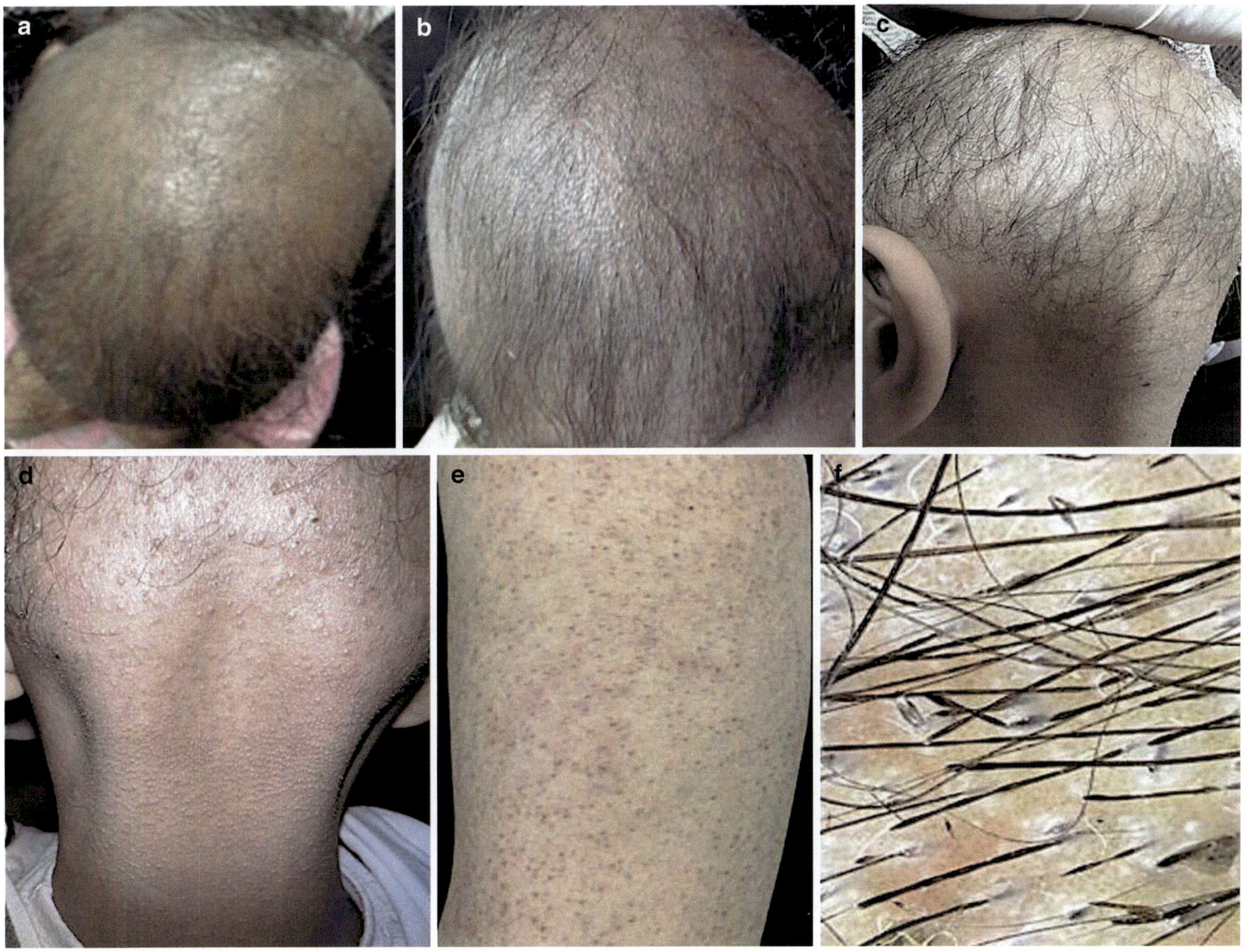

Fig. 10.12 Monilethrix. Brittle hair and hypotrichosis (**a–d**), hyperkeratotic follicular papules on occiput (**d**) and keratosis pilaris (**e**). Trichoscopy of the hair shaft demonstrating uniform elliptical nodes (containing medulla) and intermittent/periodic constrictions (no medulla) (**f**)

Atrichia with Papular Lesions (AR) [12, 13] (Figs. 10.13, 10.14, and 10.15)

- Atrichia with papular lesions (APL) is a rare form of irreversible alopecia.
- Autosomal recessive, with mutation in the Zinc finger domain of human hairless gene.
- Onset: within months after birth.
- Clinical characteristics:
  - Patients are born with irreversible hair fall.
  - Papular lesions of keratin cysts (milia like papules) on body.
- **Diagnostic criteria for atrichia with papular lesions** [13].
- **Major criteria (4 out of 5 required for diagnosis).**
  - Permanent and complete absence of scalp hair by the first few months of life.
  - Few to widespread smooth, whitish, or milia-like papules on the face, scalp, arms, elbows, thighs or knees from infancy or childhood.
  - Replacement of mature hair follicle structures by follicular cysts filled with cornified material in scalp histology.
  - Mutation(s) in the human hairless gene through genetic testing.
  - Clinical and/or molecular exclusion of vitamin D-dependent rickets.

Minor criteria (supplementary criteria).
  - Family history of consanguinity.
  - Absence of secondary axillary, pubic, or body hair growth and/or sparse eyebrows and eyelashes.
  - Normal growth and development, including normal bones, teeth, nails, and sweating.
  - Whitish hypopigmented streaks on the scalp.
  - Lack of response to any treatment modality.

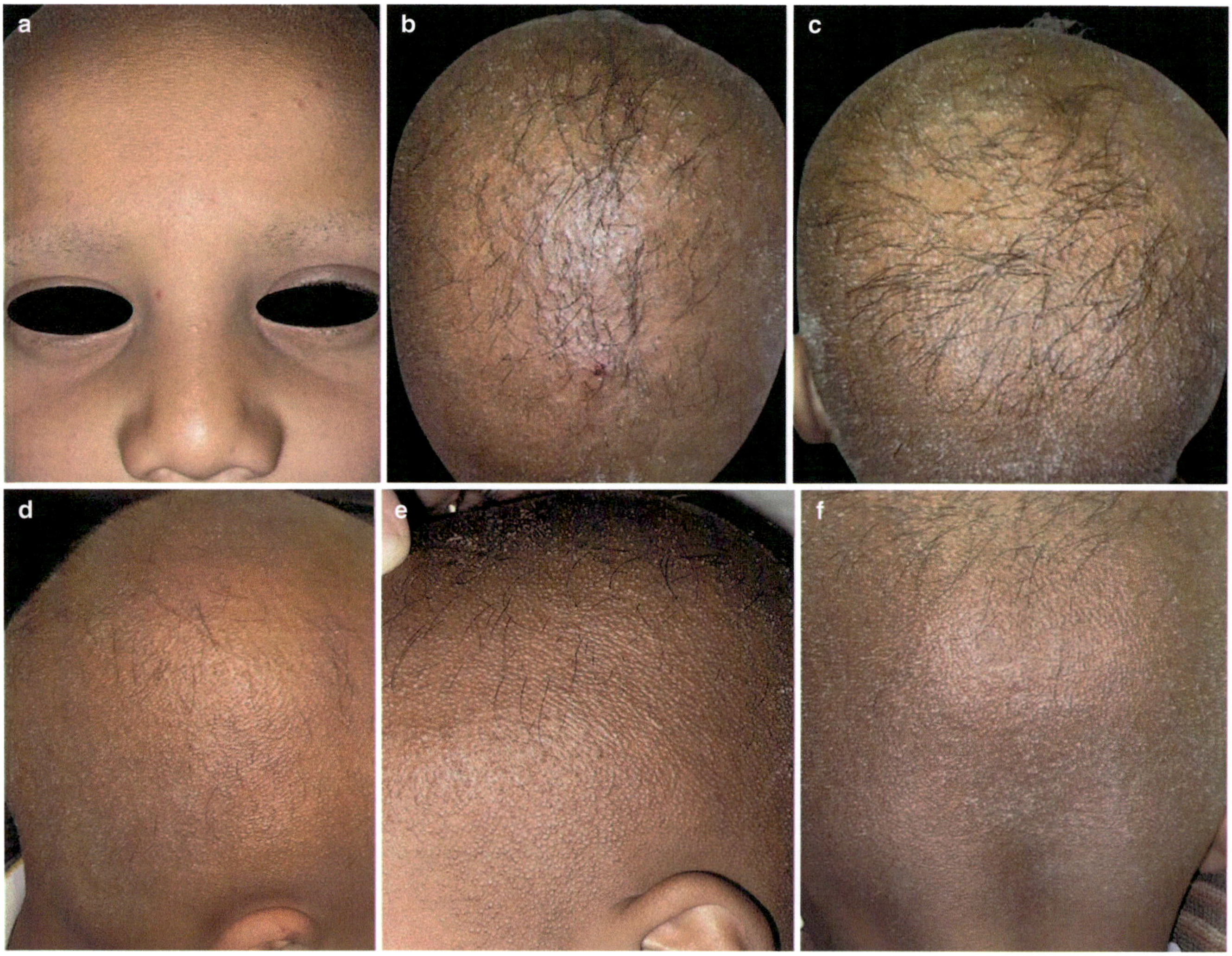

Fig. 10.13 Generalized atrichia. Brittle hair and hypotrichosis with follicular papules (**a**–**f**)

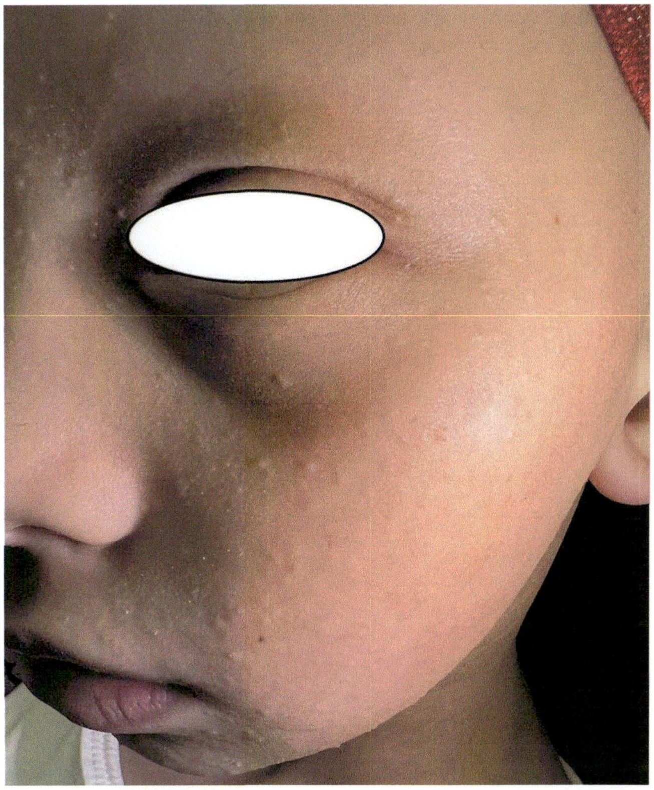

Fig. 10.14 Generalized atrichia. Generalized atrichia and milia like papules on the face

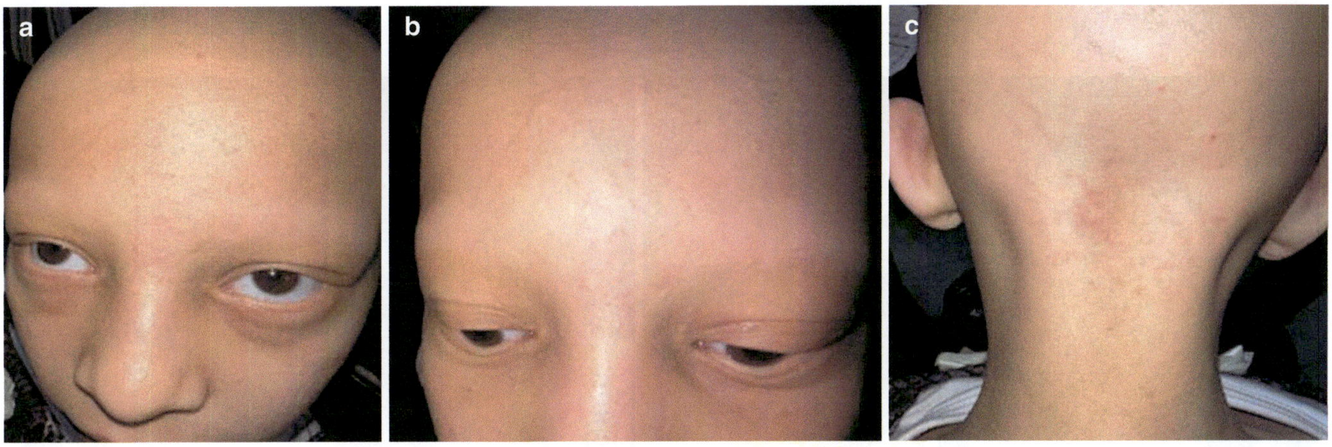

Fig. 10.15 Generalized atrichia. Generalized atrichia with follicular papules (**a**–**c**)

Uncombable Hair Syndrome (AD/AR) [14] (Fig. 10.16)

- Uncombable hair syndrome, pili trianguli et canaliculi, is a rare structural anomaly of hair shaft.
- Inheritance: autosomal dominant or recessive, with mutations in *ATP7A* [copper (Cu) transporter] gene. However, few sporadic forms may be present.
- Clinical characteristics:
  - Dry, frizzy, blond hair impossible to comb, giving a synthetic doll hair-like look.
  - Glistening appearance of hair because of altered reflection of light from grooved flattened hair shaft.

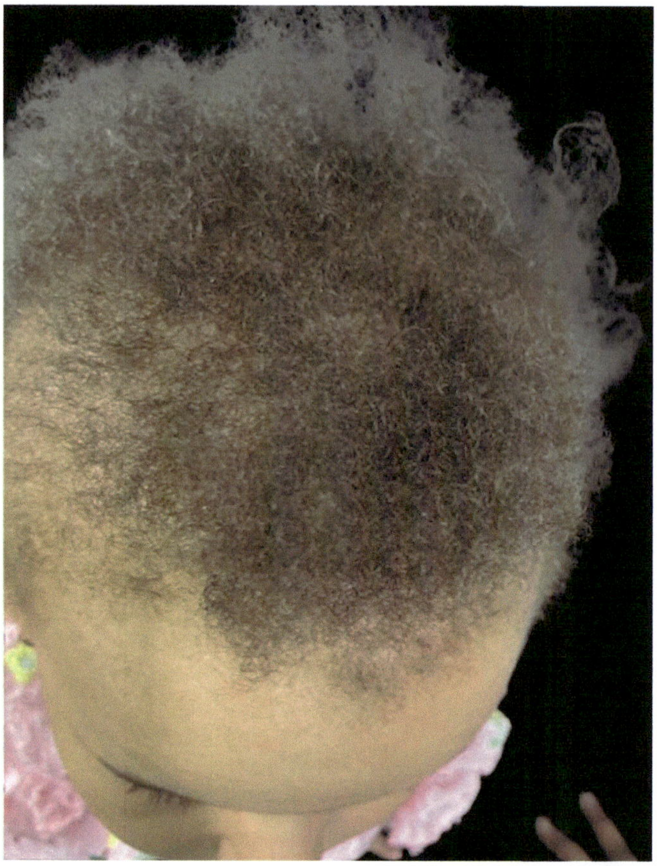

Fig. 10.16 Uncombable hair syndrome. Dry, frizy, hair impossible to comb

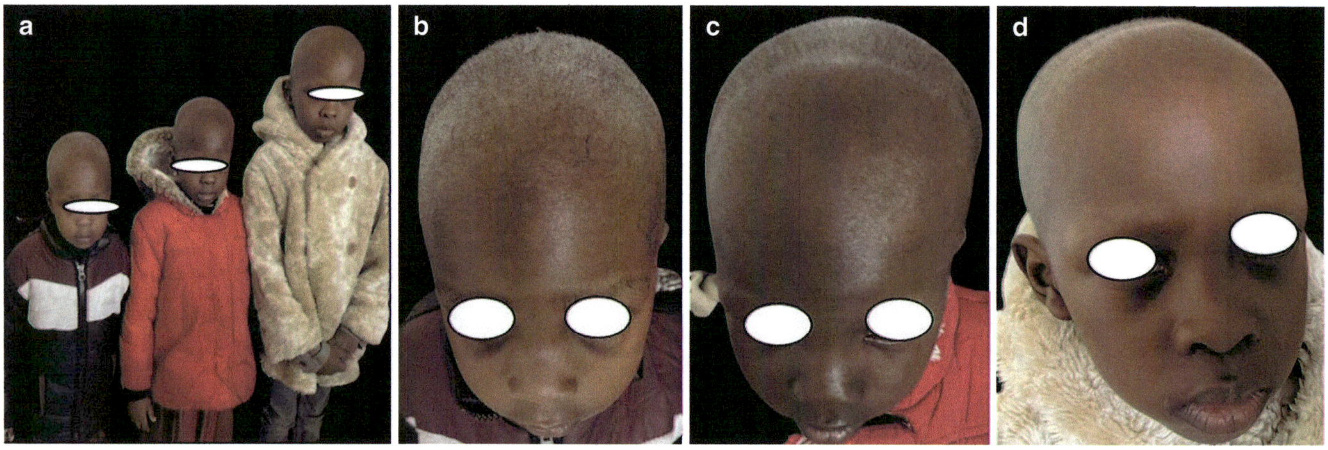

Fig. 10.17 Three Siblings of Björnstad Syndrome. Short brittle sparse hairs and deafness (**a**–**d**)

Björnstad Syndrome (AR) [15, 16] (Fig. 10.17)

- Björnstad syndrome is congenital condition showing pili torti and sensorineural deafness.
- Inheritance: autosomal recessive, with mutation in *BCS1L* gene.
- Onset: before 2 years of life.
- Clinical characteristics:
  - Pili torti (twisted hair shafts) and alopecia.
  - The present hairs (on head, eyebrows, eyelashes and others) appear dry, blonde, fragile, and coarse).
  - Sensorineural hearing loss.
  - Intellectual disabilities and hypogonadism.
- Electron microscope: hair shafts from scalp or body appear flattened and/or twisted (torti) at regular intervals.

References

1. Yavuz I, Baskan Z, Ulku R, et al. Ectodermal dysplasia: retrospective study of fifteen cases. Arch Med Res. 2006;37(3):403–9.
2. Paramkusam G, Meduri V, Nadendla LK, et al. Hereditary hypohidrotic ectodermal dysplasia: report of a rare case. J Clin Diagn Res. 2013;7(9):2074–5.
3. Chitty LS, Dennis N, Baraitser M. Hidrotic ectodermal dysplasia of hair, teeth, and nails: case reports and review. J Med Genet. 1996;33(8):707–10.
4. Arora KS, Hundal KD, Kaur RD, et al. Hidrotic ectodermal dysplasia: case report and review. J Oral Med Oral Surg Oral Pathol Oral Radiol. 2015;1(3):156–9.
5. Julapalli MR, Scher RK, Sybert VP, et al. Dermatologic findings of ankyloblepharon-ectodermal defects-cleft lip/palate (AEC) syndrome. Am J Med Genet A. 2009;149A(9):1900–6.
6. Siegfried E, Bree A, Fete M, et al. Skin erosions and wound healing in ankyloblepharon-ectodermal defect-cleft lip and/or palate. Arch Dermatol. 2005;141(12):1591–4.
7. Arora V, Agrawal KK, Mishra A. Witkop's syndrome: a case report. J Oral Bio Craniofac Res. 2016;6(1):79–81.
8. Neki AS. Hallermann-Streiff syndrome. Indian J Ophthalmol. 1993;41(2):83–4.
9. Atwa FA, Farag MMA, Mansour MN, et al. Hallermann-Streiff syndrome. A case report from Egypt. Egypt J Hosp Med. 2014;55:142–5.
10. Oliveira EF, Araripe AL. Monilethrix: a typical case report with microscopic and dermatoscopic findings. An Bras Dermatol. 2015;90(1):126–7.
11. de Lencastre A, Tosti A. Monilethrix. J Pediatr. 2012;161(6):1176.
12. Bansal M, Manchanda K, Lamba S. Atrichia with papular lesions. Int J Trichology. 2011;3(2):112–4.
13. Zlotogorski A, Panteleyev AA, Aita VM, et al. Clinical and molecular diagnostic criteria of congenital atrichia with papular lesions. J Invest Dermatol. 2002;118(5):887–90.
14. Rieubland C, de Virah PA, Addor MC. Uncombable hair syndrome: a clinical report. Eur J Med Genet. 2007;50(4):309–14.
15. Hinson JT, Fantin VR, Schönberger J, et al. Missense mutations in the BCS1L gene as a cause of the Björnstad syndrome. N Engl J Med. 2007;356(8):809–19.
16. Selvaag E. Pili torti and sensorineural hearing loss. A follow-up of Bjørnstad's original patients and a review of the literature. Eur J Dermatol. 2000;10:91–7.

11 Premature Aging Syndromes (Progeroid Syndromes)

Hereditary Conditions with Premature Aging

- **Progeria (Hutchinson-Gilford Syndrome) (AD)**
- **Adult Progeria (Werner Syndrome) (AR)**

Progeria (Hutchinson-Gilford Syndrome) (AD) [1, 2] (Fig. 11.1)

- Incidence: it is a very rare genetic disorder, which occurs approximately in 1:4,000,000 births. The ratio of females to males is 1:1.5.
- Autosomal dominant inheritance: it results from de novo heterozygous mutation of Lamin A (*LMNA*) gene encoding laminin A; however, it is actually not inherited because the patient dies before the age of reproduction.
- Onset: It could not be diagnosed at birth, but after the age of 2 years, visible and prominent symptoms can be observed.
- Clinical features:
  - Characteristic clinical facies: disproportionately large cranium with patent fontanelles and frontal bossing, protruding eyes (due to vanishing of intra-orbital and subcutaneous fat), prominent scalp veins (due to thin skin), centrofacial cyanosis, micrognathia with wrinkling around mouth and thin lips, abnormal delayed dentition with dental crowding, beaked nose, plucked bird, and prominent outer ears lacking lobules.
  - Skin: thin atrophic skin with loss of subcutaneous fat on the face and limbs, wrinkling, thickened sclerotic areas on lower trunk or thighs and progressive mottled pigmentation.
  - Nails: small, thin and dystrophic.
  - Hairs: generalized alopecia, but the few remaining hairs are pale, fine, and fuzzy, with sparse or absent eyebrows and eye lashes.
  - Skeletal abnormalities: dystrophic clavicles, coxa vulga, and progressive bone resorption and frequent fractures, with joint contractures and a shuffling gait (due to combination of joint stiffness and coxa valga).
  - Physical growth: failure to gain weight, short stature and prominent belly (due to intra-abdominal fat deposition), but with normal motor and mental development.
  - Sexual growth: underdeveloped sexual maturation with small testicles in male and striking hypoplasia (incomplete growth) of the nipples are noticed.
  - Later findings: low-frequency conductive hearing loss and highly pitched voice.
  - Death occurs between the age of 6 and 20 years, with the average life span of 13 years. The most common causes of death include atherosclerosis, cardiac disease (myocardial infarction or heart failure), cerebrovascular disease (stroke), pulmonary hypertension, and infections.

Adult Progeria (Werner Syndrome) (AR) [3, 4] (Fig. 11.2)

- It is a rare genetic disorder, in which the aging process is accelerated.
- It is caused by null mutations of the *WRN* gene (*RECQL2*), which belongs to the *RECQ* family of DNA helicases.
- Onset: patients generally develop normally until they reach adolescence (second–fourth decade).
- Clinical features:
  - Developmental growth: the first sign is the lack of a growth spurt and a relatively short stature during the early teen ages.
  - Skin: early findings (usually observed in the 20s) include skin atrophy, wrinkling, loss of subcutaneous fat, scleroderma-like skin changes and mottled pigmentation.
  - Characteristic clinical facies: a "pinched" facial appearance, thin beaked nose, graying and loss of hair, truncal obesity, thin limbs (muscle wasting and loss of subcutaneous fat) and flat feet.

N. Moftah et al., *Atlas of Common and Rare Genodermatoses*, https://doi.org/10.1007/978-3-031-60788-2_11

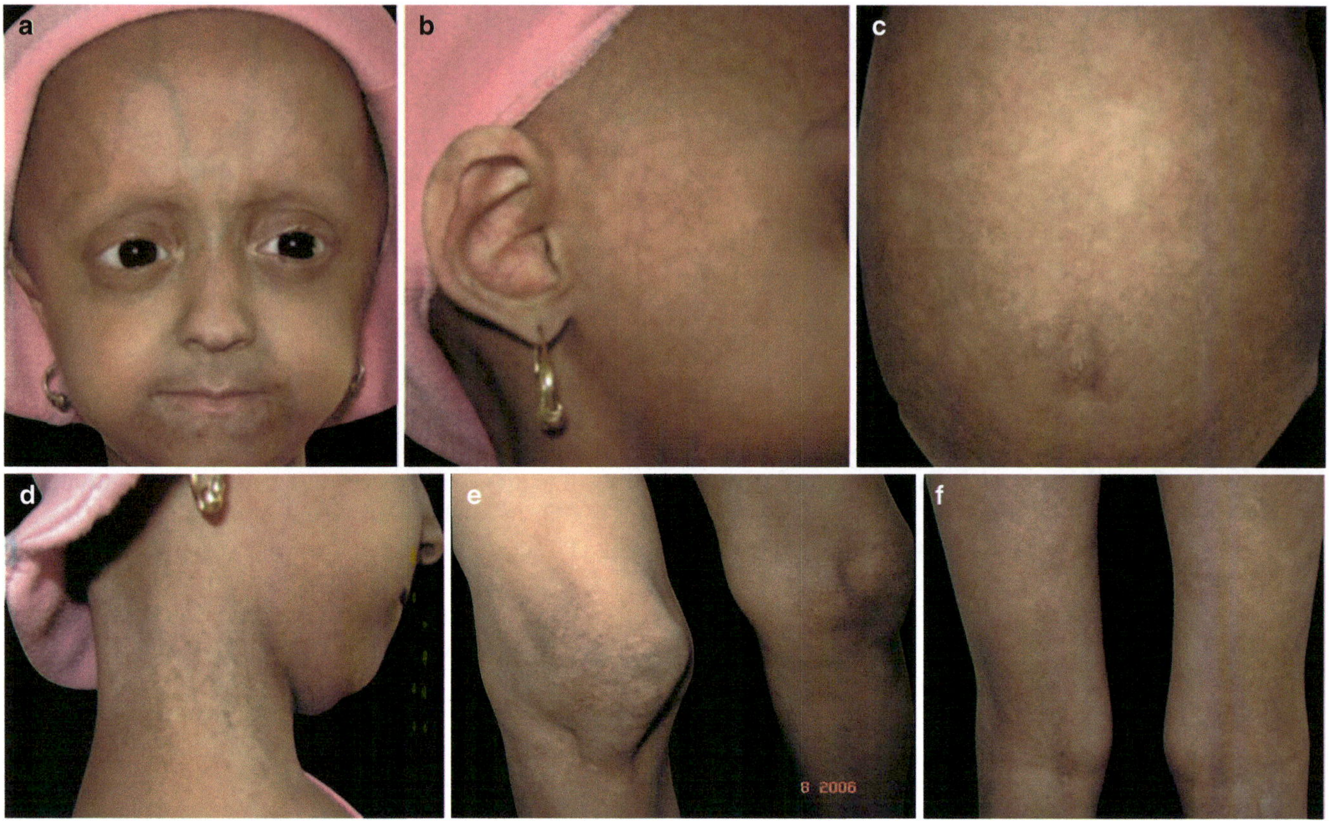

Fig. 11.1 Progeria. A 5-years-old female child with, disproportionate enlarged head, frontal bossing, beaked nose, plucked bird, micrognathia, protruding eyes, small mouth, thin lips, prominent veins, cyanosis around mouth and nasolabial folds, alopecia, loss of subcutaneous fat (**a**, **b**), prominent belly (**c**), mottled pigmentation (**d**), localized sclerodermatous changes of lower trunk and thigh and, joint distortion (**e**, **f**). (*Courtesy, Samar Ashry*)

- Indolent deep ulcerations around Achilles' tendons and, less frequently, at elbows, are almost pathognomonic. These are associated with extensive subcutaneous calcifications.
- Associated age-related disorders: bilateral cataracts, type 2 diabetes mellitus, osteoporosis, atherosclerosis in the 30s.
- Sexual maturation: hypogonadism occurs in the 30s due to interstitial fibrosis of the testes. Premature menopause occurs in females.
- Other common feature is a high-pitched hoarse voice (due to thinning of the cords and fixation of the epiglottis).
- Mental retardation and other developmental abnormalities are not features of Werner syndrome.
- Malignancies (sarcomas, meningiomas, hematological and cutaneous malignancies) are common.
- The most common causes of death are cancer and myocardial infarction, at a median age of 54.

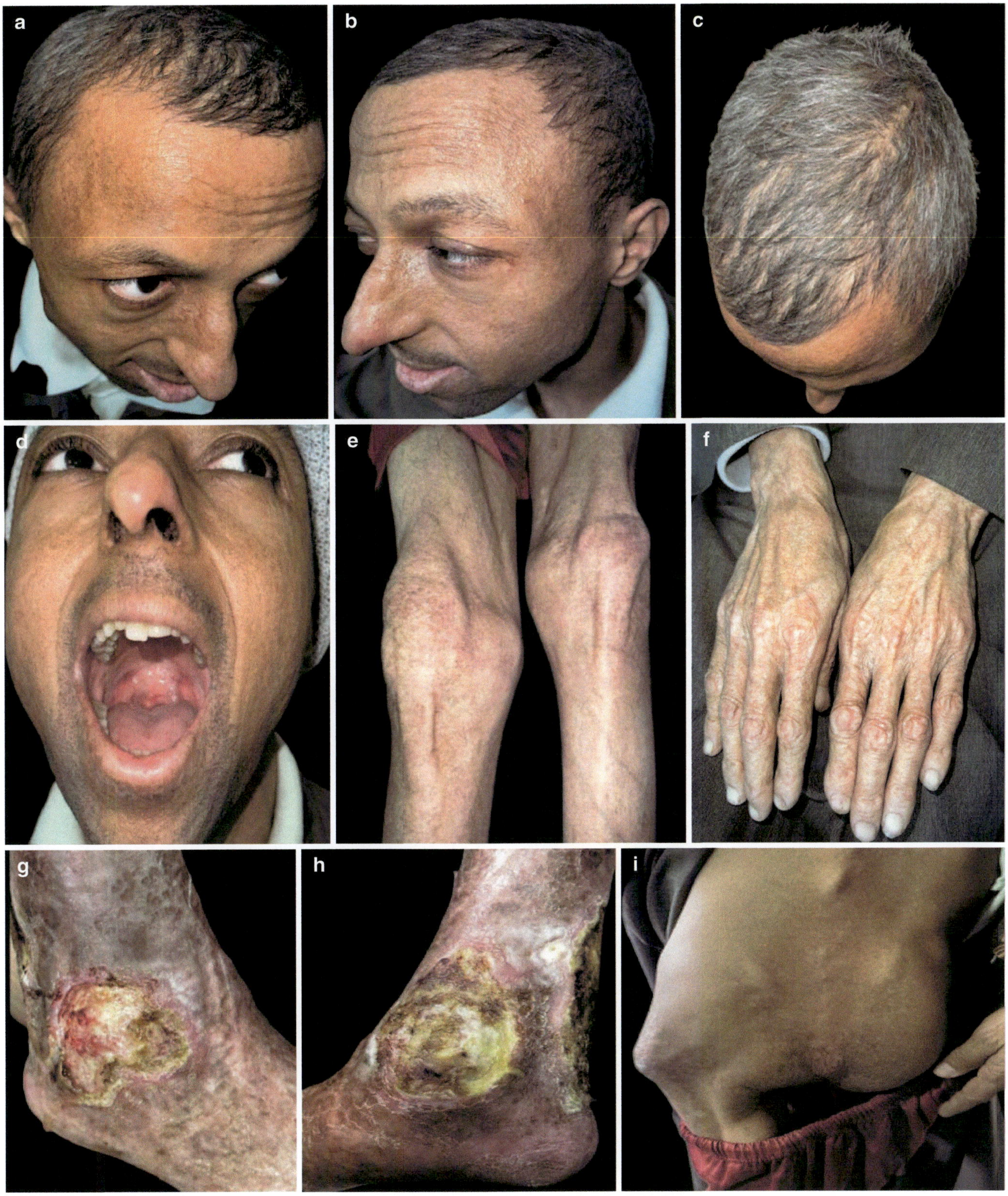

Fig. 11.2 **Werner Syndrome:** A 25-years-old male patient with thin beaked nose, small ears, protruding eyes, sclerodermoid changes (thin atrophic skin), premature graying hair, micrognathia, prominent eyes and dental crowding with oral erosions (**a–d**), thin atrophic skin, muscle wasting "thin limbs," chronic leg ulcer on joints mottled hyperpigmentation (**e–h**), dislocation of hip joint (**i**)

References

1. Sarkar PK, Shinton RA. Hutchinson-Gilford progeria syndrome. Postgrad Med J. 2001;77(907):312–7.
2. Hennekam RCM. Hutchinson–Gilford progeria syndrome: review of the phenotype. Am J Med Genet A. 2006;140(23):2603–24.
3. Oshima J, Sidorovaa JM, Monnat RJ. Werner syndrome: clinical features, pathogenesis and potential therapeutic interventions. Ageing Res Rev. 2017;33:105–14.
4. Goto M. Hierarchical deterioration of body systems in Werner's syndrome: implications for normal ageing. Mech Ageing Dev. 1997;98(3):239–54.

Genetic Immunodeficiency Disorders

12

- **Chronic mucocutaneous candidiasis (CMC) (AD/AR)**
- **Wiskott-Aldrich Syndrome (XLR)**
- **Hyper-IgE Syndrome (Job's Syndrome) (AD/AR)**

Chronic Mucocutaneous Candidiasis (CMC) (AD/AR) [1–3] (Fig. 12.1)

- Patients with CMC have inherited (familial) or acquired (late onset) T-cell deficiency, mostly T-helper (Th) 17 responses that has a critical role in immune defense against Candida.
  - Familial CMC; it starts soon after birth or in infancy. It has two forms;
    - Autosomal dominant (AD). Defect in *STAT1* gene.
    - Autosomal recessive (AR). Defect in *CARD9* and *IL17RC* genes.
  - Late onset CMC: It appears in sporadic adults secondary to HIV infection with T-cell deficiency, neoplasms, diabetes, immunosuppressive therapies (e.g., anti-cytokine blockers, antibiotic or steroid therapy).
- Heterogeneous group of abnormalities with recurrent or persistent mucocutaneous infections caused by Candida species, predominantly *Candida albicans*, affecting skin, nails, oral cavity, and genital mucosa.
- It does not represent a specific disease but rather a phenotypic presentation of a spectrum of immunologic, endocrinologic, and autoimmune diseases.
- Skin: erythematous scaly plaques or crusted granulomatous lesions (candida granuloma) on scalp, face (periorificial), intertriginous or acral areas. Scaring alopecia may occur.
- Oral involvement: oral thrush with hyperkeratotic plaque that may extend to esophagus, laryngeal mucosae, and genitalia.
- Nails involvement: they may be markedly thickened, brittle, and discolored, with edema and erythema of surrounding periungual tissues.
  - Associations:
    - Multiple and recurrent infections can occur (cutaneous dermatophyte more common), with bacterial septicemia in some cases.
    - Endocrine dysfunction; abnormalities in pituitary, adrenal, parathyroid, thyroid, and ovarian glands, in addition to diabetes mellitus.
    - Autoimmune diseases: chronic keratitis, vitiligo, and hemolytic anemia.
- Investigations.
  - KOH smear with appearance of pseudo hyphae and yeast forms.
  - Fungal culture on Sabouraud glucose agar.
  - Skin biopsy shows subcorneal pustule. However, granulomatous skin lesions show hyperkeratosis and parakeratosis, with dense mixed dermal infiltrate of lymphocytes and plasma cells. PAS stain can identify the organisms in the stratum corneum and/or dermis.
- Treatment; systemic anti-fungal agents. Treatment of any endocrinal or immunologic deficiency.

N. Moftah et al., *Atlas of Common and Rare Genodermatoses*, https://doi.org/10.1007/978-3-031-60788-2_12

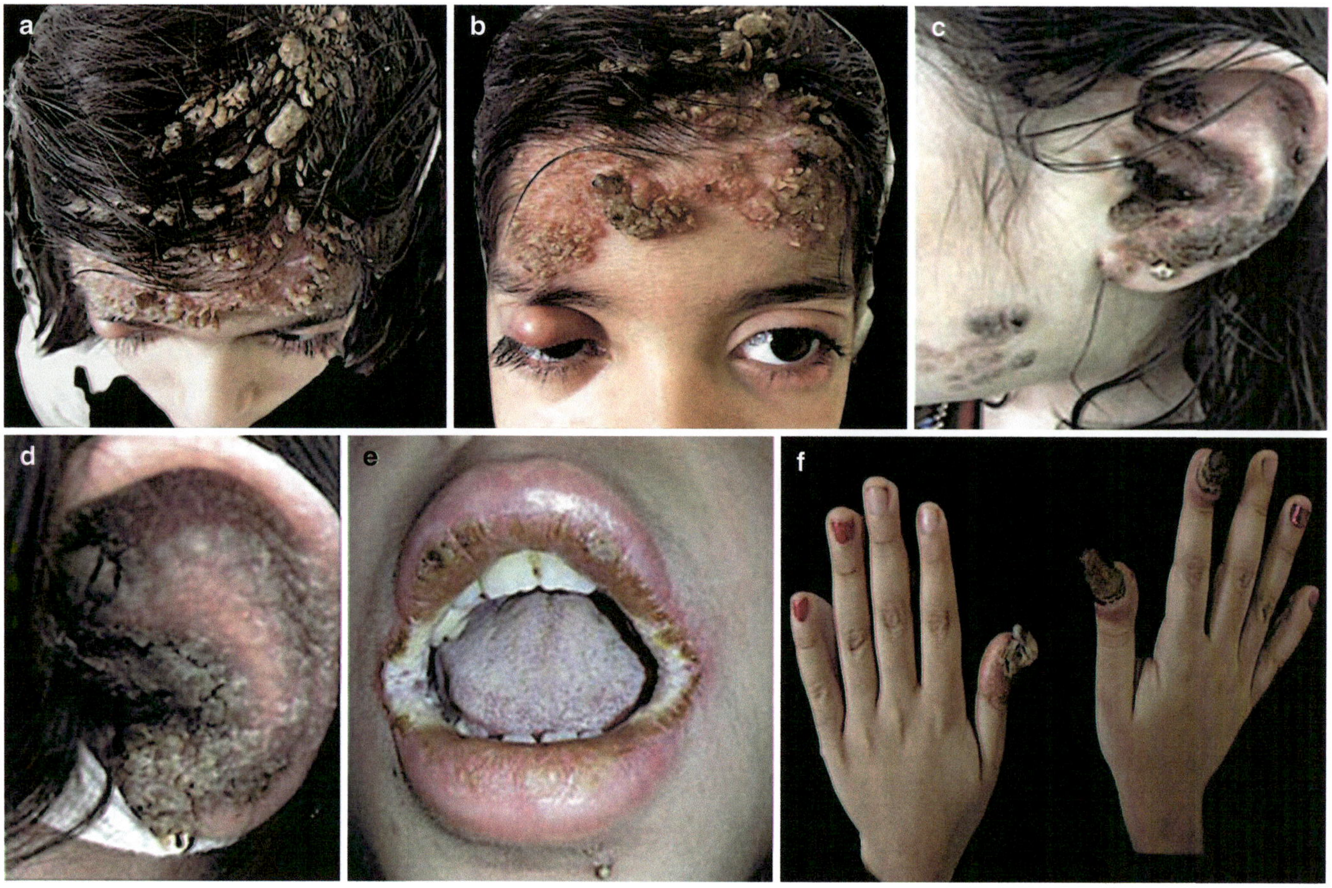

Fig. 12.1 Familial Chronic Mucocutaneous Candidiasis. Crusted granulomatous and erythematous scaly plaques on scalp, eye, and ear with eye infection (**a**–**d**), oral thrush, angular cheilitis (**e**) with paronychia, thickened and black colored nails (**f**). (*Courtesy, Samir Sabry*)

Wiskott-Aldrich Syndrome (XLR) [4, 5] (Fig. 12.2)

- Mutation in the gene encoding WAS protein (*WASp*) inducing a state of immunodeficiency, which ranged from severe phenotype (classic WAS) to milder ones [X-linked thrombocytopenia (XLT) and X-linked neutropenia (XLN)].
- Primary immunodeficiency disorder characterized by classic triad of thrombocytopenia, immunodeficiency, and eczema.
- Incidence; it is a rare genetic disorder, which occurs approximately in 1:100,000 live births. It is seen almost exclusively in males. This condition may be underreported because of misdiagnosing of mild cases as idiopathic thrombocytopenia purpura.
- Clinical features: three main clinical phenotypic manifestations:
  - Classic and severe Wiskott-Aldrich syndrome (WAS):
    Bleeding starts at birth with thrombocytopenia, and it is manifested by petechiae and prolonged bleeding from the umbilical stump or after circumcision. Purpura, hematemesis, melena, epistaxis, hematuria, and life-threatening symptoms as intracranial bleeding commonly occur.
    Immunodeficiency.
    Failure to thrive and multiple recurrent infections (otitis media, sinusitis, pneumonia, sepsis, colitis and meningitis) due to encapsulated organisms (e.g., *Haemophilus influenzae, Streptococcus pneumoniae,* and *Neisseria meningitides*).
    Susceptibility to opportunistic infections with *Pneumocystis jirovecii,* molluscum contagiosum, systemic varicella, and cytomegalovirus infection. Fungal infections are relatively rare consisting of mucocutaneous candidiasis.
    Eczema: classical atopic dermatitis of varying severity develops in approximately 50% of WAS patients during the first year of life. Eosinophilia and elevated serum levels of IgE are often accompanying signs. Allergic rhinitis, asthma, and food allergy-related diseases are also observed.
    Associations:
    - Autoimmune manifestations; hemolytic anemia, neutropenia, vasculitis (small and large vessels), inflammatory bowel disease, and renal diseases.

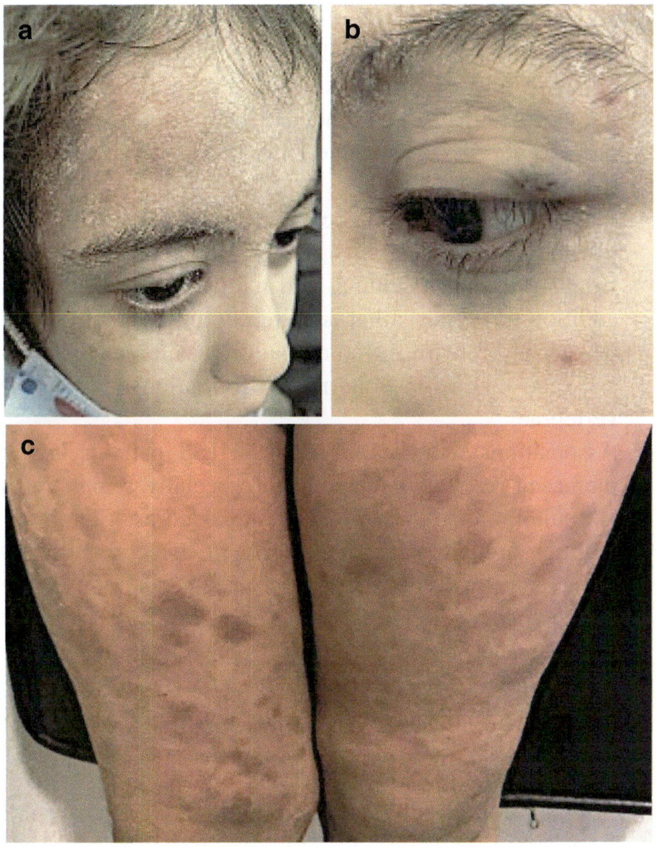

Fig. 12.2 Wiskott-Aldrich syndrome. Atopic-like dermatitis on the face (**a**) and purpuric lesions on eye lid (**b**) and lower extremities (**c**) with history of epistaxis and otitis media

  - Lymphadenopathy and hepatosplenomegaly are frequently present, especially in those WAS patients with chronic eczema.
  - Malignancies: B cell lymphoma (Epstein–Barr virus-positive) and leukemias are frequently present in adolescent and young adult males.
- X-linked neutropenia (XLN) or congenital neutropenia: these patients present with infections characteristic for neutropenia but may also develop infections associated with lymphocyte dysfunction. An elevated risk for myelodysplasia can be present.
- X-linked thrombocytopenia (XLT) or congenital thrombocytopenia: these patients generally have a benign course and good long-term survival, but still carry an increased risk (lower than that for WAS) of life-threatening infections, serious hemorrhage, autoimmune complications, and cancer.

- Diagnosis: the diagnosis of WAS should be suspected in any boy presenting with thrombocytopenia, isolated or accompanied by eczema and/or repeated respiratory infections, autoimmunity, and/or cancer. A confirmatory diagnostic workup must be required;
  - Complete blood picture: thrombocytopenia is a characteristic finding as well as anemia, neutropenia and lymphopenia, especially in the youngest patients.
  - Immune function studies: flow cytometry analysis of lymphocyte subpopulations often shows low CD8 T and B lymphocytes cell counts in children with WAS and lower proportions of memory B cells in adult WAS patients. Low levels of IgM and elevated IgA, with normal IgG concentrations.
  - WASp expression in peripheral blood leukocytes by intracellular staining and flow cytometry provide a quick way to establish a diagnosis of WAS when the result show complete lack of WASp detection.
  - Mutation Analysis in the *WAS* gene is essential for a definitive diagnosis of WAS.
- Prognosis; the prognosis of XLT is good with the life expectancy as close to the normal population, but classic WAS has a poor prognosis with decreased life expectancy due to recurrent infections, autoimmune disease, and malignancy. Bleeding is most frequently the cause of death in these patients.

Hyper-IgE Syndrome (Job Syndrome) (AD/AR) [6, 7] (Figs. 12.3, 12.4, and 12.5)

- Inheritance: Two form of hyper-IgE syndrome (HIES) have been described;
  - Autosomal dominant (AD, or type 1), associated with heterozygous mutations in the transcription factor *STAT3*.
  - Autosomal recessive (AR, or type 2), associated with *DOCK8* deficiency. Most patients with AR-HIES are from consanguineous families.
- Hyper-IgE Syndrome (HIES), previously Job's syndrome, is a rare primary immunodeficiency characterized by skin

abscesses, lung infections, recurrent eczema, eosinophilia and high serum levels of IgE (greater than 2000 IU/mL).

- Incidence; affects fewer than 1:1,000,000 population, with equal sex predilection.
- Clinical features;
  - Characteristic facies and dentition; these features evolve in AD-HIES during childhood and become more established by adolescence. There is an asymmetric facial appearance, with prominent forehead and chin, deep-set eyes, broad nose, thickened facial skin, and a high arched palate. Retention of primary teeth, even after the permanent teeth have erupted, is a consistent finding, and double rows of retained primary teeth overlaying the permanent ones are identified on panoramic X-ray views.
- Skin affection; eczema-like rashes and pustular lesions occur on the face and scalp due to infections with *Staphylococcus aureus*. Skin and nail infections with candida are common in both AD- and AR-HIES. The severity and the onset of manifestations are different according to the form of the syndrome;
  - In AD-HIES *(STAT3* mutation), lesions begin within the first 2 weeks of newborn, and cold abscess is common, with the absence of external signs of inflammation despite the presence of pus.
  - In AR-HIES (*DOCK8* deficiency) patients, lesions start early in life, although not necessarily in the newborn period. They also suffer from recurrent skin abscesses in addition to severe recurrent or persistent skin viral infections with herpes simplex, herpes zoster, and molluscum contagiosum.
- Lung affection; recurrent bacterial pneumonias are often encountered in childhood with AD-HIES due to *Staphylococcus aureus*, *Streptococcus pneumoniae*, and *Haemophilus influenzae* and fungal infections (*Aspergillus fumigatus*). These pneumonias may present with fewer symptoms; however, significant tissue damage with pneumatocele formation can occur before identification and initiation of appropriate therapy.
- Skeletal abnormalities occur only in AD-HIES and include hyperextensibility of the joints, bone fractures from insignificant trauma, and reduced bone density in addition to scoliosis that is common during adolescence or later in life with fusion of skull bones (craniosynostosis) and extra or abnormally formation of ribs or vertebrae.
- Associations; both AD- and AR-HIES patients are at increased risk for malignancies (especially lymphomas) and autoimmune diseases. Medium-sized arterial abnormalities predominate, particularly in the coronary and intracranial vasculature with ectasia and aneurysm. These are associated arterial hypertension, silent cerebral infarcts, and vasculitis. *DOCK8* deficient patients have more symptomatic neurologic diseases (facial paralysis, hemiplegia, and encephalitis) than those who have *STAT3* deficiency.
- Laboratory findings:
  - Complete blood picture: in both forms of the syndrome, high total white blood cell counts, but may not be increased during acute infection. Differential counting revealed high eosinophil numbers and neutropenia. Increased serum IgE concentrations (>2000 IU/mL), without elevation of serum IgG, IgA, and IgM, although some individuals with AD-HIES have deficiencies in one or more of these immunoglobulin subtypes.

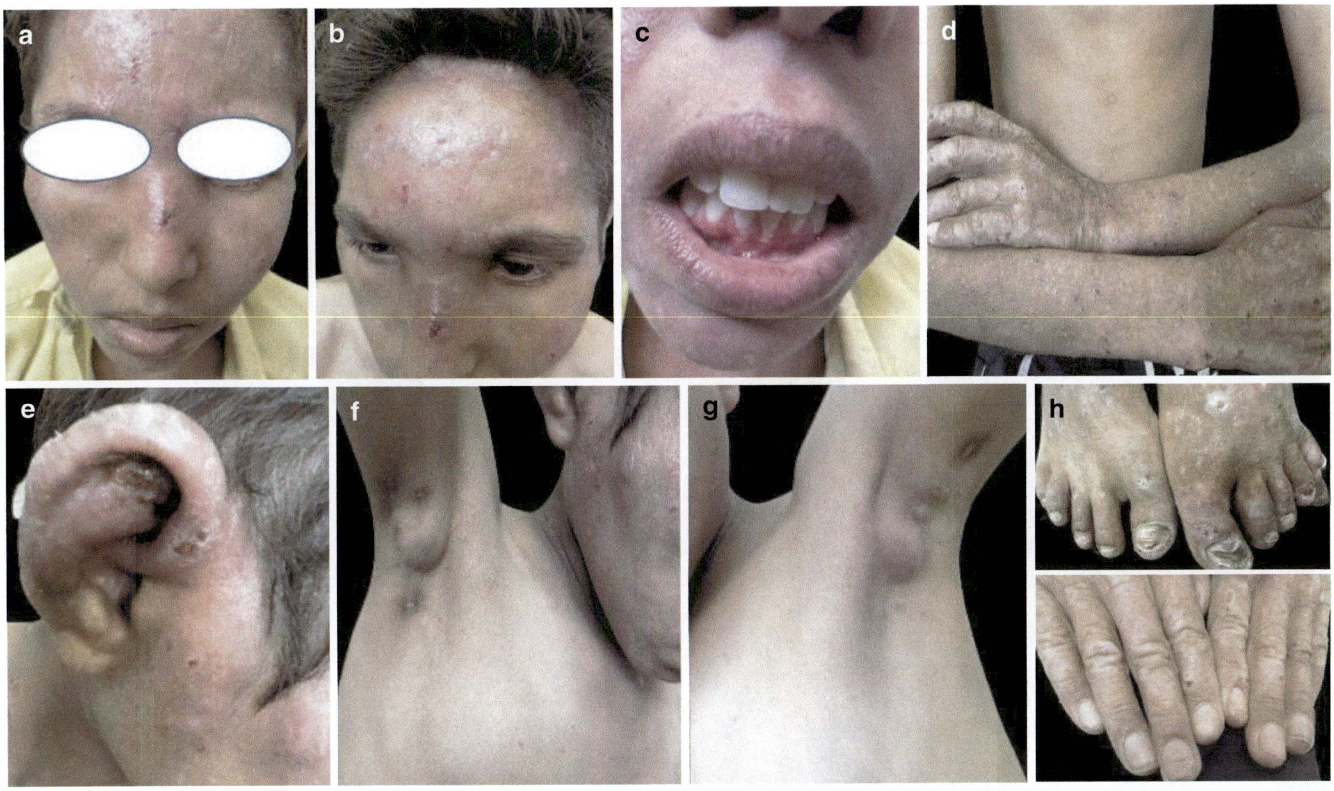

Fig. 12.3 **Hyper-IgE syndrome:** Asymmetry of the face, prominent forehead, sunken eyes, pitted scars, broad nasal bridge, wide fleshy nasal tip, prognathism (**a**–**c**), eczema-like lesions of forearms and hands (**d**), infection of ears (**e**), cold abscesses in axillae of both sides and scars of excision of previous cold abscesses (**f**, **g**) with nail dystrophy (**h**)

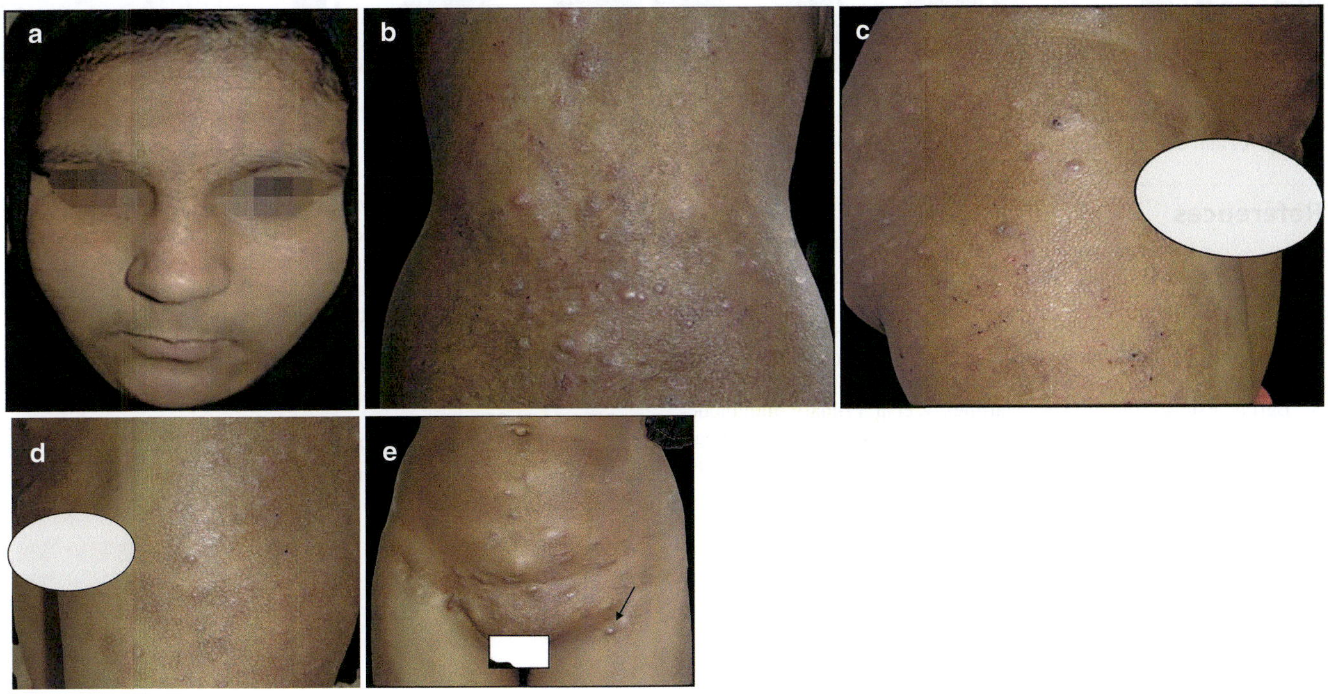

Fig. 12.4 Hyper-IgE syndrome. Sunken eyes, broad nasal bridge, wide fleshy nasal tip (**a**), eczema-like lesions on back, buttocks, and thighs (**b**–**d**), cold tender abscesses in back (**b**), lower abdomen, and genitalia with scars of excision of previous ones (**e**)

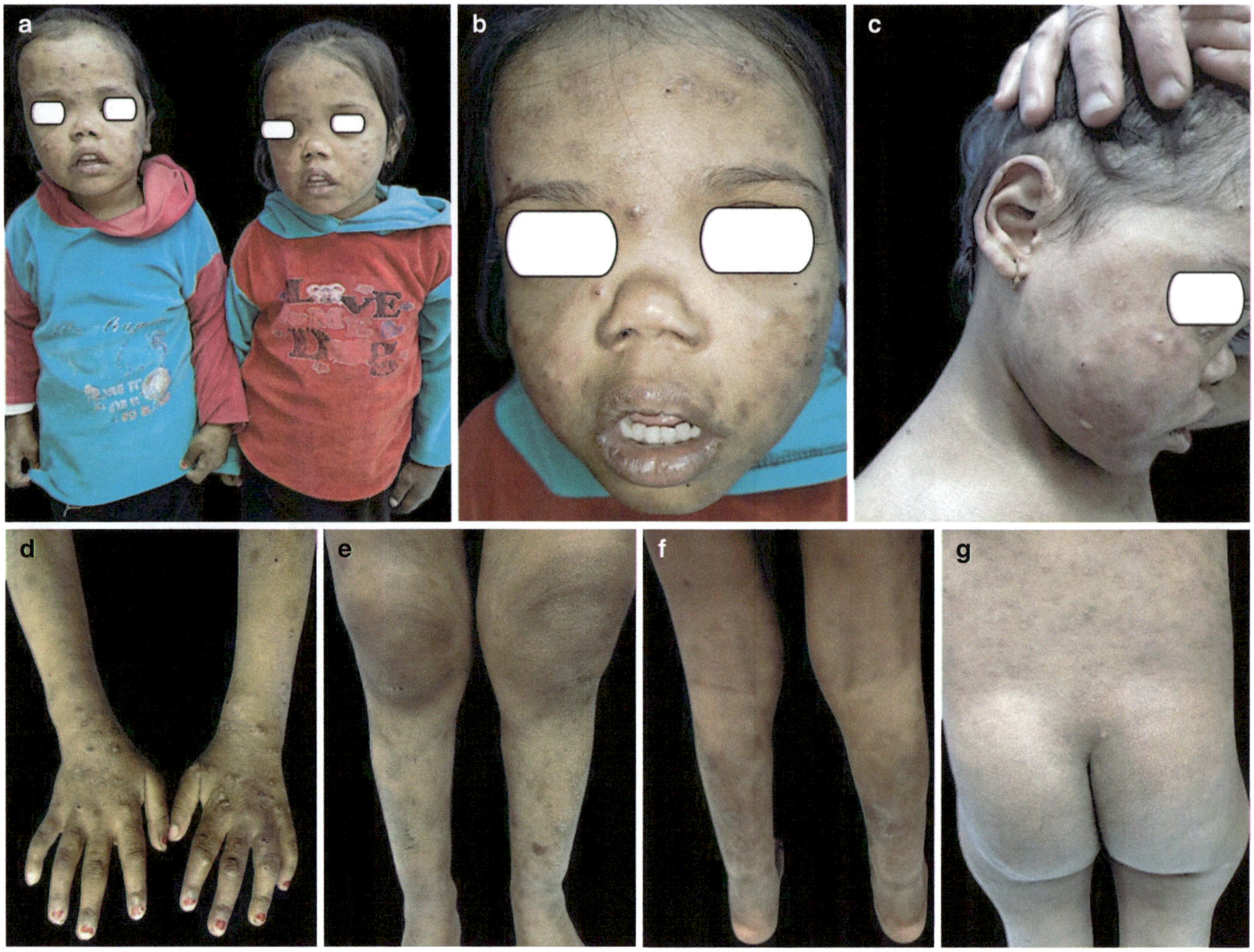

Fig. 12.5 Hyper-IgE syndrome (twins with similar presentation). Sunken eyes, broad nasal bridge, wide fleshy nasal tip, pustular lesions on the face (**a–c**) and extrimities (**d–f**) and eczema-like lesions on back, buttocks (**g**)

References

1. Kirkpatrick CH. Chronic mucocutaneous candidiasis. Pediatr Infect Dis J. 2001;20(2):197–206.
2. Puel A, Cypowyj S, Maródi L, et al. Inborn errors of human IL-17 immunity underlie chronic mucocutaneous candidiasis. Curr Opin Allergy Clin Immunol. 2012;12(6):616–22.
3. Egri N, Esteve-Solé A, Deyà-Martinez A, et al. Primary immunodeficiency and chronic mucocutaneous candidiasis: pathophysiological, diagnostic, and therapeutic approaches. Allergol Immunopathol (Madr). 2021;49(1):118–27.
4. Ochs HD, Filipovich AH, Veys P, et al. Wiskott-Aldrich syndrome: diagnosis, clinical and laboratory manifestations, and treatment. Biol Blood Marrow Transplant. 2009;15(1 Suppl):84–90.
5. Candotti F. Clinical manifestations and pathophysiological mechanisms of the Wiskott-Aldrich syndrome. J Clin Immunol. 2018;38(1):13–27.
6. Tsilifis C, Freeman AF, Gennery AR. STAT3 hyper-IgE syndrome—an update and unanswered questions. J Clin Immunol. 2021;41(5):864–80.
7. Saikia B, Rawat A, Minz RW, et al. Clinical profile of hyper-IgE syndrome in India. Front Immunol. 2021;12:1–9.

Miscellaneous

13

A very rare collection of miscellaneous group of genodermatoses is presented her which are:

- **Lesch-Nyhan syndrome**
- **GAPO syndrome**
- **Phakomatosis pigmentokeratotica**
- **Aplasia cutis congenita and membranous aplasia cutis congenita**
- **Bart syndrome**
- **Adams-Oliver Syndrome**
- **Prolidase deficiency**
- **Brauer Syndrome**
- **H syndrome**
- **Epidermodysplasia verruciformis**
- **Turner syndrome**

Lesch-Nyhan Syndrome (X-Linked Recessive) [1–3] (Fig. 13.1)

- A rare inborn error of purine metabolism characterized by absence or deficiency of the activity of hypoxanthine-guanine phosphoribosyltransferase enzyme (*HPRT*).
- Due to mutations in the *HPRT1* gene located on the X chromosome.
- Inherited in X-linked recessive pattern, most often affects males, with rare female exceptions.
- Uric acid levels are abnormally high in people with Lesch-Nyhan syndrome and sodium urate crystals abnormally accumulate in the joints and kidneys.
- Clinical characteristics: three major hallmarks: neurologic dysfunction, cognitive and behavioral disturbances including self-mutilation, and uric acid overproduction (hyperuricemia).
- Neurologic dysfunction:
  - Hypotonia and developmental delay, which are evident by 3–6 months of age.
  - Lack of speech.
  - Irritability is most often noticed along with the first signs of nervous system impairment.
  - Extrapyramidal involvement with dystonia, choreoathetosis, and opisthotonus.
  - Pyramidal system involvement, including spasticity, hyperreflexia, and extensor plantar reflexes, also occur.
- Cognitive and behavioral disturbances:
  - Uncontrollable self-injury usually begins at 3 years of age.
  - Biting of the lips and tongue then finger biting and headbanging.
  - Compulsive behaviors also occur, including aggressiveness, vomiting, spitting, and coprolalia.
- Uric acid overproduction:
  - Sand-like crystals of uric acid in the diapers of the affected infant (orange color).
  - Uric acid crystals or stones in the kidneys, ureters, or bladder.
  - Gout-like arthritis, with swelling and tenderness of the joints.
  - Hematuria, increased risk of urinary tract infection, and kidney failure by the accumulated stones.
- **Kelley-Seegmiller syndrome:** A less severe form of Lesch-Nyhan syndrome with partial HPRT deficiency and less neurological involvement but the disease still causes gout and kidney stones.
- **Diagnosis:** urate to creatinine concentration ratio in urine/activity of the HGPRT enzyme in cells from any type of tissue (e.g., blood, cultured fibroblasts, or lymphoblasts) that is less than 1.5% of normal enzyme activity confirms the diagnosis of Lesch-Nyhan syndrome.
- **Prognosis**: death is usually due to kidney failure or complications from hypotonia, in the first or second decade of life. Less severe forms have better prognosis.
- **Treatment**: mainly symptomatic/Allopurinol to control excessive amounts of uric acid/carbidopa, levodopa, diazepam, phenobarbital, or haloperidol for neurological symptoms.

N. Moftah et al., *Atlas of Common and Rare Genodermatoses*, https://doi.org/10.1007/978-3-031-60788-2_13

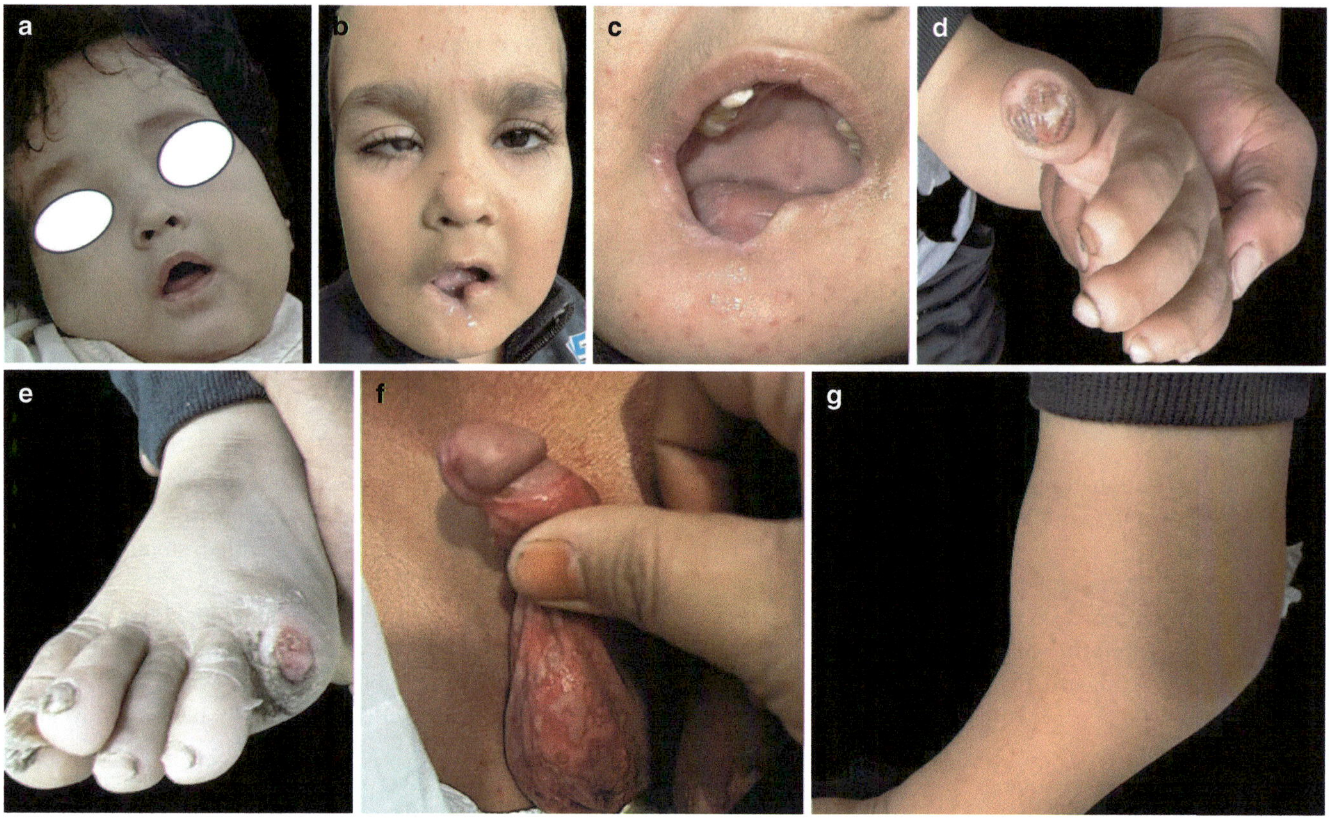

Fig. 13.1 Lesch-Nyhan syndrome. Male child was normal at birth (**a**) till 6 months where it is presented with mutilation in the lip, ocular cataract, and squint (**b**), dermatophagia with severe mutilation in the lip (**b**, **c**), fingers, toes (**d**, **e**), penis with yellow urate crystals (**f**), arthritis with swelling of elbow joint (**g**)

GAPO Syndrome (AR) [4–6] (Fig. 13.2)

- A very rare autosomal recessive disorder caused by biallelic mutations of the *ANTXR1* gene, which encodes Anthrax Toxin Receptor 1.
- The *ANTXR1* gene is critical for the creation of actin, and its disruption inhibits proper function of the actin network with subsequent buildup of extracellular matrix and degraded cell adhesions.
- The first case of GAPO syndrome was reported by Anderson and Pindborg in 1947. Another case was not recorded until 1978 by Fuks et al.
- **Clinical characteristics**: GAPO is an acronym that encompasses the predominant traits of the disorder: ***G***rowth retardation (G), ***A***lopecia (A), ***P***seudoanodontia (P), and ***O***ptic atrophy (O).
- Growth retardation, with slow skeletal bones formation (patients are below average height).
- Alopecia, the hair is typically thin and fragile, which often leads to early baldness.
- Teeth growth may be stunted, fail to emerge form the gums (pseudoanodontia) or develop normally.
- Optic atrophy occurs in approximately one-third of individuals with inhibited peripheral vision, and color blindness.
- Coarse facial features, abnormal structure of the middle portion of the face, with a large forehead, depressed nasal bridge, protruding ears, and abnormally thick lips, have been reported but are not considered unique to GAPO syndrome.
- In some patients, veins can be observed through the skin on the head, and the pulse can be heard through the scalp. Additional symptoms include loose skin, hernia, short fingers and toes, glaucoma, delayed sexual development, and brain abnormalities.
- **Prognosis**: bad with high incidence of premature death.
- **Treatment**: no available treatment. Even corrective lenses or corticosteroids failed to correct optic nerve manifestions.

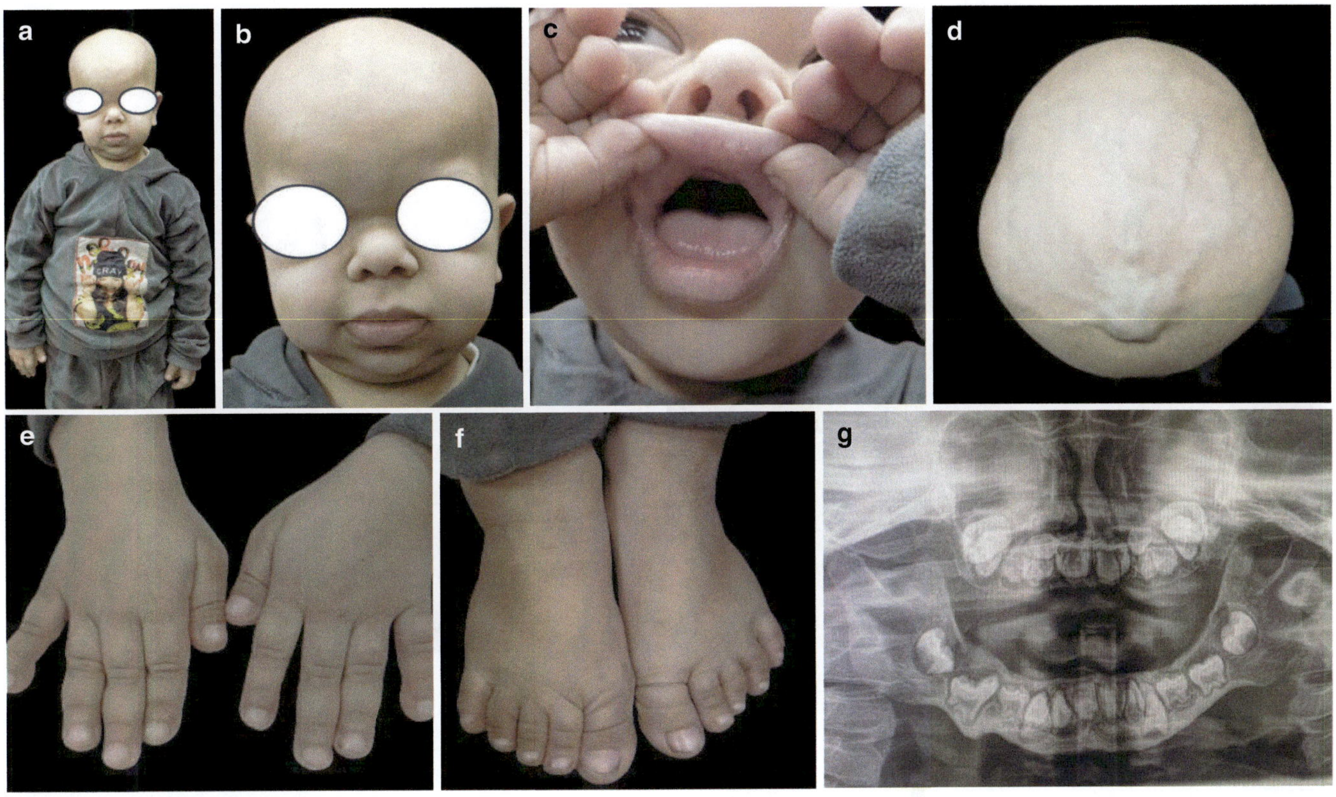

Fig. 13.2 GAPO syndrome. A 12-years-old girl with short stature (**a**), alopecia of the scalp, eye brows and lashes, coarse facial features with a large forehead, depressed nasal bridge, protruding ears, and abnormally thick lip (**b**), pseudoanodontia (**c**), dilated visible veins in the occiput (**d**), short fingers and toes (**e**, **f**). Panoramic X-ray showing the presence of non-erupted teeth (**g**). (*Courtesy, Nada Shaaban Mohamed)*

Phakomatosis Pigmentokeratotica (PPK) (AR) [7, 8] (Fig. 13.3)

- Cooccurrence of organoid nevus with sebaceous differentiation arranged along Blaschko lines, and speckled lentiginous nevus (SLN) of the papular type (papular nevus spilus) arranged in a checkerboard pattern.
- PPK is a distinct type of epidermal nevus syndrome.
- It is divided into two subgroups according to the presence or absence of extracutaneous involvements "Schimmelpenning syndrome" and "speckled lentiginous nevus (SLN)," respectively.
- PPK represented an example of the genetic mechanism "twin spotting."
- To impute "twin spotting," it is necessary for the two different recessive mutations to be located on the same chromosome.
- The chromosomes bearing these loci would then be exchanged through somatic crossing over in the early stages of embryogenesis, giving rise to two different homologous daughter cells that evolve into two different mosaic lesions.
- The common extracutaneous features include skeletal defects as bone cysts, kyphosis and scoliosis, foot and hand deformities, neurologic defects as hemimegalencephaly with contralateral motor disease, and ocular abnormalities, including coloboma and epibulbar lipodermoid. The epidermal nevi with sebaceous differentiation in PPK have greater potential to develop true basal cell carcinoma.
- The presented patient had no extracutaneous features or malignant degeneration, however, extracutaneous involvements reported in the literature indicate that we should monitor such patients carefully.

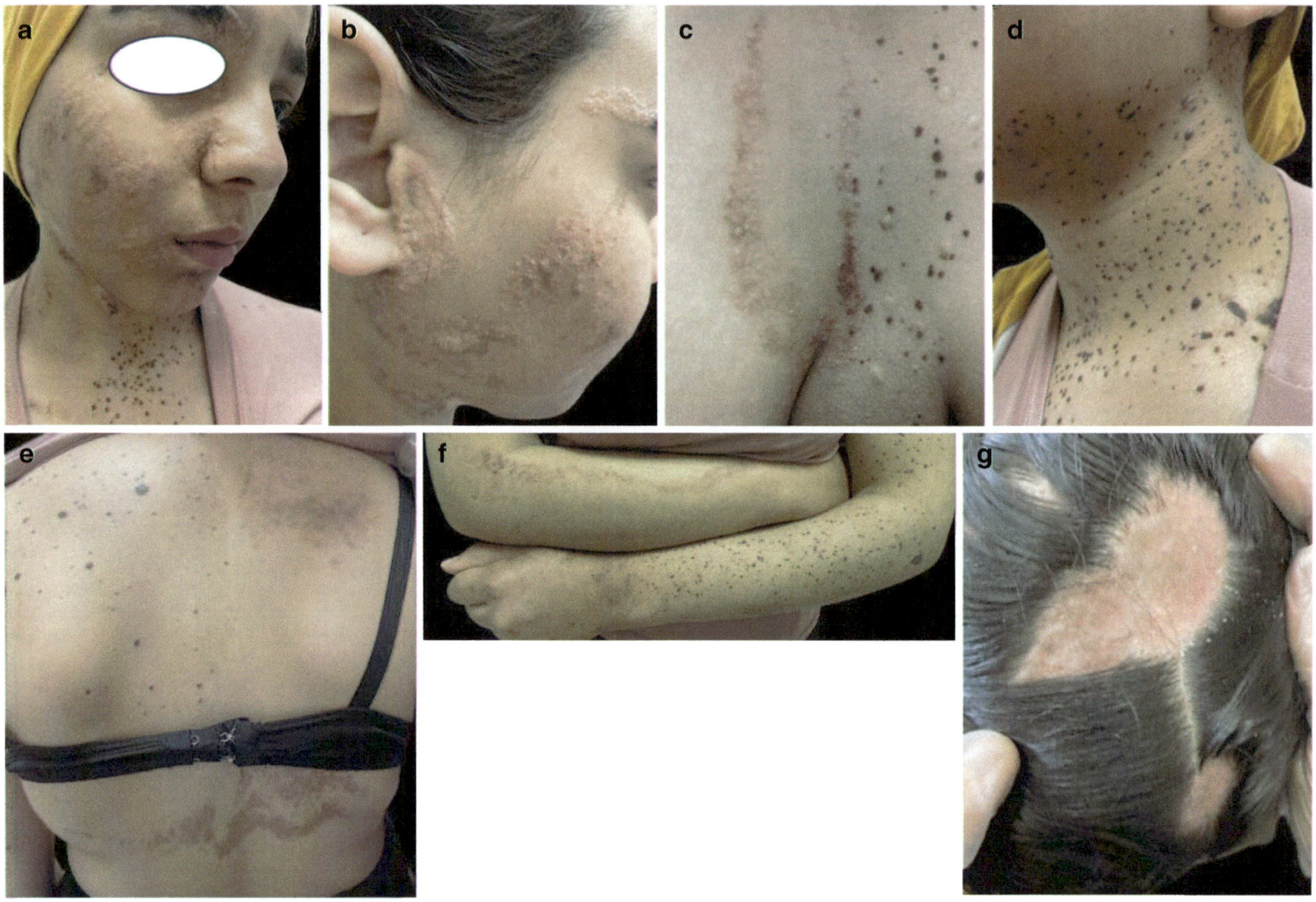

Fig. 13.3 Phakomatosis pigmentokeratotica. A 15-years-old female with epidermal verrucous nevus on the right side of the body along Blashko lines and speckled lentiginous nevus on the left side of the body (**a**–**f**). The epidermal verrucous nevus showing sebaceous differentiation on the face (**a**, **b**). Note multiple patched of nevus sebaceous in the scalp (**g**)

Aplasia Cutis Congenita (AD, AR) [9–14]

- A heterogenous group of disorders characterized by the absence of a portion of skin in a localized or widespread area at birth.
- Typically sporadic; however, autosomal dominant and, less commonly autosomal recessive cases have also been reported. Mutations in the ribosomal GTPase *BMS1* have been identified as one cause of autosomal dominant aplasia cutis congenita. Familial aplasia cutis congenita on the scalp is generally non-membranous, whereas membranous aplasia cutis congenita of the scalp is usually sporadic.
- The lesions are non-inflammatory and well-demarcated, ranging widely in size. They may be circular, oval, linear, or stellate in configuration.
- At birth, the lesions may have already healed with scarring or may remain superficially eroded to deeply ulcerated, occasionally involving the dura or the meninges. Defects in the skin that form early in gestation may heal before delivery and appear as an atrophic, membranous, bullous, or parchment-like scar with associated alopecia, whereas less mature defects present as ulcerations.
- The membranous type of aplasia cutis congenita is most common.
- Associated findings include hair collar sign, hydrocephaly, spasticity, epilepsy, cleft palate, primary optic nerve atrophy, meningeal arteriovenous fistula, corneal lipodermoid changes, cornea scleralization, nevus flammeus, and infantile hemangioma.
- Frieden [9] created a classification system for aplasia cutis congenita consisting of nine groups based on the number and location of the lesions and the presence or absence of associated malformations.

Membranous Aplasia Cutis Congenita [12–14] (Fig. 13.4)

- An abortive form of a neural tube defect.
- The hair collar sign (dome shaped hairless nodule, surrounded by hypertrichosis) regarded as a relatively specific marker for cranial neural tube closure defects, is frequently seen.
- The diagnosis is clinical and a biopsy is not needed.

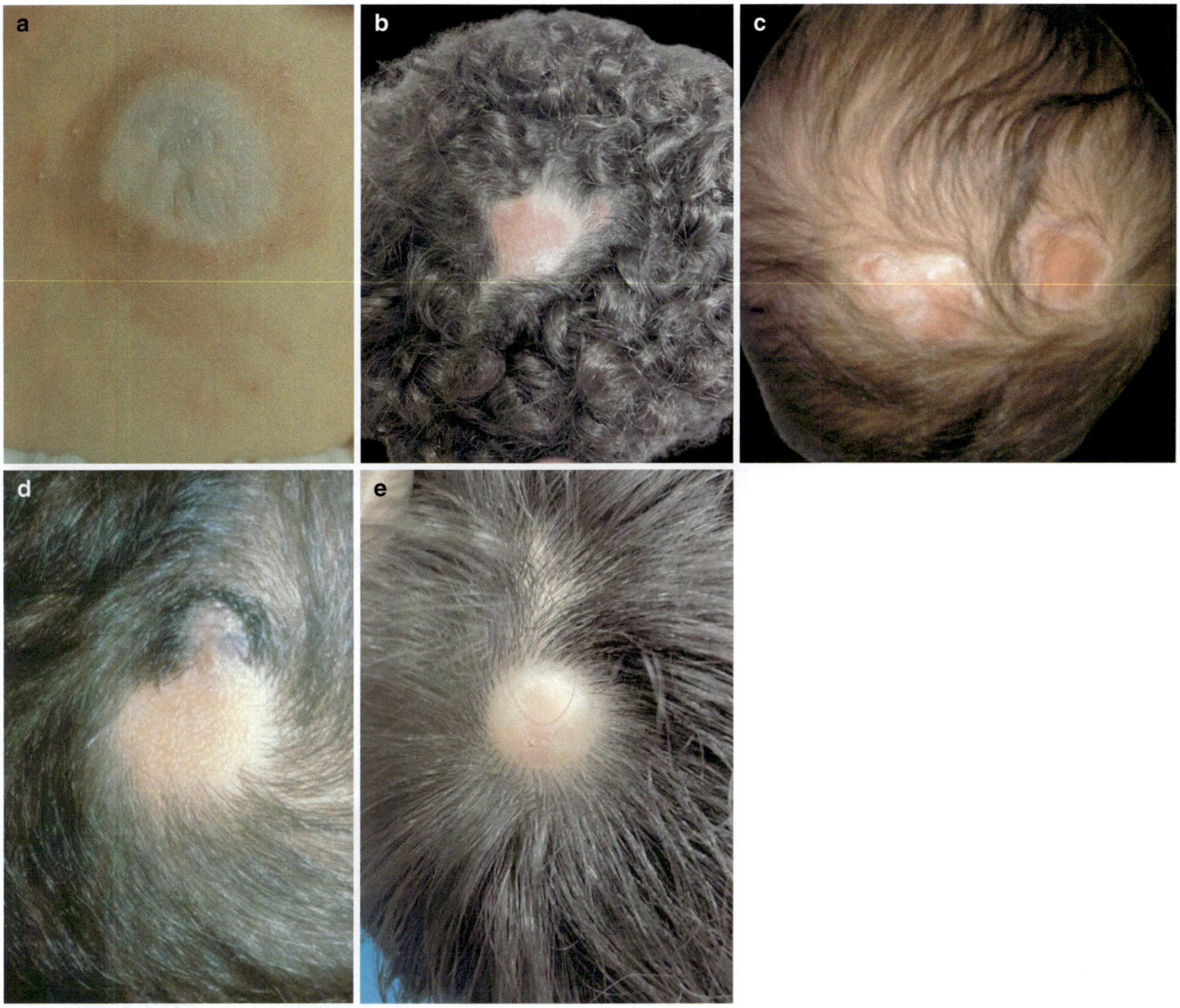

Fig. 13.4 Aplasia cutis congenita. Well-demarcated circular patch on the abdomen (**a**), Erythematous alopecic patches on the vertex of the scalp (**b**, **c**) alopecic patches with hair collar sign (**d**, **e**)

- A sonography of the lesion and a transfontanelar sonography should be done to rule out skull defects or cerebral abnormalities.
- It can be visualized on prenatal sonography as a smooth cystic lesion without flow.
- Conservative therapy is the option of choice.

Bart Syndrome [15] (Aplasia Cutis + Epidermolysis Bullosa) (Fig. 13.5)

- This is aplasia cutis congenita associated with any type of epidermolysis bullosa (simplex, junctional, or dystrophic).
- Autosomal dominant inheritance, caused by mutations in the *GJB2* gene responsible for making a protein called gap junction beta 2, more commonly known as connexin 26.
- Many reports described aplasia cutis congenita usually occurring on the lower extremities.
- A subgroup includes the association of pyloric or duodenal atresia, ureteral stenosis, renal abnormalities, craniofacial abnormalities, and nail dystrophy.

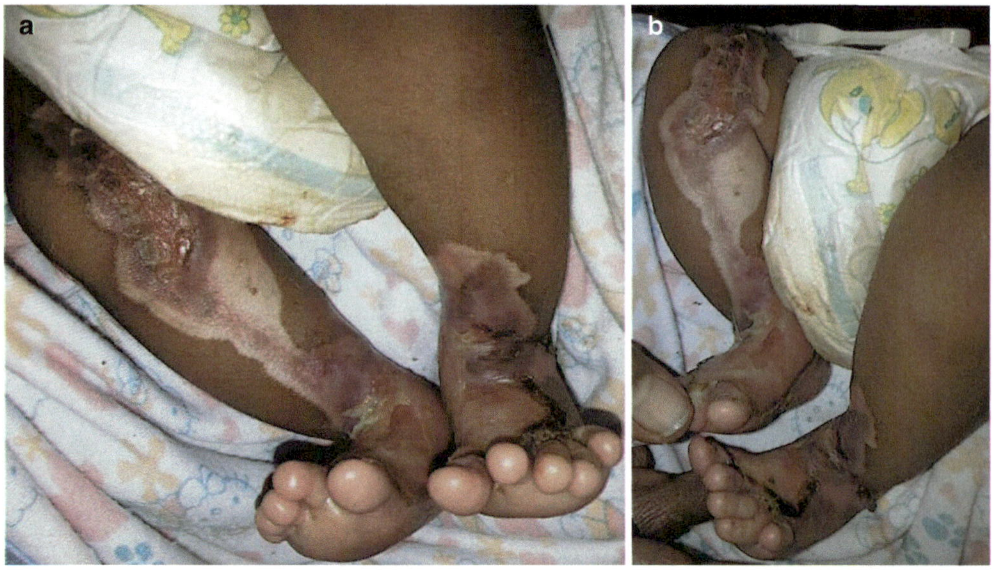

Fig. 13.5 Bart syndrome. Congenital lower limb aplasia cutis with dystrophic epidermolysis bullosa (**a**, **b**)

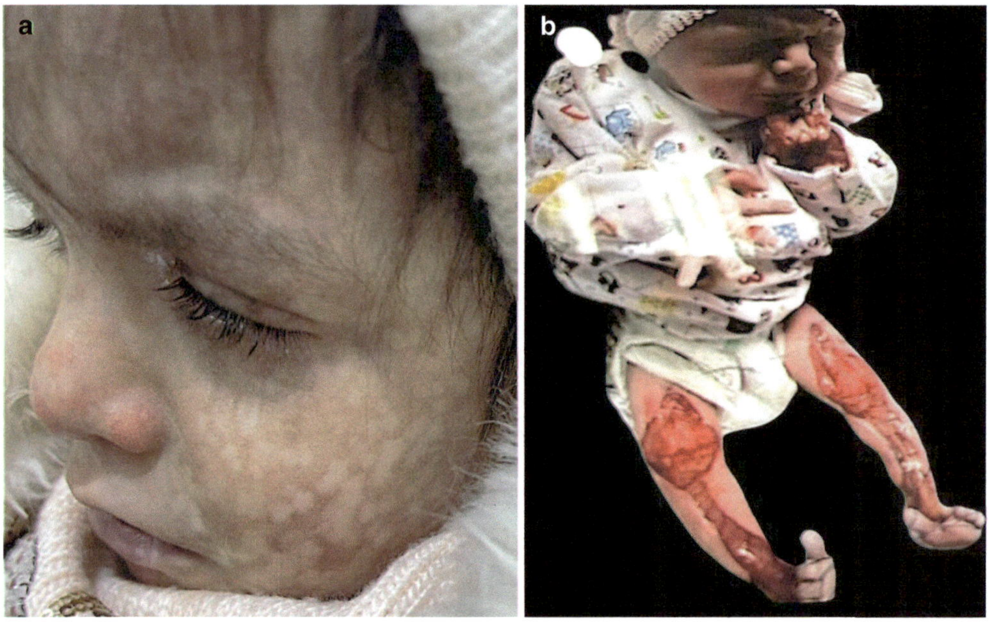

Fig. 13.6 Adams-Oliver syndrome. Facial cutis marmorata telangiectatica congenita (**a**). Severe limbs aplasia cutis (at birth) (**b**)

Adams-Oliver Syndrome (AD, AR or Sporadic) [16, 17] (Aplasia Cutis + Limb Defect) (Figs. 13.6, 13.7, and 13.8)

- A distinct disorder in which distal limb reduction abnormalities are found in association with solitary midline scalp defects.
- Mutations in the *ARHGAP31*, *DLL4*, *NOTCH1*, or *RBPJ*
- In this group of aplasia cutis congenita, the scalp lesions tend to be large. The most common limb malformation is hypoplastic or absent distal phalanges, but the severity of limb anomalies ranges from minor defects such as an absent nail or broad fingertip to more severe involvement. Limb anomalies are usually asymmetric and more commonly involve the lower extremities.
- Other anomalies may include cutis marmorata telangiectatica congenita, hemangiomas, cranial arteriovenous malformation, congenital heart defects, skin tags, supernumerary nipples, and woolly hair.

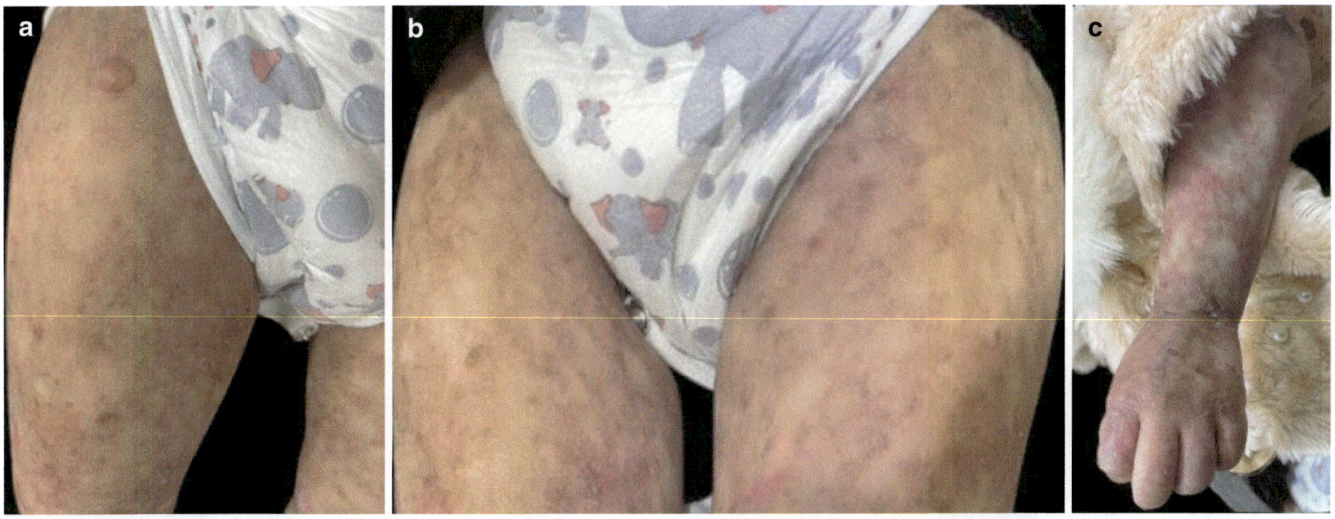

Fig. 13.7 Adams-Oliver syndrome. Cutis marmorata telangiectatica congenita (**a**–**c**) with bullous eruption in the upper thigh (**a**)

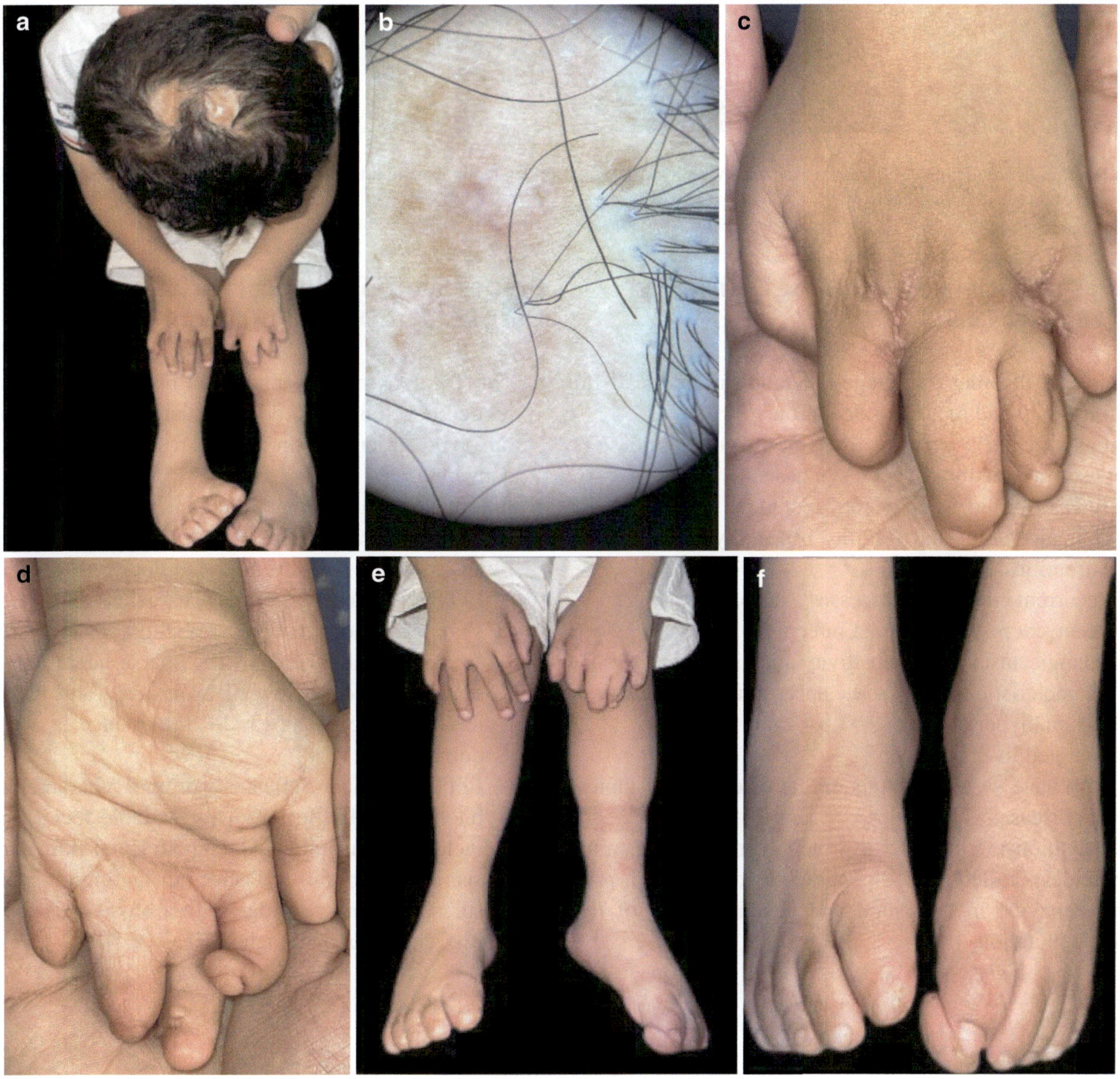

Fig. 13.8 Adams-Oliver syndrome. Midline scalp aplasia cutis (**a**), dermoscopic view of the scalp alopecic patch (**b**), left hand syndactly (**c**, **d**), and transverse terminal lower left limb reduction for which he had reconstructive surgery (**e**) and dysplastic big toe of the left foot (**f**)

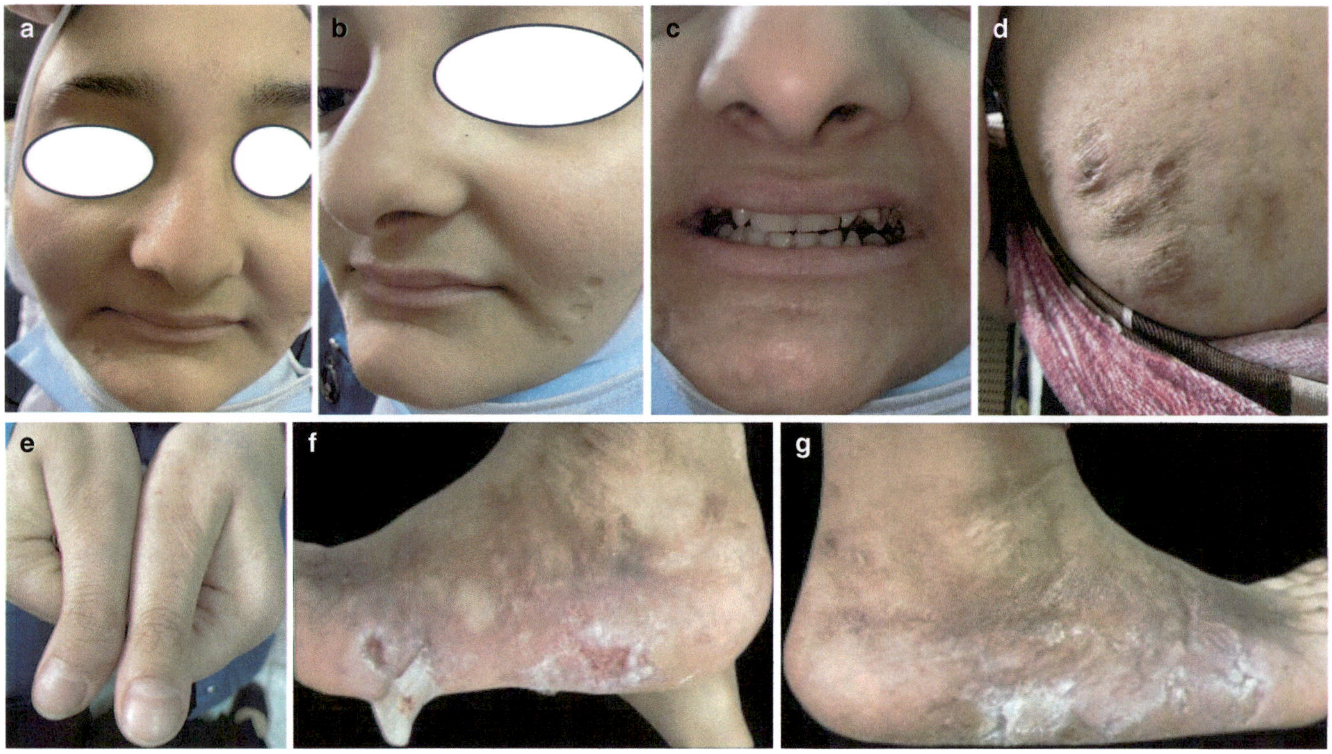

Fig. 13.9 Prolidase deficiency. Characteristic facies with hypertelorism (**a**, **b**), teeth abnormalities (**c**), scarring gluteal ulcers (**d**), skeletal abnormalities of hands (**e**), and feet ulcers (**f**, **g**)

Prolidase Deficiency (Peptidase Deficiency) (AR) [18] (Fig. 13.9)

- A rare AR disorder of collagen metabolism that leads to skin fragility and recurrent ulcerations.
- Mutation in *PEPD* gene encoding the enzyme prolidase D that uses proline for collagen synthesis.
- Features of prolidase deficiency include:
  - Skin ulceration and fragility especially of the lower extremities.
  - Recurrent cutaneous abscesses and folliculitis.
  - Recurrent respiratory tract infections.
  - Telangiectasia, photosensitivity and hirsutism.
  - Characteristic facies (saddle nose, small chin, jaw protrusion, hypertelorism).
  - Enlarged liver or spleen.
  - 10% have systemic lupus erythematosus or a lupus-like disease.
- Investigations: Urine specific proteins (proline-containing dipeptides) (called imidodipeptiduria), low levels of prolidase enzyme in the blood and genetic testing of the genetic mutation.

Brauer Syndrome (Focal Facial Dermal Dysplasia) (AD, AD) [19] (Fig. 13.10)

- The focal dermal dysplasias (FFDDs) are a group of related developmental defects characterized by bitemporal or preauricular skin lesions resembling aplasia cutis congenita.
- Inheritance is autosomal dominant.
- Cervantes-Barragan et al. [19] proposed a classification of FFDD in which there are four subtypes:
  - FFDD1 (Brauer syndrome) characterized by temporal skin depressions that resemble "forceps marks." Other facial anomalies, comprising sparse lateral eyebrows, distichiasis (extra row of eyelashes), and a flattened nasal tip, are usually mild. Inheritance is autosomal dominant.
  - FFFD2 (Brauer-Setleis syndrome) characterized by bitemporal skin lesions with variable facial findings, including thin and puckered periorbital skin, distichiasis, and/or absent eyelashes, upslanting palpebral fissures, a flat nasal bridge with a broad nasal tip, large lips, and redundant facial skin.

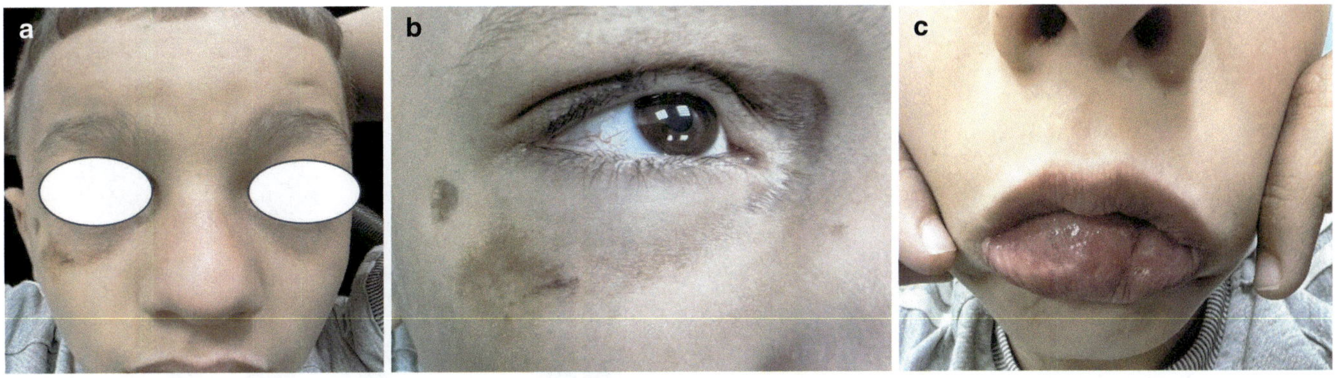

Fig. 13.10 Brauer syndrome. Periorbital hyperpigmented scar-like depressions (**a**, **b**), distichiasis (extra row of eyelashes) (**b**) and groove on the lower lip (**c**). (*Courtesy, Hayder Al-Darraji*)

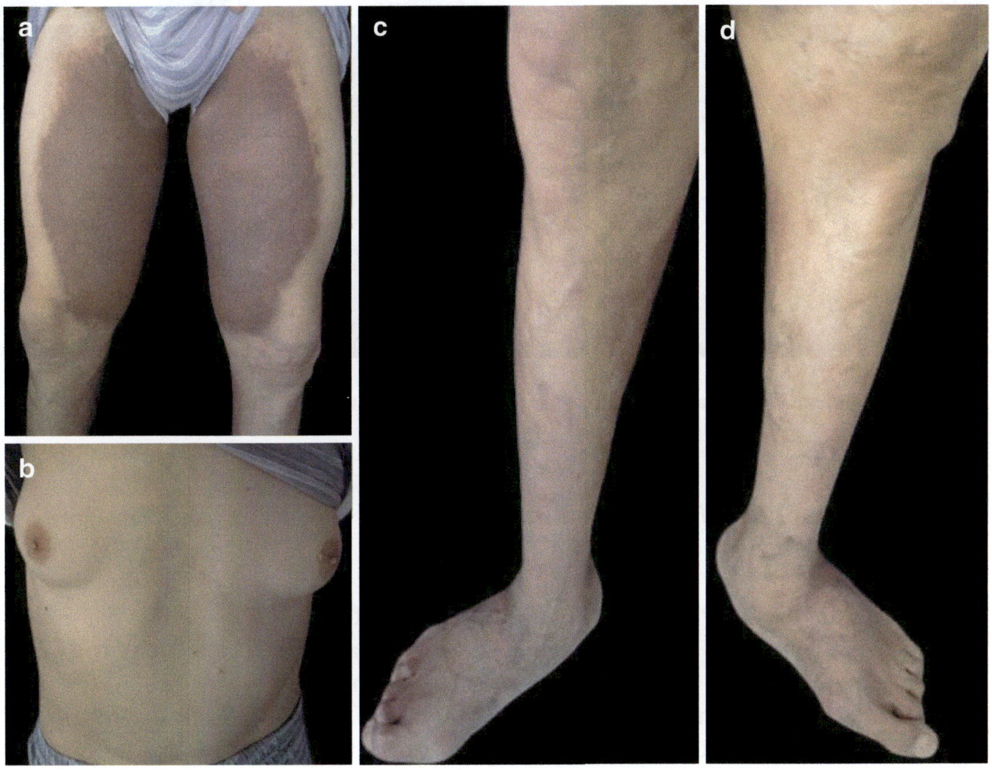

Fig. 13.11 H syndrome. Hyperpigmented, indurated symmetrical plaques on inner aspect of thigh (**a**), gynecomastia (**b**), and Hallux valgus (**c**, **d**)

- FFDD3 (Setleis syndrome) characterized by the same facial features as FFDD2, but the inheritance is autosomal recessive.
- FFDD4 characterized by isolated, preauricular skin lesions with autosomal dominant or recessive inheritance.

H Syndrome (AR) [20] (Fig. 13.11)

- A rare syndrome caused by mutations in the *SLC29A3* gene which encodes the human equilibrative nucleoside transporter 3, a protein found in endosomes, lysosomes, and mitochondria.
- It is now considered a novel form of histiocytosis.
- Features of **H** syndrome include:
  - **H**yperpigmention: Symmetrical cutaneous hyperpigmentation involving inner thighs accompanied by hypertrichosis and sclerodermatous induration are the most common features and considered hallmark of the disease.
  - **H**ypertrichosis.
  - **H**epatosplenomegaly.
  - **H**earing loss.
  - **H**eart anomalies.
  - **H**ypogonadism.
  - **H**yperglycemia.
  - **H**ypovitaminosis.
  - Low **H**eight.
  - **H**allux valgus.

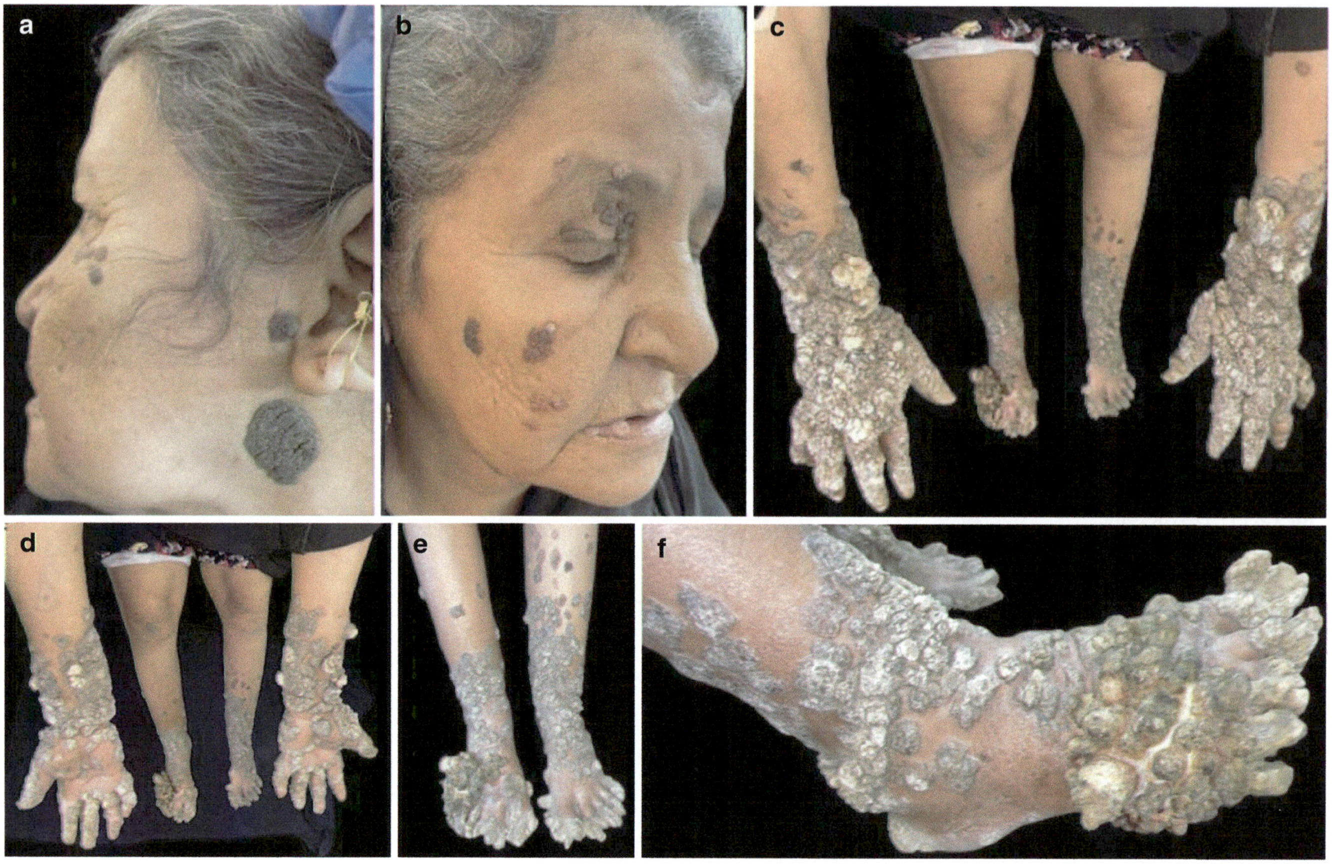

Fig. 13.12 Epidermodysplasia verruciformis (Tree-man disease). Multiple wart-like skin growths on the face (**a**, **b**), upper and lower extremities (**c**–**f**)

Epidermodysplasia Verruciformis (AR) [21] (Tree-Man Disease)

- A rare skin disorder with increased susceptibility to human papillomavirus due to mutation in genes that encode transmembrane proteins that interact with the zinc transporters affecting intracellular zinc distribution.
- Clinical features include wart-like skin growths resembling tree bark. The bark-like growths are extremely painful and disfiguring. They can become quite large, which leads to substantial disability.
- Classification is based on suspected cause:
  - Classic genetic: *EVER1/TMC6* and *EVER2/TMC8* genes mutation.
  - Non-classic genetic: *RHOH, MST-1, CORO1A,* and *ECM1* genes mutation.
  - Acquired: HIV, organ transplant drugs and lymphoma.
- The risk of malignant transformation to squamous cell carcinoma is high (Fig. 13.12).

Turner Syndrome [22] (Fig. 13.13)

- A genetic disorder that affects only females, results when one of the X chromosomes is missing or partially missing.
- The defining clinical triad is short stature, impaired sexual development, and infertility.
- Many organs may be affected with cutaneous stigmata providing critical clues for early detection.
- Skin characteristics: Lymphedema, webbed neck (resolution of cystic hygroma), multiple melanocytic nevi, keloids. It may be associated with autoimmune diseases as alopecia areata and vitiligo.

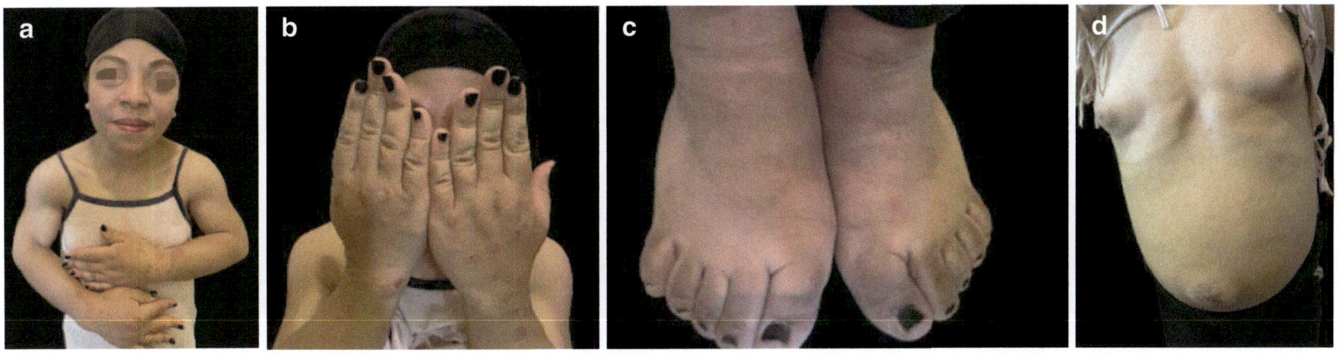

Fig. 13.13 Turner Syndrome. Short stature with skeletal abnormalities (**a**), webbed neck (**b**), bilateral broadening of hands (**c**), and feet (**d**). Broad chest with underdeveloped breast, wide spaced nipples and umbilical hernia (**d**)

References

1. Glick N. Dramatic reduction in self-injury in Lesch–Nyhan disease following S-adenosylmethionine administration. J Inherit Metab Dis. 2006;29(5):687.
2. Tewari N, Mathur VP, Sardana D, et al. Lesch-Nyhan syndrome: the saga of metabolic abnormalities and self-injurious behavior. Intractable Rare Dis Res. 2017;6(1):65–8.
3. Cauwels RG, Martens LC. Self-mutilation behaviour in Lesch–Nyhan syndrome. J Oral Pathol Med. 2005;34(9):573–5.
4. Da Silveira HE, Quadros OF, Dalla-Bona RR, et al. Dental findings in GAPO syndrome: a case report. Braz Dent J. 2006;17(3):259–62.
5. Tipton RE, Gorlin RJ. Growth retardation, alopecia, pseudo-anodontia, and optic atrophy—the GAPO syndrome: report of a patient and review of the literature. Am J Med Genet. 1984;19(2):209–16.
6. Rim PH, Marques-de-Faria AP. Ophthalmic aspects of GAPO syndrome: case report and review. Ophthalmic Genet. 2005;26(3):143–7.
7. Happle R, Hoffmann R, Restano L, et al. Phacomatosis pigmentokeratotica: a melanocytic-epidermal twin nevus syndrome. Am J Med Genet. 1996;65:363–5.
8. Tadini G, Restano L, Gonzales-Perez R, et al. Phacomatosis pigmentokeratotica: report of new cases and further delineation of the syndrome. Arch Dermatol. 1998;134:333–7.
9. Frieden IJ. Aplasia cutis congenita: a clinical review and proposal for classification. J Am Acad Dermatol. 1986;14(4):646–60.
10. Browning JC. Aplasia cutis congenita: approach to evaluation and management. Dermatol Ther. 2013;26(6):439–44.
11. Moros Pena M, Labay Matias M, Valle Sanchez F, et al. [Aplasia cutis congenita in a newborn: etiopathogenic review and diagnostic approach]. An Esp Pediatr. 2000;52(5):453–6.
12. Drolet B, Prendiville J, Golden J, et al. Membranous aplasia cutis' with hair collars. Congenital absence of skin or neuroectodermal defect? Arch Dermatol. 1995;131(12):1427–31.
13. Lozano-Masdemont B. A case of membranous aplasia cutis congenita and dermoscopic features. Int J Trichology. 2017;9(1):33–4.
14. Jelin AC, Glenn OA, Strachowski L, et al. Membranous aplasia cutis congenita: a recognizable lesion on prenatal sonography. J Ultrasound Med. 2009;28(10):1393–6.
15. Benvenuto C, Kraemer CK, Kruse RL, et al. Familial epidermolysis bullosa with aplasia cutis congenita: Bart's syndrome? Skinmed. 2003;2(5):319–21.
16. Orstavik KH, Stromme P, Spetalen S, et al. Aplasia cutis congenita associated with limb, eye, and brain anomalies in sibs: a variant of the Adams-Oliver syndrome? Am J Med Genet. 1995;59(1):92–5.
17. Temtamy SA, Aglan MS, Ashour AM, et al. Adams-Oliver syndrome: further evidence of an autosomal recessive variant. Clin Dysmorphol. 2007;16(3):141–9.
18. Alrumayyan N, Slauenwhite D, McAlpine SM, et al. Prolidase deficiency, a rare inborn error of immunity, clinical phenotypes, immunological features, and proposed treatments in twins. Allergy Asthma Clin Immunol. 2022;18:17–28.
19. Cervantes-Barragan DE, Villarroel CE, Medrano-Hernandez A, Dura'n-McKinster C, Bosch-Canto V, Del-Castillo V, Nazarenko I, Yang A, Desnick RJ. Setleis syndrome in Mexican-Nahuasibs due to a homozygous TWIST2 frameshift mutation and partial expression in heterozygotes: review of the focal facial dermal dysplasias and subtype reclassification. J Med Genet. 2011;48:716–20.
20. Meena D, Chauhan P, Hazarika N, et al. H syndrome: a case report and review of literature. Indian J Dermatol. 2018;63(1):76–8.
21. Uitto J, Saeidian AH, Youssefian L, et al. Recalcitrant warts, epidermodysplasia verruciformis, and the tree-man syndrome: phenotypic spectrum of cutaneous human papillomavirus infections at the intersection of genetic variability of viral and human genomes. J Invest Dermatol. 2022;142(5):1265–9.
22. Lowenstein EJ, Kim KH, Glick SA. Turner's syndrome in dermatology. J Am Acad Dermatol. 2004;50:767–76.

9783031607875